Ethics
for Psychologists

Dedicated to all the past and future graduate psychology students who enroll in psychology ethics classes—may you find this book engaging as you learn the professional ethics code of psychology.

Ethics for Psychologists

A Casebook Approach

Liang Tien
Antioch University

Amy Davis
Bastyr University

Thomas H. Arnold

G. Andrew F. Benjamin
University of Washington

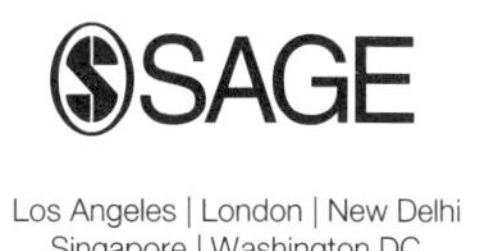

Los Angeles | London | New Delhi
Singapore | Washington DC

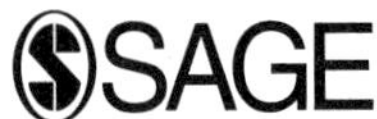

Los Angeles | London | New Delhi
Singapore | Washington DC

FOR INFORMATION:

SAGE Publications, Inc.
2455 Teller Road
Thousand Oaks, California 91320
E-mail: order@sagepub.com

SAGE Publications Ltd.
1 Oliver's Yard
55 City Road
London EC1Y 1SP
United Kingdom

SAGE Publications India Pvt. Ltd.
B 1/I 1 Mohan Cooperative Industrial Area
Mathura Road, New Delhi 110 044
India

SAGE Publications Asia-Pacific Pte. Ltd.
33 Pekin Street #02-01
Far East Square
Singapore 048763

Acquisitions Editor: Christine Cardone
Editorial Assistant: Sarita Sarak
Production Editor: Brittany Bauhaus
Copy Editors: Teresa Herlinger and Megan Markanich
Typesetter: C&M Digitals (P) Ltd.
Proofreader: Rae-Ann Goodwin
Indexer: Terri Corry
Cover Designer: Anupama Krishnan
Marketing Manager: Helen Salmon
Permissions Editor: Karen Ehrmann

Printed in the United States of America

Library of Congress Cataloging-in-Publication Data

Ethics for psychologists: a casebook approach / Liang Tien . . . [et al.].

p. cm.
Includes bibliographical references and index.

ISBN 978-1-4129-7821-7 (pbk.)

1. Psychologists—Professional ethics—Case studies. 2. Psychology—Moral and ethical aspects—Case studies. I. Tien, Liang.

BF76.4.E819 2012
174′.915—dc23 2011029055

This book is printed on acid-free paper.

11 12 13 14 15 10 9 8 7 6 5 4 3 2 1

Brief Contents

Detailed Contents

About the Authors

Liang Tien holds a BA from the University of Michigan, an MA from Antioch University, and a PsyD from the University of Denver. She is core faculty member at Antioch University Seattle's PsyD program and has a private practice. L. Tien has published and presented in the area of multicultural counseling, as well as conducted workshops on ethics. She served on the Washington State Psychological Association's Ethics Committee as a member for 7 years and as chair of the committee for 3 years, on their Ethics Hot Line for 5 years, and as a member of the Washington State Examining Board of Psychology for 2 years.

Amy Davis received her BS in health psychology from Bastyr University and her PsyD from Antioch University Seattle. Her specialized areas of training include existential/humanistic psychology and child and family systems. Her dissertation was a phenomenological exploration of suicide survivorship among lesbians. Amy currently teaches several psychology courses to undergraduate students and naturopathic doctoral students at Bastyr University.

Thomas H. Arnold is currently completing his doctoral dissertation for the Committee in the Study of Religion at Harvard University. His dissertation looks at Ludwig Wittgenstein and the idea of "experience" in the philosophy of religion. He is also coediting a book on William James and Josiah Royce. His work in philosophy of religion incorporates interests in ethics, American pragmatism, feminist theology, and cognitive science. He has taught at Harvard, Tufts University, and Stonehill College.

G. Andrew F. Benjamin, JD, PhD, ABPP, is director of the Parenting Evaluation Treatment Program (PETP) at the University of Washington. The exceptional features of Dr. Benjamin's career are the breadth of his range of professional activities and the strength of his commitment to combining the best resources of psychology and law for the benefit of adults and children enmeshed in psychopathology. While working with families engaged in high-conflict litigation and lawyers suffering from various mental health and drug abuse problems, Dr. Benjamin was named Professional of the Year by the Washington State Bar Association's Family Law Section. He was elected president of the Washington State Psychological Association, and later his colleagues there created an association award named after him for "outstanding and tireless contributions." He was honored by the Puyallup Indian Nation's Health Authority for serving as a "modern day warrior fighting the mental illnesses, drug-alcohol addictions" of the people served by the Nation's program. He has served as a member and a chair of the American Psychological Association's (APA) Committee on Legal Issues (COLI). He also has served as an elected member and chair of the APA's Policy and Planning (P&P) Board. He received the Heiser Award from APA in recognition of his record of public service and advocacy in numerous areas of professional activity.

Dr. Benjamin has published 57 peer reviewed articles in psychology, law, and psychiatry journals. He is the author of three books published by the APA: *Law and Mental Health Professionals (1995,1998); Family Evaluation in Custody Litigation: Reducing Risks of Ethical Infractions and Malpractice (2003);* and *The Duty to Protect: Ethical, Legal, and Professional Considerations for Mental Health Professionals (2009).*

Preface

Psychologists today practice in an increasingly complex world and must juggle the myriad issues and concerns of their clients while maintaining the highest standards of the profession. No matter how much rigorous training and continuing education psychologists undergo, no psychologist can anticipate all of the various dilemmas and challenges they will face in practice as a clinician, a professor, or a researcher.

There is no shortage of information about how psychologists ought to practice ethically; yet there are also consistent complaints to the regulatory boards of every state and ethics committees of professional associations about psychologists' conduct. Why, then, if we *know* the law and the contents of our own psychology's Ethics Code, that is, the *American Psychological Association's 2002 Ethical Principles of Psychologists and Code of Conduct, 2010 Amendments* do we continue to act in ways that violate them and impact public trust in our profession? How much do we understand about our own ethical decision-making process and values? How well do we understand the factors that impact our stance as psychologists? We find it curious as we have observed students in ethics classes over the years who can recite the letter and dictates of psychology's ethics code but when asked to describe *what they would actually do* their answers are at times drastically different. Why is it that we psychologists, both new and experienced, behave in ways that are different from the training we've had, and the information about the APA's *Ethical Principles of Psychologists and Code of Conduct* that in fact we understand? Perhaps in our answers to this question we bear similarities with the students who, despite their knowing the ethics codes and laws, tell us that their choices rest on their own moral values, not professional ethics.

One tendency in graduate-level education for psychologists and other mental health professionals has been to teach ethics as a structure to adhere to or comply with rather than focusing on ethics as a living, interactional system that must be carefully applied, balancing a number of different concerns. Often students can be overheard to complain at the start of a typical ethics class: "I know, I know, don't have sex with clients. Why do we need this class?" Why, indeed. As psychologists continue to be the subject of numerous ethics complaints, ranging from sexual exploitation of clients to violations of confidentiality to poor billing practices, it becomes increasingly clear that not only continued education in ethics is of critical importance for psychologists—the specific kinds of ethical education we receive should change as well. From the newest of students to the most seasoned of clinicians and researchers, we believe that our ethical decision making is not just a process of having the "right" information about what to do or not do; we believe it is a multilayered process that all psychologists, regardless of experience, can benefit from examining more explicitly.

The intersection of our legal code with our Ethics Code of ethics has resulted in a dizzying array of dos and don'ts, without much regard for the whys, and hows, as well as the implicit and explicit attitudes and values that lie at the heart of complex ethical dilemmas. We have specifically chosen dilemmas that are not obvious or egregious but more subtle, some unavoidable, and all of them pulled from our collective and actual professional experiences.

Most psychology students and professionals can spot egregious examples of misbehavior with little experience or training. What our book seeks to do instead is to create vignettes that are subtle and complex enough that almost any psychologist, from the newest student to the most seasoned psychologists, will have to struggle to resolve the issues that are raised. The premise of the book is not one of assuming malfeasance and egregious intent to harm but instead the opposite: The vignettes are written with the assumption that the psychologists within them make mistakes because of ignorance, not malevolence. We assume, therefore, the misguided actions of well-intended people to be at the center of our fictional psychologists' struggles and have created vignettes that are intentionally difficult to recognize, solve, or even fully understand at first glance. Our aim as authors is not to create clear or safe pathways through each vignette or leave you thinking "I would never do that." Instead our hope is that many of you will say, "Wow, I didn't see what was wrong with that particular situation. I might very well have done that." Or, even more powerfully, we expect that even the seasoned among you will read through some of the various dilemmas and remark to yourselves, "I *have* done that." We hope our book is educational and beneficial to *all* psychologists, regardless of experience level.

While the authors hope to teach an ethical resolution process of analysis, deliberation, and decision making within the confines of this book, we also urge you to be fully aware of the laws and codes of the states where you reside, work, and practice.

Not only does our book describe complex ethical dilemmas that any of us might encounter but our book offers many different frameworks through which to examine each dilemma: legal, moral, values-driven, and global all while offering clear and succinct commentary on the dictates of our own code of ethics. Finally, it asks you to take charge of your own learning by moving beyond simply looking up each situation and finding "the right thing to do," into a more active and participatory engagement. We hope by the end of the book that each of you understands and learns something about yourselves not only as psychologists (or psychologists-in-training) but as ethical thinkers and decision makers as well.

In this ever-changing global stage upon which psychology is now learned and practiced, it is important that psychologists be at the forefront in safeguarding the welfare of our clients, our students, the public, and ourselves. This book is a solid step in learning to answer the dictates of our own conscience, while upholding the highest ideals of society and the profession of psychology.

Such a large project is never merely the work of the authors named. Our families and friends gave us invaluable encouragement throughout our writing efforts. We also enjoyed the collegial support of many knowledgeable and outstanding collaborators who graciously contributed their time, expertise, and willingness to read parts of this manuscript at various stages of its inception and creation. The authors gratefully acknowledge the contributions and suggestions of Pat Linn, who so carefully read through every single vignette in Standard 8 and Bob Grubbs, who patiently guided us through understanding the procedures around care of animals in laboratories. We also extend our gratitude to the PsyD students in ethics classes at Antioch University Seattle who offered their commentary and feedback about the vignettes and also offered their own solutions. Finally, the authors owe a debt of gratitude that can never be repaid to Tammera Cooke our project manager, for keeping track of us, inspiring us with her ever-witty comments and observations, and blessing us with her clear-sighted vision and patience. Tammera Cooke without whom this project would never have been brought to completion, this book is gratefully dedicated to you.

Acknowledgments

The authors and SAGE would like to thank the following societies for permission for use of their ethics codes:

Texas State Board of Examiners of Psychologists

Pennsylvania State Board of Psychology

Singapore Psychological Society

Georgia State Board of Examiners of Psychologists

New Jersey State Board of Psychological Examiners

Spanish Psychological Association

Virginia Board of Psychology

Florida Board of Psychology

Massachusetts Board of Registration of Psychologists

Ohio State Board of Psychology

Canadian Psychological Association

Washington State Examining Board of Psychology

California Board of Psychology

United Kingdom British Psychological Society

New York State Board for Psychology

Psychological Society of South Africa

Arizona Board of Psychologist Examiners

Missouri State Committee of Psychologists

Czech-Moravian Psychological Society

Minnesota Board of Psychology

NIP, the Dutch Professional Association of Psychologists

Massachusetts Board of Registration of Psychologists

The New Zealand Psychological Association

Wisconsin Psychology Examining Board

Michigan Board of Psychology

Hong Kong Psychological Society

Vermont Board of Psychological Examiners

West Virginia Board of Examiners of Psychologists

Alaska Board of Psychologist and Psychological Associate Examiners

Lithuanian Psychological Society Code of Ethics

Maryland Board of Examiners of Psychologists

Illinois Clinical Psychologists Licensing & Disciplinary Committee

North Carolina Psychology Board

Oregon State Board of Psychologist Examiners

Psychology Board of Australia

Hellenic Psychological Society

Arkansas Board of Psychology

Colorado Board of Psychologist Examiners

Hawaii Board of Psychology

Idaho State Board of Psychologist Examiners

Iowa Board of Psychology Examiners

Indiana State Psychology Board

Kansas Behavioral Sciences Regulatory Board

Kentucky State Board of Examiners of Psychology

Maine Board of Examiners of Psychologists

Louisiana State Board of Examiners of Psychologists

Nebraska Board of Psychologists

State of Nevada Board of Psychological Examiners

New Hampshire Board of Mental Health Practice

New Mexico Board of Psychologist Examiners

South Carolina Board of Examiners in Psychology

South Dakota Board of Examiners of Psychologists

Tennessee Board of Examiners in Psychology

Montana Board of Psychologists

District of Columbia Board of Psychology

Oklahoma State Board of Examiners of Psychologists

Rhode Island Board of Psychology

Delaware Board of Examiners of Psychology

The authors and SAGE would also like to acknowledge the contributions of the following reviewers:

Azra Karajic Siwiec, *Walsh University*

Deborah Harris O'Brien, *Trinity Washington University*

Robert E. Doan, *University of Central Oklahoma, Edmond*

Eileen O'Neill Estes, *University of Louisville*

Erica J. Gannon, *Clayton State University*

Misty M. Ginicola, *Southern Connecticut State University*

David L. Shapiro, *Nova Southeastern University*

Sherry Dingham, *Marist College*

Introduction

Professional ethics is concerned with the proper conduct for the members of a profession. Two primary written sources addressing proper conduct for psychology as a profession exist. One source is internally generated by the profession in the form of professional associations' ethics codes. The other source is externally generated by society through the form of laws. Proper conducts specified by the profession reflect those behaviors that have been agreed upon and adopted by the members of that profession. The American Psychological Association (APA) is the primary professional association for psychologists. The APA's Ethical Principles of Psychologists and Code of Conduct 2002 (American Psychological Association [APA], 2010)—hereafter referred to as the APA Ethics Code—documents the proper conduct that has been agreed upon and adopted by the governance structure of APA. The APA Ethics Code addresses proper conduct for psychologists in their professional activities, whether the activities involve treatment, teaching, research, or administrative roles and responsibilities.

Externally driven written regulations that focus on the work of psychologists are laws. States grant psychologists licenses to practice as health care professionals. Therefore, most state laws that regulate psychologists focus on those activities involving treatment. Legal interpretations of ethical standards for psychologists—whether they occur in the form of statutes, administrative rules, administrative regulations, or judicial opinions—are substantial and varied across jurisdictions (states and provinces). Federal laws and regulations mostly address the work of psychologists involved in research.

An often invisible but ever-present source of authority is the moral values of a culture that guides and directs the formation of laws and professional ethics codes. However, as psychologists increase their sensitivity to the power of the profession, we must engage in a deeper curiousity about our assumed moral values that affect our models of professional service. "Eurocentric models may not be effective in working with other populations as well, and indeed, may do harm by mislabeling or misdiagnosing problems and treatments" (APA, 2002, p. 45). These moral values can be extrapolated through an examination of how cultures in other counties handle similar situations and through a careful questioning of our own values and rationale for any given course of action.

Our readers are invited to examine various professional situations through the three influences of the APA Ethics Code standards, state laws, and cultural values. To conduct such an examination, it is sometimes helpful to have a methodological procedure for a systematic exploration of relevant items, such as an ethical decision-making model. Many such models have been published. Next are a few examples of published models for ethical decision making. These are presented as examples and are not intended as an exhaustive listing of different models. Hopefully there are sufficient numbers of examples to provide adequate information for each reader to develop their own method for decision making.

MODELS OF ETHICAL DECISION MAKING

Koocher and Keith-Spiegal (2008) provided an ethical decision-making model that guides psychologists to engage in the following steps:

1. Determine whether the matter truly involves ethics.
2. Consult guidelines already available that might apply as a possible mechanism for resolution.
3. Pause to consider as best as possible all factors that might influence the decision you will make.
4. Consult with a trusted colleague.

5. Evaluate the rights, responsibilities, and vulnerability of all affected parties, including if relevant institutions and the general public.
6. Generate alternative decisions.
7. Enumerate the consequences of making each decision.
8. Make the decision. (p. 21)

Knapp and VandeCreek (2006) provided a five-step model that guides psychologists to engage in the following steps:

> (a) identify or scrutinize the problem to determine which moral principles appear threatened; (b) develop alternatives or hypotheses that are based on, or at least can be consistent with, general moral principles; (c) evaluate or analyze options according to a balancing or ranking of moral principles; (d) act or perform in a manner to minimize the harm to the offended principle; and (e) look back or evaluate the extent to which the actions balanced or fulfilled moral principles. (p. 43)

Fisher (2009) urged that psychologists follow steps in ethical decision making:

Step 1: Develop and sustain a professional commitment to doing what is right.

Step 2: Acquire sufficient familiarity with the APA Ethics Code General Principles and Ethical Standards to be able to anticipate situations that require ethical planning and to identify unanticipated situations that require ethical decision making.

Step 3: Gather additional facts relevant to the specific ethical situation from professional guidelines, state and federal laws, and organizational policies.

Step 4: Make efforts to understand the perspective of different stakeholders who will be affected by the decision and consult with colleagues.

Step 5: Apply steps 1 through 4 to generate ethical alternatives and evaluate each alternative in terms of moral theories, general principles, and ethical standards.

Step 6: Select and implement an ethical course of action.

Step 7: Monitor and evaluate the effectiveness of the course of action.

Step 8: Modify and continue to evaluate the ethical plan if necessary. (pp. 244–245)

Here is one more model from us. You will find that steps 2 through 5 are followed in the presentation of each standard in our book. We invite our readers to apply steps 1 and 6 through 11 on their own or with a small study group to maximize the information contained in this book.

1. Note the affective discomfort in situation and the strength of the therapeutic alliance between your client and you to help determine the accuracy of the facts you are relying upon and whether the client can assist further in delineating the facts.
2. Write down the dilemma in vignette form.
3. Identify all categories found in ethics code or state law that may be pertinent to dilemma.
4. Review each category to determine the appropriate action suggested by state laws or professional codes.
5. List all possible actions generated by the previously given list that could lead to a reasonable course of action.
6. Review the action list for inherent conflicts among the ethical standards and the state laws.
7. Reflect upon your own underlying values that guide your thinking.
8. Consult with peers who are trained similarly to you, your state's ethics panel, or a JD/PhD who offers ethical/legal consultations.
9. Determine course of action.
10. Enter a chart note with rationale for course of action.
11. Assess the course of action to determine whether further consideration is necessary.

Conduct as required by the APA Ethics Code should be the minimum level of professional conduct for any prudent psychologist. However, at times it is either not enough or impossible to meet the minimum requirements of the APA Ethics Code. Sometimes situations arise or events unfold in such a manner that different parts of the principles and/or standards appear to give conflicting directives. In short, "There is no ethics menu from which the right ethical actions can simply be selected" (Fisher, 2009, p. 241). Each of the models incorporates the notions that reflection, care, consultations, and documentation can lead to reasonable outcomes.

We invite psychologists and graduate students to derive their own method to arrive at ethical conduct via investigation of professional situations described in vignettes. Each vignette is designed to illustrate a specific standard of the APA Ethics Code. However, as in many applied situations, it is not unusual that multiple sections of the principles and standards impinge on a given set of circumstances. Therefore, following each vignette is an examination of the APA Ethics Code, state laws, and cultural specific moral values. Hopefully the exercises of working through the vignettes will assist psychologists to not only know relevant regulations but to rise above the ambiguity of divergent regulations and come to know the moral values that underpin the professional conduct.

ORGANIZATION FOR EACH STANDARD

For each standard of the APA Ethics Code examined, you will find a vignette, APA Ethics Code, state laws, cultural considerations, and action options. The vignette presents the standards in an applied context and a discussion of the issues of concern illustrated within the vignette. The APA Ethics Code section contains a discussion of relevant General Principles and a discussion of other relevant standards of the code as they may apply to the vignette. The Legal Issues section contains discussion of laws from two different states. The Cultural Considerations section contains a discussion of an ethics code from one other country and discussion of moral values based on the American culture. The final section for each standard contains an action section that reviews possible courses of action as directed by the relevant sections of the APA Ethics Code, followed by a listing of various action options that are within the parameters set by the APA Ethics Code. We urge our readers to use the possible courses of action in concert with our model regarding ethical decision making that was previously discussed whenever you are faced with a similar set of circumstances.

Standards

Each standard of the APA Ethics Code may appear deceptively simple. The full complexities of the standards come to light when examined in the context of the often multifaceted circumstances where well-intentioned competent psychologists face difficult ethical decisions. Each standard is illustrated in a vignette. All vignettes are fictional, derived from the many combined experiences of the authors. The names used in each vignette are taken in numerical order from the 2000 U.S. Census (U.S. Census Bureau, 2000) listing of the most frequently occurring first and last names. Anything in the vignettes that resemble any actual situations is purely coincidental.

A section titled "Issues of Concern" immediately follows each vignette. This section further delineates the possible ethical issues embedded in the vignette. We highlight the most apparent areas touched upon by the standard and vignette. The reader is invited and encouraged to further examine the vignettes for other possible relevant areas of practice and ethics concerns.

APA ETHICS CODE

Companion General Principles

Most psychology ethicists have pondered what core moral values psychologists should hold. Opinions differ slightly as to what these core moral values are or should be. In formulating the 2002 APA Ethics Code, psychologists collectively pondered the question of what moral values we as a profession should hold. The collective wisdom of the members of the APA generated five core values. These values are articulated in the General Principles section of the APA Ethics Code. Specifically these are (1) beneficence and nonmaleficence, (2) fidelity and responsibility, (3) integrity, (4) justice, and (5) respect for people's rights and dignity.

Our five core values of the General Principles characterize us as honest and caring. Thus a virtuous psychologist is a psychologist who is honest in all of his or her professional activities and caring of the people with whom he or she interacts in their professional role. The actions of virtuous psychologists following the principles have been characterized by others in pithy ways: "Those that fulfill the fundamental moral obligations to do good, to do no harm, to respect others, and to treat all individuals honestly and fairly" (Fisher, 2009, p. 5). "As it applies to their [psychologist] role, . . . be honest with patients, work to promote their well-being, and avoid gossiping about them" (Knapp & VandeCreek, 2006, p. 16). The General Principles of the APA Ethics Code section names specific characteristics that psychologists should hold. The explicatory text included for each General Principle specifies those attitudes, thoughts, and actions that would reflect the activities of a virtuous psychologist.

In the section titled "Companion General Principle(s)," we name those values that are relevant to the vignette. Each is followed by considerations a virtuous psychologist might examine in applying the values reflected in the five General Principles. Also included is how these values might guide the reasoning behind developing an ethical course of action in the vignette.

Companion Ethical Standard(s)

For most psychologists most of the time, appropriate conduct is clear if the dictates of the standards are followed. However, it is rarely the case in applied situations where only one standard affects a given situation. It is not uncommon for either a specific situation to arise or a course of events to evolve in such a way that different sections of the APA Ethics Code are either in conflict with each other or with the principles. These dilemmas occur for even the most ethical and virtuous of psychologists. In the section titled "Companion Ethical Standard(s)," relevant companion standards that bear on areas illustrated in the vignette are listed and examined.

STATE LAWS

Legal Issues 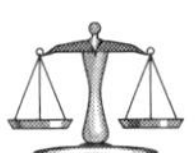

Psychologists are not only regulated by within the profession through the APA Ethics Code but also from outside of the profession, most often through state laws. The Legal Issues section examines relevant legal statutes, rules, regulations and the common law that address the issues raised by the standard and the vignette. This section is intended to illustrate the possible interplay between the APA Ethics Code and state law. Relevant laws from two different states are listed for consideration. The prudent psychologist should act in a reasonable manner to meet the requirements of law within their jurisdiction in all instances in which an ethical issue arises and law on the topic applies to the context. On occasion, conflicts between ethics/law will arise and the implementation of Standard 1.02 will be considered at that point within our text.

When first working on the beginning of the book, the laws were chosen from the 10 states where the most psychologists practiced as listed by the APA. After reviewers examined our first three chapters, we were urged to include all of the states. Starting in Standard 4, all states were then included in alphabetical order for the remaining chapters. However, those states that adopted the entire APA Ethics Code by statute or rule are only mentioned once in the book to avoid unnecessary duplication and to show the great diversity of legal writing about ethical standards that has arisen across the other jurisdictions.

State laws and court rulings are dynamic and not static. As a result, keeping up with the changing face of these legal standards regarding ethical issues is a tough challenge for psychologists. We urge our readers not to rely solely on the laws cited in this book. Instead we urge our readers to carefully seek out all laws, common-law case precedents, or licensing board opinions before acting on the law. We give one example here to illustrate the need for readers to know the state-specific laws in considering any ethical course of action. In the area of danger to others, Pabian, Welfel, and Beebe (2009) found that most of the 300 psychologists they surveyed (76.4%) were misinformed about their state laws regarding the duty to protect third parties from the violence of their clients. In states where no legal duty existed, many mistakenly believed that they were legally mandated to warn, and in states where there were legal options other than warning the potential victim, most assumed that warning was their only legal option. In addition to the inaccuracy of their knowledge, many respondents were confident that they understood the duty to protect in their own state. Nearly one third of the sample (30.6%) indicated that they were very up to date in their knowledge of this issue, and 58.9% reported that they were somewhat up to date in their knowledge (Pabian et al., 2009). In fact, many psychologists—if they had acted upon their erroneous knowledge about the duty to protect—would have violated the standards within their jurisdictions that protect confidences and subjected themselves to both malpractice risk and complaints to their licensing boards.

Psychologists' misinformation on this matter is understandable. The variability across Canada and the United States is truly daunting. For example, 23 states impose either a duty to protect or a duty to warn by statute, and 9 states have a common-law duty (i.e., a duty derived from court holdings as opposed to obligations based on law created by a jurisdiction's legislature through a statutory process or administrative rule through the licensing board rule promulgation process) as a result of court cases; 13 other states permit but do not mandate the breach of confidentiality to warn potential victims, and 7 states have not ruled on the issue. In Canada, six provinces have no statutory or common-law duty related to the issue, and seven provinces allow but do not mandate disclosure of dangerousness to third parties (Benjamin, Kent, & Sirikantraporn, 2009). Moreover, no two states or provinces have created the same law (Benjamin et al., 2009). It is important to note that in the 23 states that impose a statutory duty to protect, majorities do not specify warning as the only option to carry out the duty. Most allow hospitalization (voluntary or involuntary), and some allow intensification of outpatient treatment or other actions that appear appropriate to psychologists. Not only do laws vary across states but they also vary over time. Ohio, for example, had three different legal standards about the duty to protect in the period between 1991 and 1999, and California recently modified its duty to protect statute to a duty to warn and protect that is triggered by a family member relaying a concern about a client family member who may engage in violence (*Ewing v. Goldstein*, 2004).

Regardless of the seeming insurmountable complexities of keeping abreast of the law, we pose that it is not only possible but a duty of the prudent psychologist to know the laws of their state or province. The Association of State and Provincial Psychology Boards (ASPPB) recently has posted the statutes, rules, and regulations of most jurisdictions, and we urge our readers to refer to these postings often, as we have ourselves relied upon these postings (http://www.asppb.net/i4a/pages/index.cfm?pageid=3395). We expect that our readers, through understandings derived from reading the "Legal Issues" section of this book, will be able to read their state laws and to corroborate through peer consultation that other laws, case precedents, or licensing board opinions may not affect how to proceed in the ethical decision making regarding the particular context.

CULTURAL CONSIDERATIONS

Knapp and VandeCreek (2006) posed "Ethics should focus . . . on how all psychologists can do better at helping them [patients]. This view of ethics is called positive or active ethics. . . . Positive ethics requires a fundamental philosophical underpinning" (p. 10). We would add that most people, including psychologists, have a philosophical framework and do hold values that underpin their lives. The presence of such individual philosophical underpinnings is acknowledged in the Introduction and Applicability section of the APA Ethics Code. The last paragraph of the Introduction and Applicability section allows psychologists to follow "the dictates of their own conscience" in applying the ethics code to their professional work.

Fisher (2009) asserted, "Psychologists are not moral technocrats simply working their way through a maze of ethical rules. . . . Ethical decision making thus involves a commitment to applying the Ethics Code to construct rather than simply discover solutions to ethical quandaries" (p. 23). We think that in the construction of an ethical course of action, the influence of culture is ever present, though most of the time unarticulated and unnoticeable. Nonetheless, cultural values exert too great of an influence to remain hidden or unrecognized (Sue & Sue, 2007).

All codes of ethics for a particular profession, psychology included, can be understood to be culturally constructed documents, bound to a particular time period, and methodology of current practices. Living codes, such as our APA Ethics Code, reflect the ongoing changes of the profession, and revisions will embrace more constructs from cultures across the globe. Each country's code of ethics is a time capsule of sorts, a living, evolving document that seeks to capture and explicate each individual country's best practices for ethical decision making and behavior in the profession of psychology.

For a variety of reasons, psychologists have, for the first time, articulated moral constructs by the inclusion of the General Principles section of the 2002 APA Ethics Code. In so much as the moral constructs expressed in the APA Ethics Code's General Principles section are lists of values that ethical and virtuous psychologists should exhibit, inherent problems in virtue ethics can arise. According to Brabeck (2000), "Virtues that are community specific may promote ethnocentric atrocities" (p. 258). Indeed, engaging in the color-blind paradigm (usually unconscious behavior) results in "ignoring group differences [that] can lead to the maintenance of the status quo and assumptions that racial/ethnic minority groups share the same perspective as dominant group members" (APA, 2002, p. 21).

Further, it is suggested that a method to counter this tendency is to "systematically and continually reassess motives, perspectives, and virtues that one encourages and, more importantly, to remain open to exploring and adopting virtues other than one's own" (Brabeck, 2000, p. 258). A way to enact the safeguards proposed by Brabeck (2000) is for psychologists to look outside of our national borders and to reflect upon our own cultural morays in contrast to those of other people. The Cultural Considerations section identifies the ethical standards of different countries around the world to assist our readers in looking deeper into relevant moral values from the current American culture that are reflected by our APA Code of Ethics.

For these reasons, we include two sections that address cultural influences. One section is titled "Global Discussion" and the other is titled "American Moral Values." The Global Discussion section provides an opportunity to consider different courses of action, possibly based on different cultural values. Through noticing differences, we are providing the readers an opportunity to discover how their own values are embedded in their own culture. The American Moral Values section lists those moral questions that arise from the present American culture. Although not exclusive, the many questions listed may guide a deeper examination of one's own cultural moral values and provides another opportunity to clarify one's own moral stance.

Global Discussion

The section titled "Cultural Considerations" is meant to invite perspectives and values that reflect psychology as embedded in other nations and cultures. These psychology ethics codes from other countries are selected from a total of 89 countries currently with psychological organizations, not all of who have independent codes of ethics. These were derived from nations listed in the Directory of National Associations of Psychology (APA International Affairs). The psychological associations of these countries were contacted through e-mail, mail, or by visiting their websites for their association's ethics codes. Twenty-nine responses, including ethics codes, were received (Estonia reported adherence to the code of ethics for Scandinavian psychologists). Of these, two were not specific to psychology (Russia and China's code was for psychiatrists). In addition, seven codes were not in English. All of the foreign language translation services in metropolitan Seattle declined to provide translations, citing that the documents were extremely technical and beyond the abilities of their translators. Several countries, such as France, Germany, and Luxembourg, use one code, that of the European Federation. Thus the resulting 16 ethics codes used in this section were somewhat constrained to those of psychological societies that are recognized as enforceable, have been translated into English and were accessible to the author(s) at the time of this text's writing.

Within the scope of this book, the inclusion of a Global Discussion section was based on a question of best practices from the other perspectives of the different cultures, countries, and systems of thought. What is unfortunately tempting and seductive within the desire to include codes and perspectives of other countries is a tendency, however accidental, to inadvertently privilege the APA Ethics Code/U.S. code as being the "norm" or standard upon by which other codes are then compared—favorably, neutrally, or unfavorably. To avoid that unfair privileging of the U.S. code, sections of applicable codes from different countries were included and discussed based upon their own merits and positioning of the best practices of a psychologist wherever possible, without always drawing direct reference to the U.S. code. This enabled us to still balance the logistical requirements of text from other countries to explore, deconstruct, and on occasion, critique the U.S. code.

Many of the ethics codes of psychological associations from around the world have their origins of the APA Ethics Code. Some codes, such as those of Great Britain, South Africa, and Australia, have retained great similarity to the U.S. code, while others have deviated significantly and evolved into almost entirely different rules of professional practice. Examples of the latter would be the codes of New Zealand and Canada, in particular. Other codes, notably those of Singapore and Hong Kong, are markedly collectivistic in their approaches and philosophies and stress different aspects and assumptions about the character and intent of the behavior of a psychologist.

The Global Discussion section permitted several threads of questions: What does it mean, for example, when the demand for absolute honesty in all professional areas of a psychologists' practice is an aspirational principle in the U.S. code, versus being an enforceable standard in many other countries' codes? How do research practices vary among countries that draw no distinction between human and nonhuman animal subjects and expect their treatment to follow similar guidelines, versus in countries (including the United States) where nonhuman animals are treated differently and thought to have different rights from humans? How does the practice of psychology change in countries that equivocate regarding the use of psychological skills and services in institutions such as prisons or active military units, which may be directly or indirectly involved in acts of violence, coercion or warfare, versus countries such as Spain, which make no allowance or provision for psychologists who in any way contribute to the maltreatment of others, regardless of external justification? These were some of the questions that were hopefully addressed and explored, if not wholly answered, by the inclusion of the Global Discussion section in this text.

Some codes, such as that of South Africa in particular, are so close in content and detail to the present U.S. code that certain portions would have been unhelpful to include for any relative contrast to the U.S. code. However, substantial portions of the South African code were included where we felt the deviations from the U.S. code, particularly as they related to the ethical inclusion of different ethnicities and their needs into practice.

The code of Canada, although in many ways constructed wholly differently from that of the United States, was heavily cited in certain subject areas, such as informed consent, freedom of consent, and honesty, to name a few examples, where both the elegance of the prose and the aspirational tone of the enforceable standards are sufficiently different from our own code that they likely will prompt psychologists to pause and reflect.

The codes of Hong Kong and Singapore often spoke eloquently about the need for psychologists to understand and differentiate the external appearance of behavior, both ethical and unethical, from the internal motivations and positions for themselves and for those with whom they work. Rather than allowing adherence to rules or dictates from organizations to release a psychologist from ethical responsibility, in many cases these countries' codes demanded the psychologists decide for themselves where their allegiance(s) should lie and to follow through on their own decisions accordingly.

The code of Spain was especially striking in its discussion of the obligation of psychologists to uphold and maintain the integrity of human dignity, and the sections pertaining to a psychologist's ethical duties surrounding torture, abuse, maltreatment of persons, and a psychologist's ethical position within such circumstances stands out among all extant codes as a clarion call to action, an upholding of human rights documents dating back to the Nuremberg trials and the Geneva Convention, and a possible standard for all healing professions sincerely dedicated to the welfare of human dignity in our conflict-torn world.

It is hoped by the inclusion of this section into the text that U.S. psychologists who are unfamiliar with the codes of other countries will become more so and draw their own conclusions about best practices in psychology from a perspective situated not only within our current U.S. culture, profession, legal system, and economy but also that of a more global stage. We have the ability to learn from the collective experiences and wisdom of a number of other countries whose psychological practices have also evolved and will continue to evolve on a global, interconnected world level.

American Moral Values

The section titled "American Moral Values" is meant to invite a closer examination of American cultural moral values. The construction of the questions provides a guide for the readers to more systematically explore their own motives and flesh out their own moral stance. It is important to consider that, "psychologists do not approach the practice of psychology in a moral vacuum. They have a background of personal beliefs that they bring to their professional duties" (Knapp & VandeCreek, 2006, p. 26).

The American Moral Values section seeks to foreground for each psychologist the personal beliefs that they bring into their profession. These areas of inquiry are based on the mores most common in the current culture of the United States. This section attempts to illuminate the ethical norms, ideals, and aspirations that inform how one frames each vignette. While the questions in each section direct themselves to the particulars of each case, they employ several philosophical angles on morality and practical reasoning. These include the following:

- What principle or rule of action should one follow in this case, regardless of consequences? Would this principle hold for any psychologist who faces this situation? Questions about consequences include what kind of person the psychologist and client will become. Questions about fairness introduce ideas about equality, justice, and representation that may supplement or challenge the explicit and implicit ideals of the code.
- What kind of person, community, and society does this decision help to create? Autonomy and self-determination may compete against social integration and community service.
- What are the consequences of this action for other lives? How much pain or satisfaction will it bring about?
- What is the good life? What kind of life is worth living? Questions about what constitutes a good life, indeed what constitutes life itself, can inform decisions about pain and well-being.

The chief function of incorporating these forms of inquiry is to challenge the reader to articulate more clearly and convincingly what reasons lie behind their judgment of the vignette at hand. The other main function of the American Moral Values section is to introduce a critical yet constructive assessment of what shapes one's ethical reflection and to help the reader to recognize their cultural anchors as both resources and material for reexamination.

While reasoned argument is crucial for moral deliberation, one is bound to integrate important feelings, intuitions, cultural practices, rituals, and personal experiences in one's moral interpretations. Readers will have to think through to what degree these influences are resources to draw upon and to what degree they are unexamined obstacles to proper action. On what terms are they disowned or incorporated into well-reasoned ethical positions, as psychologist, citizen, and human being?

ETHICAL COURSE OF ACTION

Directive per APA Code

Psychology being an applied field, each professional situation holds an implicit demand for action. That is, there are demand characteristics embedded in each vignette that require the psychologist to take some type of action; even no action is a course of action. The prudent psychologist should act to minimally meet the requirements of the APA Ethics Code. Each vignette includes a section titled "Directive per APA Code" that reasons our way through the relevant sections of the APA Ethics Code to derive a course of action that can be considered minimally ethical. If conflicts between the ethical and legal standards arise in the discussion of the vignette, we also consider how to apply Standard 1.02.

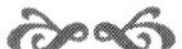

Dictates of One's Own Conscience

The title of this section is taken from the Introduction and Applicability section of the 2002 APA Ethics Code. The last paragraph of the section states the following:

> In applying the Ethics Code to their professional work, psychologists may consider other materials and guidelines that have been adopted or endorsed by scientific and professional psychological organizations and the *dictates of their own conscience* [italic added], as well as consult with others within the field. (APA, 2010)

Congruent with virtue ethics, it appears that the dictates of one's own conscience may have profound effects on activities of virtuous psychologists. Bernard and Jara (1986) found that "many psychology graduate students who reached the 'right' solution to an ethical dilemma did not intend to act on that solution" (p. 315). This is a puzzling situation that also occurred in my own teaching experience of graduate psychology students and may reflect the tendency for psychologists to follow the dictates of their own conscience, regardless of the directives of their professional association. This tendency to follow a course of action that is independent of the APA Ethics Code echoes our experience in teaching graduate level psychology ethics courses. When given ethical dilemmas, graduate students were initially unable to determine a course of action without going through a process of deliberation. Once relevant issues of concern were enumerated and the APA Ethics Code discussed, graduate students were able to derive a correct ethical course of action as defined by the standards of the APA Ethics Code and state laws. When asked, "What would you do?" the students did not consistently choose the ethical course of action. When asked, "Why would you do that instead of the action directed by the APA Ethics Code?" students often referred to their own moral values as more compelling than the directives of the APA Ethics Code.

Students, then, though unable to determine a course of action without a deliberative process, still did not consistently choose to enact the course of action derived out of an examination of the APA Ethics Code and the state laws. Again, our experiences with graduate students strongly suggested that their own moral values were influential in their decisions. The process of discovering one's own unarticulated and often unrecognized moral values may help explain and reframe what the gap is between the "correct" approach to an applied situation and the value-laden course of action one would pursue as an individual psychologist. Such reflection about one's own decision making could reshape both sides of that difference, offering critical space to rethink one's personal decision and querying the code's adequacy for the concrete example at hand.

One method to ascertain these unarticulated values is to decide on a course of action, then determine the moral value or beliefs that guided that choice. To aid readers in this process, we have listed examples of possible actions in the section titled "Dictates of One's Own Conscience." Some courses of action are clinically better than others, but all actions listed are within the wide parameters set by the APA Ethics Code and state laws. The list is not intended as endorsement for any specific action. We invite readers to take the opportunity, while working through the list of possible courses of action, to decide their most probable course of action. We recommend that readers actually choose a course of action and then review the reasons why that specific course of action(s) was selected. Once a course of action is chosen, we recommend readers to then review again the two sections under culture to articulate one's own underlying moral values that guided the decision. Readers might choose to look to the Global Discussion section to determine if one's own moral guide is reflective of a virtue that is more common in another culture.

The Dictates of One's Own Conscience section invites readers to actively engage in a dialogue between the APA Ethics Code, specifically the General Principles, the state laws, and cultural values that underline all of our behavior. Ideally the reader can articulate better reasons and arguments, with deeper considerations, than simply deciding one course of action over another. At the same time, the reader can better appreciate how moral reflection also requires the cultivation of judgments and the practice of imagination, in order that they can lay out for themselves what the critical issues are when facing a given scenario. Through such engagement, hopefully readers can resolve the differences between their own moral values and directives from the APA Ethics Code and state laws. We concur with Knapp and VandeCreek's (2006) opinion that "psychologists who have a clear sense of what they believe and why they believe it are more likely to make good ethical decisions" (p. 16).

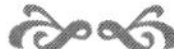

CHAPTER 1

Resolving Ethical Issues

Ethical Standard 1

CHAPTER OUTLINE

- Standard 1.01: Misuse of Psychologists' Work
- Standard 1.02: Conflicts Between Ethics and Law, Regulations, or Other Governing Legal Authority
- Standard 1.03: Conflicts Between Ethics and Organizational Demands
- Standard 1.04: Informal Resolution of Ethical Violations
- Standard 1.05: Reporting Ethical Violations
- Standard 1.06: Cooperating With Ethics Committees
- Standard 1.07: Improper Complaints
- Standard 1.08: Unfair Discrimination Against Complainants and Respondents

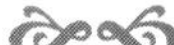

STANDARD 1.01: MISUSE OF PSYCHOLOGISTS' WORK

> If psychologists learn of misuse or misrepresentation of their work, they take reasonable steps to correct or minimize the misuse or misrepresentation.

A CASE FOR STANDARD 1.01: Innocent Oversight

Dr. Smith is a psychologist teaching health psychology at a university. Dr. Smith has published a review of the literature that points to the possibility that tai chi might be as effective for panic attacks and panic disorder as other, more traditional treatments, including pharmaceutical interventions. Her article recommends that further research be conducted before any changes in treatment can ethically be made for someone who has severe panic disorder. Dr. Smith approached the tai chi school in which she is a member to conduct research on tai chi and panic disorder. The founder of the tai chi school is an old family friend and was open to the idea of such collaboration. The partnership between the university and the tai chi school progressed to a signed "memorandum of understanding" that indicated university-supported field research at the tai chi school would occur. A few weeks later, without Dr. Smith's prior knowledge or consent, the tai chi school advertised "Stress Buster" seminars that promised to "cure" a number of conditions, including panic disorder. Dr. Smith's participation was prominently cited in their advertising flier and website. Both Dr. Smith and the university's contracts department reviewed the memorandum of understanding and noticed that the document did not include a clause that Dr. Smith or the university had to review and approve any advertisement released by the tai chi school.

Issues of Concern

It is not every day that psychologists enter into contractual agreements with private organizations for purposes of research. Though one would expect the university to have sufficient experience in forming and reviewing contracts, it can occur that some problems with the contracts may emerge later in collaboration with a contractual partner. The advertisement released by the tai chi school clearly misrepresents Dr. Smith's work since tai chi cannot "cure" anxiety or panic. However, tai chi could probably help some individuals to reduce their anxiety. Standard 1.01 directs that Dr. Smith needs to "take reasonable steps," which means Dr. Smith needs to take some sort of action. Areas of consideration may include the following questions: (1) Does Dr. Smith have the authority to change the advertisement? (2) What constitutes reasonable steps? For instance, would conducting a conversation with the tai chi school regarding the advertisement be sufficient to discharge the duty established by Standard 1.01?

APA Ethics Code

Companion General Principle

Principle A: Beneficence and Nonmaleficence

> When conflicts occur among psychologists' obligations or concerns, they attempt to resolve these conflicts in a responsible fashion that avoids or minimizes harm.

The implementation of the nonmaleficence part of Principle A can be seen in Standard 1.01, with the admonishment to correct misunderstandings. For example, if a workshop participant is left to believe that enrollment in the tai chi seminars can replace his/her medications for panic, then harm may come to the person through a panic attack. Taking steps to correct such a misunderstanding may prevent the harm caused by the mistaken belief that tai chi replaces medications.

Principle C: Integrity

> Psychologists seek to promote accuracy, honesty, and truthfulness in the science, teaching, and practice of psychology.

Allowing the advertisement to remain undisputed would not fulfill the aspirational principle of promoting accuracy, either in science or in practice.

Companion Ethical Standard(s)

Standard 5.01: Avoidance of False or Deceptive Statements

> (a) Psychologists do not knowingly make public statements that are false, deceptive, or fraudulent concerning their research, practice, or other work activities or those of persons or organizations with which they are affiliated.

Dr. Smith did not design and publish the flyer advertising the seminar. Thus, she did not knowingly make false statements. However, once discovered, if Dr. Smith does not publicly address the exaggerations of the advertisement, she may be colluding/condoning false and deceptive public statements about her research.

Standard 5.02: Statements by Others

> (a) Psychologists who engage others to create or place public statements that promote their professional practice, products, or activities retain professional responsibility for such statements.

Standard 5.02 (a) makes the distinction between public statements that are paid for by Dr. Smith and those statements that are not at Dr. Smith's request. It can be argued that since Dr. Smith did not engage the tai chi school to make public statements on her behalf that Standard 2.02 (a) does not apply.

Legal Issues 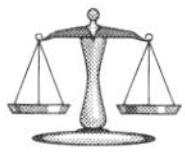

Texas

> *22 Tex. Admin. Code § 465.14(b) (2010). Misuse of licensees' services.*
>
> If licensees become aware of misuse or misrepresentation of their services . . . , they take reasonable steps to correct or minimize the misuse or misrepresentation.

Pennsylvania

> *49 Pa. Code § 41.61 (2010). Code of ethics.*
>
> *Principle 4 (a), Public Statements.* Public statements, announcements of services, and promotional activities of psychologists serve the purpose of providing sufficient information to aid the consumer public in making informed judgments and choices . . . In public statements providing psychological information or professional opinions or providing information about the availability of psychological products, publications and services, psychologists base their statements on scientifically acceptable psychological findings and techniques with full recognition of the limits and uncertainties of the evidence.

Texas's code has the same directive as the American Psychological Association (APA) Ethics Code, which directs the psychologist to "take reasonable steps" to correct the advertisement. Pennsylvania law states that a psychologist's public statements should be based on "scientifically acceptable" findings but does not give a clear directive as to what should be done in this situation. A reasonable assumption might be that a psychologist living and practicing in Pennsylvania would be expected to correct the advertisement from the tai chi school so that its effect would be "scientifically acceptable findings." Dr. Smith could engage in peer consultation with other psychologists who have a record of advertising scientifically acceptable findings, and document the consultations to establish a record that she attempted to clarify how to advertise scientifically acceptable findings in an ethical manner.

Cultural Considerations

Global Discussion

Singapore Psychological Society:
Code of Professional Ethics

> Principle 4: Misrepresentation
>
> Psychologists do not . . . permit their names to be used in connection with, any services or products in such a way as to misrepresent them, the degree of their responsibility or the nature of their affiliation.

If Dr. Smith were practicing in Singapore, Dr. Smith should immediately disassociate herself from the tai chi school by not permitting her name to be used in the misrepresentation of her work. The tai chi school would be extremely alarmed that Dr. Smith would immediately terminate all association with the school based on the advertisement.

American Moral Values

1. Dr. Smith has a relationship with both the tai chi school and the university. How does the value of her personal relationship with the tai chi school measure up to that of her professional relationship with the university? Dr. Smith may temper her reaction to the advertiser if she values the school founder as a friend and a valuable teacher for the larger community. She might not want her actions to cause the school to close, for example. On the other hand, her work as a scholar, the work of her field in general, and the reputation of her university as a scholarly institution depend on truthful claims about research. Does the tai chi school's mission of healing have greater value than the university's mission? Does that mission of healing help to excuse or offset the inaccuracies in the advertisement?

2. Dr. Smith may also consider the public effects of dissociating her research from the tai chi school. She may regard such a separation as an implicit indictment of the integrity and worth of the tai chi school, which would undermine respect for the school and tai chi in general. That kind of effect presumably conflicts with Dr. Smith's respect for tai chi's potential benefits and the school founder's personal virtue as a teacher. Dr. Smith might feel particularly torn because of tai chi's cultural status as "alternative" or "exotic" in America. If she feels such traditions have been unfairly judged by mainstream American culture, she may strive not to embarrass or delegitimize the school through her actions.

3. Dr. Smith's assessment of the tai chi school's motives will likely influence her reaction and approach to the situation. Was the tai chi school inflating the claims of a "cure" in order to increase their profit, with little concern for Dr. Smith's academic reputation? Or was the tai chi school staff instead confused by the nuance of research, with its enthusiastic advertising of research motivated by a desire to reach more people experiencing distress and panic? This moral evaluation may well guide to what degree Dr. Smith wants to work with the tai chi school moving forward (as opposed to clearing up this particular misunderstanding).

4. Dr. Smith's moral estimation of the tai chi school may involve a judgment about businesses versus the university. Does she believe the university should remain "above" the money-making necessities of a normal business? Does the advertisement corrupt the university's values of scholarship for its own sake?

Ethical Course of Action

Directive per APA Code

As directed by Standard 1.01, Dr. Smith should take "reasonable steps." The first reasonable step means to have a conversation with the tai chi school to list her concerns and determine a course of action that would rectify the misrepresentation of Dr. Smith's work.

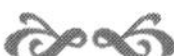

Dictates of One's Own Conscience

Beyond letting the tai chi school know of one's concerns in a conversation, which of the following might you do?

1. Approach the tai chi school to determine the source of the misunderstanding in the advertisement based on your work and the nature of data collection. Depending on the motivation behind the advertisement, act accordingly.
2. Should you be rooted in the American culture, but know that the tai chi school is expecting something akin to behavior specified in the Singapore code, you would explain that holding a conversation in which one lists the concerns is required by American ethical standards and is not intended to signal intent to withdraw from the contractual agreement with the tai chi school.
3. Should both the tai chi school and you be very much rooted in the American culture, you would ask the school to replace the advertisement. The new ad should reflect accurate information in a manner that documents how your peers have engaged in this process so that their work is never misrepresented.
4. Should both the tai chi school and you be very much rooted in the American culture, you would personally deliver to each new student of the school adequate disclosure about the current state of the research findings regarding the health benefits of tai chi and your scientific findings about the health benefits.
5. Should both the tai chi school and you be very much rooted in the American culture, you would make an offer to reimburse fees if the student decides not to continue with the school.
6. Do a combination of the previously listed actions.
7. Do something that is not previously listed.

If you practiced in Singapore, which of the following would you do?

1. Speak to a mutually trusted family friend to relay the concerns regarding the advertisement material to end the misrepresentation. In this manner, the tai chi school learns about the concerns of Dr. Smith.
2. Cease all contact with the tai chi school.

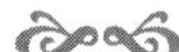

STANDARD 1.02: CONFLICTS BETWEEN ETHICS AND LAW, REGULATIONS, OR OTHER GOVERNING LEGAL AUTHORITY

> If psychologists' ethical responsibilities conflict with law, regulations, or other governing legal authority, psychologists clarify the nature of the conflict, make known their commitment to the Ethics Code, and take reasonable steps to resolve the conflict consistent with the General Principles and Ethical Standards of the Ethics Code. Under no circumstances may this standard be used to justify or defend violating human rights.

A CASE FOR STANDARD 1.02: Legal Mandate or Not?

Linda is a 16-year-old adolescent. Her parents are both police officers. Linda is seeing Dr. Johnson for therapy and carries a diagnosis of oppositional defiant disorder. In a session, Linda told Dr. Johnson that she recently made a good decision in a bad situation. During lunch she was with a group of kids when one kid, Robert, began arguing with her boyfriend, Michael. Evidently, Michael had stolen some marijuana from Robert's home. Robert threatened to tell Michael's parents so they would "kick Michael's ass!"

Michael then drove off the school grounds with Linda in the car. He drove to his house and pulled a loaded gun from his father's gun case, saying, "I'm going to get Robert after school today." Linda reported to Dr. Johnson that this is when she made a good decision: She left and told Michael he is "just too much!" Linda then said to Dr. Johnson, "Oh, well, you probably know this already since Michael comes to therapy here, too. He sees Dr. Williams."

Issues of Concern

Laws that mandate or permit psychologists to make known either to the intended victim and/or to law enforcement authorities a threat of physical harm to another person are generally referred to as "duty to protect." North American jurisdictions have diverse responses to the law stating one's duty to protect, and the laws of each jurisdiction should be checked carefully. Currently, 23 states impose a duty to protect by statute, and 9 states have a common-law duty as a result of court cases; 13 other states permit but do not mandate the breach of confidentiality to warn potential victims, and 7 states have not ruled on the issue. In Canada, six provinces have no statutory or case law related to the issue, and seven provinces allow but do not mandate disclosure of dangerousness to third parties (Benjamin, Kent, & Sirikantraporn, 2009).

Standard 1.02 obligates a psychologist to clarify the nature of the conflict between ethics and the law. In this case, depending upon which state Dr. Johnson is practicing in, the conflict may arise between the Standard 4.01 for confidentiality and a mandate to comply with the law for duty to protect. However, Michael is not Dr. Johnson's client, thus the law in some states may not apply in this case. Even so, there may still be a moral obligation of beneficence that applies, regardless of whether Michael is Dr. Johnson's client or not. Therefore, the question is as follows: Should Dr. Johnson report Michael's intent to harm Robert? Is Dr. Johnson responsible for protecting Robert from Michael based on confidential information provided by Linda?

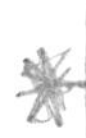

APA Ethics Code

Companion General Principle

Principle A: Beneficence and Nonmaleficence

> Psychologists strive to benefit those with whom they work and take care to do no harm.

In general, psychologists remain aware of taking any actions that might harm Linda, the identified client who is engaged in treatment. Does the principle of "do no harm" extend out to Michael, Linda's friend and client of an office colleague?

Principle B: Fidelity and Responsibility

> Psychologists establish relationships of trust with those with whom they work.

Linda's comment of "you probably know this already," seems to have an implied expectation that communication and client information is shared between psychologists in the same office suite. In most cases, clients' trust in large part is based on their knowing when and where psychologists disclose client information. Trust is not necessarily best developed from the adherence to total confidentiality. Linda's trust may increase if she thinks Dr. Johnson can keep her and her friends from harm.

Companion Ethical Standard(s)

Standard 4.01: Privacy and Confidentiality; Standard 4.04: Minimizing Intrusions on Privacy

> . . . (b) Psychologists discuss confidential information obtained in their work only for appropriate . . . professional purposes and only with persons clearly concerned with such matters.

Information obtained through Linda during a treatment session is clearly confidential. If Dr. Johnson were to discuss any information, it would "only be with persons clearly concerned." In this case, persons concerned may include Dr. Williams, school authorities, the police, Robert and his parents, Michael and his parents, and/or Linda's parents.

Standard 4.02: Discussing the Limits of Confidentiality

> . . . (b) . . . The discussion of confidentiality occurs . . . thereafter as new circumstances may warrant.

If discussions were to occur between Dr. Johnson and anyone else, Standard 4.02 (b) would direct Dr. Johnson to first have a discussion about limits of confidentiality with Linda.

Legal Issues 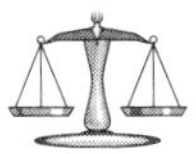

Georgia

> *Ga. Code Ann. § 43-39-16 (2008).*
>
> Client communications with psychologists "are placed upon the same basis as those provided by law between attorney and client." Georgia attorneys must maintain confidences and preserve secrets of their clients (Ga. Code. Ann. § 15-19-4(3) [2008]). Communications between attorneys and clients are not admissible in court (Ga. Code. Ann. § 24-9-21 [2008]).
>
> In light of this foundation, clients have extensive confidentiality protections. The Georgia courts have adopted

§ 319 of the Second Restatement of Torts, and have found that mental health professionals have a duty to warn or protect third persons only when the clinician has control over the client (because the client is within an inpatient setting) and knows or should know that the client is likely to harm others (*Bradley Ctr., Inc. v. Wessner*, 296 S.E.2d 693 [Ga. 1982]; *Swofford v. Cooper*, 360 S.E.2d 624 [Ga. Ct. App. 1987], *aff'd*, 368 S.E.2d 518 [Ga. 1988]; *Jacobs et al. v. Taylor et al.*, 379 S.E.2d 592 [Ga. Ct. App. 1989]) found no duty to report for generalized threats nor if the victim knew of the client's violent tendencies.

New Jersey

N.J. Stat. Ann. § 2A:62A-16 (West 2000).

A duty is imposed to warn or protect when a client communicates a threat of "imminent, serious physical violence against a readily identifiable individual or against himself and the circumstances are such that a reasonable professional . . . would believe the client intended to carry out the threat." The mental health professional discharges the duty by arranging for the client to be voluntarily hospitalized, initiating procedures for involuntary commitment, notifying law enforcement of the client's threat and the victim's identity, warning the intended victim, warning the victim's parent or guardian if the victim is under 18, or warning the client's parent or guardian if the client is under 18 and threatening suicide or "bodily injury." The duty is discharged if the psychologist takes any one of these actions, and the psychologist may also take more than one action.

Since Dr. Johnson does not treat Michael, Dr. Johnson cannot independently ascertain the validity of Linda's claim that Michael intends to harm Robert. Under the laws of Georgia and New Jersey, no duty exists because Michael is not a client.

Cultural Considerations

Global Discussion

Code of Ethics for the Psychologist: Spain

Article 65. Should a psychologist find that adverse or incompatible rules, whether in law or contained in this Code of Ethics, come into conflict in a specific case, he/she must resolve it according to his or her conscience, informing to the different parties involved and the College's Deontological Committee.

When an ethical obligation to keep client confidentiality conflicts with a duty to protect, the Spanish psychologist must seek some sort of resolution that satisfies the dictates of her own conscience, the knowledge of involved parties, and the Psychological Society of Spain. Article 65 also seems to suggest that whatever decision the psychologist comes to, she will need to communicate that resolution to Spain's Ethics Committee itself.

American Moral Values

1. Psychologists give the promise of confidentiality implicitly by holding the information divulged in treatment sessions private, and they explicitly delineate the limits of confidentiality at the onset of treatment. What is the value of the confidentiality between Dr. Johnson and Linda compared to the threat of violence between Michael and Robert? Part of Dr. Johnson's thinking may be shaped by a judgment about guns as instruments of violence. The level of violence inherent in the possession of a gun is much greater than if Michael had obtained a Swiss Army knife and made the same threats, for example. The lethal power of guns can give Dr. Johnson more urgency to prevent Michael from committing an act of violence.
2. Dr. Johnson might not break confidentiality about Michael if Linda's revelations do not seem credible. Here again, the associations with guns could play a role in the judgment, as people generally do not doubt the honesty or the accuracy of the reporter when guns are involved. On the other hand, Linda's romantic relationship with Michael may cause Dr. Johnson to wonder if Linda is observing and reporting the interactions melodramatically or from a position of overly fearful vulnerability.
3. The question of Linda's revealing her confidences can involve a moral picture of romantic relationships. A girlfriend and boyfriend might be thought to have a degree of fidelity and intimacy between them in terms of what they share together. What if Linda believes that her relationship with Michael is the only thing holding her together and helping her get through a tough time in life? For Linda to relay intimate information to Dr. Johnson may give more credence to the validity of her report and lead Dr. Johnson to feel more compelled to act. This may be especially true in the case of young love or first love, which generally carries heavier emotional weight for those involved. Thus revealing a "secret" of what was said in private could make Linda's report more believable and compelling than if Linda was a middle-aged woman.
4. Linda's offhand comment "You probably knew that already" suggested she might not know about

confidentiality as a clinical standard of practice. Would that knowledge have changed her decision in revealing that Michael's seeing Dr. Williams? Would it change how she felt about Dr. Johnson acting on her tip? Before acting on Linda's information, Dr. Johnson may want Linda to know the implications of client–therapist confidentiality so that Linda could reconsider the implications of what she has shared and what she wants to happen on that basis.

5. From what Linda has told Dr. Johnson of Michael, Dr. Johnson might consider what Michael will do if he finds out that Linda has told Dr. Johnson about the gun and that Michael sees Dr. Williams. Is Michael's danger to Robert much clearer and more urgent than any threat he poses to Linda?

Ethical Course of Action

Directive per APA Code

If you were working in Georgia or New Jersey, there would be no conflict between the standard of confidentiality and the law because Michael is not Dr. Johnson's client. The primary focus remains on the treatment relationship between Dr. Johnson and Linda. The primary topic remains one of confidentiality. As directed by Standard 4.02 (b), Dr. Johnson should reconsider with Linda the applied meaning of confidentiality.

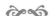

Dictates of One's Own Conscience

Beyond having a discussion to reconfirm that what Linda says in treatment stays confidential unless mandated by law, what might you do?

1. Address the secondary topic of trust—that is, whether Linda can trust you to provide protection to her boyfriend from his possible impulsive actions and protection of the relationship she has with her boyfriend.

2. Explore the situational application of Principle B: Fidelity & Responsibility that is, for you to take a course of action in such a way that does not surprise Linda or leave her to wonder why you took a certain course of action. This might mean exploring with Linda the possible implications of all parties concerned (i.e., Linda and you, Linda and Michael, Linda and her parents, Linda and Robert, Michael and his parents, Michael and Robert) should it be revealed that Linda gave consent for information to be passed on to Dr. Williams.

3. Discuss the situation with Dr. Williams based on the knowledge that Linda has provided a waiver of her confidentiality by her statement "you probably know already" and your following up with her by confirming that she expects you to talk with Dr. Williams.

4. Ask Linda for release of confidential information to talk to Dr. Williams, followed by an explanation that only with Linda's full knowledge and consent would you disclose information about Michael to Dr. Williams.

5. Invite Linda to meet with Dr. Williams and explain her concerns to Dr. Williams. You should inform Linda that by doing so she would waive her right to confidentiality about the issues that emerge during the discussion with Dr. Williams and that such a conversation may have an impact on her relationship with Michael.

6. Explore the incident further to decide if there is reason to believe someone's life is in serious danger. If yes, then discuss limits of confidentiality and duty to warn. If not, then explore future options for Linda if it may happen again—who can she report to and what can she do to keep herself safe?

7. Do a combination of the previously listed actions.

8. Do something that is not previously listed.

If you were practicing in Spain, what might you do?

1. Contact a member of the College's Deontological Committee for consultation?

2. Consider that the word *deontological* can be roughly understood to mean rules or rules for the role of psychology? You would decide which rules are the most relevant for this situation. It may be less important which rules are chosen but that the duty of the role is explicitly articulated. Decide which rules to follow, and then let everyone concerned know of your value stance.

3. Inform the College's Deontological Committee about your decision?

STANDARD 1.03: CONFLICTS BETWEEN ETHICS AND ORGANIZATIONAL DEMANDS

If the demands of an organization with which psychologists are affiliated or for whom they are working 2010 Amendment to this standard has added . . . working are in conflict with this Ethics Code, psychologists clarify the nature of the conflict, make known their commitment to the Ethics Code, and take reasonable steps to resolve the conflict consistent with the General Principles and Ethical Standards of the Ethics Code. Under no circumstances may this standard be used to justify or defend violating human rights.

A CASE FOR STANDARD 1.03: William and the Dog

William is a psychology intern in a minimum-security prison. He has been treating Barbara for about 6 months. Barbara has a history of previous trauma. Her presenting problem for treatment was trust related. In the course of treatment, Barbara repeatedly discussed how she likes her work in the prison's canine training program, but she dislikes the fellow inmates who do not know how to work with the dogs. One day Barbara was especially agitated. She decided to trust William with her real concerns and tell him an inmate abused one of the dogs. Barbara wanted William to do something to help the dog. However, fearing retaliation inside the prison, Barbara did not want William to tell anyone that she was the one who said something. In addition, Barbara would not reveal the name of the alleged abuser. William reassured Barbara the content of therapy is confidential and the situation can be taken care of without naming names.

William sought guidance from his supervisor regarding how best to proceed with an anonymous report. William's supervisor said prison policy requires immediate identification and a report of anyone who abuses the animals in the canine training program. Further, unless William identified his patient, he would be considered to be insubordinate and risk being dismissed from the internship.

Issues of Concern

Employees have a duty to uphold the policy and procedures of the employing organization. At the same time, psychologists are bound to maintain confidentiality of their clients. William would most likely feel caught between not wanting to lose Barbara's trust and damage the therapeutic relationship, the wish to protect her from the high probability of physical assault if he identifies her, and the personal wish to maintain his good standing in the internship.

APA Ethics Code

Companion General Principle

Principle C: Integrity

> Psychologists strive to keep their promises and to avoid unwise or unclear commitments . . .

Psychologists are trained to maintain client confidentiality. In line with his training, William reassured Barbara that confidentiality could be maintained. Keeping to the aspiration of Principle C: Integrity would guide William to keep Barbara's identity confidential.

Companion Ethical Standard(s)

Standard 4.05: Disclosures

> (a) Psychologists may disclose confidential information with the appropriate consent of the organizational client, the individual client/patient . . . unless prohibited by law.

Standard 4.05 directs William to reveal Barbara's identity only if he had appropriate consent from Barbara. In this case, he not only does not have consent; he actually has a explicit prohibition from Barbara against revealing her identity.

Standard 4.01: Maintaining Confidentiality

> Psychologists have a primary obligation and take reasonable precautions to protect confidential information obtained through . . . any medium, recognizing that the extent and limits of confidentiality may be . . . established by institutional rules . . .

Standard 4.05 (a) says William has the primary obligation of keeping Barbara's identity confidential. Since he is conducting treatment in a prison, Standard 4.01 also says the extent of confidentiality would be established by the policies and procedures of the prison. Standard 4.01 would lead William to reveal Barbara's identity. Standard 4.01 appears to be in conflict with the directives of Standard 1.03. Standard 4.01 obligates psychologists to recognize the limits of confidentiality as regulated by institutional rule, and would mean revealing Barbara's identity. At the same time, Standard 1.03 obligates psychologists to act in such way to be consistent with the APA Ethics Code General Principle and Ethical Standards, and to uphold Standard 4.05 (a) by not revealing Barbara's identity.

Standard 4.02: Discussing the Limits of Confidentiality

(a) Psychologists discuss with persons . . . and organizations with whom they establish a . . . professional relationship (1) the relevant limits of confidentiality and . . . (b) unless it is not feasible or is contraindicated, the discussion of confidentiality occurs at the outset of the relationship and thereafter as new circumstances may warrant.

Standard 4.02 (a) and (b) directs William to have had a discussion with Barbara about the limits of confidentiality at the onset of the therapeutic relationship and as new occasions arise. It was appropriate for Barbara to have raised the issue of confidentiality before she revealed information that was potentially dangerous to her own safety.

Standard 4.02 directs William to have discussed the limits of confidentiality before entering into any services with a client in an institutional context and memorialized in writing within the chart notes. Raising the limits of confidentiality both orally and in writing is a way to prevent any confusion and engage in sufficient informed consent to provide services. However, Standard 1.03 directs William to follow the institutional policies, regardless of whether those policies conflict with other ethics code standards.

Standard 2.01: Boundaries of Competence

(a) Psychologists provide services . . . only within the boundaries of their competence, based on their education, training, supervised experience, consultation, study, or professional experience.

William was not competent to provide treatment with a prison population by virtue of his student intern status. However, it could be argued that William was practicing within his boundaries of competency since he was under supervision of someone who knew the policies of the institution. This standard would guide William to defer to his supervisor, reveal Barbara's identity, and to request the identity of the animal abuser be revealed.

Legal Issues 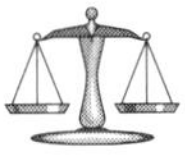

Virginia

18 Va. Admin. Code § 125-20-150(B) (2010).

. . . (5) Avoid harming patients . . . for whom they provide professional services and minimize harm when it is foreseeable and unavoidable.

. . . (7) Withdraw from, adjust, or clarify conflicting roles with due regard for the best interest of the affected party or parties and maximal compliance with these standards.

. . . (9) Keep confidential their professional relationships with patients or clients and disclose client records to others only with written consent except: (i) when a patient or client is a danger to self or others, (ii) as required under § 32.1-127.1:03 of the Code of Virginia, or (iii) as permitted by law for a valid purpose.

Florida

Fla. Admin. Code Ann. r. § 64B19-19.006 (2010). Confidentiality.

. . . Licensed psychologists in . . . subacute . . . settings should inform service users when information given to the psychologist may be available to others without the service user's written consent. Similar limitations on confidentiality may present themselves . . . in each similar circumstance, the licensed psychologist must obtain a written statement from the service user which acknowledges the psychologist's advice in those regards. This rule is particularly applicable to supervisory situations wherein the supervised individual will be sharing confidential information with the supervising psychologist. In that situation, it is incumbent upon the licensed psychologist to secure the written acknowledgement of the service user regarding that breach of confidentiality.

Both Virginia and Florida call for the limitations of maintaining confidentiality being consented to in advance of the clinical relationship. If the client provided a release, the psychologist-in-training could release her identity. It is doubtful that such a release would be given because of the likelihood of reprisals. The psychologist-in-training should maintain the confidences under the laws of both of these jurisdictions.

Cultural Considerations

Global Discussion

Singapore Psychological Society: Code of Professional Ethics

Principle 7: Client welfare.

. . . The psychologist in . . . situations in which conflicts of interest may arise among various parties, as . . . between the client and employer of the psychologist, defines . . . the nature and direction of his or her loyalties, and responsibilities and keeps all parties concerned informed of these commitments.

If William was treating Barbara in Singapore, William would be obligated to define for himself his responsibilities to both his employer, the prison, and Barbara, his client, decide the "direction of his loyalties," and communicate his intentions to all parties involved. As part of a collective culture like Singapore, William's loyalties are likely to be torn more in the direction of the benefit of the whole or larger number, rather than that being secondary to his own internship, career, or personal wishes.

American Moral Values

1. What value does William place on earning his degree and graduating as opposed to earning and keeping Barbara's trust? The value William holds in completing his internship and earning his degree seem to be set in opposition to the professional standard of confidentiality.
2. Individuals who find themselves in a highly structured environment with no realistic option for exit, such as a prison, hold a much smaller degree of freedom to form other relationships. Given Barbara's confinement, William might weigh his involvement with Barbara more seriously than if Barbara had the ability to seek out another psychologist for treatment. What will be the impact on Barbara of a ruined relationship with William?
3. William's treatment of Barbara may involve his moral image of prisoners. To the degree he believes that Barbara is most likely responsible for committing a crime, and/or rightly punished by serving in prison, he might be more inclined to think she has given up normal rights to privacy, even for reasons of personal safety.
4. William might also morally object to the way the American penal system treats prisoners. Barbara may represent a person who is trying, against the grain of prison authorities' assumptions, to improve herself. Should William go the "extra" mile to rebuild trust between Barbara and a person vested with the authority he has?
5. Does the prison policy of mandating that one report all mistreatment of the guide dogs reflect the value of individual responsibility? The dogs are not serving time for crimes committed, whereas prisoners are incarcerated as a result of their own action. Does the protection dogs deserve outweigh concerns for how prisoners may treat each other?
6. The dogs are helpless animals that cannot protect themselves against mistreatment, whereas Barbara, as a human, can protect herself more. Even though Barbara fears for her safety, can anyone else protect the dogs if he does not speak up?

Ethical Course of Action

Directive per APA Code

Following the directive of Standard 1.03, William needs to let his supervisor know of his wish to adhere to Standard 4.05 (a) disclosure and engage in an exploration of ways to resolve the situation that permits him to keep to Standard 4.05(a). As specified in Standard 1.03, psychologists then need to take reasonable steps to resolve this conflict in such a way that William is able to uphold the ethics code.

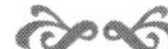

Dictates of One's Own Conscience

Standard 1.03 directs William to do something consistent with the ethics code. If you were William, what might you do?

1. Resolve to read the institutional policy and procedures manuals during initial orientation in any future jobs. The limitations for protecting the confidentiality of clients within an institutional setting should be delineated clearly in the procedures manual.
2. Reveal the identity of all parties involved to your supervisor immediately.
3. Refuse to reveal the client's identity in accordance with the ethics code.
4. Return to Barbara and explain that before any promises were made to keep the dog abuse confidential, he should have stopped her and reviewed the confidentiality policies of the prison with her, then proceed to reveal the identities of all parties involved.
5. Return to Barbara to tell her about the policies, and let her know you will be revealing the identities of all involved in order to protect the welfare of the dogs, then proceed to reveal the identities of all parties involved.
6. Ask Barbara to provide a release so that information may be revealed with Barbara's consent. If Barbara refuses to sign a release, then refuse to reveal the identity of the client to your supervisor on the grounds of confidentiality.
7. Ask Barbara to meet with the supervisor to determine some method by which to protect her identity while protecting the dog, and preventing the dog's abuser from having unfettered access to other dogs. If Barbara refuses, you would refuse to reveal the

identity of the client to your supervisor on the grounds of confidentiality.

8. Do a combination of the previously listed actions.
9. Do something that is not previously listed.

If you were practicing in Singapore, what might you do?

1. It is highly improbable that a supervisor would give the ultimatum of either breaking your promise of confidentiality or losing your internship.
2. Staying focused upon your obligation is to protect the welfare of the person with whom your work is undertaken. This means your primary obligation is to protect Barbara's welfare, secondarily to protect the welfare of the dog, and tertiarily to protect your own welfare.
3. As referenced in Singapore's Code of Professional Ethics Principle 7.1, you first define for yourself the nature and direction of your loyalties and responsibilities and then to keep all parties informed about these commitments. As you have already promised Barbara that information would be kept confidential, you have already defined the direction of your loyalty. All that is left for you to do is to let the institution and Barbara know the direction of your loyalty.

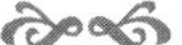

STANDARD 1.04: INFORMAL RESOLUTION OF ETHICAL VIOLATIONS

When psychologists believe that there may have been an ethical violation by another psychologist, they attempt to resolve the issue by bringing it to the attention of that individual, if an informal resolution appears appropriate and the intervention does not violate any confidentiality rights that may be involved.

A CASE FOR STANDARD 1.04: The European Vacation—Part I

Dr. Jones shares a two-office suite with three other psychologists. Mary is in treatment with Dr. Jones. Mary's daughter, 16-year-old Patricia, is in treatment with one of Dr. Jones's office mates, Dr. Brown. Dr. Jones and Dr. Brown are office mates but see each other very sporadically since they do not have overlapping office days. Mary reported that her daughter is in treatment for depression. In session, Mary talked about planning for a vacation to Las Vegas with her husband during the time her daughter Patricia was on a European vacation trip with Dr. Brown. It appears that Dr. Brown had offered to pay all expenses for Patricia to join him and his wife for this trip to Europe. Dr. Brown told Mary that this trip would build Patricia's self-esteem by allowing Patricia to give comfort to Mrs. Brown, who has been depressed since the couples' youngest child left home for college.

Issues of Concern

At face value, taking a 16-year-old patient on a European vacation is incongruent with standard practice for outpatient treatment of depression. However, Patricia is not Dr. Jones's patient, thus cannot make known her opinion regarding the European vacation. Unless Mary gives consent for Dr. Jones to discuss any aspect of the European vacation with Patricia, it is unclear whether Dr. Jones may do so without violation of Standard 4.01: Confidentiality. A question to consider in this situation is this: Does conversing with an office mate constitute violation of confidentiality rights of the client?

APA Ethics Code

Companion General Principle

Principle B: Fidelity and Responsibility

> Psychologists are concerned about the ethical compliance of their colleagues' scientific and professional conduct.

In general, psychologists are aware of our professional standing in society. Specifically, psychologists are aware of our own professional standing in the community within which we practice. In light of Principle B, Dr. Jones's professional association with Dr. Brown makes Dr. Brown's conduct of concern to Dr. Jones.

Companion Ethical Standard(s)

Standard 3.04: Avoiding Harm

> Psychologists take reasonable steps to avoid harming their clients/patients . . . and others with whom they work, and to minimize harm where it is foreseeable and unavoidable.

The primary concern in this situation is the possible harm to Patricia should she be permitted to go with Dr. Brown on his family vacation to Europe. Standard 3.04 directs Dr. Jones to take reasonable steps to avoid harm to "others with whom they work." The question here is whether Patricia or Dr. Brown falls under the category of others with whom Dr. Jones works.

Standard 4.05: Disclosures

> (a) Psychologists may disclose confidential information with the appropriate consent of the . . . individual client . . . unless prohibited by law. (b) Psychologists disclose confidential information without the consent of the individual only as mandated by law . . . (3) protect the client/patient, psychologist . . . from harm; . . . in which instance disclosure is limited to the minimum that is necessary to achieve the purpose.

Standard 4.05 (a) directs Dr. Jones to have only a discussion with Dr. Brown with the full knowledge and consent of Mary, her own client. Under circumstances specified in Standard 4.05 (b) Dr. Jones could disregard the directive of Standard 4.05 and discuss the case with Dr. Brown, regardless of the wishes of her client Mary. If Dr. Jones were to talk to Dr. Brown, she would be acting under the directive of Standard 4.05 (b) (3) "protect . . . others from harm."

Standard 2.04: Bases for Scientific and Professional Judgments

> Psychologists' work is based upon established scientific and professional knowledge of the discipline.

There is no known current scientific or professional knowledge that would justify Dr. Brown taking a client on vacation for the benefit of his wife. Thus Dr. Brown is in violation of Standard 2.04.

Legal Issues 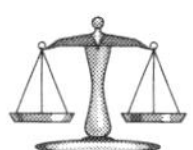

Massachusetts

> *251 Mass. Code Regs. 1.10 (2010). Ethical standards and professional conduct.*
>
> (1) The Board adopts as its standard of conduct the Ethical Principles of Psychologists and Code of Conduct of the American Psychological Association.
>
> *Mass. Ann. Laws ch. 112, § 129A (LexisNexis 2003).*
>
> All communications between a licensed psychologist and the individuals with whom the psychologist engages in the practice of psychology are confidential . . . No psychologist . . . shall disclose any information acquired or revealed in the course of or in connection with the performance of the psychologist's professional services . . . except under the following circumstances:
>
> . . . (b) upon express, written consent of the patient . . .

Ohio

> *Ohio Admin. Code 4732:17-01 (2010).*
>
> (C) Welfare of the Client:
>
> (4) Dependency.
>
> Due to inherently influential position, a psychologist . . . shall not exploit the trust or dependency of any client . . . with whom there is a professional psychological role. . .
>
> (G) Confidentiality.
>
> (1) Confidential information is information revealed by an individual . . . obtained as a result of the professional relationship between the individual(s) and the psychologist. . . Such information is not to be disclosed by the psychologist . . . without the informed consent of the individual(s).
>
> (a) When . . . interacting with other appropriate professionals concerning the welfare of a client, a psychologist . . . may share confidential information about the client provided that reasonable steps are taken to ensure that all persons receiving the information are informed about the confidential nature of the information being shared and agree to abide by the rules of confidentiality.
>
> (J) (4) Reporting of Violations to Board.
>
> A psychologist . . . who has substantial reason to believe that another licensee . . . has committed an apparent violation of the statutes or rules of the board that . . . is likely to substantially harm a person . . . when the information regarding such violation is obtained in a professional relationship with a client, the psychologist . . . shall report it only with the written permission of the client. . .

Both Massachusetts and Ohio law would preclude the informal resolution process contemplated by APA Ethics Code Standard 1.04 without an explicit release of the mother's confidential material being provided by the mother, Mary. If a release were provided, Massachusetts would permit the informal resolution process. Ohio, on the other hand, directs Dr. Jones to engage in the filing of a complaint to the licensing board if in Dr. Jones's view the behavior of Dr. Brown is likely to cause substantial harm to Patricia, the client of the offending psychologist.

In Ohio, Dr. Jones is not to approach Dr. Brown to engage in an informal conversation since it would violate confidentiality.

Cultural Considerations

Global Discussion

Canadian Code of Ethics

> Responsibility of the individual psychologist.
>
> The discipline's contract with society commits the discipline and its members to act as a moral community . . .
>
> (1) To bring concerns about possible unethical actions by a psychologist directly to the psychologist when the action appears to be primarily a lack of sensitivity, knowledge, or experience, and attempt to reach an agreement on the issue and, if needed, on the appropriate action to be taken.

If Dr. Jones was practicing in Canada, and if she assumes that Dr. Brown's actions were likely the result of a lack of sensitivity, knowledge, or experience, the code would direct her to have an immediate discussion with Dr. Brown first. Because the Canadian code charges members with accountability for the education and training of new members, it is the responsibility of both psychologists to attempt an agreement regarding what, if any, corrective action needs to be taken. "Appropriate action" would likely vary and is entrusted to the psychologists involved to decide.

American Moral Values

1. Dr. Jones's confidentiality with Mary conflicts with a possible need to intervene in Dr. Brown's decision about Patricia. What are the consequences to the client–therapist relationship if Dr. Jones breaks confidentiality? Is Mary trying to draw Dr. Jones into making a decision for her about Patricia? Dr. Jones may consider how Mary's own therapeutic needs will be affected by this situation, despite the fact that she seems fine with Patricia's vacation plan.
2. Dr. Jones must also consider whether Dr. Brown's decision could be harmful enough to Mary and Patricia to merit breaking confidentiality. Is Patricia, as a minor, old enough to make this decision? Is Dr. Brown making it for her? Should a therapist be inviting a client into a personal and familial relationship, especially given the power dynamic of a teenage client with an older therapist? Dr. Jones may feel that Patricia is in need of protection from the dysfunctional character of this vacation, whether or not Mary recognizes it.
3. Familial relations can carry a special cultural and emotional significance in terms of closeness and privacy. On the one hand, Dr. Brown seems to be eliding the boundary between his client Patricia and his own family. In particular, Dr. Jones must consider what role Dr. Brown sees Patricia fulfilling for his depressed wife. At the same time, if Dr. Jones intervenes with Dr. Brown she may also be seen as meddling in Mary and Patricia's mother/daughter relationship. As her client and Patricia's mother, does Mary need to give Dr. Jones consent before contacting Dr. Brown about the situation?
4. Dr. Jones could also consider how "standard practice" has changed over time. At one time in the history of psychological treatment, it was not out of the question for treating professionals to avoid abandoning their clients by taking them along on vacation. Is it possible that Dr. Brown's approach, regardless of how inappropriate it could seem to others, would work for Patricia?
5. Considerations of class may be appropriate for Dr. Jones's deliberation. Does Dr. Jones give a fair value to Mary's decision to go to Las Vegas, given its connotations for some educated professionals? Might Dr. Jones consider Mary's position differently if Mary had needed time away to care for a sick mother? Likewise, does Dr. Brown's choice of a European vacation change its perceived value as an experience for Patricia (given its positive associations for many Americans as an opportunity for education and self-refinement)?
6. Dr. Jones must also confront the example she and Dr. Brown could set for other psychologists, as well as the public example that could appear to the larger community. Is Dr. Brown's decision a poor example upon which others might base their opinion of psychologists, especially since news of such an unusual move might "get out" into the community? Dr. Jones might value her own professional reputation in the community in such a way as to ensure her office mates work within the usual and customary standards of practice (presumably not taking one's client on vacation).
7. Dr. Jones may value the harmonious relationship she has with her office mates (including Dr. Brown) at this point, and she may not wish to disturb the smooth running of the office by bring up difficult items based on the report of a client, which may or may not be true. What value does that collegiality and camaraderie have set against this vacation and its implication for Mary and Patricia?

Ethical Course of Action

Directive per APA Code

Standard 1.04 would guide Dr. Jones to, at a minimum, have an informal discussion with Dr. Brown. This standard directs that this conversation should occur only if such a discussion does not violate Mary's confidentiality rights. However, if Dr. Jones were practicing in Ohio, a Standard 1.02 conflict between ethics/law would arise and Dr. Jones is not to approach Dr. Brown for such a conversation since it would violate the confidentiality law.

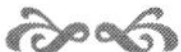

Dictates of One's Own Conscience

Beyond having a conversation with Dr. Brown, if you were practicing in Massachusetts and actions as directed by Standard 1.04, what might you do?

1. For your own deliberations regarding this situation, through casual inquiry, consider consultation with other psychologists to explore the best course of action and whether the ethical and legal standards appeared to be blurred by such a trip.
2. Obtain information about the standards of psychology practice and vacationing with one's client and then share the information which can be shared with Mary.
3. Protect the therapeutic alliance between Dr. Jones and Mary and explore with Mary the idea of holding a joint meeting with Dr. Brown. The purpose of such a joint meeting would be to raise questions about the European vacation and whether such a trip should occur.
4. Do a combination of the previously listed actions.
5. Do something that is not previously listed.

If you were practicing in Canada, what would you do?

1. Discuss the situation with Dr. Brown by first inquiring as to why Dr. Brown thinks taking Patricia on his family vacation is a good idea.
2. Endeavor to explore with Dr. Brown the scientific and professional basis for taking a patient on a family vacation.
3. Tell Dr. Brown that he has failed to identify any valid scientific and profesional basis for taking Patricia on the European vacation and that he should not do it.

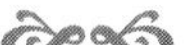

STANDARD 1.05: REPORTING ETHICAL VIOLATIONS

> If an apparent ethical violation has substantially harmed or is likely to substantially harm a person or organization and is not appropriate for informal resolution under Standard 1.04: Informal Resolution of Ethical Violations, or is not resolved properly in that fashion, psychologists take further action appropriate to the situation. Such action might include referral to state or national committees on professional ethics, to state licensing boards, or to the appropriate institutional authorities. This standard does not apply when an intervention would violate confidentiality rights or when psychologists have been retained to review the work of another psychologist whose professional conduct is in question.

A CASE FOR STANDARD 1.05: The European Vacation—Part II

Continuing from A Case for Standard 1.04: The European Vacation—Part I, Dr. Jones asked Mary for permission to discuss the matter with Dr. Brown. Mary said that Patricia is very sensitive and does not want her mother to interfere with Patricia's treatment. In addition, Mary has not had a vacation with her husband for some time and thinks this trip would very much help the marriage. Without client consent to reveal confidential information, Dr. Jones did not approach Dr. Brown. Time passes, and Mary and her husband have had a good holiday. Patricia has returned from vacation with Dr. Brown. Mary reported that the after-effect of the vacation on Patricia appears to be positive in that Patricia is not depressed anymore. However, now Patricia is defiant, and Mary thinks Dr. Brown has undermined her parental authority and positive relationship with her daughter. Mary now thinks it was a bad idea for Patricia to have gone on vacation with Dr. Brown. Mary asked Dr. Jones what can be done about what Mary now thinks is a bad relationship between Dr. Brown and her daughter, Patricia.

Issues of Concern

Dr. Jones now has an after-the-fact situation that is not amenable to informal resolution under Standard 1.04. Is there sufficient concern about unprofessional conduct for Dr. Jones to take further action or cause Mary to take further action? Is the violation of such gravity to merit contacting either the national committees on professional ethics or the state licensing board?

APA Ethics Code

Companion General Principle

Principle A: Beneficence and Nonmaleficence

> In their professional actions, psychologists seek to safeguard the welfare and rights of those with whom they interact professionally and other affected persons.

With the passage of time and further unfolding of events, Mary sees the harm from her daughter going on a European vacation with Dr. Brown. Aspirations based on Principle A would allow Dr. Jones to act in the highest good for "other affected persons," namely Patricia.

Principle B: Fidelity and Responsibility

> Psychologists are concerned about the ethical compliance of their colleagues' . . . professional conduct.

In general, psychologists are aware of our professional standing in society. Specifically, psychologists are aware of our own professional standing in the community within which we practice. Even with the passage of time and unfolding of events, Principle B still holds. Dr. Jones's professional association with Dr. Brown makes Dr. Brown's conduct of concern to Dr. Jones.

Companion Ethical Standard(s)

Standard 4.05: Disclosures

> (a) Psychologists may disclose confidential information with the appropriate consent of the . . . individual client. . .

Dr. Jones has implicit consent from Mary to break confidentiality to file a complaint or cause Mary to file a complaint against Dr. Brown.

Standard 1.04: Informal Resolution of Ethical Violations

> When psychologists believe that there may have been an ethical violation by another psychologist, they attempt to resolve the issue by bringing it to the attention of that individual, if an informal resolution appears appropriate and the intervention does not violate any confidentiality rights that may be involved.

Unlike the vignettes appearing before the European Vacation, this standard no longer applies. Informal resolution is no longer possible given the gravity of the event and the fact that Mary now wishes to file a formal complaint.

Legal Issues 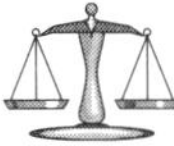

Texas

> *22 Tex. Admin. Code § 465.1 (2010). Definitions.*
>
> . . . (2) "Dual Relationship" means a situation where a licensee and another individual have both a professional relationship and a non-professional relationship. Dual relationships include . . . personal friendships, . . . family . . . ties, . . .
>
> *22 Tex. Admin. Code § 465.13 (2010). Personal problems, conflicts and dual relationships.*
>
> . . . (b) Dual relationships.
>
> (1) A licensee must refrain from entering into a dual relationship with a client . . . if such a relationship presents a risk that the dual relationship could . . . exploit or otherwise cause harm to the other party.
>
> . . . (6) A licensee in a potentially harmful dual or multiple relationship must cease to provide psychological services to the other party, regardless of the wishes of that party.

Washington

> *Wash. Admin. Code § 246-924-357 (2009). Multiple relationships.*
>
> The psychologist shall not undertake or continue a professional relationship with a client . . . because of the psychologist's present . . . social, . . . emotional, . . . with the client. . . When such relationship impairs objectivity, the psychologist shall terminate the professional relationship with adequate notice and in an appropriate manner; and shall assist the client in obtaining services from another professional.
>
> *Wash. Rev. Code Ann. § 18.130.180 (West 2010). Unprofessional conduct.*
>
> The following conduct . . . constitute[s] unprofessional conduct for any license holder under the jurisdiction of this chapter:

. . . (4) . . . malpractice which results in injury to a patient. . .

Wash. Admin. Code § 246-16-220 (2009). Mandatory reporting —How and when to report.

(1) Reports are submitted to the department of health. The department will give the report to the appropriate disciplining authority for review, possible investigation, and further action

. . . (b) . . . Reports of unprofessional conduct are submitted to the department.

In both Texas and Washington, Dr. Brown has engaged in a dual or multiple relationship with his client. Texas law has no mandatory duty to report another license holder. Washington's duty to report is necessary under the current law given the circumstances of this particular case.

Cultural Considerations

Global Discussion

Canadian Code of Ethics

Responsibility of the individual psychologist.

The discipline's contract with society commits the discipline and its members to act as a moral community . . .

. . . (2) To bring concerns about possible unethical actions of a more serious nature (e.g., actions that have caused . . . serious harm, or actions that are considered misconduct in the jurisdiction) to the . . . body(ies) best suited to investigating the situation and to stopping or offsetting the harm.

Dr. Jones has an ethical obligation in acting as an agent of a "moral community" charged with care and responsibility of others to bring matters of obviously serious misconduct to the attention of the investigating body of that province involved. While it may not be possible to stop harm as item 2 of this standard dictates, certainly harm can be offset for Mary and Dr. Brown's future clients if Dr. Jones brings her concerns to the attention of the ethics board. It does not have to be shown in this case that Mary herself has to have undergone "serious harm" if Dr. Brown's actions are egregious enough to be considered "misconduct."

American Moral Values

1. Given that Mary initially did not give consent for Dr. Jones to intervene before Patricia went on vacation with Dr. Brown, how does Dr. Jones justify intervening now that Mary is upset with the aftermath? Does her role as therapist to Mary include an attempt to address her daughter's defiance, or should Dr. Jones concentrate on Mary's own ability to confront that behavior?
2. Dr. Jones may have a less sympathetic moral assessment of Mary's complaint, since Mary seemingly placed greater value on helping her marriage with the Las Vegas trip than on protecting Patricia from a possibly harmful situation with her therapist. Is it self-serving for Mary to complain only after Patricia's defiance made life more difficult for her (as opposed to Patricia and the other people in Patricia's life)?
3. As for Patricia's treatment by Dr. Brown, Dr. Jones could consider whether the treatment did in fact work. Does Mary's complaint carry as much weight given that, by her own admission, her daughter is no longer depressed? A chief measure of efficaciousness of treatment is whether it addresses client's concerns. If Patricia's concern is conquering depression, does Dr. Brown's treatment not fulfill her therapeutic need? Or does Dr. Brown's personal behavior that violates ethical and legal standards taint the outcome?
4. As in the first segment of this vignette, the sanctity of family appears as a possible moral consideration. Despite what may seem like a self-serving complaint, does Mary see Dr. Brown as supplanting her authority as a parent? Given that he has also erased the boundary between Patricia's therapy and his own family life, should Dr. Jones more carefully consider whether Dr. Brown has assumed a parental role for Patricia? Has he assumed a more illicit role? Does this warrant more of an action than if his in-office therapy alone had seemed to produce these behavioral changes?

Ethical Course of Action

Directive per APA Code

Both Mary's request for Dr. Jones to help her file a complaint and Dr. Jones's concern regarding Dr. Brown's unprofessional standards indicate harm. Given that the European vacation has already occurred and is thus not appropriate for informal resolution, Standard 1.05 directs Dr. Jones to "take further action appropriate to the situation."

To comply with directives of Standard 1.05, Dr. Jones does need to decide further the "appropriate" action to take.

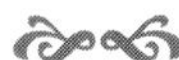

Dictates of One's Own Conscience

Given that "action appropriate to the situation" is necessary, what would you do?

1. Decide that doing nothing may be most "appropriate to the situation" since Patricia is not your client.
2. Alert Mary to the violation of state law, and provide her with contact information of the psychology licensing board.
3. If provided a release of confidentiality by Mary, file a complaint with your state psychological association, APA, and/or the state licensing board in your jurisdiction immediately.
4. Regardless of release of confidentiality from Mary, contact your state psychological association, APA, and/or the state licensing board in your jurisdiction immediately.
5. Give Mary all the necessary information for Mary to contact the state or national committees on professional ethics and/or to state licensing boards.
6. Contact Dr. Brown and discuss the situation with him only.
7. Explore with Mary relevant questions about the trip, such as her daughter's change of behavior and Dr. Brown's role in the chain of events.
8. Explore with Mary the possibility of a joint meeting with yourself and Dr. Brown to discuss the nature of Mary's concern.
9. Wait to see Dr. Brown's reaction to the knowledge of Dr. Jones's concerns and Mary's request to make a formal complaint before taking any subsequent action.
10. Contact Dr. Brown and request that he needs to stop engaging in his multiple relationships with Mary's daughter.
11. Do a combination of the previously listed actions.
12. Do something that is not previously listed.

If you were practicing in Canada, what would you do?

1. Have a conversation with Dr. Brown regarding Patricia going on a vacation with his family.
2. Let Dr. Brown know that you will be reporting his unethical behavior to the provincial psychology board.
3. Report Dr. Brown for an ethics violation without further consideration or further conversation with either Dr. Brown or with Mary.

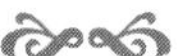

STANDARD 1.06: COOPERATING WITH ETHICS COMMITTEES

Psychologists cooperate in ethics investigations, proceedings, and resulting requirements of the APA or any affiliated state psychological association to which they belong. In doing so, they address any confidentiality issues. Failure to cooperate is itself an ethics violation. However, making a request for deferment of adjudication of an ethics complaint pending the outcome of litigation does not alone constitute noncooperation.

A CASE FOR STANDARD 1.06: Out of the Blue

It is a very busy day with almost back-to-back appointments for Dr. Miller in his outpatient forensic practice. At 4:00 p.m. he went to his waiting room for his next appointment. In the waiting room, David intercepted Dr. Miller. David said he works for the state department of licensing as an investigator and that a complaint has been filed against Dr. Miller. David requested that they speak privately for a few minutes and to instruct his front office staff to turn over all client files for review by David.

Issues of Concern

What constitutes failure to cooperate? Could Dr. Miller say, "I have a client appointment scheduled now and would you please come back later?" without being additionally accused of being uncooperative. Alternatively, could Dr. Miller say, "May I see proof of your credentials and I want to contact my attorney for advice?" without being additionally accused of being uncooperative?

APA Ethics Code

Companion General Principle

Principle A: Beneficence and Nonmaleficence

Psychologists strive to benefit those with whom they work and take care to do no harm.

To the extent possible, psychologists do not cancel client appointments. For Dr. Miller to not start a scheduled appointment with a client in order to respond to the impromptu intrusion of an investigator, at a minimum, does not benefit the client. Alternatively, if the complaint was of sexual misconduct, David's intrusion may have protected a client from Dr. Miller's unwanted sexual advances.

Principle B: Fidelity and Responsibility

> Psychologists' . . . cooperate with . . . institutions to the extent needed to serve the best interests of those with whom they work.

In the interest of cooperating with other institutions, this aspiring principle does guide Dr. Miller to at least have a dialogue with David.

Companion Ethical Standard(s)

Standard 4.01: Maintaining Confidentiality

> Psychologists have a primary obligation and take reasonable precautions to protect confidential information . . . , recognizing that the extent and limits of confidentiality may be regulated by law or established by institutional rules . . .

Standard 4.05: Disclosures

> . . . (b) Psychologists disclose confidential information without the consent of the individual only as mandated by law, or where permitted by law for a valid purpose such as to . . . (3) protect the client/patient . . . from harm . . . , in which instance disclosure is limited to the minimum that is necessary to achieve the purpose.

Complying with David's request by turning over client files would certainly be in violation of Standards 4.01 and 4.05.

Legal Issues

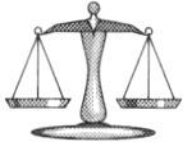

California

> *Cal. Bus. & Prof. Code § 2969(a) (West 2003).*
>
> Refusal to comply with request for medical records of patient; civil penalty; written authorization; court order.
>
> (1) A licensee who fails . . . to comply with a request for . . . records of a patient, that is accompanied by that patient's written authorization for release of records to the board, within 15 days of receiving the request and authorization, shall pay to the board a civil penalty of one thousand dollars ($1,000) per day for each day that the documents have not been produced after the 15th day, unless the licensee is unable to provide the documents within this time period for good cause.
>
> (2) Any licensee who fails or refuses to comply with a court order, issued in the enforcement of a subpoena, mandating the release of records to the board, shall be subject to a civil penalty . . .
>
> . . . (d) A failure . . . of a licensee to comply with a court order, issued in the enforcement of a subpoena, mandating the release of records to the board constitutes unprofessional conduct and is grounds for suspension or revocation of his or her license.

Ohio

> *Ohio Admin. Code 4732:17-03 (2010). Bases and procedures for disciplinary actions.*
>
> . . . (D) Pre-hearing Procedures.
>
> (1) Exchange of documents and witness lists
>
> (a) Any representative of record may serve upon the opposing representative of record a written request for a list of both the witnesses and the documents intended to be introduced at hearing. . .
>
> . . . (3) Requirements for pre-hearing exchange of information. The hearing examiner . . . shall . . . issue an order setting forth a schedule by which the parties shall exchange hearing exhibits . . .

Under the laws of both states, notice is required to be provided by the licensing boards. Dr. Miller may request that the investigator provide the licensing board documentation that specifies the notice provisions and the releases to the records under investigation.

Cultural Considerations

Global Discussion

British Psychological Society Code of Conduct, Ethical Principles & Guidelines

> (5) Personal conduct.
>
> Specifically they shall: 5.10 . . . take all reasonable steps to assist those charged with responsibility to investigate them.

What constitutes a "reasonable" step in this case? Could the psychologist first see all clients scheduled that day and turn over records at the start of the next day? Could the psychologist delay a records request until after having seen both his/her attorney and the credentials of the investigator? Would the psychologist's willingness to comply with an investigation be altered by whether a claim or complaint was knowingly fraudulent or malicious?

American Moral Values

1. Dr. Miller is confronted with a moral choice involving state regulation and personal practice. How does the value in the state's enforcement of standards for psychologists measure up to the individual duty of the practitioner to serve clients and maintain confidentiality?
2. One way Dr. Miller might frame the situation is maintaining his long-term ability to serve by keeping his license versus a short-term refusal to turn over client files for the sake of confidentiality. Does he see the principle of confidentiality as too essential to his practice to consider sacrificing it short term for a longer career of service to clients? Does he consider his current clients as only the first in a long line of clients he can have over the years, thus tempering the moral stand to protect them and risk his career?
3. How does Dr. Miller morally appraise the bureaucracy of the licensing board? Does he associate it with frivolous complaints and needless procedures or even with a self-justifying need to trump up charges with minor offenses? How will resisting the board affect the authority of that institution with other psychologists? Will it undermine its positive regulatory role in pursuing cases of real abuse? Is there a value in and of itself in being cooperative with the people on the board, especially since they are also colleagues in the field?
4. Dr. Miller should consider the character of David's particular demand to turn over files. Is giving over all his files too extreme a step to require of a psychologist? Can refusing to do so be part of a protest about the terms of that specific demand, rather than a challenge to the board per se?

Ethical Course of Action

Directive per APA Code

Standard 1.06 directs Dr. Miller to "cooperate in ethics investigations" with the caveat of "In doing so, they address any confidentiality issues." In the absence of state laws or administrative code, Dr. Miller would have to interpret the behavior operationalization of the word *cooperate.*

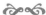

Dictates of One's Own Conscience

Given that cooperation is necessary, what would you do?

1. Cancel your next client appointment so you can make copies, and provide David with the requested documents.
2. Ask for proof of identity and signed releases of information while your next client waits in the reception room. If David provides the necessary documents, cancel your next appointment and make copies of requested files before handing over any client files.
3. Direct your office staff to contact the state department of licensing to verify David's identity, and proceed with your next clinic appointment while office staff is making contact with the state department.
4. Ask for David's full name and contact information, let David know that your lawyer will be following up with David and the state board, and then proceed with your next appointment.
5. Make known to David (as directed in Standard 1.02) your commitment to Standards 4.01 and 4.05, and do not comply with David's request. Instead ask for David's full name and contact information. Let David know that your lawyer will be following up with David and the state board and proceed to engage your next client.
6. Do a combination of the previously listed actions.
7. Do something that is not previously listed.

If you were practicing in Great Britain, the options would be no different from those previously presented.

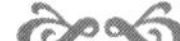

STANDARD 1.07: IMPROPER COMPLAINTS

Psychologists do not file or encourage the filing of ethics complaints that are made with reckless disregard for or willful ignorance of facts that would disprove the allegation.

A CASE FOR STANDARD 1.07: Undue Influence

Drs. Davis and Wilson, both psychologists, are in the midst of a contentious divorce from each other. One day, after having been served yet another motion, Dr. Davis went to Dr. Wilson's office. In the empty waiting room, Dr. Davis angrily complained to the receptionist about denying her entry to Dr. Wilson's office. She called Dr. Wilson a few unflattering names, swore, and walked out. Dr. Wilson later talked to the receptionist, his employee, into reporting Dr. Davis's unprofessional conduct to the state's psychology board.

Issues of Concern

What is the line between the private and professional life for a psychologist? Did Dr. Wilson encourage the receptionist to file a frivolous complaint against Dr. Davis to the state psychology board?

APA Ethics Code

Companion General Principle

Preamble: Introduction and Applicability

> (paragraph 2) This Ethics Code applies only to psychologists' activities that are part of their scientific, educational, or professional roles as psychologists.

Since Dr. Davis's visit to Dr. Wilson's office was personal, not professional, the ethics code does not apply to her conduct in Dr. Wilson's office. However, since Dr. Wilson's relationship to the receptionist is professional, the ethics code does apply to Dr. Wilson's conduct.

Principle B: Fidelity and Responsibility

> Psychologists establish relationships of trust with those with whom they work.

In this case, the relationship in question is not between Drs. Davis and Wilson. Their relationship is personal, not professional. The professional relationship in this situation is between Dr. Wilson and the receptionist in his office. If the receptionist was not inclined to make a report of Dr. Davis's conduct to the state's psychology board, then Dr. Wilson's request violated the conventional understanding of trust between an employer and employee.

Companion Ethical Standard(s)

Section 3. Human Relations; Standard 3.03: Other Harassment

> Psychologists do not knowingly engage in behavior that is harassing . . . to persons with whom they interact in their work based on factors such as . . . socioeconomic status.

Section 3. Human Relations Standard 3.08: Exploitative Relationships

> Psychologists do not exploit persons over whom they have supervisory . . . authority such as . . . employees.

Though it can be argued that Dr. Davis's behavior toward the receptionist was negative, hers was not done in the professional life of a psychologist but rather in her private life as Dr. Wilson's divorcing wife. Depending on the receptionist's willingness to participate in her employer's marital life, the receptionist may experience Dr. Wilson's request as a form of harassment. If the receptionist's sympathies lie with Dr. Davis more than Dr. Wilson, in addition to harassment, the receptionist may feel exploited in acting as an instrument of Dr. Wilson's harassment of Dr. Davis.

Legal Issues 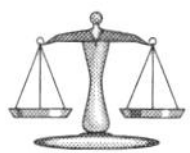

Georgia

> *Ga. Comp. R. & Regs. 510-5-.10 (2010). Aiding illegal practice.*
>
> . . . (3) Psychologists do not . . . encourage the filing of complaints that are frivolous or maliciously intended.

New York

> *N.Y. Comp. Codes R. & Regs. tit. 8, § 29.1 (2010). General provisions.*
>
> (a) Unprofessional conduct shall be the conduct prohibited by this section. . .
>
> (b)(6) willfully making or filing a false report . . . or inducing another person to do so. . .

Dr. Wilson's conduct could be considered as unprofessional in Georgia and New York as the licensing laws in both jurisdictions focus on the regulation of client/psychologist relations. In light of the circumstances of the complaint, by inducing his secretary to file a complaint with the licensing board both jurisdictions are likely to find the complaint frivolous, malicious, or false.

Cultural Considerations

Global Discussion

The Professional Board for Psychology Health Professions Council of South Africa: Ethical Code of Professional Conduct (April 2002)

> 11. Resolving ethical issues.
>
> Psychologists shall adopt an ethical attitude at all times in the conduct of their professional lives.
>
> 11.6. Improper complaints.
>
> Psychologists shall not file or encourage the filing of ethics complaints that are frivolous and are intended to harm the respondent rather than to protect the public.

If Dr. Davis was practicing in South Africa, her conduct would not be considered a violation of the ethics code as her behavior came in context of her personal, not her professional life. Dr. Wilson's behavior, however, can be considered unethical according to South Africa's ethical code due to his involvement of his employee in his own personal life.

American Moral Values

1. The contentiousness of Dr. Davis and Dr. Wilson's divorce has entered into this incident at Dr. Wilson's office. The moral consideration of what each of them is responsible for involves trying to sort where personal and professional lines needed to have been maintained. Angered by divorce proceedings, Dr. Davis's behavior at the office seems to have been aimed at the personal relationship. One may ask if her language toward the receptionist would have been aired out for others in the waiting room as a way of hurting his career, but here all we know is that Dr. Davis spoke to the receptionist in order to speak to Dr. Wilson. Are Dr. Wilson's complaints initiating a fight at the professional level?

2. Dr. Wilson may be using his professional code to inflict personal injury to Dr. Davis. In addition to the annoyance to Dr. Davis for having to take time to respond to a complaint, Dr. Davis's reputation may be tainted if she knows members of the psychology board. It is unpredictable as to what impact personal information about that divorce may have on her professional standing. What if Dr. Davis practices and lectures on treatment with couples? Might the information about her behavior during her divorce impact her livelihood, regardless of whether the complaint is investigated?

3. What are the moral dimensions to Dr. Wilson's relationship with his receptionist? Does Dr. Wilson need to accommodate Dr. Davis's visits more readily in order that the receptionist does not become involved in the conflict? Can the receptionist be expected to fulfill her normal role if put in a position between Dr. Wilson and Dr. Davis's fighting? Needless to say, the receptionist's workload will increase as well with the burden of filing all the complaints Dr. Wilson has requested. Is that a justified increase?

Ethical Course of Action

Directive per APA Code

Standard 1.07 directs psychologists not to file improper complaints. Since the complaint was filed by someone who is not a psychologist, the APA Ethics Code does not apply to the receptionist. To the extent that the receptionist is an employee of a psychologist and acted under his directive, then the APA Ethics Code does apply to Dr. Wilson's conduct. The board is likely to find the complaint frivolous, malicious, or false.

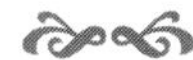

Dictates of One's Own Conscience

Given that a complaint has been filed, what would you do?

1. As Dr. Davis, file a counter-complaint against Dr. Wilson for violation of Standard 1.07.

2. As Dr. Davis, after . . . taking some time to calm down and reflect, acknowledge to the receptionist that she acted rudely and apologize to her.

3. As the receptionist, let Dr. Wilson know the level of discomfort at being used as an instrument of aggression against his wife.

4. As the licensing board member reviewing the case, send a message to Dr. Wilson that he has acted unprofessionally.

5. As Dr. Wilson, after . . . taking some time to calm down and reflect, acknowledge to the receptionist that he crossed a boundary by using his authority as an employer to foist her into filing an ethics complaint against his wife and apologize to his employee.

6. As Dr. Wilson, after . . . taking some time to calm down and reflect, apologize to his wife for involving her in a spurious complaint.

7. Do a combination of the previously listed actions.
8. Do something that is not previously listed.

If you were practicing in South Africa, chances are that you would not consider any options that are different from those previously listed since the United States and South Africa have very similar stances regarding frivolous complaints.

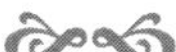

STANDARD 1.08: UNFAIR DISCRIMINATION AGAINST COMPLAINANTS AND RESPONDENTS

> Psychologists do not deny persons employment, advancement, admissions to academic or other programs, tenure, or promotion, based solely upon their having made or their being the subject of an ethics complaint. This does not preclude taking action based upon the outcome of such proceedings or considering other appropriate information.

A CASE FOR STANDARD 1.08: Privileged Versus Insider Information

Dr. Moore was appointed to her state psychology board a few months ago and has completed training to review disciplinary complaints. She returned from her first discipline case review where complaints were presented. In this phase, the board members heard the complaints without psychologists' names attached to prevent bias and to protect anonymity in case the complaint is considered frivolous or without sufficient grounds. In addition, Dr. Moore is now on rotation to receive full case reviews with all identifiers such as names and addresses of psychologists. Before leaving for the day, staff told Dr. Moore to expect to receive documents for full case review.

Dr. Moore is also faculty at a university. This year she is chairing the hiring committee for a new faculty position. The hiring has progressed through to the campus visit of the top three candidates. One of the top candidates is Dr. Taylor. The day before the hiring committee was scheduled to meet for final selection, Dr. Moore received a box from the state psychology board. In the box are documents for her first full disciplinary case review. Upon opening the box, Dr. Moore discovered the subject of the investigation is Dr. Taylor. The complaint concerns charges of unprofessional conduct for entering into multiple relationships with a client. The document contains results of the investigation undertaken in response to the complaint made against Dr. Taylor.

If Dr. Moore was not concurrently sitting on both the disciplinary committee of the state psychology board and the departmental hiring committee, the search committee would not have known of the ethics complaint against Dr. Taylor. What should Dr. Moore do with the information?

Issues of Concern

Recusing herself from chairing the hiring committee would not only undermine the university hiring but it could possibly bring unfair speculation about the professional standing of all three candidates. Recusing herself while identifying Dr. Taylor as the candidate with whom Dr. Moore has the conflict of interest would unfairly identify Dr. Taylor. Remaining on the committee and not voting for Dr. Taylor would unfairly discriminate against Dr. Taylor when no finding on the ethics complaint has been made. Remaining on the committee and disclosing the fact that an ethics complaint has been filed against Dr. Taylor might bias the committee. Remaining on the committee and reading the full disciplinary investigation file against Dr. Taylor to gain sufficient information to make an informed decision regarding a course of action would bias Dr. Moore. If Dr. Moore decided that the investigation did not hold enough evidence to support the complaint, thus moving ahead with the hiring process without revealing her own additional knowledge becomes one form of bias. Conversely, if Dr. Moore decided against Dr. Taylor, Dr. Moore could be accused of acting on bias against Dr. Taylor.

APA Ethics Code

Companion General Principle

Principle D: Justice

> Psychologists exercise reasonable judgment and take precautions to ensure that their potential biases . . . do not lead to or condone unjust practices.

As just delineated, what course of action might Dr. Moore take to achieve the aspirations of Principle D?

Companion Ethical Standard(s)

Standard 3.05: Multiple Relationships

> . . . (b) If a psychologist finds that, due to unforeseen factors, a potentially harmful multiple relationship has arisen, the psychologist takes reasonable steps to resolve it with due regard for the best interests of the affected person and maximal compliance with the Ethics Code.

The situation Dr. Moore finds herself in qualifies under "unforeseen factors." Standard 3.05 (b) directs Dr. Moore to "take reasonable steps" toward resolution. Standard 3.05 (b) also directs Dr. Moore to choose the option that would serve "the best interest of the affected person," namely, Dr. Taylor.

Legal Issues 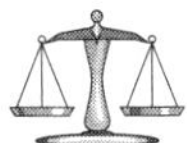

Arizona

> *Ariz. Admin. Code § R4-26-301 (2008). Rules of professional conduct.*
>
> A psychologist shall practice psychology in accordance with the ethical standards contained in standards 1.01 through 10.10 of the "Ethical Principles of Psychologists and Code of Conduct" adopted by the APA effective June 1, 2003, the provisions of which are incorporated by reference.

Missouri

> *Mo. Code Regs. Ann. tit. 20, § 2235-5.030 (2010). Ethical rules of conduct.*
>
> (2) Definitions.
>
> (A) Client—means a receiver of psychological services . . . when the objectivity or competency of the psychologist is . . . impaired because of the psychologist's present . . . administrative or . . . relationship with the client. . . If a dual relationship . . . is discovered after the professional relationship has been initiated, the psychologist shall terminate the professional relationship in an appropriate manner. . .
>
> . . . (6) Multiple relationships.
>
> . . . (B) Multiple Relationship Affecting Psychologist's Judgment. The psychologist shall not undertake or continue a professional relationship with a client . . .

In Arizona, Dr. Moore would follow the directives of Standard 1.08. If Dr. Moore was working in Missouri—and we presume the "client" in this case is the university—then Dr. Moore should act with alacrity to "terminate the professional relationship" and recuse herself from the hiring committee. If Dr. Moore also was prudent, she would consider recusing herself from Dr. Taylor's case.

Cultural Considerations

Global Discussion

Czech-Moravian Psychological Society Code of Ethics

> 4.6. Psychologists approach other psychologists in the spirit of principles of professional cooperativeness with trust and will to cooperate; they do not diminish each other's professional competence.

The directive of this portion of the Czech code is that professionals cooperate with each other, trust each other, and seek not to harm one another's professional reputation or make decisions that would knowingly harm another psychologist's professional standing. Approaching other psychologists in a "spirit of cooperativeness, with trust" requires a different approach than in the United States.

American Moral Values

1. Dr. Moore must weigh the importance of the complaint against her need to be an unbiased contributor to the search committee. Will her work on the committee be jeopardized if she makes the complaint known or even if she reads the complaint privately? What value does an objective faculty search have for Dr. Moore compared to the prospect of hiring a person who could have been guilty of clinical malpractice?
2. Would the nature of the ethics complaint affect Dr. Moore's actions? If so, could Dr. Moore trust herself to read Dr. Taylor's file and make a wise decision about how best to proceed with the hiring? If she does read the file privately and has second thoughts about Dr. Taylor, must she reveal her concerns to the committee? Would hiding her explicit concerns undermine the objectivity and transparency of the search? Or should she try to avoid prejudicing other search committee members with information to which they should not have access?
3. Dr. Moore may also have to consider the different virtues that are called for in clinical practice versus university teaching and research. Is Dr. Taylor's clinical work necessarily relevant to her

prospects as a faculty member? If the nature of the complaint was based on client financial arrangements, for example, is Dr. Taylor's action as relevant for his candidacy in a university setting (where no fees are charged)?

4. What value does Dr. Moore place on her own work and career in relation to the problem? Should Dr. Moore avoid even the possibility of impropriety in either of her two roles, even though it would jeopardize that particular faculty search? How does her decision contribute to the work of the respective institutions involved? Will licensing boards and university administrators overreact in trying to avoid future conflicts of interests for clinical psychologists?

Ethical Course of Action

Directive per APA Code

Standard 1.08 directs Dr. Moore to "not deny persons employment . . . based solely upon their being the subject of an ethics complaint." In the most concrete terms, Dr. Moore needs to assure that if Dr. Taylor is not offered a position at the university that the reasons for the denial is not based solely on the ethics complaint.

Dictates of One's Own Conscience

There are a number of ways by which Dr. Moore might comply with the directives of Standard 1.08, given that the serendipitous nature of Dr. Moore's knowledge is not congruent with the aspiration of nonpartiality of university hiring committees. To be guided by the highest aspiration of hiring committees and directive of Standard 1.08, which of the following would you do?

1. Recuse yourself from reviewing the complaint case; return the complaint documents unopened to the licensing board, citing that you have a conflict of interest in that the psychologist being investigated is known to you; and attempt to proceed with the hiring without mentioning Dr. Taylor's status with the licensing board investigation.
2. Read the complaint documents to determine whether the nature of the complaint is relevant to a faculty's duty at the university, and attempt to proceed with the hiring without mentioning Dr. Taylor's status with the licensing board investigation.
3. Assume a managerial role only as chair of the committee in directing the committee's business without venturing any personal opinions about the three candidates. In this way, the knowledge of the ethics complaint does not inadvertently affect your behavior and meets Standard 1.08.
4. Recuse yourself from reviewing the complaint case, return the complaint documents unopened to the licensing board, and cite that you have a conflict of interest in that the psychologist being investigated is known to you. Also recuse yourself from the hiring committee without giving any reason associated with the hiring process, and do not make any disclosure to the hiring committee about knowledge about the ethics complaint.
5. Do a combination of the previously listed actions.
6. Do something that is not previously listed.

If you were practicing in Czech-Moravian, what would you do?

1. Request that the hiring committee postpone the selection meeting until you have made further inquiry into Dr. Taylor's references.
2. Have a conversation with Dr. Taylor, and ask her about the ethics complaint made against her.
3. Invite the committee to listen to Dr. Taylor's further explanation to a general question about whether there have been any complaints made against her work.

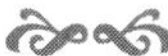

CHAPTER 2

Competence

Ethical Standard 2

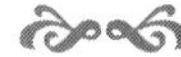

CHAPTER OUTLINE

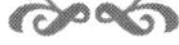

STANDARD 2.01: BOUNDARIES OF COMPETENCE

(a) Psychologists provide services, teach, and conduct research with populations and in areas only within the boundaries of their competence, based on their education, training, supervised experience, consultation, study, or professional experience.

A CASE FOR STANDARD 2.01 (A): Good Citizen in One's Agency

Dr. Collins is three months out of graduate school. In his first postgraduate, pre-licensure job, he works at a church-based counseling agency under the direct supervision of a newly licensed clinical psychologist. Three months ago, the agency decided not to replace a therapist due to budgetary shortfall. This has meant not only an increasing workload but also a more varied caseload for Dr. Collins. One patient, Jane, was assigned to him with a diagnosis of bipolar disorder. In the process of working with Jane, Dr. Collins was contacted by Jane's family regarding their increasing concern over Jane's noncompliance with treatment for her diabetes. Dr. Collins had no prior knowledge of Jane's diabetes, nor did Dr. Collins have experience in working with diabetic patients. Before Dr. Collins was able to staff the case with a physician, Jane fell into a deep depression, failed to take her insulin properly, and went into a medical emergency. Dr. Collins received two phone calls—one from the hospital requesting consultation and one from Jane's family.

Issues of Concern

In difficult budgetary times, it is not unusual for agencies to reduce staff size, thus requiring existing personnel to take on more work and cases that are not necessarily within their established competency range. Dr. Collins is still in the postdoctoral stage of training, thus not licensed to practice independently. Should Dr. Collins decline to consult with the hospital based on his level of competency?

Should Dr. Collins not have accepted the case based on his supervisor's areas of competency? Was it possible for Dr. Collins to have declined the case given his employment situation? Should Dr. Collins have requested supervision or consultation with a health psychologist before taking on the case or as soon after knowledge of the medical complications as possible?

APA Ethics Code

Companion General Principle

Principle A: Beneficence and Nonmaleficence

> Psychologists strive to benefit those with whom they work and take care to do no harm. In their professional actions, psychologists seek to safeguard the welfare and rights of those with whom they interact professionally and other affected persons . . . When conflicts occur among psychologists' obligations or concerns, they attempt to resolve these conflicts in a responsible fashion that avoids or minimizes harm.

Acting for the highest good of the client, the first two sentences of Principle A would direct Dr. Collins to do what he could at this point in order to do the most good for Jane, and to act in such a way as to minimize whatever harm might have been done through his own lack of full competence in the area of medical psychology.

The third sentence of Principle A suggests that Dr. Collins would have a conversation with his supervisor and others in the agency about the dangers of providing services outside one's area of competency without adequate support.

Principle B: Fidelity and Responsibility

> Psychologists consult with, refer to, or cooperate with other professionals and institutions to the extent needed to serve the best interests of those with whom they work.

Principle B guides psychologists to practice as members of the health care profession and to cooperate with the hospital as the hospital struggles to care for Jane. Thus, aspiring to the highest principles of Fidelity and Responsibility, Dr. Collins would return the phone call from the hospital as soon as possible.

Companion Ethical Standard(s)

Standard 1.03: Conflicts Between Ethics and Organizational Demands

> If the demands of an organization . . . for whom they are working conflict with this Ethics Code, psychologists clarify the nature of the conflict, make known their commitment to the Ethics Code, and to the extent feasible, resolve the conflict in a way that permits adherence to the Ethics Code.

While Principle A would suggest that Dr. Collins address the problems in this situation based on organizational demands, Standard 1.03 would direct Dr. Collins to raise these problems with the agency, and the conflicts they pose with the ethics code. Demanding that Dr. Collins take on treatment cases that are outside of both his supervisor's and his areas of competency is problematic, regardless of budgetary constraints. While Standard 1.03 directs Dr. Collins to dialogue with the agency, it invites resolution only "to the extent feasible" for the agency and Dr. Collins.

Standard 4.05: Disclosures

> (a) Psychologists may disclose confidential information with the appropriate consent of . . . the individual client/patient, or another legally authorized person on behalf of the client/patient unless prohibited by law.
>
> . . . (b) Psychologists disclose confidential information without the consent of the individual only as mandated by law, or where permitted by law for a valid purpose such as to . . .
>
> . . . (1) provide needed professional services; . . . (2) obtain appropriate professional consultations; . . .

In the absence of a signed release of information from Jane to family members, Standard 4.05 (a) would direct Dr. Collins not to return the phone call from Jane's family. Additionally, in the absence of a signed release of information from Jane, Standard 4.05 (b) directs Dr. Collins to review the laws of his state regarding release of information without Jane's specific consent. If the state law allows for disclosure in a medical emergency, Standard 4.05 (b) (2) would direct Dr. Collins to return the call from the hospital.

Standard 3.09: Cooperation With Other Professionals

> When indicated and professionally appropriate, psychologists cooperate with other professionals in order to serve their clients/patients effectively and appropriately.

Standard 3.09 provides operational definitions of both Fidelity and Responsibility. It extends the duty beyond Standard 4.05 where psychologists are permitted to contact other health care providers. Standard 3.09 directs psychologists to cooperate when appropriate. In this case, with a hospital treating a depressed client for a medical emergency, most psychologists would deem it appropriate for Dr. Collins to return the call from the hospital for continuity of care.

Standard 4.06: Consultations

> . . . (2) Psychologists . . . disclose information only to the extent necessary to achieve the purposes of the consultation.

Standard 4.06 gives directives to Dr. Collins as to what should be disclosed about Jane when he converses with the hospital.

Legal Issues

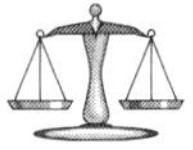

Texas

> *22 Tex. Admin. Code § 465.9 (2010).*
>
> (a) Licensees provide only services for which they have the education, skills, and training to perform competently.
>
> . . . (d) Licensees provide services in an unfamiliar area . . . only after first undertaking appropriate study and training, including supervision, and/or consultation from a professional competent to provide such services.
>
> . . . (f) Licensees are responsible for ensuring that all individuals practicing under their supervision are competent to perform those services.
>
> . . . (h) Licensees who lack the competency to provide particular psychological services to a specific individual must withdraw and refer the individual to a competent appropriate service provider.
>
> *22 Tex. Admin. Code § 465.12 (2010).*
>
> (a) Licensees utilize business practices and provide services in a manner that safeguards the privacy and confidentiality of patients and clients.
>
> . . . (e) Licensees disclose confidential information without the consent of a patient or client only in compliance with applicable state and federal law. [Under HIPPA, 45 CFR 164.508, a valid written authorization must exist before Personal Health Information (PHI) can be released.]

Minnesota

> *Minn. R. 7200.4600 (2010). Competence.*
>
> *Subpart 1. Limits on practice.* A psychologist shall limit practice to the areas of competence in which proficiency has been gained through education and training or experience and which have been stated in writing to the board by the psychologist.
>
> . . . *Subpart 3. Consultation with other professionals.* In cases in which a new . . . specialty is developing, a psychologist shall engage in ongoing consultation with other psychologists or similar professionals as skills are developed in the new area and shall seek continuing education which corresponds to the new area.
>
> *Subpart 4. Referrals.* A psychologist shall recognize that there are other professional . . . resources available to clients and make referrals to those resources when it is in the best interests of clients to be provided with alternative or complementary services.
>
> *Minn. R. 7200.4700 (2010). Protecting the privacy of clients.*
>
> *Subpart 1. In general.* A psychologist shall safeguard the private information obtained in the course of practice. . . With the exceptions listed in subparts 2, 4, 5, 10, and 12 [none of these subparts apply to the facts of the case discussed above], private information is disclosed to others only with the informed written consent of the client.

In both jurisdictions, upon learning of the diabetic condition of his client, unless the supervisor of Dr. Collins is competent in this area of psychology, Dr. Collins should withdraw from the case and refer his client to a professional within his agency competent to provide treatment. In addition, both jurisdictions preclude his violating the confidences of his client without obtaining a release of information.

Cultural Considerations

Global Discussion

Czech-Moravian Psychological Society
Code of Ethics

> Principle 1: Competence, responsibility.
>
> Psychologists must attempt to ensure, maintain and develop their professional competence including supervision and recognize and maintain the limits of their competence.
>
> 1.1. Psychologists shall practice only within the area of their field for which they have got the appropriate preparation and achieved qualifications.

Dr. Collins's supervisor could be out of compliance with the Czechoslovakian code if he was not qualified with adequate health psychology training to supervise Dr. Collins in this case. The Czechoslovakian code specifies "appropriate preparation and . . . qualifications," which Dr. Collins did not have. This code would next direct Dr. Collins to train and improve his own competence through supervision, which in this case he did not have time to do.

American Moral Values

1. Jane's family is calling on Dr. Collins during a life-threatening situation. Does providing assistance in such a situation, in whatever manner possible, supersede the approach normally taken when someone's life is not at stake? Would Dr. Collins be abandoning the family at a critical time if he did not return their call?
2. What difference does it make to Dr. Collins that a client's family is calling, rather than the client herself? What kind of value does a clinical psychologist put on establishing or maintaining a relationship with the family member of his/her client? Does the value change depending on the psychologist's theoretical views of how families work?
3. What value does the psychologist place on a life, especially during the time of a medical emergency for a life-threatening situation? How does the value of a life and a potentially fatal medical illness put the questions of confidentiality in a different frame?
4. What are the moral considerations for the patient when the psychologist is practicing beyond his/her area of competency? Does Dr. Collins's untrained service outweigh the standard of competence, given that upholding that standard might well have denied Jane help? What if Jane cannot afford any other form of service?
5. How does Dr. Collins take into account Jane's ability to afford care elsewhere (with someone who was qualified)? Does the church-based agency's sliding scale represent Jane's only chance to afford mental health care?
6. What is the moral context for a church-based agency providing these services? Would the family expect spiritual support/expertise from Dr. Collins due to his working there? How does the church-based orientation affect Dr. Collins's relationship with the family and his thinking about confidentiality?
7. What does Dr. Collins owe the hospital as Jane's treating psychologist? Is there any help he should impart beyond confessing to be out of his area of expertise? Should he share anything else that might help her? At what point does he owe it to himself to protect his own career in terms of what he might share with authorities?

Ethical Course of Action

Directive per APA Code

Standard 2.01 would have allowed Dr. Collins to accept and treat Jane if his supervisor was competent to provide treatment and supervision for health psychology in addition to treatment for adults. But if Dr. Collins's supervisor was not competent, Standard 1.03 would direct Dr. Collins to raise the question of adequate competency either through training or by supervision. Regardless of occurrences before the present emergency, once having accepted Jane into his caseload, Standard 4.05 directs Dr. Collins not to return the phone call to the family member. Standard 4.05 would allow Dr. Collins to return the phone call from the hospital emergency room only if state law permits such a breach of confidentiality.

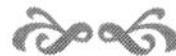

Dictates of One's Own Conscience

If the state you practice in allows for returning the phone call to the emergency room without the signed consent for release of information from your client, knowing the problems that emerged from this case, what might you do?

1. Regardless of whether breaching confidentiality is "mandated by law or where permitted by law" in the state you practice, you would call the hospital to give assistance with psychological knowledge.
2. Regardless of whether breaching confidentiality is "mandated by law or where permitted by law" in the state you practice, you would call the family to give comfort and assistance with psychological knowledge.
3. Call the hospital to say that you are not a trained health psychologist and thus cannot provide any assistance.
4. Call the family to say that you are not a trained health psychologist and thus can provide assistance only about the management of the depression.
5. You would not call the hospital because the client has failed to sign a release of information.
6. You would not call the family on the grounds that client has not signed a release of information.
7. Resolve to refuse onto your caseload any client for whom you are not competent by training or supervision to serve, but given the gravity of the present situation, call both the family and the hospital.
8. Consult your supervisor before taking any action. Then proceed to contact the hospital and the family if the supervisor suggests this course of action.
9. Resolve to seek out, complete, and receive specialized training in health psychology or an allied specialty that would allow competent care of clients such as Jane before taking on any more clients with physical health related disorders, and notify your supervisor of this resolve.
10. Refer Jane to your supervisor if he/she is competent for health psychology and refer the hospital phone call to the agency staff physician. Ask your supervisor and/or agency staff physician to return the phone calls to the hospital and the family.
11. Ask to be transferred to another supervisor, one who was closer to being trained as a clinical health psychologist, and then follow the direction of this new supervisor.
12. Do a combination of the previously listed actions.
13. Do something that is not previously listed.

If you were Dr. Collins working in Czechoslovakia, what might you do?

1. Consult your supervisor before taking any action.
2. Proceed to contact the hospital and the family if the supervisor suggests this course of action.

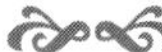

STANDARD 2.01: BOUNDARIES OF COMPETENCE

. . . (b) Where scientific or professional knowledge in the discipline of psychology establishes that an understanding of factors associated with age, gender, gender identity, race, ethnicity, culture, national origin, religion, sexual orientation, disability, language, or socioeconomic status is essential for effective implementation of their services or research, psychologists have or obtain the training, experience, consultation, or supervision necessary to ensure the competence of their services, or they make appropriate referrals, except as provided in Standard 2.02, Providing Services in Emergencies.

A CASE FOR STANDARD 2.01 (B): The N-Word

Sarah is a psychologist-in-training in her practicum placement at a social services center. Sarah is an African American female born and raised in an urban metropolitan city on the West Coast. Her supervisor is Dr. Stewart.

Sarah's client of approximately one month, Betty Ann, has a multitude of problems including a history of drug and alcohol dependence. In supervision with Dr. Stewart, Sarah reported the following events in her last session with Betty Ann. Betty Ann came into therapy complaining about an altercation she had just had at the bus stop on her way to the session. Betty Ann said, "And I gave that nigger a piece of my mind. Who does he think he is talking to a white woman like that? Oh, but honey, you are not like that." Sarah reported this incident to Dr. Stewart in supervision and asked Dr. Stewart how best to handle such incidences in therapy with Betty Ann.

Issues of Concern

If Sarah, an African American, was not competent to provide services to Betty Ann, a white female who is possibly racist, then Standard 2.01 (b) directs Sarah to seek out supervision to develop such competency. In this situation,

Sarah is in compliance with the dictates of Standard 2.01 (b) by engaging in supervision with Dr. Stewart.

The primary area of focus is whether Dr. Stewart is competent to provide supervision to Sarah, a non-white student who is treating white clients with a cultural background of race discrimination. Although it is possible the racist remark by Betty Ann may be personally and morally repugnant, the racist remark Betty Ann made toward Sarah is a clinically significant issue. What is of issue here is the supervisor's approach to Sarah: Is Dr. Stewart competent as a non–African American to consult and supervise in this context? Does her "whiteness" make her vulnerable to engaging in micro-aggressions or somehow lead her to collude with the client in making Sarah feel invisible in that the client's remark is somehow excusable or viewed as not racist? Or, does her whiteness allow her to supervise Sarah with regard to how best to address issues of race and discrimination in therapy, presuming the supervisor has done some personal investigation into the areas of racism and privilege?

How can the supervisor take necessary steps to ensure that the supervisee receives or has received proper training to treat this client, as well as providing a safe space during supervision to describe honestly whether she (Sarah) is comfortable treating the client?

APA Ethics Code

Companion General Principle

Principle A: Beneficence and Nonmaleficence

> Psychologists strive to benefit those with whom they work.

In this case, it is the supervisor's obligation to see to her trainee's education and the benefits from working with her client Betty Ann.

Principle B: Fidelity and Responsibility

> Psychologists establish relationships of trust with whom they work.

In this case, it is the obligation of the supervising psychologist's to form a trusting role with her supervisee.

Principle E: Respect For People's Rights and Dignity

> Psychologists are aware of and respect cultural . . . differences, including those based on . . . race, ethnicity . . . and consider these factors when working with members of such groups. Psychologists try to eliminate the effect on their work of biases based on those factors, and they do not knowingly participate in or condone activities of others based upon such prejudices.

Adhering to Principle E in the provision of competent supervision would guide Dr. Stewart to be aware of Sarah's cultural values, beliefs, and practices about racist white people like Betty Ann. Along the same line, Principle E in the provision of competent treatment would guide Sarah to be aware of Betty Ann's cultural values, beliefs, and practices. As Sarah's supervisor, Dr. Stewart would need to direct Sarah, an African American, to respect the culturally based racist behavior of Sarah's client, Betty Ann.

Principle D: Justice

> Psychologists recognize that fairness and justice entitle all persons to access to and benefit from the contributions of psychology and to equal quality in the processes, procedures, and services being conducted by psychologists. Psychologists exercise reasonable judgment and take precautions to ensure that their potential biases, the boundaries of their competence, and the limitations of their expertise do not lead to or condone unjust practices.

Adhering to Principle E in which psychologists respect the client's cultural practices would also lead psychologists into direct conflict with that section of Principle D in which psychologists are to "ensure . . . [they] . . . do not . . . condone unjust practices." Adhering to Principle E where Sarah respects Betty Ann's racist cultural practices would mean condoning the oppression of Sarah as an African American by a white female in the therapy session. The supervisor must balance her need to see her trainee stay emotionally safe with the client's right to receive services even if the client presents with anger and prejudiced beliefs.

Companion Ethical Standard(s)

Standard 2.01 (a): Boundaries of Competence.

> (a) Psychologists provide services, teach . . . with populations and in areas only within the boundaries of their competence, based on their education, training, supervised experience, consultation, study, or professional experience.

Is Dr. Stewart's competency based on training, study, or professional experience, to provide supervision for African American students who must handle race discrimination from their clients? Should Dr. Stewart consider whether the trainee is competent to treat this client, even under supervision, given the complexities of overlapping diagnoses coupled with possible apparent hostility toward the trainee's ethnic background?

Standard 2.05: Delegation of Work to Others

> Psychologists who delegate work to . . . supervisees . . . take reasonable steps to . . . (2) authorize only those responsibilities that such persons can be expected to perform competently on the basis of their education, training, or experience, either independently or with the level of supervision being provided; and (3) see that such persons perform these services competently.

Dr. Stewart must be certain that Sarah is competent to treat Betty Ann; competence here also refers to maintaining sufficient objectivity on Sarah's part such that she can continue treating Betty Ann in a way that benefits Betty Ann. How can Dr. Stewart take necessary steps to ensure that Sarah receives or has received proper training to treat Betty Ann, as well as provide a safe space during supervision to describe honestly whether Sarah is comfortable treating the client?

Standard 3.01: Unfair Discrimination

> In their work-related activities, psychologists do not engage in unfair discrimination based on . . . race, ethnicity, culture, . . . socioeconomic status, or any basis proscribed by law.

If Dr. Stewart becomes indignant when hearing Betty Ann's comments, this might cause Sarah to form a negative judgment of Betty Ann. Racism and unfair discrimination would then enter both the therapeutic and supervision alliances and possibly perpetuate bias in both relationships.

> Guidelines on Multicultural Education, Training, Research, Practice, and Organizational Change for Psychologists (American Psychological Association [APA], 2003)
>
> Guideline 1. Psychologists are encouraged to recognize that, as cultural beings, they may hold attitudes and beliefs that can detrimentally influence their perceptions of and interactions with individuals who are ethnically and racially different from themselves.

Sarah provides psychological treatment to Betty Ann. As suggested under Guideline 1, Sarah is to recognize that her own beliefs influence her bias about Betty Ann's culture. Through such awareness, Sarah would not necessarily move to condemn Betty Ann's attitude toward "that nigger."

Dr. Stewart provides supervision to Sarah, and as suggested under Guideline 1, Dr. Stewart would also work to recognize her own beliefs that influence her bias about both Sarah and Betty Ann's culture.

Legal Issues 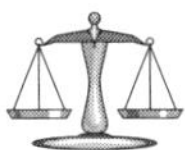

California

> *Cal. Bus. & Prof. Code § 2915(i) (West 2003). Practice outside fields of competence.*

(i) A psychologist shall not practice outside his or her particular field or fields of competence as established by his or her education, training, continuing education, and experience.

> *Cal. Bus. & Prof. Code § 2960(p) (West, 2003). Causes for disciplinary action.*
>
> . . . (p) Functioning outside of his or her particular field or fields of competence as established by his or her education, training, and experience.

Virginia

> *18 Va. Admin. Code § 125-20-150(B) (2010). Standards of practice.*
>
> . . . B. Persons licensed by the board shall:
>
> 1. Provide and supervise only those services and use only those techniques for which they are qualified by training and appropriate experience. Delegate to their . . . supervisees . . . only those responsibilities such persons can be expected to perform competently by education, training and experience. Take ongoing steps to maintain competence in the skills they use.
>
> . . . 5. Avoid harming patients or clients, . . . students . . . , for whom they provide professional services and minimize harm when it is foreseeable and unavoidable. . .
>
> *18 Va. Admin. Code § 125-20-160 (2010). Grounds for disciplinary action or denial of licensure.*
>
> The board may take disciplinary action or deny a license for any of the following causes:
>
> . . . 5. Performing functions outside areas of competency;
>
> . . . 7. Failure to comply with the continued competency requirements set forth in this chapter; or

> (a) Violating or aiding and abetting another to violate any statute applicable to the practice of the profession regulated or any provision of this chapter. . .

California law is silent about the specific duties of the supervisor, but the general standard that applies to all psychologists would charge Dr. Stewart to develop and sustain competency to provide such services. Virginia provides more concrete direction under the law. Not only must Dr. Stewart be competent to provide supervision but also she must not harm Sarah during the supervision. Sarah also owes the duty to not harm Betty Ann. Even though the law is silent, the APA Multicultural Guidelines provide a foundation for each jurisdiction to assess whether either Dr. Stewart or Sarah lack competence when providing their psychological services. Both Dr. Stewart and Sarah would be expected to develop and sustain multicultural competency in the evaluation and treatment of clients and supervisees.

Cultural Considerations

Global Discussion

Code of Ethics: Netherlands

III. 2. Respect; III. 2.1.3. Non-discrimination.

> The psychologist takes into account and respects individual and cultural diversity resulting from differences in race, . . . ethnicity. . . He makes an effort that, despite these differences, all persons are granted equal opportunities under equal circumstances. Discrimination on these or any other grounds is prohibited.

Nowhere in the Netherlands' code does it discuss whether clients may make racist or discriminatory statements to the psychologist treating them—only that treatment of clients may not be different based on any identity variable. However, it would not be acceptable to advise Sarah that Betty Ann be treated any differently based on her racist remark. Discrimination from the psychologist based on differences in race is prohibited.

American Moral Values

1. Does Dr. Stewart find it better to respond to Sarah more as a person than strictly as a professional by morally objecting to the racial slur, for example: "I'm sorry that you had to be exposed to that"?
2. Does Dr. Stewart, keeping in mind her status as a white figure of authority, express her solidarity with Sarah by saying that it was not acceptable for Betty Ann to have used the N-word?
3. Does Dr. Stewart place a greater value on her role as supervisor by not expressing her own personal opinion, instead focusing on Sarah's development as a therapist by talking to Sarah about how she could best maintain her professional stance? Would ignoring the slur be the strategy she would recommend?
4. How should Dr. Stewart, as an educated white professional, speak about Betty Ann, if at all? Should she defend whites "as a whole"? Should she try not to put down this client for acting as "white trash"? Is Dr. Stewart tempted to distance herself as a white person from Betty Ann?
5. If Dr. Stewart responds aggressively about Betty Ann's comment, has she framed Sarah as primarily a victim of racial discrimination? Does that deny Sarah authority as a young therapist? Does it insinuate that Sarah needs protection rather than just encouragement to deal with it on her own? How can Dr. Stewart avoid patronizing Sarah?
6. Will Dr. Stewart have reenacted racial discrimination and be party to racial oppression by not allowing Sarah to craft an intervention in which she is the primary agent? Will Sarah even be able to execute Dr. Stewart's instruction as an African American with Betty Ann as her client?

Ethical Course of Action

Directive per APA Code

Standard 2.01 directs Dr. Stewart to "have or obtain the training, experience, consultation, or supervision necessary to ensure the competence of services, or make appropriate referrals" when dealing with "factors associated with age, gender, gender identity, race, ethnicity, culture, national origin, religion, sexual orientation, disability, language, or socioeconomic status." This means Dr. Stewart is to refer Sarah for supervision to someone else unless Dr. Stewart is competent to supervise African Americans on how to treat white clients who hold racist beliefs.

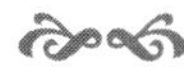

Dictates of One's Own Conscience

If Dr. Stewart is like most psychologists, she would not have received any special training on how, as a white female, to supervise an African American student on providing culturally sensitive treatment to a white racist. You might say to yourself, "Good thing I don't practice outside of my competence and thus would never have taken on Sarah as a supervisee." However, if you were Dr. Stewart and you had not received specific training by education or supervision on providing supervision to African American students, what might you do?

1. Ask Sarah how she feels, and explore Sarah's countertransference to Betty Ann.
2. Ask Sarah what else was going on in the session and not address the racial slur.
3. Direct Sarah to tell Betty Ann that the comment "Oh, but honey, you are not like that" is racist and offensive.
4. Become indignant on behalf of Sarah, and talk about how inappropriate it is for anyone to hold such an old-fashioned racist attitude.
5. Say to Sarah that the focus of treatment is not Betty Ann's racist attitudes but her bipolar symptoms. As such, psychologists have to let many things slide in session in the service of treatment for the primary symptoms.
6. Explore with Sarah whether it is possible for a person from a minority race to conduct psychotherapy with a white person. After exploration, encourage Sarah to transfer Betty Ann to a psychologist who is not a person of color.
7. Explore with Sarah how any clinical psychologist responds to clients who either question overtly or covertly the psychologist's authority as a way to undermine the treatment, and point out that in this case the challenge happens to be racially based.
8. Do a combination of the previously listed actions.
9. Do something that is not previously listed.

If you were Dr. Stewart practicing in the Netherlands, the previously listed options would still apply since the guideline for nondiscrimination is substantially the same as the one listed by the APA Ethics Code.

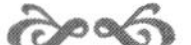

STANDARD 2.01: BOUNDARIES OF COMPETENCE

> . . . (c) Psychologists planning to provide services, teach, or conduct research involving populations, areas, techniques, or technologies new to them undertake relevant education, training, supervised experience, consultation, or study.

A CASE FOR STANDARD 2.01 (C): Overconfident

Lisa and Charles are in treatment with Dr. Morris. Their presenting complaint is difficulty with communication. Lisa has an extensive trauma history, with both emotional and physical abuse in her past. After five sessions, Dr. Morris suspected the communication problems were being exacerbated by an undiagnosed personality disorder for Lisa. Lisa is also in school and has been recently struggling with one of her classes. Dr. Morris referred Lisa for academic testing to explore possible reasons for her school failure. Due to Lisa's limited funds, she went to her school's student counseling clinic.

Dr. Morris held a clinical associate faculty appointment at the school Lisa attends. For training purposes and in consultation with the student's supervisor, Dr. Morris agreed to a joint feedback session. Members present for the feedback session were the student who conducted the testing, Dr. Morris, Lisa, and Charles. It was expected that the assessment feedback session would help Lisa and Charles understand how Lisa's possible impairment may be contributing to her academic failure, overall stress, and difficulties communicating.

During the feedback session, Wayne, the graduate student who administered the assessment, reported that he had initially scheduled the Wechsler Adult Intelligence Scale-IV (WAIS-IV), and the Delis -Kaplan Executive Function System (D-KEFS) for comparative purposes. However, due to reported time constraints, only the WAIS-IV was administered. The results of the WAIS-IV indicated an estimated Full Scale Intelligence Quotient (FSIQ) of 100, a Verbal Comprehension Index (VCI) of 125, and Processing Speed Index (PSI) of 81: Wayne then went on to say to Lisa, "You have a right-hemisphere deficit syndrome, most likely caused by being born premature and being in a neonatal unit for 3 weeks." Dr. Morris is well aware that a learning disability cannot be accurately assessed with only one assessment measure and a clinical interview. He is also aware that this diagnosis is premature at best; inaccurate and misleading at worst. Lisa, however, seems relieved at this news and reports feeling that "finally things make sense." At this point, Dr. Morris cautioned that results are not final until the report with the supervisor's signature is issued.

Upon debriefing, Dr. Morris queried the student regarding his academic training and the extent of supervision he received on this case. The student reported that he is in training for neuropsychology, has had an assessment course, has discussed the case with his clinical supervisor (not his neuropsychology professor), and felt he is competent to undertake cases such as Lisa's.

Issues of Concern

Wayne thinks he has undertaken appropriate training and is now competent to provide services. Wayne's supervisor must have been under the impression that proper and appropriate supervision had been provided in order to prepare Wayne to conduct a feedback session. The question is at what point a psychologist is considered to have undertaken "relevant education, training, supervised experience, consultation, or study" sufficient to reach a competency level necessary to participate in a client feedback session?

APA Ethics Code

Companion General Principle

Principle A: Beneficence and Nonmaleficence

> Psychologists strive to benefit those with whom they work and take care to do no harm . . .

Wayne has done harm to Lisa by providing an inaccurate assessment of her possible disability. Dr. Morris has inadvertently done harm by participating in a process that has provided Lisa with inaccurate information.

Principle B: Fidelity and Responsibility

> Psychologists establish relationships of trust with those with whom they work. . . Psychologists uphold professional standards of conduct, clarify their professional roles and obligations, accept appropriate responsibility for their behavior, and seek to manage conflicts of interest that could lead to exploitation or harm. Psychologists consult with, refer to, or cooperate with other professionals and institutions to the extent needed to serve the best interests of those with whom they work. They are concerned about the ethical compliance of their colleagues' scientific and professional conduct.

Presumably Dr. Morris, being the treating psychologist, has established a relationship of trust with Lisa and Charles. In cooperating with the doctoral training program and by his presence in the room with Wayne, Dr. Morris lends a certain degree of trust to Wayne. At the same time, Principle B exhorts Dr. Morris to uphold professional standards, which in this case means confronting Wayne's behavior.

Companion Ethical Standard(s)

Standard 3.04: Avoiding Harm

> Psychologists take reasonable steps to avoid harming their clients/patients, students, . . . and to minimize harm where it is foreseeable and unavoidable.

It appears that Wayne is unaware of the harm he has done by his overzealous interpretation of the assessment results which was inadequately supervised and insufficient. Concurrently, Standard 3.04 guides Dr. Morris, who is aware of the harm, to take steps that will minimize the effects of Wayne's inaccurate interpretation and assessment of Lisa.

Standard 7.06: Assessing Student and Supervisee Performance

> (a) In academic and supervisory relationships, psychologists establish a timely and specific process for providing feedback to students and supervisees. Information regarding the process is provided to the student at the beginning of supervision. (b) Psychologists evaluate students and supervisees on the basis of their actual performance on relevant and established program requirements.

Wayne is not supervised by Dr. Morris, is not in a position to be graded by Dr. Morris, and has no other direct relationship with Dr. Morris. Given that Dr. Morris is associated with the training program as faculty and Dr. Morris conducted the joint feedback session in his capacity as an adjunct faculty, Standard 7.06 (b) guides Dr. Morris to give feedback to both Wayne and to the training program regarding Wayne's conduct.

Legal Issues 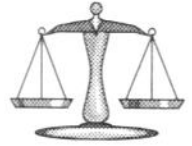

Massachusetts

> *Mass 251 Mass. Code Regs. CMR 1.10 (2010). Sanctions. Ethical standards and professional conduct.*
>
> . . . (6) In addition to acts prohibited by the *Ethical Principles of Psychologists and code of Conduct* referenced in 251 CMR 1.10(1) . . . ; the following acts are deemed to be grounds for disciplinary action, pursuant to M.G.L. c. 112, § 128:
>
> . . . (c) Jeopardizing the physical or emotional security of a patient or client by engaging in inappropriate diagnostic or treatment procedures . . .

Ohio

Ohio Admin. Code 4732:17-01 (2010).

. . . (B) Negligence.

(1) A psychologist . . . shall be considered negligent if his/her behaviors toward his/her clients, . . . or students, in the judgment of the board, clearly fall below the standards for acceptable practice of psychology. . .

(C) Welfare of the client.

. . . (2) Sufficient professional information. A psychologist . . . rendering a formal professional opinion or recommendation about a person shall not do so without substantial professional client information.

(3) Informed client. A psychologist . . . shall give a truthful, understandable, and reasonably complete account of a client's condition to the client. . .

(F) Testing and test interpretation.

(1) Assessment procedures.

. . . (c) A psychologist . . . shall include in his/her report of the results of a test or assessment procedures any reservations regarding the possible inappropriateness of the test for the person assessed. . .

(3) Test interpretation.

. . . (b) Test results or other assessment data used for evaluation or classification are communicated . . . in such a manner as to guard against misinterpretation or misuse. . .

(H) Competence.

(1) Limits on practice. A psychologist . . . shall limit his/her professional practice to those specialty areas in which competence has been gained through education, training, and experience. If important aspects of the client's problem fall outside the boundaries of competence, then the psychologist . . . assists his/her client in obtaining additional professional help.

. . . (6) Referrals. A psychologist or school psychologist shall make or recommend referral to other professional, . . . when such referral is in the best interests of the client.

In both jurisdictions, Wayne's failing to provide an appropriate diagnostic assessment and Dr. Morris's failing to provide adequate supervision about the limitations of the evaluation would violate the laws. Dr. Morris should have recognized that he was acting outside his area of competence, called into question Wayne's interpretation of the data, and referred Lisa to further testing by someone competent to perform the neuropsychological assessment.

Cultural Considerations

Global Discussion

New Zealand Psychological Society Code of Ethics

2.1. Competence and accountability.

Psychologists recognize the boundaries of their own competence and provide only services for which they are qualified by training and experience. They refer matters outside their areas of competence to appropriately qualified persons.

When Dr. Morris invited Wayne into the therapy setting to discuss the results of the assessment, he assumed responsibility for that feedback; that it came from a student practicing outside the bounds of competence and was inaccurate is now assumed to be under Dr. Morris's license. If the situation occurred in New Zealand, Dr. Morris needed to be competent to conduct assessments for learning disorders specifically and possibly neuropsychological ones as well. If Dr. Morris had not requested the feedback session as part of a therapy session but simply referred Lisa to an outside psychologist or psychometrist who was "appropriately qualified," he would have provided services for which Dr. Morris was qualified and would not then be responsible for this breach occurring.

American Moral Values

1. Given Wayne's inadequate training and the significance of his diagnosis, should Dr. Morris tell Lisa that she should wait for more diagnostic assessment before accepting the testing results being reported by Wayne? Does Dr. Morris have a duty to let Lisa know the truth about the need for further assessment, even if an unsubstantiated diagnosis makes her feel better? Should Dr. Morris disclose that the diagnostic assessment engaged in by Wayne exceeds his level of competence?
2. Will the trust between Dr. Morris, Lisa, and Charles be broken if Dr. Morris initially supports the work of the assessment before raising the limitations about the findings of the assessment? Lisa and Charles could question why Dr. Morris brought Wayne into a joint session. What is the cost of dismissing the student's evaluation as insufficient? What is the cost of not pointing out Wayne's naïveté? Should Dr. Morris express regret to Lisa in having participated in this feedback session without adequate assurance of Wayne's competence?

3. How useful is it to support the results (regardless of the accuracy of the testing and interpretation) if Lisa finds it comforting? Will the explanation Wayne offers affect Lisa's treatment or long-term outlook? What effects justify dispelling that illusion?
4. What is Dr. Morris's responsibility toward Wayne? Does being a senior member of the profession and/or a professor associated with the training program encumber Dr. Morris with authority and responsibility for a problematic student? How should he engage in an appropriate professional interaction in light of the ethical standards and the law of the jurisdiction? Does Wayne need better supervision? Will Dr. Morris be worried about his own professional reputation because of Wayne's actions?

Ethical Course of Action

Directive per APA Code

Wayne is clearly in violation of Standard 2.01 if he proceeded with the feedback session without the full knowledge or consent of his supervisor. However, the issue of concern in this vignette is whether Dr. Morris was competent to take on a quasi-supervisory role with regard to Wayne. Given how the session with Lisa and Charles unfolded, it is doubtful whether Dr. Morris was competent to provide oversight for the interpretation session. Dr. Morris needed to be practicing within the limits of his competence in order to provide supervision/oversight of Wayne's work, and is in violation of Standard 2.01.

To be in compliance with Standard 2.01, Dr. Morris would have had to speak to Wayne before the joint session and have obtained from Wayne the full contents of the completed assessments and the results of the tests. Dr. Morris should have consulted with a colleague about the measures and findings of the evaluation. Finally, Dr. Morris needed to determine what Wayne intended to say to Lisa and temper the remarks so that they would disclose the limitations of the measures and the need for more a sophisticated evaluation.

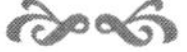

Dictates of One's Own Conscience

Regardless of how carefully each of us conducts our practice and how hard we strive to practice within the area of our competence, every once in a while some area catches us by surprise. If you somehow were caught off guard in a joint session with another psychologist, like Dr. Morris, what might you do?

1. Stop the discussion as soon as it goes wayward and defer further discussion about the assessment results until Wayne, his supervisor, and you can come to an agreement about how to provide appropriate disclosures about the findings of the assessment.
2. Let Wayne know that you will be discussing his performance with his academic program.
3. Schedule another session with clients Lisa and Charles and with Wayne's supervisor for the case after the full write-up is complete with supervisor signatures.
4. Lodge a complaint with the psychology program, taking to task both the neuropsychology and clinical supervisors for allowing Wayne to conduct a feedback session before everything had been verified.
5. Ascertain whether the training program has had previous problems with Wayne and, if so, recommend that Wayne be formally disciplined.
6. Do a combination of the previously listed actions.
7. Do something that is not previously listed.

If you were Dr. Morris practicing in New Zealand, the previously listed options would still apply since the guidelines for practicing within one's own competence are not substantially different from those listed by the APA Ethics Code.

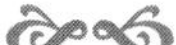

STANDARD 2.01: BOUNDARIES OF COMPETENCE

> . . . (d) When psychologists are asked to provide services to individuals for whom appropriate mental health services are not available and for which psychologists have not obtained the competence necessary, psychologists with closely related prior training or experience may provide such services in order to ensure that services are not denied if they make a reasonable effort to obtain the competence required by using relevant research, training, consultation, or study.

A CASE FOR STANDARD 2.01 (D): A Change of Circumstances

Dr. Rogers, working in a community health clinic, inherited Nancy, a chronically mentally ill client who exhibits symptoms of schizophrenia with fixed delusions of persecution and who has been steadfast in her refusal to take any psychotropic medications. Dr. Rogers likes working with the chronically mentally ill clients and during the course of several months had been successful in encouraging Nancy to engage with her case manager and psychiatrist for medication. As medication took effect and the delusional symptoms cleared, Nancy started reporting intrusive memories of childhood sexual abuse, usually followed by long periods of blank memory. In one session, Dr. Rogers noticed a marked change in Nancy's demeanor. Upon inquiry, the client announced, "Nancy is not here. I'm Karen. I come when Nancy can't handle it anymore."

Dr. Rogers does not necessarily think dissociative identity disorder (DID) is a legitimate diagnosis, has not been trained in the treatment of DID, and does not consider himself competent in treating clients with reported symptoms of DID.

Issues of Concern

At the time that Dr. Rogers began working with Nancy, Dr. Rogers was working well within the boundaries of his competency. However, as the case unfolded, the situation moved outside of Dr. Rogers's area of competency. It can be argued, per Standard 2.01 (a), that at the point where Nancy is stabilized on appropriate medication and Nancy's presenting problem shifts outside of Dr. Rogers's area of competency, Dr. Rogers now should refer Nancy to someone who is competent to work with DID or at least competent to assess whether the diagnosis of DID is warranted.

If Dr. Rogers were able to establish a therapeutic alliance so solid that Nancy was able to engage in treatment that included psychotropic medication, then more likely than not Nancy would expect and ask that her treatment continue with Dr. Rogers. Although the APA Ethics Code would support Dr. Rogers in transferring Nancy to a competent treatment provider of DID, would Nancy experience such a transfer as abandonment? Would a client feel betrayed and abandoned under certain circumstances, even as clinical psychologists move to comply with psychology ethical standards?

APA Ethics Code

Companion General Principle

Principle B: Fidelity and Responsibility

> Psychologists establish relationships of trust with those with whom they work.

Aspiring not only to establish but also to keep the trust with those with whom we work, Principle B guides Dr. Rogers to build Nancy's trust. In this situation, would Dr. Rogers's retention of Nancy as a client, even in an area of practice in which he is not competent, best enable Dr. Rogers to uphold Principle B?

Principle A: Beneficence and Nonmaleficence

> Psychologists strive to benefit those with whom they work and take care to do no harm.

Aspiring to practice in such a way as to provide benefit to Nancy, Dr. Rogers is faced with deciding how best to uphold Principle A. By keeping to Standard 2.01 (a) as the best way to uphold Principle A, Dr. Rogers may harm Nancy through creating a sense of abandonment. By aligning to the value of Fidelity as the best way to uphold Principle B and not transferring Nancy to another psychologist for treatment, Dr. Rogers may harm Nancy by providing services in an area in which he is not competent.

Companion Ethical Standard(s)

Standard 2.04: Bases for Scientific and Professional Judgments

> Psychologists' work is based upon established scientific and professional knowledge of the discipline.

Although DID is a controversial diagnosis, it is recognized in the *Diagnostic and Statistical Manual of Mental Disorders* (*DSM-IV*) as a mental disorder (Piper & Merskey, 2004). There has been debate about the diagnostic criteria for DID (Davidson & Foa, 1993; Dell, 2001; Spiegel, 2001). Individual psychotherapy is the treatment of choice for individuals suffering from any type of dissociative disorder and emphasizes the integration of the various personality states into one, cohesive whole personality (International Society for Study of Dissociation, 2005; Kluft, 1999).

Since individual psychotherapy is the treatment of choice, Dr. Rogers appears to be well situated to provide such service. Per Standard 2.01 (d), Dr. Rogers may continue treatment of Nancy if he undertakes "training, consultation or study" to obtain the necessary competency.

Standard 2.01: Boundaries of Competence

> . . . (e) In those emerging areas in which generally recognized standards for preparatory training do not yet exist,

> psychologists nevertheless take reasonable steps to ensure the competence of their work and to protect clients/patients . . . from harm.

Dr. Rogers might argue that since he does not necessarily think DID is a substantiated diagnosis, thus no adequate course of treatment is yet known. Standard 2.01 would counter such argument with directive that Dr. Rogers take reasonable step to ensure that this work with Lisa was done competently so to ensure treatment does not cause Lisa harm.

Legal Issues 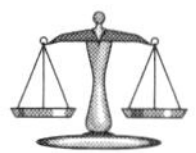

Wisconsin

> *Wis. Admin. Code Psy. § 5.01 (2010). Professional conduct.*
>
> The practice of psychology is complex and varied and, therefore, allows for a broad range of professional conduct. The following acts constitute unprofessional conduct by applicants for licensure and licensees of the board and are prohibited. Complaints regarding these acts shall be investigated and may lead to disciplinary proceedings.
>
> . . . (4) Performance of professional services inconsistent with training, education, or experience.

Missouri

> *Mo. Code Regs. Ann. tit. 20, § 2235-5.030 (2010). Ethical rules of conduct.*
>
> . . . *(3) Competence.*(A) Limits on Practice. The psychologist shall limit practice and supervision to the areas in which competence has been gained through professional education, training derived through an organized training program and supervised professional experience. If important aspects of the client's problems fall outside the boundaries of competency, then the psychologist shall assist his/her client in obtaining additional professional consultation.

In both jurisdictions, Dr. Rogers may be engaging in practice outside of his level of competence. Missouri more clearly establishes the path to avoid violating the law. Dr. Rogers should obtain consultation from a fellow psychologist competent in the evaluation and treatment of DID. His client should be involved in this process so that Dr. Rogers will not seem as if he is abandoning his client. It is likely that both jurisdictions would view this approach as sufficient for engaging in the continued care of his client.

Cultural Considerations

Global Discussion

Canadian Code of Ethics for Psychologists

> Principle II: Responsible caring; competence and self-knowledge.
>
> II.8. Take immediate steps to obtain consultation or to refer a client to a[n] . . . appropriate professional, whichever is more likely to result in providing the client with competent service, if it becomes apparent that a client's problems are beyond their competence.

The code states that once it is clear a client's problems are beyond a psychologist's experience or competence, the client may either be referred or sufficient consultation should occur. The course chosen should be whichever seems most likely to provide the client with more competent service.

American Moral Values

1. How does Dr. Rogers view the act of referring Nancy to someone trained to treat DID? Is he abandoning his client? Will Nancy view it as abandonment, threatening the progress she has made with medication?
2. What kind of responsibility does Dr. Rogers feel for Nancy? Does he take responsibility for her taking medication and beginning to exhibit symptoms of DID? Does he want to "follow through" with the effects that have emerged from his treatment recommendations (regardless of whether they were foreseeable)?
3. Does Dr. Rogers consider the good and bad effects that staying with Nancy might have on his career? Will she give him valuable experience? Assuming she does command such an interest, should Dr. Rogers consider whether his reluctance to let her go might be due to his professional interest in her case?
4. Does Dr. Rogers think he has a provider trained in DID who could establish rapport with Nancy? Will that provider be able to maintain her willingness to take medication? Is Nancy's ability to pay, given her reliance on a community health clinic, a problem for such a referral?

Ethical Course of Action

Directive per APA Code

Standard 2.01 (d) directs what to do when psychologists find themselves needing to practice outside their competency. Standard 2.01 also holds that the psychologist is being "asked to provide services for whom appropriate mental health services are not available." If Dr. Rogers was practicing in a city, it is very doubtful that appropriate mental health services through a psychologist competent in treating DID would not be available. Thus, Standard 2.01 would direct Dr. Rogers to transfer Nancy to another psychologist. Now let us presume that based upon the case history, Dr. Rogers, his supervisor, and the agency management believe in the argument that no other psychologist has been able to make a therapeutic working alliance with Nancy, thus other "appropriate mental health services are not available." In this case, Standard 2.01 directs Dr. Rogers to acquire the competency through using "relevant research, training, consultation, or study." This might include taking CE workshops, reviewing the published literature or seeking consultation from someone who is competent to treat DID.

Dictates of One's Own Conscience

It is not unusual for cases to evolve as treatment progresses and thus psychologists are faced with some new area of treatment necessity. The arguments for transfer are as sound as arguments for not transferring a client when treatment evolves away from the original presenting complaint. What would you do?

1. Discuss the matter with the agency director and do whatever the agency decides.
2. Uphold Standard 2.01 and do the following:
   a. Refer the client to the most knowledgeable person in treatment of DID within a 25-mile radius, regardless of where this person works or whether she has transportation.
   b. Refer the client to someone else within the agency who is better trained in DID.
3. Protect the value of the therapeutic alliance by continuing treatment with Nancy, but do the following:
   a. Obtain a new supervisor who is knowledgeable about DID.
   b. Obtain peer group consultation and collectively take on the study of DID.
   c. Read a book on DID and develop another treatment plan from the details of the book.
   d. Attend continuing education (CE) workshops on DID.
4. Monitor self-level of competence, discuss with the client the pros and cons of transferring, and develop steps to evaluate and treat the possible emergence of DID in consultation with a supervisor competent in the area of DID.
5. Do a combination of the previously listed actions.
6. Do something that is not previously listed.

If you were Dr. Rogers practicing in Canada, would you refer the client to another therapist who is competent to treat DID as the Canadian code specifies that Dr. Rogers is to take whichever course of action is more likely to result in providing the client with competent service?

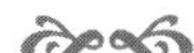

STANDARD 2.01: BOUNDARIES OF COMPETENCE

> . . . (e) In those emerging areas in which generally recognized standards for preparatory training do not yet exist, psychologists nevertheless take reasonable steps to ensure the competence of their work and to protect clients/patients, students, supervisees, research participants, organizational clients, and others from harm.

A CASE FOR STANDARD 2.01 (E): Touch?

Dr. Reed is a clinical psychologist in partnership with Dr. Cook, a naturopathic physician. Dr. Reed has signed a partnership agreement with Dr. Cook that in-office referrals for psychotherapy, including "alternative and complementary modalities" will be part of her expected work contract. Both professionals practice in a jurisdiction that by law permit health care providers with different scopes of practices to engage in a business partnership. As part of a team treatment plan, Angela has been referred to Dr. Reed. Angela has revealed to Dr. Cook that she has emerging memories of being sexually abused as a child, based on significant gaps in her memory, a series of progressively more violent and bizarre dreams, emergent anger at her family members, and current physical pain and feelings of panic during sexual relations with her partner. During Angela's first session with Dr. Reed, Angela focused on the physical pain during sexual intercourse. Dr. Reed recommended "somatic therapy" for treatment of the pain. When

Angela inquired about the nature of somatic therapy, Dr. Reed said it's proven to be helpful and she has successfully treated many patients with Angela's complaints when she was a massage therapist.

Issues of Concern

Dr. Reed holds two licenses, one as a massage therapist and one as a psychologist. Dr. Reed has gained additional knowledge and expertise by virtue of her licensure as a massage therapist. Unquestionably, skills and knowledge from previous training transfer to subsequent training. However, does holding two different licenses give permission for Dr. Reed to blend the two practices in such a manner that is not generally recognized by either psychology or massage therapy? Could Dr. Reed argue that somatic therapy is an emerging treatment specialty or a treatment art form only for those select practitioners who are dually licensed in massage and psychology?

APA Ethics Code

Companion General Principle

Principle C: Integrity

> Psychologists seek to promote accuracy, honesty, and truthfulness in the science, teaching, and practice of psychology. In these activities psychologists do not . . . engage in . . . intentional misrepresentation of fact.

Aspiring to Principle C, Dr. Reed would endeavor to describe somatic therapy accurately and say nothing that could be interpreted as intentional misrepresentation of fact. This means that Dr. Reed would need to let Angela know that somatic therapy is neither a standard nor proven course of treatment for pain during intercourse. Dr. Reed's saying "it's proven to be helpful" is misleading given that she is now a clinical psychologist and Angela was referred to her in her role as a clinical psychologist, not as a massage therapist. As a psychologist who has read the literature from both fields, Dr. Reed can accurately characterize any limitations in the methodology of studies that have emerged about somatic therapy. Such limitations would likely lead to a more circumspect description of the efficacy of somatic therapy.

Principle A: Beneficence and Nonmaleficence

> Psychologists . . . take care to do no harm.

As directed by Standard 2.01 (e) when providing treatment in "emerging" areas, the overarching principle that should guide psychologists as we do our work is Principle A: Nonmaleficence. In aspiring to uphold Principle A, Dr. Reed would endeavor to continually monitor the treatment progress to assure no harm comes to Angela as a result of the somatic therapy treatment.

Companion Ethical Standard(s)

Standard 3.10: Informed Consent

> (a) When psychologists . . . provide . . . therapy . . . they obtain the informed consent of the individual . . .
> (d) Psychologists appropriately document written or oral consent . . .

In providing treatment that is outside of standard and customary services, it is especially important for Dr. Reed to inform Angela of the nature of treatment and obtain consent from Angela for somatic therapy. Standard 3.10 (d) directs Dr. Reed to document such consent.

Standard 10.01: Informed Consent to Therapy

> (a) When obtaining informed consent to therapy . . . psychologists inform clients/patients as early as is feasible in the therapeutic relationship about the nature and anticipated course of therapy . . .
>
> . . . (b) When obtaining informed consent for treatment for which generally recognized techniques and procedures have not been established, psychologists inform their clients/patients of the developing nature of the treatment, the potential risks involved, alternative treatments that may be available, and the voluntary nature of their participation.

Building on Standard 3.10 (a) and (d) Standard 10.01 (a) directs Dr. Reed to explain somatic therapy at the beginning of the treatment relationship. This means that when Dr. Reed introduced the idea of somatic therapy and Angela inquired about the nature of it Dr. Reed should thoroughly explain the treatment and any methodological concerns that warrant viewing such an approach as nonstandard. Standard 10.01 (d) directs such an explanation and the potential risks and possible alternative treatments available to Angela.

Standard 2.04: Bases for Scientific and Professional Judgments

> Psychologists' work is based upon established scientific and professional knowledge of the discipline.

Having followed the directives of Standard 10.01 and 3.10, Dr. Reed can proceed following the directives of Standard 2.04. Standard 2.04 directs Dr. Reed to proceed with the experimental somatic therapy based on her knowledge of the standards of the profession and the established scientific knowledge.

Legal Issues 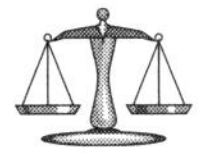

Michigan

> *Mich. Admin. Code r. 338.2515 (2010). Prohibited conduct.*
>
> *Rule 15.* Prohibited conduct includes, but is not limited to, the following acts or omissions by any individual covered by these rules:
>
> . . . (c) Taking on a professional role when . . . professional, . . . relationships could impair the exercise of professional discretion or make the interests of a patient, . . . secondary to those of the licensee.

Oregon

> *Or. Admin. R. 858-010-0075 (2010). Code of professional conduct.*
>
> The Board adopts for the code of professional conduct of psychologists in Oregon the American Psychological Association's "Ethical Principles of Psychologists and Code of Conduct" effective June 1, 2002.

Both jurisdictions would likely find that Dr. Reed engaged in ethical violations. If Dr. Reed indicated to Angela the methodological concerns that warranted viewing such an approach as nonstandard and provided her the opportunity to check with other health care professionals about the purposed approach, then if Angela had consented to proceed, Dr. Reed could engage in the nonstandard treatment. To further protect against the licensing boards finding ethical violations had occurred, Dr. Reed also could engage in ongoing consultation with another psychologist so that accurate appraisals of the efficacy of the nonstandard approach could be documented.

Cultural Considerations

Global Discussion

Lithuanian Psychological Society Code of Ethics

> . . . e) Psychologist shall not use the techniques that have not been fully developed yet, or that do not answer basic methodological requirements; but in case Psychologist does use them, he/she shall not overlook their experimental character and avoid making conclusion that are not guaranteed by said techniques.

If Dr. Reed combined two separate disciplines in a new way that is outside both scopes of practice, she is clearly working with an approach of an experimental nature. In Lithuania, if Dr. Reed chooses to practice somatic therapy with her client, she must make her client aware both of the experimental nature of the intervention and possible risks as well as benefits.

American Moral Values

1. Is it right to use massage therapy while working under contract as a psychologist, both for Angela and for her partner Dr. Cook? Would Dr. Cook have understood "alternative modalities" to include a practice like "somatic" touch therapy? Does their contract implicitly give Dr. Reed the authority to judge whether such a therapy is appropriate?
2. Do the regulations governing licensing, as well as her particular contract with Dr. Cook, override the clinician's desire to find a successful treatment for Angela? Does professional integrity require Dr. Reed to treat Angela within the scope of both of her licenses, or should she refer her client to another competent somatic therapist?
3. Does the practice of clinical psychology pay enough attention to the "body" in relation to the mind? Does Dr. Reed feel that massage therapy has not been given enough respect by the field? Could she use it to treat Angela on the principle that it is an as-yet-unrecognized complementary modality?
4. What is the moral importance of transparency for the client in terms of knowing her psychologist's qualifications? Can Dr. Reed let Angela make the decision, based on a full understanding of Dr. Reed's separate training and qualifications for both licenses?
5. Does Dr. Reed risk undermining Angela's trust in Dr. Cook, given that Angela was referred by Dr. Cook to Dr. Reed as a psychologist? Is Dr. Reed undermining either Angela or Dr. Cook's trust in the profession of psychology?
6. How does Dr. Reed handle the ambiguous status of emerging practices, where no definite system of accountability and supervision exists? Should she obtain supervision as a way of being accountable to her patient and herself?

Ethical Course of Action

Directive per APA Code

Given that she is combining the knowledge from two disciplines, where the treatment is not standard for either profession, Dr. Reed has stepped into an emerging area of treatment. Standard 2.01(e) directs Dr. Reed to "take reasonable steps to ensure the competence of their work and to protect clients/patients . . . from harm." This means Dr. Reed should probably take extra measures to ensure the competence of her work, perhaps by arranging for extra consultation with both the naturopath, colleagues who are practicing massage therapists as well as other psychologists.

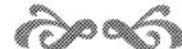

Dictates of One's Own Conscience

Having explained somatic therapy to Angela, what would you then proceed to do?

1. Proceed with treatment at the point where the vignette leaves off.
2. Provide an opportunity for Angela to understand what she is giving consent to by asking that Angela go home and think about the nature and limitations of somatic therapy and consult with her other health care providers before starting treatment.
3. Try to persuade Angela by bringing in additional supporting literature.
4. Refer Angela back to Dr. Cook for further consultation.
5. Inspire credibility by proceeding to provide treatment with confidence.
6. Assemble a supervision team consisting of a massage therapist and a psychologist to jointly supervise the treatment of Angela and then proceed with somatic therapy.
7. Do a combination of the previously listed actions.
8. Do something that is not previously listed.

If you were Dr. Reed dually licensed and practicing in Lithuania, what would you do? Beyond those already listed, the additional activities would include the following:

1. Explain to Angela that the treatment has potential to help, not that it has been successfully used in the past.
2. Regardless of whether treatment was successful or not for Angela, you would avoid ascribing positive or negative attributes to the technique or generalizing to other similar situations, without further study.

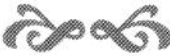

STANDARD 2.01: BOUNDARIES OF COMPETENCE

. . . (f) When assuming forensic roles, psychologists are or become reasonably familiar with the judicial or administrative rules governing their roles.

A CASE FOR STANDARD 2.01 (F): Lesbian No More

Melissa referred herself to Dr. Morgan for depression. Melissa has decided to divorce her husband because she believes herself to be gay and is no longer willing to be married to a man. She told Dr. Morgan that this has been a tremendously difficult situation and that she is afraid of losing custody of her two small children because her husband will accuse her of being "sick" or "evil." Melissa reported that her marriage has been otherwise "fine" and that her husband has not been abusive or unfaithful and is very loving and devoted to her. Dr. Morgan stated that many gay people do not have the same parental or custodial rights as heterosexual people and that she will likely lose the support of her church, putting her at risk for increased stress and depression. He cited current research showing that gay people are at greater risk for depression, substance abuse, suicidality, and discrimination. He suggests Melissa undergo conversion therapy, at the conclusion of which Dr. Morgan would submit a parenting custody evaluation on her behalf.

Dr. Morgan negotiates a forensic role from the start of his treatment relationship with Melissa in which his sole focus in treatment is to enable him to act as a positive force in the forensic arena. In the course of treatment leading up to his writing a parenting custody evaluation, he referred Melissa to publications that reported on the successful treatment of homosexual tendencies. Dr. Morgan's conceptualization of the case is that the source of Melissa's suffering is related to her fears of committing more fully to her marriage, her low self-esteem about herself as a wife and a mother, and depression that is unrelated to her desires to explore relationships with other women. Further Dr. Morgan contextualized the field's negative stance on conversion therapy as being based on political correctness, not on helping clients suffering from homosexuality.

After Melissa successfully underwent conversion therapy, she decided not to divorce her husband and at that point ended treatment with Dr. Morgan. Shortly afterward, she joined a local conversion therapy support group. Listening to other members of the group, she came to understand the nature of the controversy. She decided to go into psychotherapy with another psychologist who has expertise in gay and lesbian identity concerns. After a few sessions, Melissa contacted Dr. Morgan again, told him how she feels betrayed by him, and is considering reporting him for malpractice.

Issues of Concern

Dr. Morgan assumes a forensic role from the very start of a professional relationship with Melissa because the totality of the treatment is for the purpose of writing a custody parenting evaluation. Regardless of what Dr. Morgan assumes, the question is whether Dr. Morgan engaged in both a therapeutic and a forensic role with Melissa. Standard 2.01 (f) directs Dr. Morgan to be "familiar with the judicial or administrative rules governing their roles." Dr. Morgan would refer to the rules in the state he is both licensed and practicing.

APA Ethics Code

Companion General Principle

Principle A: Beneficence and Nonmaleficence

> Psychologists strive to benefit those with whom they work and take care to do no harm.

It can be argued that Dr. Morgan thinks his treatment plan was the best course of action to not only help Melissa with her depression but also ultimately help Melissa live a normal and productive life. In his conceptualization of Melissa, Dr. Morgan formulated a treatment plan that aspires to Principle A.

Principle E: Respect for People's Rights and Dignity

> Psychologists are aware of and respect . . . differences, including those based on . . . sexual orientation, . . . and consider these factors when working with members of such groups.

Dr. Morgan's conceptualization of Melissa's problem did not uphold Principle E in that he did not respect Melissa's sexual orientation. His treatment was aimed at altering Melissa's sexual orientation by having her undergo conversion therapy.

Companion Ethical Standard(s)

Standard 2.04: Bases for Scientific and Professional Judgments

> Psychologists' work is based upon established scientific and professional knowledge of the discipline.

Homosexuality per se is not a mental disorder as evidenced by the absence of diagnosis in the *DSM-IV* (American Psychiatric Association, 2000). The APA's Task Force on Appropriate Therapeutic Responses to Sexual Orientation found no studies of adequate scientific rigor to conclude whether or not recent sexual orientation change efforts (SOCE) do or do not work to change a person's sexual orientation (APA Task Force on Appropriate Therapeutic Responses to Sexual Orientation, 2009).

Dr. Morgan's suggestion of conversion therapy violated Principle A: Nonmaleficence in two ways. Harm came from Dr. Morgan's suggestion of an unproven treatment, conversion therapy. Harm also came from Dr. Morgan suggesting treatment for a condition that is considered within the normal range of human behavior. By treating Melissa's homosexuality, Dr. Morgan has violated Principle E: Respect for People's Rights and Dignity which includes a person's sexual orientation

Standard 3.05: Multiple Relationships

> (a) A multiple relationship occurs when a psychologist is in a professional role with a person and . . .
>
> . . . (1) at the same time is in another role with the same person. . . A psychologist refrains from entering into a multiple relationship if the multiple relationship could reasonably be expected to . . . risks . . . harm to the person with whom the professional relationship exists. Multiple relationships that would not reasonably be expected to cause impairment or risk exploitation or harm are not unethical.

Melissa has sought out treatment services from Dr. Morgan. Dr. Morgan inserts a forensic evaluative role into the treatment relationship. Dr. Morgan is engaged in a multiple relationship as defined by Standard 3.05 (a) (1). Though Standard 3.05 does not categorically prohibit multiple relationships, it does caution against such relationship if it is expected to harm the client in some way. As time passes and Melissa becomes more knowledgeable about her own condition and comes to understand the unsubstantiated treatment merit of conversation therapy, it appears that she thinks she has been harmed. It appears that Dr. Morgan is in violation of Standard 3.05.

Legal Issues 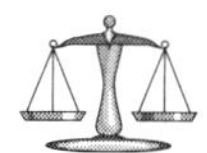

Washington

Wash. Admin. Code § 246-924-359 (2009). Client welfare.

. . . *(3) Stereotyping.* In their work-related activities, psychologists do not engage in unfair discrimination based on . . . sexual orientation . . .

Wash. Admin Code § 246-924-445 (2009). Parenting evaluations—Standards.

Psychologists may be called upon to evaluate members of a family to assist in determining an appropriate residential arrangement, parental duties, or parental relationship with respect to a minor child. These rules establish minimum standards for conducting parenting evaluations. The psychologist must perform the evaluation focusing on the best interest of the child. . .

. . . (3) In conducting parenting evaluations, the psychologist shall not discriminate based on . . . sexual orientation. . .

. . . (7) The psychologist shall not have provided therapeutic services to any party involved in the evaluation. . .

Florida

Fla. Admin. Code Ann. r. 64B19-18.007 (2010). Requirements for forensic psychological evaluations of minors for the purpose of addressing custody, residence or visitation disputes.

. . . (3) It is a conflict of interest for a psychologist who has treated . . . any of the adults involved in a custody or visitation action to perform a forensic evaluation for the purpose of recommending with which adult the minor should reside, which adult should have custody, or what visitation should be allowed. Consequently, a psychologist who treats . . . any of the adults involved in a custody or visitation action may not also perform a forensic evaluation for custody, residence or visitation of the minor. . .

Dr. Morgan's engaging in therapy with Melissa then writing a letter to the courts is considered two separate professional roles: first that of a treating psychologist and the other a forensic psychologist. According to Washington and Florida laws, Dr. Morgan's conduct is in violation of their administrative codes. Evaluation for a child custody case would be viewed as an unethical infraction under each jurisdiction's rules. In Washington, Dr. Morgan also would be viewed as stereotyping his client and engaging in unethical treatment on the basis of his personal prejudice rather than any research findings that are supported by methodologically sound research.

Cultural Considerations

Global Discussion

The Professional Board for Psychology Health Professions Council of South Africa: Ethical Code of Professional Conduct (April 2002)

2.6 Multiple relationships.

2.9.1. A multiple relationship occurs when the psychologist is in a professional role with a person/organisation and (1) at the same time is/was in another role with the same person. . .

2.9.2. Psychologists shall refrain from entering into a multiple relationship if the multiple relationships could reasonably be expected to impair the psychologists' objectivity, competence, or effectiveness in performing their functions as psychologists. . .

7. Psycho-legal activities; 7.5. Conflicting roles.

In most circumstances, psychologists shall avoid performing multiple and potentially conflicting roles in psycho-legal matters. When psychologists may be called on to service in more than one role in a legal proceeding (for example, as consultant or expert for one party or for the court and as a fact witness) they shall clarify role expectations and the extent of confidentiality in advance to the extent feasible, in order to avoid compromising their professional judgment and objectivity.

If Dr. Morgan was practicing in South Africa, he would be in violation of their ethics code by assuming a dual role with his client and secondly by not clarifying the expectations of each role, as well as the limits to confidentiality to his client at the outset of their work together. Because Dr. Morgan appointed himself to this dual role, rather than having it court ordered or mandated by law, he is in violation of the boundary of competence. Dr. Morgan's dual role as both treating and forensic psychologist, as well as his use of the controversial technique of conversion therapy, can be considered a significant enough impairment to his professional objectivity and effectiveness as to risk potential harm to his client, Melissa.

American Moral Values

1. Can Dr. Morgan uphold his promised primary role as a forensic psychologist while suggesting conversion therapy as a more conventionally therapeutic role? Is the therapeutic device a form of blackmail—that is, he will only write the letter if the therapy is accepted? Or is he following his conscience in setting out a condition for his letter to be written?
2. What is Dr. Morgan's moral view of homosexuality, and how does that relate to his therapeutic view of why homosexuality is harmful to Melissa's mental health? Is his moral judgment influencing his recommendation for conversion therapy? Is his evidence for conversion therapy enough to demand Melissa's participation? Is the citation of "many gay people" not having equal parenting rights sufficient evidence for Melissa's decision? How does Dr. Morgan interpret the selected "current research" that he believes shows mental health problems for homosexuals? Could the society's oppressive attitudes and practices (perhaps like those of Dr. Morgan himself) help account for those statistics?
3. Do Dr. Morgan's arguments about homosexuality and depression have validity? Or does his treatment represent the type of behavior that makes life for homosexuals more difficult to begin with? Can one argue for conversion therapy without being homophobic?
4. How does Dr. Morgan's view of women factor into his recommendations? Are women uniquely committed to children and spouses, disposed to low self-esteem without them?
5. How should Dr. Morgan consider Melissa's fears about her husband? Is she in an abusive marriage if she fears being called "sick" and "evil"?
6. What is the moral implication of the term *political correctness*? What is the importance of fighting political correctness, and when is it an excuse to air views without apology or reasoning?

Ethical Course of Action

Directive per APA Code

As directed by Standard 2.01, it is clear that Dr. Morgan was not "reasonably familiar with the judicial or administrative rules governing their roles." One would hope that Dr. Morgan has a consultation group with whom he discusses cases and is obtaining guidance that would help him avoid future threats of grievances. Having provided treatment to Melissa that violated Standard 2.01 and other standards, Dr. Morgan is vulnerable to findings of unethical behavior should Melissa decide to proceed with her grievance.

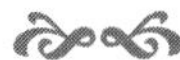

Dictates of One's Own Conscience

If you were Dr. Morgan and faced with an angry ex-client, what would you do?

1. Offer Melissa a free session to tell you more of what is on her mind.
2. Reason that since Melissa decided not to go through with the divorce and you did not write a custody evaluation that Melissa has no grounds for a successful complaint.
3. Thinking that Melissa is angry about the conversion therapy, continue to defend the recommendation and to say that it was ultimately Melissa's decision to engage in conversion therapy.
4. When Melissa calls, apologize to her for having caused her additional pain if between the end of Melissa's treatment and the time of the phone call your teenage son comes home from college and said, "Dad, I have to tell you something. I found out that I am gay." Having lived through the many discussions with your son, you have changed your mind about conversion therapy.
5. Do a combination of the previously listed actions.
6. Do something that is not previously listed.

If you were Dr. Morgan practicing in South Africa, the previously listed options would still apply since the guidelines for treatment and forensic practice are not substantially different from those listed by the APA Ethics Code.

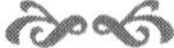

STANDARD 2.02: PROVIDING SERVICES IN EMERGENCIES

> In emergencies, when psychologists provide services to individuals for whom other mental health services are not available and for which psychologists have not obtained the necessary training, psychologists may provide such services in order to ensure that services are not denied. The services are discontinued as soon as the emergency has ended or appropriate services are available.

A CASE FOR STANDARD 2.02: First Responder

Dr. Bell is employed full-time as an associate professor in a small undergraduate liberal arts college. Of the three psychology faculty at the college, she is the only licensed psychologist while others are nonclinical psychologists. Her training and dissertation is in gifted adolescents with learning disabilities. The college is located in a very small rural township in the Midwest and is a 2-hour drive from the nearest town.

On Sunday, the campus awoke to the news that one of the fraternity houses had an all-night party and a freshman woman was found dead. Dr. Bell is asked by the president of this small college to enter into the fraternity house and freshman dormitory that day to conduct crisis grief counseling for the students.

Issues of Concern

Does Standard 2.02 allow for, or direct, Dr. Bell to coordinate a response in the absence of any other service providers who are competent to provide a comprehensive crisis response? Would the possibility of Dr. Bell's potential mishandling of the situation, including the risk of more trauma for members of the community, guide Dr. Bell to decline the college president's request?

APA Ethics Code

Companion General Principle

Principle B: Fidelity and Responsibility

> They are aware of their professional and scientific responsibilities to society and to the specific communities in which they work.

Aspiring to uphold Principle B, Dr. Bell would consider herself as holding a professional responsibility to the university community in which she works. This means that Dr. Bell should provide any assistance she could in this situation. Since she appears to be the only trained clinical psychologist within a 2-hour radius, her professional responsibility would extend to the work of helping coordinate and provide direct crisis intervention to the students in the college.

Principle A: Beneficence and Nonmaleficence

> In their professional actions, psychologists seek to safeguard the welfare and rights of those with whom they interact professionally and other affected persons.

Sentence two of Principle A would guide Dr. Bell to proceed with awareness on safeguarding the welfare of the students, faculty, and staff of the university.

Companion Ethical Standard(s)

Standard 2.01: Boundaries of Competence

> (a) Psychologists provide services . . . in areas only within the boundaries of their competence, based on their education, training, supervised experience, consultation, study, or professional experience.

Clearly, crisis response and grief work is not within Dr. Bell's areas of competence. Thus to follow the dictates of Standard 2.01 (a), Dr. Bell would be required to decline the president's request to take a leadership role in the campus response to the tragedy of a young woman's death.

Standard 2.01: Boundaries of Competence

> . . . (d) When psychologists are asked to provide services to individuals for whom appropriate mental health services are not available and for which psychologists have not obtained the competence necessary, psychologists with closely related prior training or experience may provide such services in order to ensure that services are not denied if they make a reasonable effort to obtain the competence required by using relevant research, training, consultation, or study.

Standard 2.02 appears to focus the psychologist's attention on the emergency and indicates that temporarily Standard 2.02 supersedes the requirement for competency as required in Standard 2.01 (a) and (d).

The difference between Standards 2.02 and 2.01 (a)/(d) is the temporary nature of providing assistance in an emergency.

Standard 3.05: Multiple Relationships

> . . . (c) When psychologists are required by . . . extraordinary circumstances to serve in more than one role in . . . administrative proceedings, at the outset they clarify role expectations and the extent of confidentiality and thereafter as changes occur.

In this situation, with the request of the university president, it can be construed that Dr. Bell is required by extraordinary circumstances to serve in more than one role. The extraordinary circumstance is the death of a young woman in a very remote college town. The multiple roles involve the role of faculty, the role of administrator responding to tragic circumstances, and the role of a clinical psychologist providing direct treatment. Standard 3.05 directs Dr. Bell to clarify the extent of confidentiality. This may allow Dr. Bell to avoid possible future problematic dilemmas including any necessary actions she may have to take should she learn from the students that the death was not accidental and information that may directly lead to the identification of the perpetrator(s).

Standard 3.07: Third-Party Requests for Services

> When psychologists agree to provide services to a person or entity at the request of a third party, psychologists attempt to clarify at the outset of the service the nature of the relationship with all individuals or organizations involved.

This clarification includes the role of the psychologist (e.g., therapist, consultant, diagnostician, or expert witness), an identification of who is the client, the probable uses of the services provided or the information obtained, and the fact that there may be limits to confidentiality (see also Standard 3.05: Multiple Relationships and Standard 4.02: Discussing the Limits of Confidentiality).

It behooves Dr. Bell to have a conversation with the university president (considered the third party in the language of Standard 3.07) to clarify not only her role but also the possible use of the information revealed by the students should she be providing direct treatment and intervention.

Standard 4.02: Discussing the Limits of Confidentiality

> (a) Psychologists discuss with persons . . . and organizations with whom they establish a . . . professional relationship (1) the relevant limits of confidentiality and (2) the foreseeable uses of the information generated through their psychological activities. . .
>
> . . . (b) Unless it is not feasible or is contraindicated, the discussion of confidentiality occurs at the outset of the relationship and thereafter as new circumstances may warrant.

As directed by Standard 4.02, at the onset of contact with students, Dr. Bell is to discuss with them the following items: how the university might use any information revealed to Dr. Bell by students and under what circumstances Dr. Bell may reveal confidential information told to her in either private or group sessions in regards to the death of the student.

Standard 10.03: Group Therapy

> When psychologists provide services to several persons in a group setting, they describe at the outset the roles and responsibilities of all parties and the limits of confidentiality.

More likely than not, should Dr. Bell take a leadership role in the university's response to the tragedy, she would find herself holding group sessions where students discuss their reactions and future implications of the tragedy and of the circumstances surrounding a fellow student's death. As in any case where treatment is provided, clarification of roles and limits of confidentiality are required by Standard 4.

Legal Issues 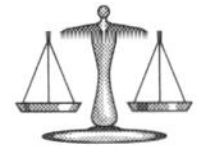

New Jersey

> *N.J. Admin. Code § 13:42-10.4 (2010). Professional responsibilities to . . . the public.*
>
> . . . (d) A licensee shall maintain competence consistent with professional responsibilities, including the following:
>
> . . . 5. A licensee shall practice only in his or her area of competence, consistent with his or her training, experience, education or supervision, and shall make appropriate referrals to practitioners of related or other professions.

California

Cal. Code Regs. tit. 16, § 1396 (2010). Competence.

A psychologist shall not function outside his or her particular field or fields of competence as established by his or her education, training and experience.

The laws of both jurisdictions would preclude the psychologist conducting such crisis intervention in light of her lack of training and experience. Neither state permits providing services, probably even in emergencies, that are beyond a psychologist's competence.

Cultural Considerations

Global Discussion

British Psychological Society Code of Conduct, Ethical Principles and Guidelines

1. Competence.

2.4. If requested to provide psychological services, and where the services they judge to be appropriate are outside their personal competence, give every reasonable assistance towards obtaining those services from others who are appropriately qualified to provide them.

If Dr. Bell was practicing in Britain, the code clearly guides her to put her energy toward finding psychologists or other mental health providers trained to provide crisis counseling for the college students, rather than assuming such a role herself.

American Moral Values

1. How does Dr. Bell weigh the importance of treating others within one's area of competence against her academic community's need to grieve and mourn a death? Does a crisis involving death and communal grief mandate a more involved response by Dr. Bell than she would otherwise attempt? How does the context of grief and death affect Dr. Bell's professional assessment of her abilities and proper role? Would acting outside of her competence, even if there were no qualified specialists able to lead grief counseling, be more harmful for the college than if no counseling were offered at all?
2. How does Dr. Bell evaluate the community's need to come together in order to heal after death? Is the mutual support and emotional cohesion of the community important enough to risk unqualified leadership in grief counseling? Would Dr. Bell's attempt itself, as a gesture witnessed by the community, be more constructive than them seeing a licensed psychologist refuse to lead?
3. What is Dr. Bell's responsibility for representing psychology and other psychologists to the university? Will her actions have magnified consequences for how the university community thinks about the field and its practitioners? Does this underscore the importance of having a well-trained psychologist lead the counseling?
4. Does Dr. Bell see her choice as between acting (leading) and not-acting (declining the invitation to lead)? How does this relate to the APA principle of "First, do no harm"? Does that imply being more cautious instead of gambling for a greater "help"? Or is noncompetent intervention a more reckless act, both in the present and as an example, than restraint?

Ethical Course of Action

Directive per APA Code

Standard 2.02 allows for Dr. Bell to respond affirmatively to the university president's request. It states that a psychologist "may" provide . . . The word *may* is a permissive stance, not a directive stance as would be implied in the use of the words *must* or *shall*. Thus Dr. Bell is free to decide whether to take on a leadership role and/or direct service role in the campus emergency, at least until either the emergency ends or such time as other appropriate services are available. However, if the university were located in New Jersey, California, or Great Britain, Dr. Bell would be in violation of the law if she were to provide services of any kind in her current professional capacity.

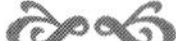

Dictates of One's Own Conscience

Standard 2.02 does not give clear directives as to whether Dr. Bell should or should not step into the situation as requested by the university president. Thus Dr. Bell needs to decide based on circumstances and her own moral values as to how best to position herself in the campus community. If you were Dr. Bell, what would you do?

1. Consider it important to be an involved citizen, and provide aid in whatever manner possible; say yes to the president's request, and take whatever action you deem appropriate.
2. Be ever-mindful of the advantages of compliance to authority or at least the disadvantages of crossing someone in authority, decide to say yes to the president's request, and hold a few meetings in the dormitories with whichever students decide to attend.
3. Align with the British code, and decide to give "reasonable assistance" by immediately driving the 2 hours to the nearest town and return with qualified mental health professionals.
4. Get on the Internet and do a very quick read-up on the best practices for emergency response to death in a community, and proceed to follow the directions for best practice.
5. Call a colleague who has some expertise in the area and ask for assistance, then follow whatever instructions given by the colleague.
6. Find someone with expertise, and give the name of this psychologist to the president.
7. Tell the university president it's against your ethics code to practice outside your competency and go back to bed.
8. Proclaim incompetence, make it known that you are ethically bound not to practice outside your area of competency but should the university president order it you would do your best (per Standard 1.03), thus absolving yourself of any responsibility for negative consequences of your actions.
9. Do a combination of the previously listed actions.
10. Do something that is not previously listed.

If you were Dr. Bell teaching in England, what would you do?

1. Tell the president of the university that you will make contact with psychologists who are competent to handle such situations and will get back to him shortly.
2. Contact your colleague who is an expert in crisis mental health, and arrange for this colleague to teleport into the community to organize response effort.
3. Under no circumstances would you attempt to provide services yourself.

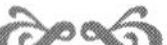

STANDARD 2.03: MAINTAINING COMPETENCE

> Psychologists undertake ongoing efforts to develop and maintain their competence.

A CASE FOR STANDARD 2.03: I Meant to Do It (Really, I Did)

Dr. Murphy, being a bit overwhelmed by his very busy schedule, renewed his state psychology licensure without checking for documentation but knew surely that he had attended and acquired the necessary CE credits in the past year. Unluckily, his renewal was randomly drawn to submit proof of CE credits. Dr. Murphy was alarmed to discover that he actually had not accumulated the required number of CE credits through attendance at CE events. However, Dr. Murphy reasoned that he has done enough reading of self-help books to qualify for self-guided CE credits.

Issues of Concern

Not checking to make sure one has accumulated sufficient CE credits to maintain licensure is sloppy practice but a mistake that ethical psychologists may make. Does Dr. Murphy's next step of retroactively claiming reading of commercial self-help books meet either the spirit or the letter of the requirement to maintain competence? Has Dr. Murphy lied by claiming self-guided CE learning?

APA Ethics Code

Companion General Principle

Principle C: Integrity

> Psychologists seek to promote accuracy, honesty, and truthfulness in the . . . practice of psychology. In these activities psychologists do not . . . engage in fraud . . . or intentional misrepresentation of fact.

Does Dr. Murphy's action constitute intentional misrepresentation of fact? Does such a "white lie" harm any of Dr. Murphy's clients? Responding to the inquiry by claiming readings in such a way that it appears he fulfilled the CE requirement, Dr. Murphy misrepresents how many CE credits he has accumulated and thus is in violation of Principle C.

Principle B: Fidelity and Responsibility

> Psychologists . . . accept appropriate responsibility for their behavior, and seek to manage conflicts of interest that could lead to exploitation or harm.

Aspiring to the spirit of Principle B, Dr. Murphy would respond to the inquiry with a statement that indicates he has not accumulated sufficient CE workshops. He would uphold Principle B if he reported reading of self-help books and inquired whether such effort fulfills the CE requirement. If not, he must be willing to undertake whatever remedial actions his state licensing board advises.

Companion Ethical Standard(s)

No other relevant or conflicting standards apply in this situation.

Legal Issues 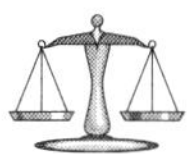

Virginia

> *Va. Code Ann. § 54.1-3606.1 (West 2009).*
>
> Continuing Education.
>
> A. The board shall promulgate regulations governing continuing education . . . such regulations shall require the completion of the equivalent of fourteen hours annually in board-approved continuing education courses for any license renewal or reinstatement after the effective date.
>
> . . . C. . . Applicants for renewal or reinstatement of licenses issued pursuant to this article shall retain for a period of four years the written certification issued by any course provider.
>
> *18 Va. Admin. Code § 125-20-160 (2010). Grounds for disciplinary action or denial of licensure.*
>
> The board may take disciplinary action or deny a license for any of the following causes:
>
> . . . 7. Failure to comply with the continued competency requirements set forth in this chapter. . .

Pennsylvania

> *49 Pa. Code § 41.59 (2010). Continuing education.*
>
> . . . (b) Continuing education requirement for biennial renewal.
>
> As a condition of biennial license renewal, a psychologist shall have completed during the preceding biennium a minimum of 30 contact hours (3 CEUs) of continuing education in acceptable courses, programs or activities which shall include at least 3 contact hours per biennium in ethical issues. . .
>
> . . . (c) Reports to the Board.
>
> A psychologist shall certify to compliance with the contact hours requirement at the time of biennial renewal. A psychologist shall retain for at least two bienniums, certificates, transcripts or other documentation showing completion of the prescribed number of contact hours. These records are subject to audit by the Board.
>
> . . . (e) Home study.
>
> A psychologist may accrue up to 15 of the required contact hours in home study courses offered by approved sponsors as long as the course has specific learning objectives and the sponsor evaluates the extent of learning that has taken place.
>
> . . . (k) Curing deficiencies.
>
> A psychologist with a deficiency in contact hours may apply to the Board in writing for leave to make up the contact hours in arrears. The request shall include an explanation of why the deficiency occurred and a plan, along with the estimated time needed, for curing it. Requests will be evaluated by the Board on a case-by-case basis and will be approved or disapproved at its discretion.
>
> *49 Pa. Code § 41.61 (2010). Code of ethics.*
>
> Principle 2. Competency.
>
> . . . (d) Psychologists accurately represent their competence, education, training and experience.

In both Virginia and Pennsylvania, Dr. Murphy has failed to meet the standards for amassing sufficient CE credits. Pennsylvania has a formal procedure for curing a deficiency. For both jurisdictions the reading of self-help books without engaging in testing from license board approved vendors will be viewed as insufficient CE.

Cultural Considerations

Global Discussion

Lithuanian Psychological Society

> Preamble.
>
> . . . A Psychologist must avoid losing his/her high professional competence, understand that it is necessary to

> learn and to continually refresh possessed knowledge, to grasp and to adapt everything that is new and progressive in his/her professional line, and to seek his/her colleagues, advice if needed.

The Lithuanian psychologist is charged with refreshing their existing knowledge, to learn what is new in the field, and to uphold the prestige and dignity of the profession of psychology as a whole. The Lithuanian code does not direct the means of grasping new knowledge and suggests that it can come from professional colleagues.

American Moral Values

1. What is Dr. Murphy's assessment of the CE requirement's value? Is it a valuable requirement for psychologists or is it a bureaucratic hurdle that is not worth honoring? Is one's "self-help" reading a good enough substitute for those credits, making it more permissible to lie about the credits? How do these self-help books measure up to actual psychology courses, on Dr. Murphy's view?
2. What does Dr. Murphy think about misrepresenting his education? Could that threaten his career? Does he not want to follow a bad precedent for other psychologists, or does he count himself a worthwhile exception? What other form of defying regulatory bureaucracies would Dr. Murphy endorse, and of which would he still disapprove?
3. Independent of the specific question of CE credits, does Dr. Murphy frame his decision as one about "lying"? Does lying about the CE credits nag at his own self-image, both as a person and as a psychologist? Can he imagine it being a burden to his conscience?
4. If Dr. Murphy is a newly licensed psychologist—and thus just out of school—does he justify or feel entitled to claim personal reading as CE credits, in light of having only recently been out of classes? Does the expense of doctoral-level tuition and texts in psychology, as well as monthly loan repayments, "entitle" Dr. Murphy to feeling as though he has very recently done more than sufficient work to claim CE credits?

Ethical Course of Action

Directive per APA Code

Both Standard 2.03 and state laws make it imminently clear that Dr. Murphy was to have completed CE hours. Inherent in Dr. Murphy's dilemma, it is evident that he knows he should have made sure he completed all of his required CE hours. Aspiring to uphold Principle C: Integrity and be ever truthful about what he has done, and to enact Principle B: Fidelity and Responsibility to accept any consequences of his actions, Dr. Murphy should make clear to the licensing board the exact nature and extent of his CE activities in the last licensing period.

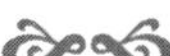

Dictates of One's Own Conscience

If, given the very busy nature of a full-time practice, the sometimes prohibitive cost of CE, and possibly not aspiring to practice in new areas of competency, and believing that you may have upheld the spirit of Standard 2.03 and the state CE requirement, what course of action might you take?

1. Respond with a claim that though you have met the spirit of CE requirement, you admit to a lack of sufficient credit hours documented by any external entity.
2. Respond with accurate accounts of the CE hours attended and the list of books read. Argue that the books constitute sufficient new learning as to meet the CE requirements.
3. Respond with accurate accounts of the CE hours attended, list some scholarly books that you had read several years ago, and do not list the self-help books you read.
4. Respond with a confession of insufficient CE hours accumulated in the last year, and lay out a plan of action for making up the deficiency in CE credits within a reasonable period of time.
5. Do a combination of the previously listed actions.
6. Do something that is not previously listed.

If you were Dr. Murphy practicing in Lithuania, faced with a request for CE hours, would you respond with a confession of insufficient CE hours accumulated in the last year and lay out a plan of action for making up the deficiency in CE credits within a reasonable period of time?

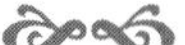

STANDARD 2.04: BASES FOR SCIENTIFIC AND PROFESSIONAL JUDGMENTS

> Psychologists' work is based upon established scientific and professional knowledge of the discipline.

A CASE FOR STANDARD 2.04: But Does It Work?

Daniel, a 22-year-old male, is in treatment with Dr. Bailey in order to work on the many ramifications of his identity as a homosexual male. Daniel reported that his parents did not react well to their discussion regarding his sexual identity and that, as always after a visit with his parents, he was feeling depressed and thoughts of wishing to die crossed his mind. Upon hearing Daniel's suicidal ideation, Dr. Bailey immediately proceeded to have Daniel complete a signed suicide contract wherein Daniel promised not to attempt suicide. Dr. Bailey also then inquired as to whether Daniel had considered conversion therapy.

Issues of Concern

Standard and customary practice when a client expresses suicidal ideation is to engage the client in signing a suicide contract. Conversion therapy, though controversial, is a treatment that some psychologists might argue may be appropriate for Daniel, especially in light of the fact that death by suicide is one of the leading causes of death in young gay males (D'Augelli et al., 2005; Kitts, 2005).

However, neither suicide contracts nor conversion therapy are supported by "established scientific and professional knowledge." Exploration into the effectiveness of suicide contracts as an intervention method to prevent suicide attempts indicates that the presence of a suicide contract with a therapist does not deter suicide attempts (Werth, Welfel, & Benjamin, 2009). Use of conversion therapy is experimental, and the recent APA statement on conversion therapy does not support this experimental treatment. The following resolution was adopted by the APA in August 2009: http://www.apa.org/about/governance/council/policy/sexual-orientation.aspx

APA Ethics Code

Companion General Principle

Principle A: Beneficence and Nonmaleficence

> Psychologists strive to benefit those with whom they work and take care to do no harm.

Dr. Bailey is upholding Principle A, to benefit those with whom [they] work, by taking action that would prevent Daniel from committing suicide. Dr. Bailey is addressing the immediate harm posed by Daniel's suicidal ideations. Dr. Bailey also likely believes he is addressing the underlying cause of the suicidal ideation, Daniel's homosexuality.

Principle E: Respect for People's Rights and Dignity

> Psychologists are aware of and respect . . . differences, including those based on . . . sexual orientation . . . and consider these factors when working with members of such groups.

Dr. Bailey's suggestion of conversion therapy violates the spirit of Principle E in regards to Daniel's sexual orientation.

Companion Ethical Standard(s)

Standard 3.04: Avoiding Harm

> Psychologists take reasonable steps to avoid harming their clients/patients . . . and to minimize harm where it is foreseeable and unavoidable.

Standard 3.04 is the operationalization of Principle A. Beneficence and Nonmaleficence. Assuredly Dr. Bailey does not intend to harm his patients, thus upholding the value of nonmaleficence. However, by not keeping up with and practicing with the established scientific and professional knowledge, psychologists may, with the best of intentions, be harmful to their clients. Dr. Bailey, by not keeping up with current knowledge, is in violation of Standard 3.04.

Standard 2.01: Boundaries of Competence

> . . . (e) In those emerging areas in which generally recognized standards for preparatory training do not yet exist, psychologists nevertheless take reasonable steps to ensure the competence of their work and to protect clients/patients . . . from harm.

Standard 2.01 (e) gives further specification to the value of Nonmaleficence and Standard 3.04, Avoiding Harm, by requiring that should Dr. Bailey work in areas that are considered "emerging" then he should take reasonable steps to acquire competence. Standard 2.01 (e), at a minimum, would require Dr. Bailey to be knowledgeable about the experimental nature and the specifics of the controversy regarding conversion therapy before he recommends such treatment to Daniel. If Dr. Bailey made recommendation for conversion therapy without such knowledge, then he would be in violation of Standard 2.01 (e).

Standard 10.01: Informed Consent to Therapy

> . . . (b) When obtaining informed consent for treatment for which generally recognized techniques and procedures have not been established, psychologists inform their clients/patients of the developing nature of the treatment, the potential risks involved, alternative treatments that may be available, and the voluntary nature of their participation.

Enacting the value of Principle E to respect Daniel's right to self-determination, Standard 10.01 requires that Dr. Bailey inform Daniel of the current level of knowledge regarding conversion therapy as well as suicide contracts. It appears that Dr. Bailey is in violation of Standard 10.01 in the area of suicide contracts and may be in violation as well in the area of conversion therapy.

Legal Issues 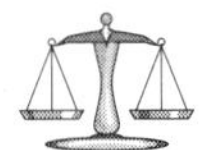

Georgia

> *Ga. Comp. R. & Regs. 510-4-.02 (2010). Code of ethics; APA ethical standards.*
>
> . . . (2) Competence
>
> . . . (d) 2.04 Bases for . . . Professional Judgments. Psychologists' work is based upon established scientific and professional knowledge of the discipline.

Maryland

> *Md. Code Ann., Health Occ. § 18-313 (West 2009). Denials, reprimands, suspensions, and revocations—grounds.*
>
> . . . (20) Does an act that is inconsistent with generally accepted professional standards in the practice of psychology.
>
> *Md. Code Regs. 10.36.05.04 (2010). Competence.*
>
> A. Professional Competence. A psychologist shall . . .
>
> . . . (4) Use intervention . . . techniques only when the psychologist knows that the circumstances are appropriate applications of those interventions and techniques, supported by reliability, validation, standardization, and outcome studies . . .

In both jurisdictions, engaging in therapeutic practices that are not adequately substantiated scientifically would be viewed as ethical infractions under the jurisdictions' rules. Both practices have been called into question by solid methodological research and should not be used under the laws of either jurisdiction.

Cultural Considerations

Global Discussion

Lithuanian Psychological Society Code of Ethics

> . . . a) in the course of investigation, Psychologist shall try to create the situation in which [the client] can feel that the interaction answers his/her interests; the basic principle is to make [the client] interact of his/her free will; b) Psychologist shall not use his/her professional knowledge or knowledge relating to [clients] in order to harm [clients] or make [clients] suffer needlessly.

In this case of conversion therapy, Dr. Bailey could be seen as violating Daniel's free will as Daniel did not request this treatment. Dr. Bailey is also engaging in professional behavior that would make Daniel "suffer needlessly." Therefore, Dr. Bailey must carefully consider how "free will" and suicidal ideation intersect, whether that will is compromised by a wish to die, and what would cause greater suffering to Daniel: imposing a scientifically unfounded suicide contract and the use of an at-best controversial treatment (conversion therapy) or allowing Daniel to exercise his own free will and possibly choose death by suicide?

American Moral Values

1. How does Dr. Bailey choose conversion therapy as a response to Daniel's situation? Is homosexuality being singled out as the problem that threatens Daniel's life? Does that indicate an unstated moral condemnation of homosexuality on Dr. Bailey's part? Or does Dr. Bailey take sexuality in general to be an

area to "fix" in order to save one's life? How does Dr. Bailey see sexuality fitting into a life worth living?

2. What is the evidence that conversion therapy works? What are the possible repercussions of a failed conversion therapy on Daniel's state of mind?
3. Is the reaction of Daniel's parents problematic? Could Dr. Bailey single out Daniel's relationship with his parents as a problem? Does Dr. Bailey grant the parents too much authority and respect by default? Could Dr. Bailey address Daniel's need for their support in other ways? What if the parents remain unsupportive about Daniel's sexual life and romantic choices?
4. How does a "suicide contract" work? Does it serve Daniel to believe that his desire to honor a contract will override his suicidal feelings and disappointment over his parents' disapproval? What must Dr. Bailey assume about Daniel's trust in him to think this contract will work? Is this contract for Daniel's sake or Dr. Bailey's?

Ethical Course of Action

Directive per APA Code

Standard 2.01 requires that Dr. Bailey keep current regarding best practice treatment for clients who are struggling with problems secondary to sexual identity. Best practices, which are based on established scientific and professional knowledge of the discipline, as required by Standard 2.04, for those whose sexual identity is not heterosexual, does not indicate the use of conversion therapy. Additionally, best for those with suicidal ideation does not indicate the use of suicide contracts. To be in compliance with Standard 2.04, Dr. Bailey is not to use suicide contracts in response to Daniel's report of suicidal ideation nor suggest conversion therapy.

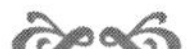

Dictates of One's Own Conscience

Faced with a young man who is part of a high-risk group for suicide and who is expressing suicidal ideation, might you not also seek any means to keep your client safe? In this case, what would you do?

1. Explain to Daniel that being gay puts him in a very high-risk group for death from suicide, and because of this fact, Daniel must promise you that he will not kill himself.
2. Explain to Daniel that the source of his miseries is his homosexuality and that there are many human conditions for which we do not yet have effective treatment, but it may help to discuss the causes of homosexuality, thus treating the cause of his depression.
3. Explain to Daniel that his homosexual identity is not the source of his suicidality but society's (and his family's) response to his homosexuality is the likely source of his depression. Thus it may be helpful to explore Daniel's wish for his parents to be more supportive, thus treating the cause of his depression.
4. Explain to Daniel that being able to explore his depressed feelings and suicidal thoughts allows a release, like a pressure valve exists to allow a release of built-up tension. Thus, you would encourage Daniel to talk about the suicidal thoughts.
5. Explain to Daniel that it is against the law to kill himself and you must take measures to stop him. Further, you would warn Daniel that you are obligated to hospitalize him unless he promises not to break the law by signing a promissory note, as in a suicide contract, that allows you not to hospitalize him.
6. Do a combination of the previously listed actions.
7. Do something that is not previously listed.

If you were Dr. Dr. Bailey working in Lithuania, what might you do?

1. Explain to Daniel that being able to explore his depressed feelings, suicidal thoughts, and his parents' reaction to his sexual identity allows a release like a pressure valve exists to allow a release of built-up tension.
2. Encourage Daniel to talk about the suicidal thoughts.

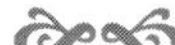

STANDARD 2.05: DELEGATION OF WORK TO OTHERS

Psychologists who delegate work to employees, supervisees, or research or teaching assistants or who use the services of others, such as interpreters, take reasonable steps to (1) avoid delegating such work to persons who have a multiple relationship with those being served that would likely lead to exploitation or loss of objectivity; (2) authorize only those responsibilities that such persons can be expected to perform competently on the basis of their education, training, or experience, either independently or with the level of supervision being provided; and (3) see that such persons perform these services competently.

A CASE FOR STANDARD 2.05 (2): Software Ghosts

Dr. Rivera noticed that his office is receiving insurance payments for client sessions that did not occur. Dr. Rivera spoke to his part-time bookkeeper, Sandra, who does general office work, client billing, and filing of insurance claims. Sandra claimed that she never submitted insurance claims for the treatment sessions in question but that she would certainly contact the insurance company to see what she could find out. After contacting the insurance company, Sandra reported that Christopher, the tech support for the insurance software that Sandra has been using, was the generator of the insurance claims for the erroneous sessions in question. Sandra also said that she had been having some difficulties with the new claims software's electronic interface with the insurance company so she had been working with Christopher to work out these problems.

Issues of Concern

It is not unusual for psychologists in practice to have access to and to delegate administrative tasks, like insurance work, to support staff. Standard 2.05 holds Dr. Rivera responsible for hiring and supervising someone competent to perform the work delegated. And indeed, as directed by Standard 2.5 (2), it appears that Dr. Rivera has delegated the work to someone who can perform the assigned task competently in that Sandra contacts appropriate support personnel when she encounters barriers. In this case, it is the software company who has hired someone who appears to be either incompetent or dishonest. Is Dr. Rivera responsible for the actions of Christopher?

Regardless of who performs the administrative tasks or who files insurance claims, would the insurance company hold Dr. Rivera responsible for the claims? Since the claims are for sessions that were never held, is Dr. Rivera exposed to the charge of fraud?

APA Ethics Code

Companion General Principle

Principle C: Integrity

> . . . Psychologists to not steal, cheat, or engage in fraud, subterfuge, or intentional misrepresentation of fact.

Though unintentional, unbeknownst to Dr. Rivera, fraudulent claims were sent under his license. Not only were claims sent but also insurance made payment on these fraudulent claims. The resultant exchange of money indicates that Dr. Rivera has violated the intent of Principle C: Integrity.

Companion Ethical Standard(s)

P.L. 104-191 Health Insurance Portability and Accountability Act (HIPAA) of 1996. Section 1173

> . . . (d) Security standards for health information.
>
> . . . (2) Safeguards. Each . . . who . . . transmits health information shall maintain reasonable and appropriate . . . safeguards (A) to ensure the integrity and confidentiality of the information; (B) to protect against any . . . (ii) unauthorized uses or disclosures of the information; . . .

Per U.S. P.L. 104-191, section 1173 of HIPAA, it is clear that Dr. Rivera is responsible for ensuring compliance with security of the individual health information, regardless of whether it is intentionally or unintentionally transmitted by entities other than himself. It can be argued that since the individual health information was provided through Dr. Rivera's office, it was Sandra who was in violation of ensuring security of the information. Since Sandra is an employee of Dr. Rivera, this section of HIPAA stipulates that Dr. Rivera is thus responsible for the breach of security.

Standard 4.01: Maintaining Confidentiality

> Psychologists have a primary obligation and take reasonable precautions to protect confidential information obtained through or stored in any medium . . .

Per P.L. 104-191 Section1171 (6), the information contained in the electronic transmission from Christopher at the software company is considered individual health care information. As such, psychologists are directed by Standard 4.01 to protect the insurance billing information.

Standard 4.05: Disclosures

> ... (b) Psychologists disclose confidential information without the consent of the individual ... where permitted by law for a valid purpose such as to ... (2) obtain appropriate professional consultations ...

Per Standard 4.05 (b) (2), it could be argued that Dr. Rivera's office released confidential information with the consent of the client was for a valid purpose of obtaining "appropriate professional consultation." The caveat in such an argument is the stipulation of "where permitted by law." The law, as stipulated by HIPAA, does not permit such a release. Thus Dr. Rivera's office was in violation of Standard 4.05.

Standard 6.02: Maintenance, Dissemination, and Disposal of Confidential Records of Professional and Scientific Work

> (a) Psychologists maintain confidentiality in creating, storing, accessing, transferring, and disposing of records under their control, whether these are written, automated, or in any other medium.

Standard 6.02 directs Dr. Rivera to maintain confidentiality in "accessing" and "transferring" of his client insurance information. His office released the confidential information without client consent, thus violating Standard 6.02, when Sandra gave Christopher files with live data.

Standard 6.06: Accuracy in Reports to Payors and Funding Sources

> ... Psychologists take reasonable steps to ensure accurate reporting of the nature of the service provided...

Standard 6.06 directs and places responsibility for accuracy of insurance charges on Dr. Rivera. Also, Standard 2.05 makes it clear that regardless of whether the insurance filing was done with or without Dr. Rivera's awareness or whether they were submitted from his office or by the software company that Dr. Rivera holds ultimate responsibility for the accuracy of all reporting, including insurance billing.

Standard 6.04: Fees and Financial Arrangements

> ... (c) Psychologists do not misrepresent their fees.

Standard 6.04 directs Dr. Rivera to not misrepresent their fees, which includes charges submitted to insurance companies. The submission of charges for work he has not done constitutes misrepresentation.

Legal Issues 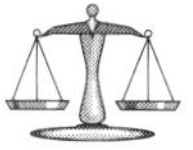

Illinois

> *225 Ill. Comp. Stat. Ann. 15/15 (West 2007). Disciplinary action; grounds.*
>
> The Department may ... suspend, or revoke any license ... for any one or a combination of the following reasons:
>
> ... (6) Professional connection or association with any person ... holding himself, herself, themselves, or itself out in any manner contrary to this Act.
>
> ... (14) Willfully making or filing false records or reports, including but not limited to, false records or reports filed with State agencies or departments.
>
> *Ill. Admin. Code tit. 68, § 1400.80 (2010). Unethical, unauthorized, or unprofessional conduct.*
>
> The Department may suspend or revoke a license, refuse to issue or renew a license or take other disciplinary action, based upon its finding of "unethical, unauthorized, or unprofessional conduct" ... to include, but is not limited to, the following acts or practices:
>
> ... j) Submission of fraudulent claims for services to any health insurance company or health service plan or third party payor...

New York

> *N.Y. Comp. Codes R. & Regs. tit. 8, § 29.1 (2010). General provisions.*
>
> a. Unprofessional conduct shall be the conduct prohibited by this section.
>
> ... 6. willfully making or filing a false report ...
>
> ... 10. delegating professional responsibilities to a person when the licensee delegating such responsibilities knows or has reason to know that such person is not qualified, by training, by experience or by licensure, to perform them ...

In both jurisdictions, the insurance submission would likely be investigated by the licensing boards as a fraudulent act. Since it is generated from Dr. Rivera's patient list and the reimbursement was paid to Dr. Rivera, he would be named the person who committed a fraudulent act. If Dr. Rivera was practicing in Illinois, he would be subjected to disciplinary proceedings. If Dr. Rivera were practicing in New York, the filing may not be considered fraudulent since New York makes a distinction between willfully making a report and those not done with intention. In this case, neither Dr. Rivera nor Sandra willfully or intentionally caused the fraudulent report to be filed.

Cultural Considerations

Global Discussion

The Professional Board for Psychology Health Professions Council of South Africa: Ethical Code of Conduct (April 2002)

> Professional competence.
>
> Psychologists shall accept that they are accountable for professional actions in all domains of their professional lives.
>
> 1.6. Delegation of work.
>
> Psychologists who delegate work to employees . . . shall take reasonable steps to (2) authorise only those responsibilities that such persons can be expected to perform competently on the basis of training or experience, and (3) see that such persons perform these services competently.

In South Africa, Dr. Rivera needs to delegate work to persons who are trained and can perform it competently; regardless, he is still accountable for all "professional actions" in the domain of clinical practice as a psychologist. Therefore, even if Dr. Rivera's hiring of an employee and training of her on a new software program was done correctly, regardless of whether the employee knowingly did anything wrong, Dr. Rivera is still accountable for the actions originating from his clinical practice.

American Moral Values

1. How does Dr. Rivera understand the mistaken insurance claims? Is this an honest mistake on Sandra's part? Was it not her fault at all but rather an accident on the part of Christopher? Or was it a deliberate and illegal act on the part of one or both of them?
2. Based on those possible scenarios, what is the best way to make it right? Should Dr. Rivera retrain Sandra on the process of filing claims? Should Dr. Rivera request that Christopher not come again and then establish a protocol for Sandra regarding computer assistance? Or does Dr. Rivera need to question Sandra and Christopher further, possibly calling the authorities to assist in the investigation?
3. How does Dr. Rivera understand his own responsibility for the problem? Did he adequately train Sandra? Does he see himself as a leader who is expected to be responsible for the office's overall performance? Is Sandra's performance a reflection on him?
4. What is Dr. Rivera's view of insurance companies and the laws surrounding insurance claims? Does he see this as a minor matter rather than full-blown fraud? Is it worth firing Sandra or even questioning her on the basis of this mistake? Or is this office's unity worth more to patients than strict bookkeeping laws?

Ethical Course of Action

Directive per APA Code

Standard 2.05 and all other cited standards and federal laws in this section place the responsibility of the fraudulent insurance claim on Dr. Rivera. Guided by Principle B to "accept appropriate responsibility for their behavior," it behooves Dr. Rivera to do something to right this fraudulent act.

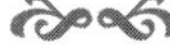

Dictates of One's Own Conscience

If you were in Dr. Rivera's position, understanding that a fraudulent act has been committed and knowing you need to act, what would you do?

1. Personally contact the insurance company to rescind the insurance filings, and request that the already reimbursed funds be applied to future filings.
2. Personally contact the insurance company to rescind the insurance filings, and refund the total sum of the reimbursed fees to the insurance company.
3. Personally contact each of the patients to notify them that a breach of security has occurred.
4. Conduct an investigation to assess whether the filings of his employee occurred because of poor training or because of criminal intent.

5. Set up disciplinary action for Sandra in the form of remediation program for software or more supervision to determine whether further filings are accurate.
6. Decide that Sandra was and is not competent beyond what can be remediated, thus terminate her employment.
7. Report the case to the police.
8. Assist the police in the investigation of the fraudulent claims.
9. Seek professional consultation to assess whether the release of information from Sandra to Christopher was due to lack of training or because criminal behavior occurred.
10. Seek a professional consultation with an independent claims specialist or with a defense lawyer who specializes in insurance fraud to look at the record.
11. Keep meticulous notes of his own investigative process, consultation received, and any subsequent actions taken to show that Dr. Rivera acted in a prudent and reasonable manner to rectify the inaccurate filings and the errant employee's behavior.
12. Redesign your office procedures in such as way that all incoming funds pass through your hands.
13. Contact the software company to obtain assurance that your private confidential information is not used in any manner by the software company.
14. File a complaint against the software company for unauthorized use of confidential information.
15. Switch to a different software insurance billing company.
16. Do a combination of the previously listed actions.
17. Do something that is not previously listed.

If you were Dr. Rivera practicing in South Africa, the previously listed options would still apply since the responsibility for work delegated to others is not substantially different from those listed by the APA Ethics Code.

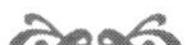

STANDARD 2.06: PERSONAL PROBLEMS AND CONFLICTS

(a) Psychologists refrain from initiating an activity when they know or should know that there is a substantial likelihood that their personal problems will prevent them from performing their work-related activities in a competent manner.

A CASE FOR STANDARD 2.06 (A): Temporary Impairment

Dr. Cooper has a very busy day with four clients in the morning and an additional three scheduled after lunch. Toward the end of his half hour lunch break, as he was chatting with office mates, the building swayed from an earthquake. Turning on the radio, a severe regional earthquake is confirmed. Dr. Cooper also learned the epicenter of the quake is near his home and the elementary school his children attend. In the next treatment session, Dr. Cooper is preoccupied with how to find his children to assure himself of their safety. Dr. Cooper is unable to track his client's conversation.

Issues of Concern

If Dr. Cooper were sick with the flu, he would surely cancel his afternoon appointments. Most of us are aware of our own physical illnesses that cause temporary impairment. Many psychologists would, more likely than not, miss the temporary situations that cause us to be less-than-fully present for our clients. In this case, should Dr. Cooper have known that being so preoccupied and distracted with the welfare of his children would interfere with his ability to perform work-related duties adequately? Has he violated the directives of Standard 2.06 (a) by continuing to work without knowing that his children are safe? Should he have cancelled the next session so that he had the time to ascertain the safety of his children?

APA Ethics Code

Companion General Principle

Principle A: Beneficence and Nonmaleficence

> Psychologists strive to be aware of the possible effect of their own physical and mental health on their ability to help those with whom they work.

Understandably, Dr. Cooper is unable to be fully present for his clients while he is concerned for the safety of his children. Aspiring to uphold Principle A, what might

Dr. Cooper have done to be more aware of the effects of his distractibility on his patient?

Companion Ethical Standard(s)

Standard 2.06: Personal Problems and Conflicts

> . . . (b) When psychologists become aware of personal problems that may interfere with their performing work-related duties adequately, they take appropriate measures, such as . . . determine whether they should . . . suspend . . . their work-related duties.

Once aware of his distractibility, Standard 2.06 (b) directs Dr. Cooper to take appropriate measures, which in this case may be to have either delayed or cancelled his next appointment.

Legal Issues 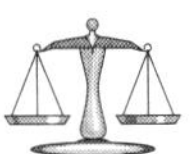

California

> *Cal. Code Regs. tit. 16, § 1396.1 (2010). Interpersonal relations.*
>
> It is recognized that a psychologist's effectiveness depends upon his or her ability to maintain sound interpersonal relations, and that temporary . . . problems in a psychologist's own personality may interfere with this ability. . . A psychologist shall not knowingly undertake any activity in which temporary . . . personal problems in the psychologist's personality integration may result in inferior professional services or harm to a patient or client. If a psychologist is already engaged in such activity when becoming aware of such personal problems, he or she shall seek competent professional assistance to determine whether services to the patient or client should be continued or terminated.

Massachusetts

> *251 Mass. Code Regs. § 1.10 (2010). Ethical standards and professional conduct.*
>
> (1) The Board adopts as its standard of conduct the *Ethical Principles of Psychologists and Code of Conduct* of the American Psychological Association, except as that code of ethics in any way deviates from the provisions of 251 CMR 1.00 or M.G.L. c. 112, §§ 118 through 129A.

In both jurisdictions, Dr. Cooper has a duty to reschedule the appointment until he can provide the level of attention that a reasonably prudent psychologist must give to clients. Clients would likely understand his distress and appreciate his transparency. In either jurisdiction, if he fails to reschedule the appointment, he could be disciplined for violating the standard of care expected of psychologists.

Cultural Considerations

Global Discussion

The Professional Board for Psychology Health Professions Council of South Africa:
Ethical Code of Conduct (April 2002)

> 1.5. Personal impairment.
>
> 1.5.1. Psychologists shall refrain from undertaking professional activities when there is the likelihood that their personal circumstances (including mental, emotional . . .) may prevent them from performing such professional activities in a competent manner.
>
> 1.5.2.1. Psychologists shall be alert to signs of, and obtain appropriate professional assistance for, their personal problems at an early stage in order to prevent impaired performance.
>
> 1.5.3. When psychologists become aware of personal circumstances that may interfere with their performing professional duties adequately, they shall take appropriate measures, . . . and determine whether they should limit, suspend, or terminate their professional duties.

If Dr. Cooper were practicing in South Africa, it would be incumbent upon him to recognize his temporary impairment and take actions to alleviate or eliminate their effects upon his clients. As this is a situation of temporary impairment, he must first recognize it as such and take immediate steps to suspend or terminate his client's session until source of the impairment (worry about the welfare of his children) can be successfully addressed or managed.

American Moral Values

1. Is Dr. Cooper serving his client adequately in this session? Should Dr. Cooper cancel the session because he is too worried and preoccupied to listen to his client? What harm would the client suffer by having an inattentive therapist?
2. Would cancelling the appointment be abandoning his client? Would Dr. Cooper see himself as a weak

or fragile therapist? Does his identity as a male affect how he chooses, either in trying to be professional or in being a "protector" of his family? Would a female therapist have the same attributions of "protector" made to her, either in support or criticism? Does Dr. Cooper have female colleagues who are facing the same situation as parents?

3. How different is this type of cancelling from cancelling because one has a contagious illness? Could cancelling depend on whether Dr. Cooper has had to cancel other appointments with the client recently?

4. Does Dr. Cooper need to leave to make sure his family is OK, or does he just need to clear his head? Is there other work he could do at the office until he hears that the authorities have restored public safety? What actions would Dr. Cooper take if he subsequently learns that one or both of his children have been injured or are missing?

5. Would it make a difference if his client started panicking over the earthquake? Would cancelling send that client into further panic?

6. Does the character of the area around Dr. Cooper's home and his child's school make a difference to his decision? Is it a "safe" area, or would security be more of a concern after this type of event? How does the socioeconomic status of the neighborhood play into that consideration? If the school building was dilapidated, would it change Dr. Cooper's thinking?

7. What is Dr. Cooper's responsibility to his children? Are the children old enough to use a cell phone or have their own mode of transportation? Are they old enough to understand how dangerous earthquakes are? What will their feeling be in the wake of the earthquake?

Ethical Course of Action

Directive per APA Code

Standard 2.06 directs Dr. Cooper to postpone or cancel his next therapy session if Dr. Cooper knew he would not be able to concentrate. But going into the session, Dr. Cooper did not know that he could not focus. The consideration in regards to Standard 2.06 is whether he *should* have known. Depending on the age of his children, location of the children's school, his level of trust in the school's competency in handling emergencies, and the age of the school building, it may have been unreasonable to think that Dr. Cooper should have known he was thus preoccupied.

Dictates of One's Own Conscience

If you found yourself in a similar situation where you were worried about the safety of a loved one, or worried about any personal problems that call your attention away from the client in the session, regardless of whether you should have known going into the session that you might be distracted, what would you do?

1. See all your scheduled clients, and make phone calls between sessions.
2. Cancel all scheduled clients, and go home to look for your kids.
3. Call your partner to have him/her go home.
4. Direct your administrative assistant to contact the school or to call your partner.
5. Discuss with your client the possibility that you might be interrupted by a phone call to update you about your children post earthquake, then proceed with the session.
6. Obtain consent from the client to engage in the treatment session, saying that both of you may be a bit preoccupied with the earthquake that just happened.
7. Talk about the earthquake in session, inquire whether your client has children who might be affected, and then jointly make calls to schools.
8. Stop the next session halfway through once you realized your preoccupation and reschedule your client's session.
9. Do a combination of the previously listed actions.
10. Do something that is not previously listed.

If you were Dr. Cooper working in South Africa, the previously listed options would still apply since the directive for handling personal problems is not substantially different from those listed by the APA Ethics Code.

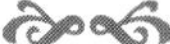

STANDARD 2.06: PERSONAL PROBLEMS AND CONFLICTS

> . . . (b) When psychologists become aware of personal problems that may interfere with their performing work-related duties adequately, they take appropriate measures, such as obtaining professional consultation or assistance, and determine whether they should limit, suspend, or terminate their work-related duties.

A CASE FOR STANDARD 2.06 (B): A Divorce

Dr. Richardson is a newly licensed psychologist who has relocated in order to join a group practice. Instead of moving to join her in the new city, as planned, her husband asked for a separation and filed for divorce. Dr. Richardson has been distraught and shocked by this turn of events. She has not had time to develop any new friendships. She is reluctant to discuss her personal life with any of her work colleagues and does not have her own consulting group or personal psychotherapist. For the past 2 weeks, she has become increasingly depressed, anxious, and is constantly tearful when not at work. At night, she has begun to drink several glasses of wine before bed instead of her usual one and hasn't been able to sleep for more than two to three hours per night. Seeking support, she called a former school classmate, now also a licensed psychologist, for advice. Her friend listened to her story and told her not to worry too much, that she is competent to practice, but should probably "get out more" and try to "get some sleep."

One day in a couples' session, a client disclosed that he was having an extramarital affair and wanted to end the marriage. Dr. Richardson felt herself becoming angry, outraged, and then tearful during the session at the male of the couple, and rather than continue, she ended the session early. She now finds herself wondering whether her partner was having an affair and if that is why he chose to file for divorce.

Issues of Concern

Dr. Richardson was clearly aware of the fact that she had personal problems, thus satisfying the conditions for Standard 2.06 to be in effect. Per Standard 2.06, Dr. Richardson did take measures to determine her best course of action. It is questionable as to whether consulting a friend, even when the friend is a psychologist, in the face of symptoms of depression with increased use of alcohol would be considered taking appropriate measures. The resultant events in the couple's session is clear evidence that the measures Dr. Richardson took to address her personal problems were not appropriate and did not prevent them from interfering with her work performance. Unfortunately, unsuccessful attempts to address her emotions in a trying situation do not satisfy the directives of Standard 2.06.

APA Ethics Code

Companion General Principle

Principle A: Beneficence and Nonmaleficence

> Psychologists strive to be aware of the possible effect of their own physical and mental health on their ability to help those with whom they work.

The ultimate goal of monitoring and managing one's own personal problems in such a way so as not to interfere with one's work is for the benefit of clients and to assure to the best of one's ability that psychologists guard against inflicting harm on others. Dr. Richardson does aspire to uphold Principle A through consultation with her friend.

Principle B: Fidelity and Responsibility

> Psychologists uphold professional standards of conduct, clarify their professional . . . obligations, accept appropriate responsibility for their behavior, and seek to manage conflicts of interest that could lead to exploitation or harm.

Regardless of the actions taken by Dr. Richardson in managing her own personal problems, Principle B guides Dr. Richardson to take responsibility for whatever negative effects her problems have had on the couple in treatment with her.

Companion Ethical Standard(s)

Standard 3.04: Avoiding Harm

> Psychologists take reasonable steps to avoid harming their clients/patients . . . and to minimize harm where it is foreseeable and unavoidable.

Standard 3.04, the implementation of Principle A, directs Dr. Richardson to take steps to avoid harming her clients, in this case the couple in treatment. Standard 3.04 does not specify what should be done once harm has already occurred, which is most likely the case due to Dr. Richardson's reaction and early termination of the session.

Standard 10.10: Terminating Therapy

> (a) Psychologists terminate therapy when it becomes reasonably clear that the client/patient . . . is being harmed by continued service.

At this point of treatment, does Dr. Richardson need to follow the directives of Standard 10.10 and terminate treatment with the couple because Dr. Richardson can no longer assure that her currently ineffective management of her personal problems would not bring harm to this specific couple? Perhaps she is still competent to provide treatment for those clients who are not struggling with marital problems.

Legal Issues 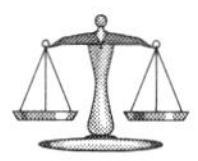

Georgia

> *Ga. Comp. R. & Regs. 510-4-.02 (2010). Code of ethics; APA ethical standards.*
>
> (2) Competence.
>
> . . . (f) 2.06 Personal problems and conflicts.
>
> 1. (a) Psychologists refrain from initiating an activity when they know or should know that there is a substantial likelihood that their personal problems will prevent them from performing their work-related activities in a competent manner.
>
> 2. (b) When psychologists become aware of personal problems that may interfere with their performing work-related duties adequately, they take appropriate measures, such as obtaining professional consultation or assistance, and determine whether they should limit, suspend, or terminate their work-related duties. (See also Standard 10.10, Terminating Therapy)

Ohio

> *Ohio Admin. Code 4732:17-01 (2010). General rules of professional conduct pursuant to section 4732.17 of the revised code.*
>
> (C) Welfare of the client.
>
> . . . (12) Practicing while impaired.
>
> A psychologist . . . shall not undertake or continue a professional psychological role when the judgment, competence, and/or objectivity of the psychologist or . . . is impaired due to mental, emotional, . . . conditions. If impaired judgment, competence, and/or objectivity develops after a professional role has been initiated, the psychologist . . . shall terminate the professional role in an appropriate manner, shall notify the client or other relevant parties of the termination in writing, and shall assist the client, supervisee, or evaluee in obtaining appropriate services from another appropriate professional.

In both jurisdictions, Dr. Richardson has to address her impairment and protect her clients. In Georgia, Dr. Richardson can obtain professional consultation or assistance to determine the steps she would take to protect her clients. In Ohio, she must terminate the clinical relationships in writing and help her clients obtain appropriate services.

Cultural Considerations

Global Discussion

Singapore Psychological Society:
Code of Professional Ethics

> 3. The psychologist especially in clinical work recognizes that effectiveness depends in good part upon the ability to maintain sound interpersonal relations and that, temporary or more enduring aberrations in the psychologist's own personality may interfere with this ability or distort the appraisal of others. The psychologist refrains from undertaking any activities in which personal problems are likely to result in inferior professional services or harm to a client; or if the psychologist is already engaged in such an activity and then becomes aware of such personal problems, competent professional assistance to determine whether to continue or terminate psychological services to the client should be sought.

To satisfy this part of Singapore's code, Dr. Richardson would be directed to immediately address the potential harm caused to her clients by ending the session early and consider transferring them to another couples therapist. It would then be imperative for her to consider, with the help of a "competent professional," such as a supervisor or consultation group, rather than a well-meaning psychologist friend, whether she should take on any new clients at all until her personal situation has stabilized.

American Moral Values

1. How is Dr. Richardson's personal life affecting the quality of her therapy? Which problems are the most urgent for her to take care of in order to maintain an acceptable level of performance? Is it her reaction to divorce? Alcohol usage? Lack of friends?
2. Is Dr. Richardson bringing her own moral judgment into the counseling session without explanation? Can a therapist ever use discussions in therapy as a possible aid to their own personal relationships? When does that violate one's duty to a client? What did her ending the session early do to the client-therapist relationship? Does she need to take steps to address those effects, for example explaining her related personal issues?
3. How can Dr. Richardson alleviate her increasing distress, in particular her newfound suspicion of infidelity? If she is triggered by her client's infidelity, can she continue as their therapist? Can she maintain this relationship while seeing another therapist about her own feelings of betrayal?

Ethical Course of Action

Directive per APA Code

Once Dr. Richardson becomes aware of a personal problem that interferes with her work, Standard 2.06 directs Dr. Richardson to make some type of change in her work-related duties. In this case, Dr. Richardson, per Standard 2.06, should have obtained professional consultation or assistance. Regardless of whether a personal friend happens to be a licensed psychologist, a friend is biased and is unlikely to be effectively able to make objective assessment of Dr. Richardson's level of impairment. At this point in time, Standard 2.06 directs Dr. Richardson to seek professional consultation or assistance to make a determination as to her practice and Principle B would guide Dr. Richardson to repair the harm done to her couples' client.

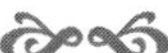

Dictates of One's Own Conscience

If you were Dr. Richardson, having realized that your personal problems have interfered with your professional work and possibly inflicted harm to your couples' client, what next step would you do?

1. After due consideration, you decide that the difficulty is not in your conclusion but the management of your own emotions. After obtaining firmer control over your emotions, you tell the wife to divorce her husband during the next scheduled treatment session.
2. After due consideration, you decide that the difficulty is not in your conclusion but the management of your own emotions. After obtaining firmer control over your emotions, you describe to the husband your reaction in the previous session, state that such a severe emotional reaction is typical, and that his wife is also having the same reaction you did to the news of his infidelity. Thus the husband needs to abandon the affair, apologize to his wife before treatment could proceed.
3. Realize that your reaction was indicative of how important your marriage was to you and thus decide to quit your job and move back to attempt reconciliation with your husband.
4. Call up your husband and berate him for causing you to lose a patient. Say that his presence is absolutely necessary to your ability to work, thus he needs to come immediately.
5. Take a vacation.
6. Rely on your former classmate as a friend but not for professional consultation and continue your practice.
7. Enter into personal psychotherapy immediately and continue your practice.
8. Engage in extra supervision and continue your practice.
9. Engage in peer consultation with office mates and continue your practice.
10. Enter into personal psychotherapy immediately, and curtail your practice to working with individuals only.
11. Engage in extra supervision, and curtail your practice to working with individuals only.

12. Engage in peer consultation with office mates, and curtail your practice to working with individuals only.
13. Enter into personal psychotherapy immediately, and temporarily stop providing treatment altogether.
14. Engage in extra supervision, and temporarily stop providing treatment altogether.
15. Engage in peer consultation with office mates, and temporarily stop providing treatment altogether.
16. Refund payment or not charge for the couple's session that was ended early.
17. Do a combination of the previously listed actions.
18. Do something that is not previously listed.

If you were Dr. Richardson and practicing in Singapore, what would you do?

1. Drinking too much wine and failing to seek help is a temporary impairment that any reasonable psychologist might make. Making the decision to be consoled by the reassurances of a friend and former classmate, instead of an unbiased professional, and failing to seek further consultation, shows a possible deeper problem, one that may be considered "more enduring aberrations in the psychologist's own personality" than a passing situation. As such, might you decide to leave the business of treatment and maybe take on other aspects of professional work?
2. Enter into personal psychotherapy immediately, and curtail your practice to working with individuals only.
3. Engage in extra supervision, and curtail your practice to working with individuals only.
4. Engage in peer consultation with office mates, and curtail your practice to working with individuals only.

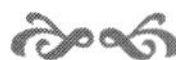

CHAPTER 3

Human Relations

Ethical Standard 3

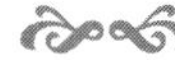

CHAPTER OUTLINE

STANDARD 3.01: UNFAIR DISCRIMINATION

In their work-related activities, psychologists do not engage in unfair discrimination based on age, gender, gender identity, race, ethnicity, culture, national origin, religion, sexual orientation, disability, socioeconomic status, or any basis proscribed by law.

A CASE FOR STANDARD 3.01: I Can't Understand Her English

Dr. Powell sat on the screening committee for psychology interns. Some students were invited for an interview, in person or by phone, only after an extensive review of their files had occurred. The internship has an excellent program and reputation and so receives applications from exceptional students. One applicant, Ruth, stood out;

she was coming from a strong doctoral program, has obtained good letters of recommendation, and had published a peer reviewed article in a solid psychology journal. On the scheduled date of the interview, Ruth called into the committee for a phone interview. It is obvious that although fluent Ruth's English is heavily accented.

At the screening committee meeting to select the slate of interns, two of three committee members spoke emphatically against offering a seat to Ruth on the grounds that the clients would not be able to understand Ruth's accented English.

Issues of Concern

Standard 3.01 would guide the psychologists sitting on the internship selection committee to "not engage in unfair discrimination based on" national origin. The screening committee argues that Ruth speaks English, but with a heavy accent. They believe that given their client population, Ruth would not be able to engage in the necessary therapeutic work and would not be appropriate for the internship site. Is the screening committee justified in setting standards for selection which include English proficiency? Or does the demand for unaccented spoken English disguise discrimination based on national origin or race?

APA Ethics Code

Companion General Principle

Principle E: Respect for People's Rights and Dignity

> Psychologists respect the dignity and worth of all people ... Psychologists are aware of and respect ... differences, including those based on ... language, and ... consider these factors when working with members of such groups. Psychologists try to eliminate the effect on their work of biases based on those factors, and they do not knowingly participate in or condone activities of others based upon such prejudices.

Aspiring to the highest principle of respecting people's rights, psychologists do not engage in prejudicial acts based upon language. Thus, if Dr. Powell and the internship selection committee were to act in accordance with Principle E, Ruth's accented English would not have emerged as a selection criterion.

Principle D: Justice

> Psychologists recognize that fairness and justice entitle all persons ... to equal quality in the processes, procedures, and services being conducted by psychologists. Psychologists exercise reasonable judgment and take precautions to ensure that their potential biases, the boundaries of their competence, and the limitations of their expertise do not lead to or condone unjust practices.

Aspiring to the highest principle of fairness, Ruth would be entitled to serious consideration for the internship position if all psychology-related selection criteria were excellently met. Dr. Powell might caution the internship selection committee members to "exercise reasonable judgment" by considering Ruth's qualifications independent of her ability to speak Standard English.

Companion Ethical Standard(s)

Standard 3.03: Other Harassment

> Psychologists do not knowingly engage in behavior that is ... demeaning to persons with whom they interact in their work based on factors such as ... language.

Standard 3.03 translates the aspirational principles D and E to enforceable standards, giving a directive for psychologists not to engage in behavior that is demeaning. However, unlike sexual harassment in Standard 3.02, the American Psychological Association (APA) Ethics Code does not specify the types of behavior that are considered demeaning. It is not necessarily clear from reading Standard 3.03 whether or not the internship selection committee's disparaging view of Ruth's verbal proficiency in Standard English is demeaning.

Standard 2.01: Boundaries of Competence

> (a) Psychologists ... teach ... with populations and in areas only within the boundaries of their competence, based on their education, training, supervised experience, consultation, study, or professional experience.

Standard 2.01 directs psychologists to engage only in areas within the boundaries of our competency. As such, it can be argued that the internship selection committee members are acting in such a way as to protect the profession from someone who is not capable of gaining competence since language fluency is not an area that the internship is able to provide training in for Ruth.

Thus, the internship selection committee is upholding and ensuring Standard 2.01.

Standard 7.02: Descriptions of Education and Training Programs

> Psychologists responsible for education and training programs take reasonable steps to ensure that there is a current and accurate description of the program content (including participation in required course- or program-related counseling, psychotherapy, experiential groups, consulting projects, or community service), training goals and objectives, stipends and benefits, and requirements that must be met for satisfactory completion of the program. This information must be made readily available to all interested parties.

Standard 7.02 directs the internship program to have a description of their program that includes requirements for satisfactory completion. If Standard English was a required minimal requirement for satisfactory completion of the internship program, Standard 7.02 directs the program to have such requirements clearly stated. Eliminating a candidate based on selection criteria that were not stated in the program description violates the spirit of Principle D as well as directives of Standard 7.02.

Legal Issues 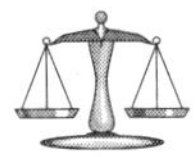

Massachusetts

> *251 Mass. Code Regs. 1.10 (2010). Ethical standards and professional conduct.*
>
> (1) The Board adopts as its standard of conduct the Ethical Principles of Psychologists and Code of Conduct of the American Psychological Association.

Georgia

> *Ga. Comp. R. & Regs. 510-4-.02 (2010). Code of ethics; APA ethical standards.*
>
> 3. Human relations.
>
> (a) 3.01 Unfair discrimination. "In their work-related activities, psychologists do not engage in unfair discrimination based on . . . race, ethnicity, culture, national origin. . ."

In both jurisdictions, it appears that discriminating against Ruth because of her accent may be viewed as a violation of their ethical standards. Dr. Powell should advise her colleagues that she cannot condone their behavior and that they should reconsider their decisions in light of their needing to stay within the confines of the law. In Massachusetts, Dr. Powell would engage in the Standard 1.04: Informal Resolution of Ethical Violations and attempt to resolve the issue by bringing it to the attention of the individual psychologists.

Cultural Considerations

Global Discussion

Canadian Code of Ethics for Psychologists

> Principle I: Respect for the dignity of persons.
>
> In these contacts, psychologists accept as fundamental the principle of respect for the dignity of persons; that is, the belief that each person should be treated primarily as a person or an end in him/herself, not as an object or a means to an end. In so doing, psychologists acknowledge that all persons have a right to have their innate worth as human beings appreciated and that this worth is not dependent upon their . . . nationality, ethnicity, . . . or any other preference or personal characteristic, condition, or status.
>
> *General Respect.*
>
> I.5. Avoid or refuse to participate in practices disrespectful of the legal, civil, or moral rights of others.

If the selection committee was overseeing internship sites in Canada, it is likely their actions would need to attend to the subtlety of a "status-based" versus a "skill-based" factor of discrimination. English language proficiency is a skill-based discriminating factor in placing interns who work with English speakers. The issue becomes harder to separate when it is at the juncture of where a skill-based factor (language proficiency) intersects with a status-based variable (race, ethnicity, nationality). The Canadian code does not address skill-based discrimination. If the English proficiency was used to cover up for the race-based discrimination, then Canadian Standard 1.5 would admonish any psychologist to "Avoid or refuse to participate in" the selection committee because the committee would have engaged in "practices [that are] disrespectful of the . . . civil . . . rights of" the applicant.

American Moral Values

1. Is Ruth's accent a fair criterion for disqualifying her? Or is a clinical psychologist's speech the equivalent of a surgeon's hand so that any speech irregularity jeopardizes treatment? What is the threshold of understanding beyond which a therapist is ineffective for her client?

2. What is the accent that Ruth speaks with? Are all accents really equivalent—a thick Irish or German accent as opposed to a Spanish or Chinese or Jamaican accent? Would someone from France be given more leeway than someone from Mexico? Are there cultural assumptions about Ruth made on the basis of the accent that could be in play here? Is there an insinuated cultural divide between Ruth and the clients the committee has in mind? Does speaking English without an accent indicate a cultural superiority as well?
3. What is the importance of Ruth's other qualifications? How can Ruth's prior work be built upon if she is turned down by the internship for having an accent? Is there a way the committee could still select Ruth based on those considerations and still address their concerns with Ruth?
4. What does rejecting Ruth mean for the larger field of clinical psychology? What message will be sent to academic and professional institutions by this decision? Does the committee have a responsibility not to discourage applicants of different national origins, cultures, races, etc., from believing their merits will not be enough?
5. Is Ruth's proficiency in the languages she speaks listed? If not, why not? What other languages does she speak? Is there a better way to classify and describe language proficiency within the profession to consider about the effect of accents in better context? Is the United States provincial in how it deals with this qualification?

Ethical Course of Action

Directive per APA Code

Standard 3.01 admonishes psychologists to "not engage in unfair discrimination based on . . ." what appear to be status-based variables instead of skill-based variables. For clinical psychology and psychotherapy, language is equivalent to a surgeon's steady hand. Therefore, language-based selection criteria are not necessarily a violation of Standard 3.01. In the absence of knowing whether the same selection committee has denied someone an internship based on, for example, a Welsh accent, it is not possible to determine whether the discrimination in this situation is based on national origin. If this same training center has had a history of treating other European-based accents more favorably than non-European based accents, then Dr. Powell and the internship screening committee would be in violation of Standard 3.01. If the selection committee is basing their decision purely on the skill of spoken English, regardless of the type of accent, than consideration of language proficiency does not violate Standard 3.01.

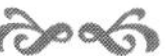

Dictates of One's Own Conscience

At issue is whether discrimination is ever "fair" to consider, if language proficiency is a justifiable reason to bar entry into an internship program, or if other means of placing this intern are obligatory for the psychologists. Stating language requirements clearly in the placement advertisement, whatever they may be, might be one way to preserve both the dignity of applicants and the criteria for the placement itself.

If you were Dr. Powell on the selection committee, what might you say to the selection committee?

1. Advocate for Ruth by disputing the assumption that her English is not understandable and to reiterate her other very fine qualities.
2. Suggest that the organization take advantage of a bilingual internship to make some outreach effort to the local ethnic community, therefore viewing Ruth's accented English as an asset instead of a liability.
3. Question the committee member's erroneous assumption that clients would be unable to understand her.
4. Perform a combination of the previously listed actions.
5. Do something that is not previously listed.

If you were Dr. Powell on the selection committee, having practiced in Canada for a period of time and knowing the background issues between skill-based factors such as language proficiency and status-based variables such as national origin, what additional comments might you make to the selection committee?

1. Raise the issue of fairness in advertisements, and suggest that since the program did not specify a level of language fluency that an internship selection committee should not consider language as a factor in deliberations about Ruth.
2. Raise the question of whether discrimination is ever "fair" or if language proficiency is a justifiable reason to bar entry into an internship program.
3. Make a request to the appropriate department in the organization to request that language requirements be clearly added to the placement advertisement.

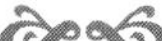

STANDARD 3.02: SEXUAL HARASSMENT

> Psychologists do not engage in sexual harassment. Sexual harassment is sexual solicitation, physical advances, or verbal or nonverbal conduct that is sexual in nature, that occurs in connection with the psychologist's activities or roles as a psychologist, and that either (1) is unwelcome, is offensive, or creates a hostile workplace or educational environment, and the psychologist knows or is told this or (2) is sufficiently severe or intense to be abusive to a reasonable person in the context. Sexual harassment can consist of a single intense or severe act or of multiple persistent or pervasive acts.

A CASE FOR STANDARD 3.02: A Therapist Revealed, a Client Feels Unsafe

Dr. Long and Dr. Patterson are coworkers in the same mental health clinic. Dr. Long is identified lesbian. Dr. Patterson identifies gay. Dr. Patterson is not open about his sexual identity, whereas Dr. Long is much more open about her sexual identity. Dr. Patterson periodically makes sexually explicit remarks to Dr. Long at work and asks questions such as whether Dr. Long is the "man" in her relationship or whether she is "out" to her clients. One day during lunch outside of the office, Dr. Long said, "You need to be a bit more open about your sexual identity, or stop making sexual comments to me that can be misinterpreted as sexual come-ons or harassment." As Drs. Long and Patterson walked back into the clinic's waiting room, Dr. Patterson said, "Do you use sex toys when you have sex with your girlfriend?" At that moment, Dr. Long saw that her next client appeared startled, as if she overheard the comment. Dr. Long's client is a young woman who is struggling to understand her own sexual identity.

Issues of Concern

Dr. Long has approached Dr. Patterson informally to request that he stop the sexual comments. Yet Dr. Patterson continues with questions that were explicitly sexual. Are sexual comments with no intention of eliciting sexual contact sufficient to constitute sexual harassment? What harm can occur to a therapeutic relationship when clients unexpectedly learn personal information, such as the sexual orientation of their psychologist?

APA Ethics Code

Companion General Principle

Introduction and Applicability

> This Ethics Code applies only to psychologists' activities that are part of their scientific, educational, or professional roles as psychologists . . . These activities shall be distinguished from the purely private conduct of psychologists, which is not within the purview of the Ethics Code.

Are one's comments to a colleague of a personal nature, such as sexual identity or religion, considered within the purview of professional conduct? It can be argued that one's sexual identity is not "part of their scientific, educational, or professional role as psychologist." Therefore, as such, Dr. Patterson's comments to Dr. Long are outside the purview of their professional roles.

Principle A: Beneficence and Nonmaleficence

> Psychologists strive to benefit those with whom they work and take care to do no harm. When conflicts occur among psychologists' obligations or concerns, they attempt to resolve these conflicts in a responsible fashion that avoids or minimizes harm.

"Take care to do no harm . . ." applies not only to client and research subjects but also to coworkers. The aspiration of Principle A is that "psychologists strive to benefit those with whom they work," which encompasses the relationship between Drs. Long and Patterson. Sexual harassment comes in many forms and can harm more than one person. If Dr. Long considered Dr. Patterson's behavior as offensive, then this constitutes sexual harassment. Even if Dr. Long does not herself find Dr. Patterson's behavior offensive, would the comment still be considered sexual harassment if someone else within hearing distance found it offensive?

Principle E: Respect for People's Rights and Dignity

> Psychologists are aware of and respect . . . sexual orientation . . . and consider these factors when working with members of such groups.

Dr. Patterson's comments in relation to Dr. Long's sexuality do not indicate respect, regardless of whether both are homosexual. Aspiring to Principle E of respect for all people, Dr. Patterson should refrain from making comments containing sexual references to coworkers.

Companion Ethical Standard(s)

Standard 1.04: Informal Resolution of Ethical Violations

> When psychologists believe that there may have been an ethical violation by another psychologist, they attempt to resolve the issue by bringing it to the attention of that individual . . .

Dr. Long considered the relationship with Dr. Patterson as professional in nature, in as much as both are psychologists working in the same agency with no other non-work-related interactions. Standard 1.04 would guide Dr. Long to bring her concerns to Dr. Patterson informally.

Standard 5.01: Advertising and Other Public Statements; Standard 5.01: Avoidance of False or Deceptive Statements

> (a) Public statements include but are not limited to paid or unpaid advertising, product endorsements, grant applications, licensing applications, other credentialing applications, brochures, printed matter, directory listings, personal resumes or curricula vitae, or comments for use in media such as print or electronic transmission, statements in legal proceedings, lectures and public oral presentations, and published materials.
>
> . . . Psychologists do not knowingly make public statements that are false, deceptive, or fraudulent concerning their research, practice, or other work activities or those of persons or organizations with which they are affiliated.

Statements in any form to a client regarding a psychologist's personal life may or may not have significant impact. Information such as religion, political affiliation, and/or sexual identity may be of more therapeutic significance then a psychologist's hobbies or favorite food. In the American culture at the present time, sexual identity is generally considered significant. However, keeping with the stance of the ethics code applying solely to a psychologist's professional life, Section 5 does not speak to personal information. Thus, the ethics code is silent on the matter of personal information crossing into professional work.

Regardless of guidance from the ethics code, would the client consider the sexual identity of his/her psychologist to be private and nonprofessional information? What is the line between private and professional in terms of personal information such as religion, sexual identity, political affiliation?

Standard 10.01: Informed Consent to Therapy

> (a) When obtaining informed consent to therapy . . . psychologists inform clients/patients as early as is feasible in the therapeutic relationship about the nature and anticipated course of therapy, fees, involvement of third parties, and limits of confidentiality and provide sufficient opportunity for the client/patient to ask questions and receive answers.

Statements in any form to a client regarding psychologist's personal lives may or may not have significance. Information such as religion, political affiliation, and/or sexual identity may be of more therapeutic significance and for some clients on par with information about fees and theoretical orientation. In the American culture at the present time, sexual identity is generally considered significant. If one keeps to the stance that sexual identity is personal, like marital status, and keeping with the position, that the ethics code only applies to a psychologist's professional life, then Dr. Patterson was inappropriate to have revealed personal information to Dr. Long's client.

However, if one considers sexual identity, like race and gender, to be significant information for clients to have in order to develop a more informed stance for treatment consent, then Dr. Long's sexual identity should have been revealed to the client at the onset of treatment. Thus the situation of Dr. Patterson's inappropriate comment would have had very little therapeutic effect.

Legal Issues 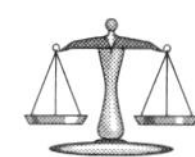

New Jersey

> *N.J. Admin. Code § 13:42-10.9 (2010). Sexual misconduct.*
>
> (a) As used in this section, the following terms have the following meanings unless the context indicates otherwise: . . .
>
> "Sexual harassment" means . . . verbal . . . conduct that is sexual in nature, and . . . occurs in connection with a licensee's activities . . . and that is . . . unwelcomed . . . and the licensee . . . is told this. . . "Sexual harassment" may consist of . . . multiple acts, and may include, but is not limited to, conduct of a licensee with a . . . co-worker . . . whether or not such individual is in a subordinate position to the licensee.
>
> . . . (d) A licensee shall not engage in sexual harassment in a professional setting (including, but not limited to, an office . . .) or outside of the professional setting.

Texas

> *22 Tex. Admin. Code § 465.33 (2010). Improper sexual conduct.*
>
> (a) "Sexual Harassment" includes . . . verbal . . . conduct consisting of . . . multiple persistent . . . acts by a licensee toward another individual that are sexual in nature and occur in connection with licensee's professional activities and that are unwelcome . . .

The law of both jurisdictions may lead a licensing board to conclude that Dr. Patterson has engaged in sexual harassment of Dr. Long. His verbal comments are highly offensive to Dr. Long and would likely be viewed by the licensing boards as sexual harassment. Most telling from a licensing board's point of view would be Dr. Patterson's remark was made in front of a witness, and in fact, a client.

Cultural Considerations

Global Discussion

Canadian Code of Ethics for Psychologists

> Definition of terms for the code.
>
> a. Sexual harassment includes either or both of the following: (ii) Engaging in deliberate and/or repeated unsolicited sexually oriented comments . . . if such behaviors: are offensive and unwelcome; create an offensive, hostile, or intimidating working, learning, or service environment; or, can be expected to be harmful to the recipient.
>
> Principle I: Respect for the Dignity of Persons.
>
> *General respect.*
>
> (I.2) Not engage publicly (e.g., . . . with clients) in degrading comments about others, . . . based on such characteristics as . . . sexual orientation. (I.3) Strive to use language that conveys respect for the dignity of persons as much as possible in all written or oral communication. (I.4) Abstain from all forms of harassment, including sexual harassment.

The Canadian code prohibits comments that are harassing toward anyone. Because comments about Dr. Long's sexual identity and personal life were made publicly and specifically mentioned aspects of private sexual activities that presumably Dr. Long does not discuss with others, Dr. Patterson has engaged in harassment and therefore a violation of the Canadian code. According to the Canadian code, even if Dr. Long herself did not find the comments offensive or harmful, it can be argued that for a client to overhear such remarks may constitute the co-creation of an "offensive, hostile or intimidating service environment" and as such may be harmful to Dr. Long's therapeutic relationship with her client.

American Moral Values

1. Do Dr. Patterson's remarks hurt Dr. Long's performance? Are they just personally disturbing? How could they affect Dr. Long's client, who overheard his remark and is herself struggling with her sexual identity? Are they helpful for Dr. Patterson himself and his sexual identity?
2. Dr. Long may feel sympathy for Dr. Patterson's hesitancy to be open about his sexual identity. Would a sexual harassment complaint force his homosexuality into becoming public information? How could she balance her sympathy for his struggles with her self-defense against continuing sexual harassment?
3. Does Dr. Long value Dr. Patterson as a friend and colleague, aside from this kind of remark? Would she hesitate to pursue charges against him because she does not want to betray him or threaten his career? Would Dr. Patterson harass other people in the future if he is not adequately opposed by Dr. Long?
4. What will be the reaction of the office and larger community to this charge if it moves forward? Will Dr. Long be attacked for being too sensitive and threatening Dr. Patterson's career? Does Dr. Long have the support necessary to withstand that pressure?
5. Would the client consider the sexual identity of his/her psychologist to be private and nonprofessional in nature? Would that disclosure help or hinder Dr. Long's therapy? What is the line between private and professional in terms of personal information, such as religion, sexual identity, political affiliation, etc.?

Ethical Course of Action

Directive per APA Code

Standard 3.02 defines sexual harassment as unwelcome conduct that is sexual in nature occurring in the work environment. Dr. Long was explicit with Dr. Patterson in that any reference to sexual identity was unwelcome. Thus, as directed by Standard 3.02, Dr. Patterson should have ceased making comments that were sexual in nature after Dr. Long talked to him at lunch. Dr. Patterson's hallway comment after lunch clearly violates Standard 3.02.

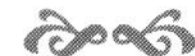

Dictates of One's Own Conscience

Because the remarks were repeated in a professional environment, it would fall upon Dr. Long to seek informal resolution again with Dr. Patterson and raise the concern therapeutically with her client. Having tried the route of informal resolution to no effect, if you were Dr. Long, what would you do?

1. Try again to seek informal resolution with Dr. Patterson by talking to him.
2. Explore with your client what she understood of the overheard comment, and tell her that you have a very casual relationship with Dr. Patterson that allows for mutual comments regarding personal lives.
3. Explore with your client what she understood of the overheard conversation; share with her that your relationship with Dr. Patterson has taken an unexpected and troubling turn and that such comments about personal lives of psychologists are an unwelcome deviation rather than a common occurrence.
4. Explore with your client what she understood of the overheard conversation, and inquire as to her reaction to it.
5. Raise the concern therapeutically with your client about the fact that your sexual identity is homosexual.
6. Tell Dr. Patterson that his constant sexual remarks are inappropriate and that you feel harassed by him.
7. Tell Dr. Patterson that your client overhead his comment, and then stop talking to Dr. Patterson.
8. Tell Dr. Patterson that he revealed her sexual identity to the client, and that unless he ceases all sexual comments immediately, you will start revealing his sexual identity to select coworkers, file a complaint with the licensing board, and submit a written record of the dates and contents of the harassing remarks.
9. Make a casual inquiry to determine if your client actually heard Dr. Patterson's comment, and if heard, that she actually made a connection between you and Dr. Patterson's comment and you.
10. Address your client immediately in session with something like the following: "I'm checking in with you to see how it was for you to hear the conversation just now in the lobby." Then proceed from there. Speak with Dr. Patterson privately and directly request that he refrain from all personal remarks in the workplace, especially sexually charged ones. Let him know that a failure to do so will not be treated informally. Suggest several groups for Dr. Patterson to go to or Internet resources and books on sexual identity and coming out.
11. Perform a combination of the previously listed actions.
12. Do something that is not previously listed.

If you were Dr. Long practicing in Canada, the previously listed options would still apply since the guideline for sexual harassment is not substantially different from those listed by the APA Ethics Code.

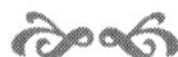

STANDARD 3.03: OTHER HARASSMENT

> Psychologists do not knowingly engage in behavior that is harassing or demeaning to persons with whom they interact in their work based on factors such as those persons' age, gender, gender identity, race, ethnicity, culture, national origin, religion, sexual orientation, disability, language, or socioeconomic status.

A CASE FOR STANDARD 3.03: Leading a Class Discussion

Dr. Hughes is an assistant professor in a professional psychology program. Dr. Hughes included a section on non-Western concepts of mind/body and health in his psychophysiology class. During the in-class discussion of traditional versus alternative treatment, Michelle, a student in the class, stated that she has had much healing from acupuncture, spiritual work such as sweat lodges, and some forms of prayer. George, another student in the class, responded with the following: "Those things are unscientific, unproven, and equivalent to working with rattles and feathers. Unless psychologists want to be in the same category as witch doctors, these things should not be discussed in a respected psychology program." Michelle stated that her family heritage includes indigenous blood. She asked George to refrain from using cultural references like "rattles and feathers" as insults. He is unapologetic, explaining that he used to work in an area with a large Native population and that no one else has been offended by his remarks. Besides, George pointed out to Michelle, she hardly looks like she has Native ancestry. How was he supposed to know?

Issues of Concern

Was it inappropriate for Michelle to bring claims of success with treatments that are not evidence-based into the psychophysiology classroom? Was it appropriate for George to challenge such a claim? Standard 3.03 would direct George to handle Michelle's comments in a manner that is not culturally demeaning, such as using rattles and feathers with a negative connotation.

Depending on how Dr. Hughes handles the situation, it is possible Michelle will leave the classroom feeling demeaned and harassed for her cultural heritage and George may feel justified in defending psychology on the grounds of evidence-based practice. What does Dr. Hughes say to Michelle, George, and the class about culture and healing practices, both traditional and nontraditional? Do both views allow for scholarly analysis, cross-cultural competence, and respect?

APA Ethics Code

Companion General Principle

Principle A: Beneficence and Nonmaleficence

> Psychologists strive to benefit those with whom they work and take care to do no harm. When conflicts occur among psychologists' obligations or concerns, they attempt to resolve these conflicts in a responsible fashion that avoids or minimizes harm.

The aspiration of Principle A—"take care to do no harm . . . "—also applies to students. It seems that Michelle felt harmed while George felt justified in defending science. Acting on the highest aspiration of nonmaleficence, Dr. Hughes is called upon to negotiate a constructive dialogue between Western science and indigenous medicine while at the same time facilitating a discussion that has turned very personal.

Principle E: Respect for People's Rights and Dignity

> Psychologists respect the dignity and worth of all people . . . Psychologists are aware of and respect . . . cultural, . . . and role differences, including those based on . . . ethnicity . . . religion . . . and consider these factors when working with members of such groups. Psychologists try to eliminate the effect on their work of biases based on those factors, and they do not knowingly participate in or condone activities of others based upon such prejudices.

The aspiration of Principle E is to respect all individuals and treat each with dignity. Dr. Hughes, to uphold the aspirations stated in Principle E, needs to create a safe learning environment with due respect for both George's individualistic culture of mechanistic science, as well as Michelle's culture of indigenous medicine.

Companion Ethical Standard(s)

Standard 7.04: Student Disclosure of Personal Information

> Psychologists do not require students . . . to disclose personal information in course . . . related activities, either orally or in writing, regarding . . . relationships with parents. . .

In our teaching, Standard 7.04 directs professors to not require self-disclosure. This means that students are expected to self-monitor their own level of comfort with disclosure and to take responsibility for what and when personal information is disclosed. In this case, it appears that the class topic of treatment models does not explicitly nor implicitly require students to self-disclose their personal history of health-seeking behavior. Thus Dr. Hughes has acted in accordance with the directive of Standard 7.04.

Guidelines on Multicultural Education, Training, Research, Practice, and Organizational Change for Psychologists (APA, 2003)

Guideline 3

> As educators, psychologists are encouraged to employ the constructs of multiculturalism and diversity in psychological education.

This APA (2003) guideline notes that "all interactions are cross-cultural and, by extension, all classroom interactions are multicultural" (p. 31). "Thus the challenges . . . to ensure a safe learning environment, an ability to know the course content, and to manage emotions that emerge" (APA, 2003, p. 34). Indeed, Dr. Hughes finds himself with an emotionally charged cross-cultural class discussion. Dr. Hughes may find guidance on handling the type of classroom exchange typified by those between George and Michelle by following the recommendations outlined in this APA guideline. Recommendations include, but are not limited to, the necessity for Dr. Hughes to become knowledgeable about different learning and philosophical models and to be informed by research findings on the topic.

Standard 7.06: Assessing Student and Supervisee Performance

> ... (b) Psychologists evaluate students ... on the basis of their actual performance on relevant and established program requirements.

Dr. Hughes has the responsibility of assessing Michelle and George's performances in class. If Dr. Hughes has included classroom behavior as one of the criteria upon which students' course grades are based, then he has the responsibility to let both Michelle and George know how their exchange effects their course grade and/or the program's annual review of students.

Legal Issues 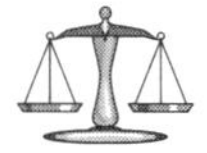

Pennsylvania

> *49 Pa. Code § 41.61 (2010). Code of ethics.*
>
> Principle 3. Moral and legal standards.
>
> ... (b) As teachers, psychologists are aware of the fact that their personal values may affect the selection and presentation of instructional materials. When dealing with topics that may give offense, they recognize and respect the diverse attitudes that students may have toward materials.

Virginia

> *18 Va. Admin. Code § 125-20-150 (2010). Standards of practice.*
>
> A. ... Psychologists respect the rights, dignity and worth of all people, and are mindful of individual differences.

If Dr. Hughes was licensed and teaching in either Pennsylvania or Virginia, he is directed to respect diverse attitudes. APA Code of Conduct 3.01 and the laws of both states also would direct him to give due respect to both Michelle's and George's distinctly different attitudes.

Cultural Considerations

Global Discussion

Canadian Code of Ethics for Psychologists

> Principle I: Respect for the dignity of persons.
>
> *General respect.*
>
> I.2. Not engage publicly ... in degrading comments about others, including demeaning jokes based on such characteristics as culture, ... ethnicity ... religion, ...
>
> I.3. Strive to use language that conveys respect for the dignity of persons as much as possible in all ... oral communication.
>
> I.4. Abstain from all forms of harassment ...

If George made these remarks in a Canadian classroom, regardless of the proven nature of indigenous healing practices as evidence-based or not, clearly, he has transgressed from critical argument of science versus spirituality into comments that were based on religion and culture, which likely caused harm to Michelle. Regardless of whether someone is phenotypically a minority, psychologists are compelled by the Canadian code to abstain from public remarks that degrade others, including classmates.

American Moral Values

1. What is Dr. Hughes's guiding value in discussing non-Western approaches to body and mind? What kind of respect does he feel these ideas deserve? How much does he want that respect to be a topic for debate? Have George's comments crossed a line in terms of intellectual respect for class material, or does Dr. Hughes welcome those kinds of comments as material for correction and edification? Could the tone, word choices, and the dramatic impact of his remarks be modified so that they convey the intellectual challenge but in a manner that is less likely to be perceived as patronizing and offensive?
2. How does Michelle's reaction affect Dr. Hughes's assessment of George's comments? Does he believe that George is creating a hostile environment for students like Michelle, indeed any student who wishes to learn about non-Western culture? Does he believe Michelle needs defending and protecting, or does he allow Michelle to respond to George and defend herself the way she sees fit? Does he need to show support to Michelle in front of the class to send a message about respect for other cultures? How does he engage in the support of Michelle's position, particularly in light of George's response, without patronizing Michelle?
3. What does Dr. Hughes owe to George as a student in the class? What should George take from the discussion, and what approach will help him learn it and become a more productive member in the class? Does George need to be led, Socratic style, through some of the assumptions his remarks betray?
4. For instance, what is the relevance of working on a reservation in determining what is offensive? Does

George have a position to stand on? If not, why not? How has George determined empirically that these practices are "unscientific" and don't work? Why should Michelle looking one way or another determine whether his comments were justified? Are comments about indigenous cultures all right as long as no member of such groups is present in the class?

5. How does the particular remark of "rattles and feathers" affect how this situation is handled? Is there a particular character to the practices mentioned that elicits more or less sympathy than those of other religious traditions? What if the practice were clitorectomy in African indigenous religion, or Muslim-inspired traditions of hymen reconstruction, or a Christian evangelical one of speaking in tongues? What cultures seem insightful about mind–body connections and why?
6. Is there a way to demand evidence without dismissing possible effective cultural practices with insults? Is Michelle's testimony some kind of evidence, albeit not as strong as a double-blind study? Does George's experience on the reservation count as evidence?
7. What is the line between respecting culture and condoning superstition? How can Dr. Hughes promote critical evaluation of claims while not indulging in stereotypes? Does he need to explain historical context for how non-Western traditions are represented within Western science?

Ethical Course of Action

Directive per APA Code

Standard 3.03 directs psychologists not to engage in behavior that is demeaning. George's remark, regardless of the subject matter, was said in such a way that is demeaning. Dr. Hughes, following the directive from Standard 3.03, might lead a discussion on how best to constructively engage in discourse that does not involve demeaning or harassing language.

If the professor stays silent and does not intervene in this exchange, there is concern that the takeaway message is that psychology has no room for indigenous healing practices and/or nonwhite females are not to challenge white males. Regardless of which message is salient, Michelle will feel harassed based on gender, culture, and/or religion.

If the professor does anything that implies George's response is not appropriate, there is concern that the takeaway message is that psychology dares not venture into discussion of cultural practices. The fear of being politically incorrect may be experienced by some as harassment by individuals who are nonwhite.

It is difficult to disentangle conduct from subject matter. To make such differentiation clear, it is worth taking the time to guide the class in a discussion about American belief systems regarding body and mind and about the current research on the interconnections between faith/body/illness/healing. To lead such a discussion that is not demeaning has the potential to enact Standard 3.03 and more fully meet the aspiration of respecting differences.

Dictates of One's Own Conscience

Recognizing that there are always pressures in a classroom setting due to lack of time, the desire to fully cover an array of complex course material, and that having to manage one problematic student interchange can take considerable resources, if you were Dr. Hughes, what would you do?

1. Keep in mind that George's remark may be crafted to intentionally demean native cultures based on his past history of working with the tribes. George may not have been aware of Michelle's cultural heritage, thus thought it was acceptable to make disparaging remarks. Hold a discussion to focus on the danger of keeping to "political correctness."
2. Acknowledge that although it was an unintentional oversight on his part, may want to George provide Michelle with an apology for his demeaning comment.
3. Acknowledge that although it is a difficult topic for some people to discuss, Michelle may not want to bring her personal family history into a classroom discussion.
4. Make a formal request to the department head that as a program that touts "multicultural competence" as one of the most important facets of clinical practice that a class on multicultural and indigenous practices should be created and offered as soon as is reasonably feasible.
5. Acknowledge that the difficult interpersonal exchanges do not take away from the substance of discussing course material.
6. Ignore the interchange and proceed with a general discussion about various healing practices, noting

that no undue privilege should be afforded any one treatment method solely because it is commonly used among the majority culture, nor solely because of a desire to be "politically correct" and thereby less controversial.

7. Suggest that the efficacy of a particular treatment, regardless of it's origin, can be evaluated and critically discussed without demeaning or disrespectful language being used by anyone.
8. Dismiss the class for a short break for everyone to cool down.
9. Invite George and Michelle to do research and present short lectures in the next class on each other's preferred modalities as a way of fostering scholarly dialogue and multicultural flexibility.
10. Perform a combination of the previously listed actions.
11. Do something that is not previously listed.

If you were Dr. Hughes practicing in Canada, the previously listed options would still apply since the guideline for harassment is not substantially different from those listed by the APA Ethics Code.

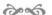

STANDARD 3.04: AVOIDING HARM

> Psychologists take reasonable steps to avoid harming their clients/patients, students, supervisees, research participants, organizational clients, and others with whom they work, and to minimize harm where it is foreseeable and unavoidable.

A CASE FOR STANDARD 3.04: Confidentiality or Personal Harm

Dr. Flores has been treating a 12-year-old boy, Kenneth, to help him with problem behaviors at school and at home. Kenneth was physically abused in the past. One day after a session, as Kenneth was walking out of the outer door of Dr. Flores's office, Kenneth turned around, smiled at Dr. Flores, and waved goodbye with Dr. Flores's wallet in his hand. He then raced out of the building. At the next break in his schedule, Dr. Flores called Kenneth's house with the intent of confronting Kenneth about taking the wallet. Kenneth's father answered the phone and said that Kenneth was still not home and that he was 2 hours late for dinner. The father said, "You would only call if something were wrong. What is it?"

Issues of Concern

There are several ways that Kenneth could be harmed by Dr. Flores's action at this juncture. Based on the history of past physical abuse, Dr. Flores may have cause to believe that if the parents knew of the wallet theft, then there would be a high probability of a severe altercation that may lead to psychological and physical abuse. Standard 3.04 would have guided Dr. Flores not to have called Kenneth's home. However, having made the phone call, Standard 3.04 would guide Dr. Flores not to respond to the father's inquiry. Contradictorily, by not taking action, Dr. Flores has allowed a 12-year-old boy on the loose with money and credit cards. To avoid this type of harm, Standard 3.04 would guide Dr. Flores to take immediate action to locate Kenneth, such as by calling his home, and to take steps to prevent anyone from using the contents of his wallet. Which is the lesser of possible harms?

Regardless of the potential for harm, state law may preempt this consideration if Kenneth is a minor, thus Dr. Flores may not have a choice in regards to answering questions by Kenneth's father.

APA Ethics Code

Companion General Principle

Principle A: Beneficence and Nonmaleficence

> Psychologists . . . take care to do no harm.

Principle A is the aspirational basis for the enforceable Standard 3.04. Aspiring to foster nonmaleficence may be difficult in this situation. Ideally, the course of action to do no harm is preventative; we hope that all psychologists set up their offices securely enough to prevent temptation. Kenneth, having succumbed to temptation, can come to harm in a number of different ways, including by necessitating Dr. Flores's phone call home, which could jeopardize Kenneth's safety, regardless of what Dr. Flores discloses.

Principle B: Fidelity and Responsibility

> Psychologists establish relationships of trust with those whom they work.

Trust holds multifaceted dimensions in this situation. Steeped in the cultural expectation of individualism and privacy, Kenneth may deem Dr. Flores untrustworthy if Dr. Flores is unable to confine and resolve conflicts just between the two of them. Additionally, Kenneth may deem Dr. Flores not trustworthy if Dr. Flores fails to keep him safe from his own impulses of stealing and harmful activities once he has money. Kenneth may also deem Dr. Flores untrustworthy if Dr. Flores is unable to keep him safe from his (Kenneth's) father.

Principle C: Integrity

> Psychologists strive to keep their promises and to avoid unwise or unclear commitment.

The principle of integrity guides Dr. Flores to follow through with whatever agreements have been made about communication with Kenneth's parents. If the established understanding is for Dr. Flores to convey the content of the treatment sessions to Kenneth's parents and then uphold the principle of integrity, Dr. Flores would tell Kenneth's father about the stolen wallet.

Companion Ethical Standard(s)

Standard 3.06: Conflict of Interest

> Psychologists refrain from taking on a professional role . . . [that] . . . could reasonably be expected to, (1) impair their objectivity, competence, or effectiveness in performing their functions as psychologists . . .

Standard 3.06 directs Dr. Flores to weigh the consequences of various actions he might take following Kenneth's theft of the wallet. What kind and how much information may be provided to the parents in light of the possibility that Kenneth may be punished severely by his father and use the money and credit cards to run away from home.

Standard 4.02: Discussing the Limits of Confidentiality

> (a) Psychologists discuss with persons (including, to the extent feasible, persons who are legally incapable of giving informed consent and their legal representatives) . . .
>
> . . . (1) the relevant limits of confidentiality and . . .
>
> . . . (2) the foreseeable uses of the information generated through their psychological activities . . .
>
> . . . (b) . . . the discussion of confidentiality occurs at the outset of the relationship and thereafter as new circumstances may warrant.

Standard 4.02 directs Dr. Flores to have had a conversation with either Kenneth, if he is considered at the age of majority, and/or Kenneth's parents, if Kenneth is considered a minor, regarding what kind and how much information may be provided to the parents. Guided by the principles of integrity and fidelity, Dr. Flores is now directed to enact the terms of the initial agreement with Kenneth and his parents.

Standard 4.05: Disclosures

> . . . (b) Psychologists disclose confidential information without the consent of the individual only as mandated by law, or where permitted by law for a valid purpose such as to . . . (3) protect the client/patient, psychologist, or others from harm . . .

Standard 4.05 directs Dr. Flores to answer Kenneth's father's question if Dr. Flores practices in a state that does not consider 12 to be age of the majority for the purposes of receiving health care.

Standards 3.04 and 4.05 (3) guide Dr. Flores to disclose information to Kenneth's parents in order to protect Kenneth from harm if the harm is from possessing the contents of his wallet.

Standards 3.04 and 4.05, however, also guide Dr. Flores *not* to disclose information to the parents if the harm is from possible abuse by the parents. On the grounds that psychologists need not give up his/her social rights, such as protection from theft, Standard 4.05 (3) simultaneously allows Dr. Flores to take measures to protect himself from harm, in this case this harm that results from having his wallet stolen.

Standard 10.02: Therapy Involving Couples or Families

> (a) When psychologists agree to provide services to several persons who have a relationship (such as . . . parents and children), they take reasonable steps to clarify at the outset . . . (2) the relationship the psychologist will have with each person. This clarification includes the psychologist's role and this probable uses of the services provided or the information obtained.

Standard 10.02 directs Dr. Flores to have had a conversation to clarify how information will be shared between Kenneth and his parents. If that initial agreement was for total confidentiality, then Dr. Flores is directed to respond with "I can't tell you why I am calling" to the father's inquiry.

Standard 10.10: Terminating Therapy

> . . . (b) Psychologists may terminate therapy when . . . endangered by the client . . .

Standard 10.10 further allows Dr. Flores to protect himself by terminating therapy with Kenneth following the theft of his wallet.

Legal Issues

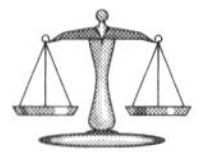

Maryland

> *Md. Code Regs. 10.36.05.07 (2010). Client welfare.*
>
> *A. A psychologist shall:*
>
> 1) Take appropriate steps to disclose to all involved parties conflicts of interest that arise, with respect to a psychologist's clients, in a manner that is consistent with applicable confidentiality requirements. . .

Arizona

> *Ariz. Admin. Code § R4-26-301 (2008). Rules of professional conduct.*
>
> A psychologist shall practice psychology in accordance with the ethical standards contained in standards 1.01 through 10.10 of the "Ethical Principles of Psychologists and Code of Conduct" adopted by the American Psychological Association effective June 1, 2003, the provisions of which are incorporated by reference. This incorporation does not include any later amendments or editions of the incorporated matter. . .

An appearance of conflict may have emerged in this case as a dilemma has emerged—Dr. Flores's desire to keep his client safe from his father's wrath and his judgment about whether to talk to the father about whether Kenneth has used the contents of his wallet to engage in unsafe behavior. Dr. Flores must evaluate what he knows about Kenneth's past behavior to determine the course to take in light of the current events, and what course of action will lead to less harm to Kenneth. Such a course may involve disclosing actions that emerged during the confidential therapeutic relationship. The evaluation should detail his thinking and record his plan of action to follow. It also is an instance where contemporaneous consultation with a trained colleague would help both licensing boards find that Dr. Flores did not violate the ethical standards. A peer consultation would show that all the facts were considered and weighed in an reasonable manner.

Cultural Considerations

Global Discussion

Code of Ethics: Netherlands

> III.4.3 Prevention of harm.
>
> III.4.3.1 Negative experiences.
>
> The psychologist does not expose those involved . . . to any potentially harmful experience, unless this is strictly necessary to achieve professional objectives . . . In such cases, he will do his utmost to minimize or to counterbalance the harmful effect of such experiences on those involved.
>
> III.4.3.2 Far-reaching indirect consequences of the professional acting.
>
> The psychologist takes into account that, apart from direct consequences of his professional acting, far reaching indirect consequences may occur. If this happens, he acts according to the above-mentioned stipulation.

If Dr. Flores is practicing in the Netherlands, he must consider the possible long-term impact of disclosing the wallet theft to Kenneth's parents. He must also consider other "indirect" consequences of his decision and balance that with the "far-reaching" consequences of a decision *not* to inform Kenneth's parents about the theft. Exposing Kenneth to harm by revealing the theft may not fall under the domain of being "strictly necessary to achieve professional objectives"—it is to prevent personal harm to himself. Not disclosing the wallet theft to Kenneth's parents and raising the issue instead with Kenneth could have the far-reaching indirect consequence of an enhanced therapeutic relationship between them, or it could result in Dr. Flores deciding to no longer treat Kenneth.

American Moral Values

1. What is the likelihood of Kenneth being abused for stealing Dr. Flores's wallet? Is the wallet and possibly sending Kenneth a message about stealing worth risking abuse from his parents?
2. Would including Kenneth's father in the discussion about what Kenneth might do with the contents of the wallet increase Kenneth's safe return to his home?

3. If Kenneth's father is told, how will this affect Kenneth's relationship with Dr. Flores and their prospects for successful treatment? Are the possible negative consequences of his father's involvement offset by Kenneth destroying trust by taking the wallet? Is this an incident to use to illustrate the nature of that trust and how to work through the consequences of violating trust?
4. Is Kenneth's class relevant for taking action about the wallet? Does Kenneth have a monetary need, or is this a gratuitously mischievous act? How will this affect Dr. Flores's approach?

Ethical Course of Action

Directive per APA Code

Standard 3.04 directs Dr. Flores to take a course of action to avoid harm to his client. In this situation, Standard 3.04 intersects with both theoretical orientation, state law on age of majority, and Standard 4 posing an interesting question: What is harm? If one takes the directive from Standard 3.04 in combination with Standard 4.02, the course of action that leads to the least amount of harm to the therapeutic relationship is to enact whatever was agreed upon among Dr. Flores, Kenneth, and his parents.

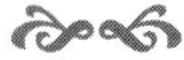

Dictates of One's Own Conscience

If, for some reason, you had not obtained consent to treatment that encompassed the question of confidentiality, what would you do now?

1. Ask Kenneth's parents to have Kenneth contact you.
2. Cancel your credit cards, and discuss the theft with Kenneth in your next session.
3. Tell Kenneth's father about the theft of your wallet, and request that both parents and Kenneth attend the next scheduled therapy session.
4. Tell Kenneth's father about the theft of your wallet, and terminate the therapeutic relationship.
5. Tell Kenneth's father that you needed to reschedule an appointment.
6. Call the police to report the theft of your wallet, and report Kenneth's absence so that Kenneth is found.
7. Perform a combination of the previously listed actions.
8. Do something that is not previously listed.

If you were practicing in the Netherlands and had not obtained consent to treatment that encompassed the question of confidentiality, the previously listed options would still apply since the guideline for nonmaleficence is not substantially different from those listed by the APA Ethics Code.

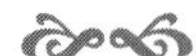

STANDARD 3.05: MULTIPLE RELATIONSHIPS

(a) A multiple relationship occurs when a psychologist is in a professional role with a person and (1) **at the same time is in another role with the same person,** (2) at the same time is in a relationship with a person closely associated with or related to the person with whom the psychologist has the professional relationship, or (3) promises to enter into another relationship in the future with the person or a person closely associated with or related to the person.

A psychologist refrains from entering into a multiple relationship if the multiple relationship could reasonably be expected to impair the psychologist's objectivity, competence, or effectiveness in performing his or her functions as a psychologist, or otherwise risks exploitation or harm to the person with whom the professional relationship exists.

Multiple relationships that would not reasonably be expected to cause impairment or risk exploitation or harm are not unethical.

A CASE FOR STANDARD 3.05 (A) (1): Split Fidelity

Dr. Washington has a busy practice with a specialty in treating women with extensive childhood history of sexual abuse. Kimberly has been in treatment with Dr. Washington for at least a year. Kimberly has been estranged from her family of origin despite the fact that Kimberly's family lives in the same city. In the course of treatment, Kimberly has decided to ask her mother about some childhood events and contacts her mother to request a visit.

Also on Dr. Washington's caseload is Deborah, who has been in treatment with Dr. Washington for about 3 months. During one session Deborah talked about concern for her parents because an estranged sister had recontacted the family. Deborah mentioned the name of Kim as the troubled sister who now wants to stir up problems for the family. Given a few further details of the family situation and physical description, Dr. Washington realized that Kimberly and Deborah are sisters, each having taken their husband's last name.

Issues of Concern

By no design on Dr. Washington's part, she is "at the same time" Kimberly's therapist and Kimberly's sister's therapist. Given that Kimberly and Deborah are both married and took their husbands last names, and they do not live in the same household, there was no way for Dr. Washington to have known of the two women were related to each other. The last sentence of Standard 3.05 (a) allows Dr. Washington to continue treatment of both Kimberly and Deborah provided the situation would not cause impairment. In the given situation, it is unimaginable that Dr. Washington's judgment of either sister or of the family situation would not be influenced by simultaneous information from Kimberly and Deborah, which means that Dr. Washington's objectivity would be compromised. Thus, though allowable, this standard would guide Dr. Washington not to continue treating both sisters.

The difficulty lies in how Dr. Washington can best extricate herself from either therapeutic relationship without either harming the client by rejecting her or by giving a reason for the termination that would compromise the confidentiality of one or both of her clients.

APA Ethics Code

Companion General Principle

Principle A: Beneficence and Nonmaleficence

> When conflicts occur among psychologists' obligations . . . , they attempt to resolve these conflicts in a responsible fashion that avoids or minimizes harm.

Dr. Washington is obligated to provide the best treatment she can to both of her clients. Given the multiple relationship, it is not possible for Dr. Washington to provide service that is objective and unbiased. In such an event, Principle A guides Dr. Washington to act in such a way as (1) to be responsible, (2) to resolve the conflict, and (3) to avoid or minimize harm.

Principle B: Fidelity and Responsibility

> Psychologists establish relationships of trust with those with whom they work.

> Common usage and understanding of Fidelity is loyalty, in this case loyalty to one's client. In any ordinary circumstance, had Dr. Washington known of Deborah's relationship to an existing client, Dr. Washington would remain loyal to the first client and thus not take on Deborah as a client. In this current situation, both clients have equal claim of loyalty from Dr. Washington. Should the sisters find out that the other sister was also a client before Dr. Washington figures out how to resolve this dilemma, there may be feelings of betrayal.

Principle D: Justice

> Psychologists recognize that fairness and justice entitle all persons to access to and benefit from the contributions of psychology and to equal quality in the . . . services being conducted by psychologists. Psychologists exercise reasonable judgment and take precautions to ensure that their potential biases . . . do not lead to . . . unjust practices.

Biases may occur when a psychologist favors one family member over another. Regardless of the genesis of bias, Principle D entreats psychologists to guard against the negative effects of their biases.

The principle of justice entitles both sisters to equal benefit. Should Dr. Washington decide to end treatment with one of the sisters in order to eliminate the multiple relationship or the potential bias, Dr. Washington would have unfairly denied one person the benefit of uninterrupted treatment.

Principle E: Respect for People's Rights and Dignity

> Psychologists respect the dignity and worth of all people, and the rights of individuals to privacy, confidentiality . . .

Client's rights to privacy and confidentiality are central to psychologist's clinical work. Both of the sisters have a right to confidentiality, which includes not having Dr. Washington tell anyone that she is in treatment. Aspiring to this principle would guide Dr. Washington not to reveal the fact that either sister is in treatment with her.

Companion Ethical Standard(s)

Standard 4.01: Maintaining Confidentiality

> Psychologists have a primary obligation . . . to protect confidential information obtained through . . . any medium, recognizing that the extent and limits of confidentiality may be . . . established by . . . professional . . . relationship.

Standard 4.01 directs Dr. Washington to keep all client information confidential. It is a breach of confidentiality for Dr. Washington to tell either Kimberly or Deborah of their mutual client status on Dr. Washington's caseload. One would normally not disclose the identity of one's clients to other clients.

Standard 10.10: Terminating Therapy

> (a) Psychologists terminate therapy when it becomes reasonably clear that the client/patient . . . is being harmed by continued service.

If and when either Kimberly and/or Deborah discover that they are in treatment with the same psychologist, might they feel betrayed? Thus both Kimberly and Deborah may be harmed by continued treatment with Dr. Washington. If Dr. Washington were to keep with the principle of fidelity to the first relationship, which is with Kimberly, then Dr. Washington would move to terminate treatment with Deborah. However, to terminate without explanation, in most circumstances, would cause harm.

Standard 10.02: Therapy Involving Couples or Families

> (a) When psychologists agree to provide services to several persons who have a relationship . . . , they take reasonable steps to clarify at the outset (1) which of the individuals are clients/patients and (2) the relationship the psychologist will have with each person. This clarification includes the psychologist's role and the probable uses of the services provided . . .

Given the relationship between Kimberly and Deborah, it would be reasonable to look toward Standard 10.02 for guidance. However, this standard does not apply in this case because Dr. Washington did not agree to provide services to several persons from the same family. Therefore, Dr. Washington could not clarify from the outset the nature of her own role and the limits of confidentiality, nor could she obtain full consent from both clients.

Standard 3.06: Conflict of Interest

> Psychologists refrain from taking on a professional role . . . [that] . . . could reasonably be expected to . . . (1) impair their objectivity, . . . in performing their functions as psychologists . . .

Treating two members of the same family calls for extreme care in navigating from an unbiased position. Having two family members who, unbeknownst to each other, are telling the same story to Dr. Washington is bound to affect Dr. Washington's objectivity. Standard 3.06 directs Dr. Washington not to put herself in such a position.

Standard 3.05: Multiple Relationships

> . . . (b) If a psychologist finds that, due to unforeseen factors, a potentially harmful multiple relationship has arisen, the psychologist takes reasonable steps to resolve it with due regard for the best interests of the affected person and maximal compliance with the Ethics Code.

Once discovered, as directed by Standard 3.05 (b), Dr. Washington must take steps to resolve the multiple relationship.

Legal Issues 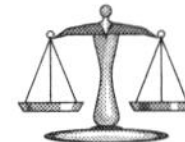

Washington

> *Wash. Admin. Code § 246-924-357 (2009). Multiple relationships.*
>
> The psychologist shall not . . . continue a professional relationship with a client when the objectivity . . . of the psychologist is impaired because of the psychologist's present . . . relationship with the client or a person associated with or related to the client. When such relationship impairs objectivity, the psychologist shall terminate the professional relationship with adequate notice and in an appropriate manner . . . and shall assist the client in obtaining services from another professional.

Massachusetts

> *251 Mass. Code Regs. 1.10 (2010). Ethical standards and professional conduct.*
>
> . . . (6) In addition to acts prohibited by the Ethical Principles of Psychologists and Code of Conduct.
>
> . . . (c) Jeopardizing the physical or emotional security of a patient or client . . . by unauthorized disclosure or communication of confidential information.

If Dr. Washington was practicing in Washington, state law mandates Dr. Washington to terminate the relationship with either or both Kimberly and Deborah. Massachusetts's law also directs that Dr. Washington would have to terminate the relationship with either or both sisters. It also focuses on not jeopardizing the emotional security of the client(s) by disclosing any confidential information during the transition to the termination(s). In both jurisdictions, the question becomes how to terminate the relationships without creating harm and making appropriate referrals for both of Dr. Washington's clients.

Cultural Considerations

Global Discussion

Ethical Code of Canadian Psychologists

> Principle III: Integrity in relationships.
>
> *Values statement.*
>
> As public trust in the discipline of psychology includes believing that psychologists will act in the best interests of members of the public, situations that present real or potential conflicts of interest are of concern to psychologists. It is the responsibility of psychologists to avoid dual or multiple relationships . . . when . . . possible. When such situations cannot be avoided . . . , psychologists have a responsibility to declare that they have a conflict of interest, to seek advice, and to establish safeguards to ensure that the best interests of members of the public are protected.
>
> *Avoidance of conflict of interest.*
>
> III.34. Manage dual or multiple relationships that are unavoidable . . . in such a manner that bias, lack of objectivity . . . are minimized. This might include obtaining ongoing supervision or consultation for the duration of the dual or multiple relationship, or involving a third party in obtaining consent . . .
>
> III.35. Inform all parties, if a . . . conflict of interest arises, of the need to resolve the situation in a manner that is consistent with Respect for the Dignity of Persons (Principle I) and Responsible Caring (Principle II), and take all reasonable steps to resolve the issue in such a manner.

It is clear that Dr. Washington could not have avoided being in a multiple relationship with the two sisters and as such needs to find a way to manage it without bias or impairment of her objectivity. It is likely that because of the nature of doing therapy with both sisters without their prior consent or current knowledge, that this is problematic at best. The Canadian code does not specify actions to be taken in this instance. It is reasonable to assume that "reasonable steps" of resolution in keeping with the aforementioned Principles I and II would include possibly terminating one or both therapeutic relationships with her clients. Conversely, Dr. Washington could consult with a supervisor.

American Moral Values

1. Now that she knows they are sisters, can Dr. Washington provide the same quality of treatment to Deborah and Kimberly as she would have before? If not, how does she decide between them? Should Dr. Washington go with the client who has been with her the longest (seniority, loyalty to longer relationship) or the client whom she feels she can help the most (trying to achieve the most good with chosen client)? Or does transferring one of the sisters still result in the loss of objectivity?
2. How does Dr. Washington weigh the effects of the two sisters finding out Dr. Washington has treated both of them? Would maintaining confidentiality and continuing to treat both constitute a deception or betrayal of Deborah and/or Kimberly's trust? Is Kimberly's particular situation of exploring possible abuse and reestablishing contact with her family relevant to whether Dr. Washington feels ready to commit?
3. If Dr. Washington discontinues her work with one client, will she have to fear charges of betrayal for not telling the other sister why she could no longer see her? Would that fear ever be strong enough to consider not treating either sister?

Ethical Course of Action

Directive per APA Code

Standard 3.05 (a) is multifaceted. Central to Standard 3.05 (a) is a caution to avoid engaging in multiple relationships and to extricate when avoidance is not possible. For Dr. Washington, it is not possible to avoid the multiple relationship. Whichever way she turns, potential harm appears unavoidable.

Standard 3.05 (a) also states that multiple relationships in and of themselves are not unethical. It is only those multiple relationships that would cause "impairment or risk exploitation or harm," which are unethical. One way to guard against bias, the potential basis for harm, if Dr. Washington continues to treat both sisters is for her to receive ongoing supervision.

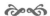

Dictates of One's Own Conscience

One would never wish for such a situation like this. However, many circumstances befall the professional life of a psychologist. Should you find yourself in the same, or similar, situation as Dr. Washington, which would you do?

1. Continue care with Kimberly and terminate treatment with Deborah, as the therapeutic relationship of 12 months is most likely better established than the therapeutic relationship of 3 months with Deborah.
   a. Find another psychologist of equal training, focus so there would not be a diminishment in the standard of care, and transfer/refer Deborah to that therapist with no explanation.
   b. Let Deborah know that the transfer of care has nothing to do with her; rather some other issues came up.
2. End treatment with both Kimberly and Deborah.
   a. Let both know that the transfer of care has nothing to do with either of them; rather some other issues came up.
   b. Tell them to ask each other as to the reason for termination of treatment.
3. Continue treatment with both Kimberly and Deborah, and obtain really good supervision to guard against likely or possible effects of bias.
4. Discuss the concepts of loyalty, promise, and betrayal in preparation for the eventual discovery that the other sister had been/is a client with the same therapist.
5. Schedule the sisters back-to-back in the hope that they meet in the waiting room. Many therapists may have a fleeting thought on this possibility. This course of action is not one that is the most considerate for avoidance of harm.
6. Perform a combination of the previously listed actions.
7. Do something that is not previously listed.

Should you be practicing in Canada and find yourself in the same, or similar, situation as Dr. Washington, you would inform all parties that a conflict has arisen and seek additional supervision to safeguard against harm.

STANDARD 3.05: MULTIPLE RELATIONSHIPS

(a) A multiple relationship occurs when a psychologist is in a professional role with a person and (1) at the same time is in another role with the same person, (2) **at the same time is in a relationship with a person closely associated with or related to the person with whom the psychologist has the professional relationship,** or (3) promises to enter into another relationship in the future with the person or a person closely associated with or related to the person.

A psychologist refrains from entering into a multiple relationship if the multiple relationship could reasonably be expected to impair the psychologist's objectivity, competence, or effectiveness in performing his or her functions as a psychologist, or otherwise risks exploitation or harm to the person with whom the professional relationship exists.

Multiple relationships that would not reasonably be expected to cause impairment or risk exploitation or harm are not unethical.

A CASE FOR STANDARD 3.05 (A) (2): Daughter's New Business

Dr. Vasquez is practicing in a rural county. Mr. Juan was referred by his family physician for psychological assessment and treatment of anxiety and panic symptoms. Initially reluctant, Mr. Juan accepted the referral after his disorder began to take on agoraphobic features and to limit his functioning. He acknowledged that had Dr. Vasquez not been Mexican American (and the only Mexican American psychologist in the area), Mr. Juan would not have been willing to engage in treatment. Treatment has been cognitive–behavioral, with 3 months of weekly sessions. Significant remission of symptoms has been achieved, but treatment is not yet complete. One day, Mr. Juan came in reporting that he would be starting a new job next month, with better salary and more opportunity for advancement. He feared with more stress associated with the new job that there would be a return of anxiety and panic symptoms. In addition, Mr. Juan wanted to discuss issues related to his new work-role identity. With further exploration, Dr. Vasquez realized that Mr. Juan's new employer is his (Dr. Vasquez's) eldest daughter, who recently established a small business marketing organic produce.

Issues of Concern

Dr. Vasquez, being simultaneously the treating psychologist for Mr. Juan and the father of Mr. Juan's boss, is unwittingly in a multiple relationship. Standard 3.05 would guide Dr. Vasquez to first refrain from entering into such a relationship. Dr. Vasquez was not in danger of entering into a multiple relationship with Mr. Juan when he originally accepted Mr. Juan as a client. Given that Dr. Vasquez now does not have the option to refrain from this multiple relationship, Standard 3.05 guides Dr. Vasquez to evaluate the chances that being the father of Mr. Juan's new boss would impair his objectivity.

Dr. Vasquez's privileged information regarding Mr. Juan's new boss might greatly assist Mr. Juan in navigating a successful work experience, thus from Mr. Juan's possible perspective continued treatment with Dr. Vasquez would not reasonably be expected to cause harm to Mr. Juan.

This situation is occurring in a rural setting. Two applicable factors about rural practice apply in this situation, namely, that resources are not as widely available, thus referrals are difficult or impossible to make, and that multiple relationships are normal everyday occurrences in rural practice. These facts influence and alter the application of Standard 3.05.

APA Ethics Code

Companion General Principle

Introduction and Applicability

> This Ethics Code applies only to psychologists' activities that are part of their . . . professional roles as psychologists. . . These activities shall be distinguished from the purely private conduct of psychologists, which is not within the purview of the Ethics Code.

Unlike the previous vignette with Dr. Washington where the psychology rules and regulations applied to all parties concerned, in this vignette, the professional rules and regulations only apply in the interaction between Dr. Vasquez and Mr. Juan.

Principle A: Beneficence and Nonmaleficence

> When conflicts occur among psychologists' obligations . . . , they attempt to resolve these conflicts in a responsible fashion that avoids or minimizes harm.

Dr. Vasquez is obligated to provide the best treatment he can to his client Mr. Juan, and an appearance of conflict of loyalties has emerged. Aspiring to enact Principle A, Dr. Vasquez would now need to resolve the conflict between his loyalty to his client and loyalty to his daughter in such a way that avoids harm only to his client Mr. Juan.

Principle B: Fidelity and Responsibility

> Psychologists establish relationships of trust with those with whom they work.

Dr. Vasquez's relationship with his daughter is not professional, thus not subject to the rules and regulations applied to his relationship with Mr. Juan. Principle B would guide Dr. Vasquez to be trustworthy and to remain loyal to his client.

Principle D: Justice

> Psychologists recognize that fairness and justice entitle all persons to access and to benefit from the contributions of psychology . . . Psychologists exercise reasonable judgment and take precautions to ensure that their potential biases . . . do not lead to . . . unjust practices.

Principle D cautions psychologists to guard against bias. In this case, there is an expectation of nepotism with bias going in favor of one's daughter.

Principle E: Respect for People's Rights and Dignity

> Psychologists respect the dignity and worth of all people, and the rights of individuals to privacy, confidentiality . . .

Enacting Principle E, Dr. Vasquez would be expected not to reveal Mr. Juan's client status to his daughter. But since the relationship between Dr. Vasquez and his daughter is not professional, the privilege of confidentiality does not extend to his daughter. This means Dr. Vasquez is able to reveal that Mr. Juan's new boss is Dr. Vasquez's daughter.

Companion Ethical Standard(s)

Standard 3.04: Avoiding Harm

> Psychologists take reasonable steps to avoid harming their clients . . . and to minimize harm where it is foreseeable and unavoidable.

Whatever steps Dr. Vasquez takes, Standard 3.04 directs Dr. Vasquez to use, as a central guiding value, the idea of avoiding harm to Mr. Juan.

Standard 3.06: Conflict of Interest

> Psychologists refrain from taking on a professional role . . . [that] . . . could reasonably be expected to (1) impair their objectivity, . . . in performing their functions as psychologists . . .

One could reasonably expect Dr. Vasquez to have impaired objectivity due to a conflict of interest when providing treatment to his daughter's employee. Standard 3.06 exhorts Dr. Vasquez not to take on a professional role with Mr. Juan. However, Standard 3.06 does not give a directive with regard to an existing and continuing relationship.

Standard 10.10: Terminating Therapy

> (a) Psychologists terminate therapy when it becomes reasonably clear that the client/patient . . . is being harmed by continued service.

Standard 10.10 directs Dr. Vasquez to end treatment with Mr. Juan should it become clear that Mr. Juan is being harmed by continuing treatment. In the current situation, no harm has yet occurred, just the fear of potential harm based on a multiple relationship. So it is unclear as to whether Standard 10.10 applies at this time and whether Dr. Vasquez is supported by dictates of the ethics code should he decide to terminate treatment with Mr. Juan.

Legal Issues 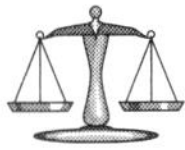

Ohio

> *Ohio Admin. Code 4732:17-01 (2010). General rules of professional conduct pursuant to section 4732.17 of the Revised Code.*
>
> . . . (C) Welfare of the client.
>
> . . . (13) Unforeseen multiple relationships.
>
> If a psychologist . . . determines that, due to unforeseen factors, a prohibited multiple relationship has developed, he or she shall take reasonable steps to resolve it with due regard for the welfare of the person(s) with whom there is . . . a professional psychological role.

New Jersey

> *N.J. Admin. Code § 13:42-10.13 (2010). Conflicts of interest; dual relationships.*
>
> . . . (d) A licensee shall not enter into any dual relationship. . .
>
> (e) A licensee who recognizes the existence of a conflict of interest or dual relationship shall take action to terminate the conflict or the dual relationship.

If Dr. Vasquez was practicing in New Jersey, he would need to move to terminate treatment with Mr. Juan. However, if he was practicing in Ohio, where the language of the APA Ethics Code has been adopted, there is not a clear mandate to terminate treatment. The Ohio mandate is to resolve the multiple relationship but not necessarily to terminate.

Cultural Considerations

Global Discussion

Ethical Code of Canadian Psychologists

> Principle III: Integrity in relationships.
>
> *Avoidance of conflict of interest.*
>
> III.34. Manage dual or multiple relationships that are unavoidable . . . in such a manner that bias . . . are minimized. This might include obtaining ongoing supervision or consultation for the duration of the dual or multiple relationship. . .
>
> III.35. Inform all parties, if a . . . conflict of interest arises, of the need to resolve the situation in a manner that is consistent with Respect for the Dignity of Persons . . . and Responsible Caring . . .

Because Mr. Juan's therapeutic relationship with Dr. Vasquez is in great part due to their shared ethnic heritage, simply referring Mr. Juan is difficult and potentially harmful. Refusing to treat Mr. Juan is harmful professionally, therapeutically, and probably also damaging within both men's membership in a small rural Hispanic community. While the Canadian code is not specific with how to resolve such a situation, it clearly mandates that the psychologist, Dr. Vasquez, is the party responsible for informing all involved and taking "reasonable steps" to resolution, using respect for the dignity of persons and responsible caring as his guides.

American Moral Values

1. How does Dr. Vasquez balance the value of his treatment of Mr. Juan with a transparency about a family member who is employing his client? Are the effects of stopping the treatment more costly than Mr. Juan feeling his therapist will side with his boss?

2. How does Dr. Vasquez judge Mr. Juan's ability to separate his own therapy from his workplace? Does he underestimate Mr. Juan's ability to put his boss's identity aside during his therapy?

3. How does Dr. Vasquez consider his own racial/cultural background in deciding whether to continue treatment of Mr. Juan? Is it important that, given where they are, Mr. Juan might not find another therapist with Dr. Vasquez's cultural competency? Does this keep Dr. Vasquez from ending the relationship because of an appearance of a conflict of interest?

4. If a problem arose between Mr. Juan and Dr. Vasquez's daughter, how will Dr. Vasquez's biases and judgments affect his relationship to both? What does Dr. Vasquez owe his daughter in terms of treating her employee?

Ethical Course of Action

Directive per APA Code

Standard 3.05 (a) (2) defines Dr. Vasquez and Mr. Juan's relationship within the confines of multiple relationships. Standard 3.05 directs Dr. Vasquez to refrain from entering into such a relationship. But if Dr. Vasquez thinks he can continue treatment of Mr. Juan in the current context without causing harm to Mr. Juan, Standard 3.05 (a) does not prohibit or condemn such a move. Considering the directives of Standard 3.05 (a) within the context of the whole code as being only applicable to psychologist's professional activities and not to a psychologist's private life, Dr. Vasquez could refrain from entering into this multiple relationship with Mr. Juan by revealing the fact that Mr. Juan's new employer is Dr. Vasquez's daughter.

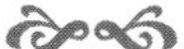

Dictates of One's Own Conscience

If you were in Dr. Vasquez's situation and had the instant awareness that revealing the nature of your multiple relationships with Mr. Juan could be done without violation of ethics and you had done so, what might you do next? And what moral value guides you to choose your course of action?

1. Refer Mr. Juan to another Mexican American therapist, although he may have to drive farther.

2. Discuss the situation with Mr. Juan, and offer the client an option of seeing another Latino psychologist, if one was readily available.

3. Discuss the situation, and offer to continue treatment with the client with full awareness of the relationship between yourself and his new employer.

4. With Mr. Juan's permission, hold a joint meeting among Mr. Juan, the daughter/employer, and you, so all are able to air and discuss their concerns; and Mr. Juan could make an informed transparent decision together.

5. Keep quiet about the multiple relationships, do not agree to work beyond the anxiety and panic; and then terminate treatment as early as feasible.

6. Do a combination of the previously listed actions.

7. Do something that is not previously listed.

If you were treating Mr. Juan in Canada, would you discuss with Mr. Juan the situation regarding he and your daughter, and include your daughter in the conversation so that all involved persons can make an informed and transparent choice together?

STANDARD 3.05: MULTIPLE RELATIONSHIPS

(a) A multiple relationship occurs when a psychologist is in a professional role with a person and (1) at the same time is in another role with the same person, (2) at the same time is in a relationship with a person closely associated with or related to the person with whom the psychologist has the professional relationship, or (3) **promises to enter into another relationship in the future with the person or a person closely associated with or related to the person.**

A psychologist refrains from entering into a multiple relationship if the multiple relationship could reasonably be expected to impair the psychologist's objectivity, competence, or effectiveness in performing his or her functions as a psychologist, or otherwise risks exploitation or harm to the person with whom the professional relationship exists.

Multiple relationships that would not reasonably be expected to cause impairment or risk exploitation or harm are not unethical.

A CASE FOR STANDARD 3.05 (A) (3): Once a Client, Always a Client?

Dr. Simmons is a 55-year-old psychologist living and practicing in rural coastal Oregon. As part of a new, comprehensive fitness program recommended by her physician, she has begun taking kayaking lessons. Dr. Simmons quickly developed significant enthusiasm, though more limited skill, for this activity. She experienced it as both psychologically and physically beneficial. At the beginning of a new module, the kayak center hired a new instructor. The instructor is a former client, Terry. Terry suggested that they team up to offer a "Kayaking for Seniors" program, with Terry providing the kayaking expertise and Dr. Simmons providing the "face validity" for taking up kayaking later in life. Terry suggested that Dr. Simmons could provide the orientation and instruction in basic skills for the class while Terry would assess individual needs and abilities and provide instruction in more advanced techniques.

Issues of Concern

Being a former client defines the first relationship between Dr. Simmons and Terry. Considering being business partners in this kayaking venture is a "promise to enter into another relationship" with Terry. Standard 3.05 would guide Dr. Simmons to refrain from entering into this new relationship. However, since Standard 3.05 more clearly pertains to current clients, it is unclear as to whether an ex-client is defined as a "professional role." By extension, it is not clear whether entering into a business relationship with an ex-client is a situation that is addressed in Standard 3.05.

Aside from the exact wording of Standard 3.05, the problematic concern is one of power. The central question is whether it is possible for an ex-client to have an equal power relationship with their former treating clinical psychologist.

APA Ethics Code

Companion General Principle

Principle A: Beneficence and Nonmaleficence

> When conflicts occur among psychologists' obligations . . . , they attempt to resolve these conflicts in a responsible fashion that avoids or minimizes harm.

Not yet engaged in a business relationship with Terry, Dr. Simmons has no conflicting obligations to Terry. Being a student of Terry may pose as concern, depending on why Terry sought out psychological services from Dr. Simmons. If Terry had difficulties of any kind with authority, Dr. Simmons's presence in Terry's class might cause harm to Terry.

Principle B: Fidelity and Responsibility

> Psychologists uphold professional standards of conduct, clarify their professional roles and obligations, accept appropriate responsibility for their behavior, and seek to manage conflicts of interest that could lead to exploitation or harm.

Should Dr. Simmons decide to go into business with Terry—and there is a power differential evident in the relationship—then the business arrangement may lead to exploitation. The exploitation that is of concern is the possibility of Dr. Simmons taking advantage of Terry based on her greater knowledge of Terry and that somehow using this knowledge may lead to Terry being harmed.

Companion Ethical Standard(s)

Standard 3.04: Avoiding Harm

> Psychologists take reasonable steps to avoid harming their clients . . . , and to minimize harm where it is foreseeable and unavoidable.

Standard 3.04 is the enactment of Principle A: Beneficence and Nonmaleficence. In this case, would it do more harm not to engage in the proposed business relationship, for example by Terry feeling rejected, than to engage in the business relationship? Depending on the nature of Terry's prior treatment problem, it might do Terry more good to have prolonged exposure to Dr. Simmons in a setting outside of the treatment room or at least would not be of likely harm to Terry.

Standard 3.08: Exploitative Relationships

> Psychologists do not exploit persons over whom they have . . . authority such as clients . . .

The assumption behind the cautionary note regarding multiple relationships in Standard 3.05 (a) is that psychologists, in fact, have power over clients. As such, Standard 3.08 directs psychologists not to exploit persons over whom they have such power.

Dr. Simmons, having had the role of treating psychologist for Terry has a great deal of information regarding Terry, and for that reason, she is in a position to exploit Terry, should they choose to engage in other types of relationships.

Legal Issues

Texas

> *22 Tex. Admin. Code § 465.1 (2010). Definitions.*
>
> . . . (2) "Dual Relationship" means a situation where a licensee and another individual have both a professional relationship and a non-professional relationship. Dual relationships include, but are not limited to . . . business or financial interactions . . .
>
> *22 Tex. Code § 465.13 (2010). Personal problems, conflicts and dual relationships.*
>
> . . . (b) dual relationships.
>
> . . . (2) A licensee must refrain from a professional relationship where pre-existing . . . professional, . . . relationships have the potential to . . . harm or exploit the other party.

Virginia

> *18 Va. Admin. Code § 125-20-150 (2010). Standards of practice.*
>
> B. 6. Avoid dual relationships with patients . . . that could . . . compromise their well-being. . .
>
> . . . 7. Withdraw from, adjust or clarify conflicting roles with due regard for the best interest of the affected party or parties and maximal compliance with these standards. . .

Texas law would view a business relationship with an ex-client as a dual (multiple) relationship. Virginia law does not make this literal distinction. Nevertheless, it is quite likely that the licensing boards of both jurisdictions would sanction Dr. Simmons for entering such a business relationship with a former client.

Cultural Considerations

Global Discussion

Singapore Psychological Society:
Code of Professional Ethics

> Principle 7. Client welfare.
>
> The psychologist respects the integrity and protects the welfare of the person . . . with whom work is undertaken.
>
> 1. The psychologist in . . . situations in which conflicts of interest may arise among various parties, . . . defines for . . . herself the nature and direction of . . . her loyalties, and responsibilities and keeps all parties concerned informed of these commitments.
>
> Principle 8. Client relationship.
>
> The psychologist informs a prospective client of the important aspects of the potential relationship that might affect the client's decision to enter the relationship.
>
> Psychologists do not normally enter into a professional relationship with . . . [those] . . . whose welfare might be jeopardized by such a dual relationship.

A psychologist in Singapore would not be automatically prohibited from entering into a professional relationship with a former client. Assuming that a former client still necessitates the same standards of relationship and protection as a current client, Dr. Simmons should inform Terry of the "important aspects" that might affect her. The Singapore code allows for the psychologist to define and determine the "nature of her own loyalties" but charges her also with the responsibility to keep all involved parties informed of possible ramifications of her actions and decisions. If the psychologist in Singapore has reason to believe that such a relationship with a former client might jeopardize Terry's welfare, then she might decide to forgo the professional venture with her former client. If the psychologist decides that the power differential between herself and her former client Terry is negligible or absent, she might decide to discuss her concerns with her ex-client and move ahead with their joint venture.

American Moral Values

1. Does a therapist have a conflict of interest in being a business partner with an ex-client? Will the issues addressed in Terry's therapy affect how she and Dr. Simmons work together? Could Dr. Simmons's presence hamper Terry's ability to perform independently? Could the business relationship itself stir up therapeutic problems Terry would otherwise not have had to confront?
2. Is this partnership more viable given Terry's more supervisory role, handling more advanced instruction? Will Dr. Simmons be willing to accept correction and instruction from Terry? Will Dr. Simmons and Terry be able to build a rapport that does not depend on their previous relationship for its expectations and patterns?

3. How much is Dr. Simmons's decision based on a desire to help Terry's career? Does a business partnership enmesh Dr. Simmons too closely with Terry's success or failure in this business?

Ethical Course of Action

Directive per APA Code

Standard 3.05 (a) (3) directs Dr. Simmons not to enter into a business relationship with Terry should Terry be a current client. However, Standard 3.05 (a) is silent in regards to previous clients. Some theoretical orientations hold to the axiom that a therapeutic relationship never ends because of the possibility that clients may return to treatment and, more importantly, the power differential between therapist/client always exerts an undue influence on the former client. Given that Dr. Simmons is not yet in a business relationship with Terry, the clinically prudent course of action might be to refrain from entering into this multiple relationship.

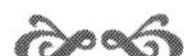

Dictates of One's Own Conscience

Knowing that the course of treatment with Terry was very brief and the nature of the problem situational and bearing in mind this is a rural community, if you were Dr. Simmons, what would you do?

1. Kindly decline the invitation, and continue in the kayak course.
2. Decline the invitation, and withdraw from the kayak course.
3. Talk with Terry about the predicament (e.g., how this would impact the ability to resume therapeutic work together, this being an issue of professional ethics rather than being a personal issue with Terry).
4. Explore all foreseeable future difficulties with Terry, urge that Terry consult a lawyer to consider the possible difficulties before signing a disclosure statement about the difficulties, and then decide to enter into the business partnership with Terry.
5. Do a combination of the previously listed actions.
6. Do something that is not previously listed.

If you were Dr. Simmons practicing in Singapore, you would hopefully decide that the nature and direction of your loyalty is first toward the profession. Having thus determined the direction of your loyality, then take the responsibilities to inform Terry of your commitment to the profession of psychology; decline her invitation for a business venture.

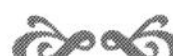

STANDARD 3.05: MULTIPLE RELATIONSHIPS

> . . . (b) If a psychologist finds that, due to unforeseen factors, a potentially harmful multiple relationship has arisen, the psychologist takes reasonable steps to resolve it with due regard for the best interests of the affected person and maximal compliance with the Ethics Code.

A CASE FOR STANDARD 3.05 (B): "But, Dad, She's Not My Client. I Want to Go!"

Dr. Foster specializes in treatment of adolescents with histories of prolonged sexual abuse. Dr. Foster's middle-school-aged child told him that she is overjoyed and is ready to leave for a specialized 10-day, overnight horseback riding camp, which was already paid for in full. Dr. Foster found out at work that Barbara, a client, would be absent from treatment for the next month because she will be working as a camp counselor at this very horseback riding camp Dr. Foster's child will be attending. Barbara is a high functioning adolescent who has experienced an eating disorder and who was sexually abused once by her uncle. Barbara will be the lead counselor and possibly the only counselor for the horseback riding portion of this camp; there would be no way for Dr. Foster's child, Dr. Foster, and Barbara not to interact at this camp.

Issues of Concern

Though not yet in place, a potential harmful multiple relationship has arisen between Dr. Foster, Dr. Foster's child, and Dr. Foster's client. Standard 3.05 directs Dr. Foster to resolve the situation "with due regard for the best interest of the affected person." The affected person, for the purpose of Dr. Foster's professional relationship, is Barbara. Withdrawing Dr. Foster's daughter from camp would be in compliance with all elements of the ethics code and would be in the best interest of Barbara. However, a psychologist does not live in the vacuum of the treatment room and it would not be in the best interest of Dr. Foster's home life to disappoint his daughter based on possible harm to a client. The relationship with a client is relatively transient whereas a relationship with a daughter is for life.

Standard 3.05 (b) specifies that the resolution of the situation needs to occur with "due regard for the best interests of the affected person." Though Dr. Foster's daughter does not have a professional relationship with him, she is one of the "affected persons" in this situation.

APA Ethics Code

Companion General Principle

Introduction and Applicability

> This Ethics Code applies only to psychologists' activities that are part of their scientific, educational, or professional roles as psychologists... These activities shall be distinguished from the purely private conduct of psychologists, which is not within the purview of the Ethics Code.

Multiple relationships often involve people who are in the psychologist's private life, as in this vignette with Dr. Foster and his home life.

Principle A: Beneficence and Nonmaleficence

> When conflicts occur among psychologists' obligations or concerns, they attempt to resolve these conflicts in a responsible fashion that avoids or minimizes harm.

Dr. Foster, aspiring to Principle A: Beneficence, would need to consider the situation through the lens of benefiting the client, not necessarily benefiting people in his private life. If he cannot steer a course of action that would be of benefit to Barbara, then he should do something that would, at a minimum, not damage Barbara.

Principle B: Fidelity and Responsibility

> Psychologists establish relationships of trust with those with whom they work.

Psychologists' private lives and personal relationships are not subject to the rules and regulations applied to work relationships. Principle B: Fidelity invites Dr. Foster to act in a trustworthy manner toward his client, Barbara. The aspirational principles are silent on whether his professional relationships, when in conflict with his personal responsibility as a father, should take precedence—that when loyalties are split that a psychologist should choose professional loyalty over personal fidelity to a child.

Principle D: Justice

> Psychologists recognize that fairness and justice entitle all persons to access to and benefit from the contributions of psychology... Psychologists exercise reasonable judgment and take precautions to ensure that their potential biases . . . do not lead to . . . unjust practices.

Principle D cautions psychologists to guard against bias. In this case, there may be bias against Barbara in the service of protecting his young daughter.

Companion Ethical Standard(s)

Standard 3.04: Avoiding Harm

> Psychologists take reasonable steps to avoid harming their clients . . . , and to minimize harm where it is foreseeable and unavoidable.

Standard 3.04 is the enactment of Principle A: Nonmaleficence. In this case, allowing Barbara to discover that Dr. Foster's daughter is attending the camp may not necessarily harm Barbara. However, depending on Dr. Foster's assessment of Barbara, allowing his daughter to be a resident under Barbara's supervision may be harmful to his young daughter. Though Standard 3.04 does not apply to Dr. Foster's relationship with his dependent daughter, the duties and expected inclination of a father is to be protective of one's daughter to assure that no harm comes to her.

Standard 10.10: Terminating Therapy

> . . . (b) Psychologists may terminate therapy when threatened or otherwise endangered by the client/patient or another person with whom the client/patient has a relationship.

One way to follow the guidance of Standard 3.05 (b) is to extricate oneself from the relationship. Depending on Dr. Foster's assessment of Barbara, he may consider his daughter to be endangered by the multiple relationship of Barbara being his client and camp counselor to his daughter. Since it is not reasonable to expect Dr. Foster to extricate himself from his relationship with his daughter, the other course of action open to him is to extricate himself from his relationship with Barbara. The consideration for termination with

Barbara is the risk of violating Standard 3.04 with the possibility that Barbara may feel abandoned, thus harmed.

Legal Issues 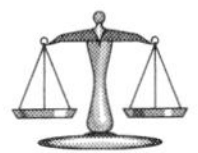

Michigan

Mich. Admin. Code r. 338.2515 (2010). Prohibited conduct.

> Rule 15. Prohibited conduct includes, but is not limited to, the following acts or omissions by any individual covered by these rules:
>
> . . . (b) Involvement in a multiple relationship with a current . . . patient . . . when there is a risk of harm . . . to the patient. As used in this rule, "multiple relationship" means a relationship in which a licensee is in a professional role with an individual and 1 of the following occurs at the same time:
>
> (i) The licensee is in another role with the same individual. (ii) The licensee is in a relationship with an individual closely associated with or related to the individual with whom the licensee has the professional relationship.

North Carolina

21 N.C. Admin. Code 54.1608 (2010). Ethical violations.

> The Board shall use those policies, publications, guidelines, and casebooks developed by the American Psychological Association in determining whether violations of the Ethical Principles of Psychologists have occurred. In addition, publications, guidelines, policies, and statements provided by the Association of State and Provincial Psychology Boards . . . may be used in interpreting the Ethical Principles of Psychologists.

N.C. Gen. Stat. § 90-270.15 (2009). Denial, suspension, or revocation of licenses and health services provider certification, and other disciplinary and remedial actions for violations of the Code of Conduct; relinquishing of license.

> (a) Any . . . person licensed . . . under this Article shall have behaved in conformity with the ethical and professional standards specified in this Code of Conduct and in the rules of the Board.
>
> . . . (10) Has been guilty of immoral, dishonorable, unprofessional, or unethical conduct as defined . . . in the then-current code of ethics of the American Psychological Association, except as the provisions of such code of ethics may be inconsistent and in conflict with the provisions of this Article, in which case, the provisions of this Article control;
>
> (11) Has practiced psychology in such a manner as to endanger the welfare of clients or patients . . .

As defined in Standard 3.05 (b) and under Michigan law, a multiple relationship has arisen. Dr. Foster must take reasonable steps to resolve the multiple relationship, "with due regard for the best interests of the affected person and maximal compliance with the Ethics Code." Standard 3.05 (a) does state that it is not unethical to continue in the multiple relationship if such a relationship would not cause impairment, risk exploitation, or harm a client. So the question for Dr. Foster to address in both jurisdictions is whether harm could occur to Barbara. Dr. Foster would have to assess whether harm would more likely occur if his daughter was withdrawn or continued to attend the camp. The assessment should be written up and checked through a peer consultation to help determine if all the facts were considered and weighed in an appropriate manner.

Cultural Considerations

Global Discussion

Canadian Code of Ethics for Psychologists

> Principle III: Integrity in Relationships.
>
> *Values statement.*
>
> It is the responsibility of psychologists to avoid dual or multiple relationships . . . when appropriate and possible. When such situations cannot be avoided . . . psychologists have a responsibility to declare that they have a conflict of interest, to seek advice, and to establish safeguards to ensure that the best interests of members of the public are protected.
>
> Principle III: Avoidance of conflict of interest.
>
> III.35. Inform all parties, if a . . . conflict of interest arises, of the need to resolve the situation in a manner that is consistent with Respect for the Dignity of Persons . . . and Responsible Caring . . . , and take all reasonable steps to resolve the issue in such a manner.

This situation cannot be avoided and would in fact be "inappropriate" to avoid both because of the potential harm to his client and his own daughter's well-being, provided that both are considered "members of the public" whom the psychologist is obligated to protect. It is unclear from this section of code if the daughter here has the same rights as the psychologists' client.

American Moral Values

1. What are the important conflicts between Dr. Foster's roles of therapist and father? Will allowing his daughter to attend Barbara's camp serve either person?
2. How would withdrawing his daughter affect Dr. Foster's work with Barbara? Should one consider the effect of Barbara finding out about the withdrawal? Would she interpret this as a lack of confidence in her abilities as a counselor?
3. How does Barbara being the only counselor affect Dr. Foster's decision? Is Barbara competent enough to run a camp for teens?
4. How will withdrawing affect Dr. Foster's relationship with his daughter? Is this important enough for the daughter that she would hold it against Dr. Foster for a long time? Does his daughter understand his work as clinician? Does this situation require that Dr. Foster explain more of what his job entails to her?
5. Would it be preferable to end treatment with Barbara, since client relationships are more temporary than family ties? Would Barbara treat his daughter worse at the camp because of his ending treatment?

Ethical Course of Action

Directive Per APA Code

As defined in Standard 3.05 (b), a multiple relationship has arisen, certainly due to unforeseen factors that are outside of Dr. Foster's control or influence. Standard 3.05 directs Dr. Foster to takes reasonable steps to resolve the multiple relationship, "with due regard for the best interests of the affected person and maximal compliance with the Ethics Code." If we interpret the parameters of "affected person" broadly, then we could include Dr. Foster's daughter as one of the affected person(s) in this situation.

Standard 3.05 (a) does state that it is not unethical to continue in the multiple relationship if such a relationship would not cause impairment, risk exploitation, or harm a client. If Dr. Foster decides that the risk of his daughter having a bad experience at camp due to Barbara's mishandling of any potential situation is limited or negligible, he could decide to allow the situation to go forward and unfold without his intervention.

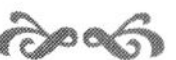

Dictates of One's Own Conscience

If you were in a similar situation as Dr. Foster—you had paid a thousand dollars for this summer camp and you did not want to negatively impact your daughter's life—what would you do?

1. Do nothing; let events unfold and hope for the best.
2. Explain the situation to your spouse; say that it is best if Barbara does not learn of the relationship between Dr. Foster and one of the campers, thus your spouse would handle all interactions and attend all parent functions during summer camp.
3. Terminate treatment with Barbara to avoid the multiple relationship.
4. Tell your daughter that she cannot go to camp, and try to make it up to her in some other way.
5. Do a combination of the previously listed actions.
6. Do something that is not previously listed.

If you were Dr. Foster practicing in Canada, to satisfy the dictates of the Canadian code, you must declare a conflict of interest, possibly with a supervisor or outside uninterested consulting psychologist, seek advice, and establish safeguards for all concerned: himself, his client, and his child.

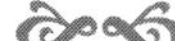

STANDARD 3.05: MULTIPLE RELATIONSHIPS

> . . . (c) When psychologists are required by law, institutional policy, or extraordinary circumstances to serve in more than one role in judicial or administrative proceedings, at the outset they clarify role expectations and the extent of confidentiality and thereafter as changes occur.

A CASE FOR STANDARD 3.05 (C): The Two Selves

Dr. Gonzales volunteers as an examiner for the state's licensing oral examinations. This year she is with a team of four psychologists, all male. Dr. Bryant is the team leader. Over the course of the day, Dr. Gonzales noticed herself being cut off by Dr. Bryant and outvoted at every turn. In one incident, Dr. Gonzales thought the team was excessively harsh toward a nonwhite immigrant applicant. Dr. Gonzales wondered if racial bias may have been a factor in the team's 4 to 1 vote to deny licensure. Later in the day, the team members seemed excessively conciliatory with a tearful attractive white female applicant who clearly did not know state law. Dr. Bryant and the other members said, "She was so nervous and tearful that she could not think straight. I am sure that she knows the state law." The vote was again 4 to 1, this time to grant her licensure. Over the course of the next few weeks, Dr. Gonzales became increasingly distressed as she considered the implications and consequences of the oral examination. Eventually Dr. Gonzales decided to write a letter of complaint to the state department regarding the apparent racial and gender biases exhibited by the oral examination team.

Earlier in the year, Dr. Gonzales had applied for a seat in the state's licensing board. Knowing that the government and the governor's office takes months to decide on board members, Dr. Gonzales went on with her work without much thought about the fate of her application. A month after the oral examination incident, Dr. Gonzales received an appointment letter to the psychology licensing board. The appointment team was unaware of the complaint letter. The investigation team was unaware of Dr. Gonzales's appointment to the psychology board of licensing.

Since Dr. Gonzales's complaint letter involved the oral examination process, it meant that every one of the board members was accused of engaging in wrongful conduct. When the investigative team reported this case to the board as a whole, Dr. Gonzales found herself in the unlikely position of being both the accuser and the defendant of racial and gender discrimination charges.

Issues of Concern

A multiple relationship occurs, as defined in Standard 3.05 (c), when one person serves in two different roles. In this particular case, Dr. Gonzales is in the difficult position of being both the protector of psychologists against institutional authority through her act of a written a letter of complaint, as well as the representative of the institutional authority from whom psychologists must be protected in her role as a board member. By definition, Dr. Gonzales is now in a multiple relationship. Standard 3.05 (c) does not require that Dr. Gonzales extricate herself from the situation. Instead, Dr. Gonzales is required to clarify "role expectations." What is her role as the person who is accusing the state board of racial discrimination? What is her role as a board member charged with oversight of the investigation? What is her role as a board member who may need to defend herself against an accusation of racial discrimination?

APA Ethics Code

Companion General Principle

Principle B: Fidelity and Responsibility

> They [Psychologists] are aware of their professional . . . responsibilities to society and to the specific communities in which they work. Psychologists uphold professional standards of conduct, clarify their professional roles and obligations, accept appropriate responsibility for their behavior, and seek to manage conflicts of interest that could lead to exploitation or harm . . . They are concerned about the ethical compliance of their colleagues' scientific and professional conduct.

As a member of the board of licensure, Principle B: Fidelity and Responsibility guides Dr. Gonzales to be aware of her professional responsibility to society. As specified in Principle B, these responsibilities include protecting the public from incompetence, such as by not awarding licenses to those who are not competent; concern about nonethical behavior of other psychologists, as in filing complaints when there is evidence of racial and gender discrimination; and clarifying role responsibilities.

Principle D: Justice

> Psychologists recognize that fairness and justice entitle all persons to access to and benefit from the contributions of psychology and to equal quality in the processes, procedures, and services being conducted by psychologists.

Principle D: Justice underlies and supports Dr. Gonzales's decision to write a letter of complaint in response to what appeared to be evidence of racial and gender discrimination.

Companion Ethical Standard(s)

Standard 3.01: Unfair Discrimination

> In their work-related activities, psychologists do not engage in unfair discrimination based on . . . race.

Standard 3.01 is the companion to Principle D. Both Principle D and Standard 3.01 require that Dr. Gonzales not engage in discrimination that is based on a person's status. In the oral examination, it appeared that the other examining team members may have been voting based on the applicant's race and sex.

Standard 1.05: Reporting Ethical Violations

> If an apparent ethical violation has substantially harmed . . . a person . . . and is not appropriate for informal resolution . . . or is not resolved properly in that fashion, psychologists take further action appropriate to the situation.

Standard 1.05 directs Dr. Gonzales to "take further action appropriate to the situation" when she determined that the examination team may have been unfairly discriminatory to the two applicants. It is reasonable to assume that Dr. Gonzales voiced her opinion to the other oral examination team members and obviously voiced her objection by registering the dissenting vote. These informal interventions were not sufficient to have prevented the possible harm of not granting license to someone who was probably competent and granting license to someone who may have not been competent. As directed by Standard 1.05, Dr. Gonzales took further action by filing a letter of complaint.

Legal Issues 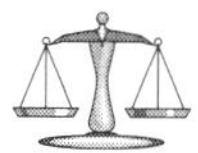

Pennsylvania

> *49 Pa. Code § 41.61 (2010). Code of Ethics.*
>
> Principle 6. Welfare of the consumer.
>
> (a) Psychologists respect the integrity and protect the welfare of the people and groups with whom they work
>
> . . . (b) Psychologists are continually cognizant of their . . . inherently powerful position . . . in order to avoid exploiting their trust and dependency. Psychologists make every effort to avoid dual relationships.

Oregon

> *Or. Admin. R. 858-010-0075 (2010). Code of professional conduct.*
>
> The Board adopts for the code of professional conduct of psychologists in Oregon the American Psychological Association's "Ethical Principles of Psychologists and Code of Conduct" effective June 1, 2002.

In both jurisdictions, Dr. Gonzales must clarify role expectations upon appointment to the licensing board, and the conflicting roles that will emerge because of her complaint against members of the licensing board for their behavior during oral examinations. In light of due process rights of those that are accused, Dr. Gonzales should recuse herself as one of the hearing examiners regarding the complaint, if asked to serve in such a role.

Cultural Considerations

Global Discussion

Code of Ethics for the Psychologist: Spain

> ***Article 15.*** When faced with a conflict between personal and institutional interests, psychologists must strive to act with the greatest impartiality. Providing their services in institutions does not exempt psychologists from giving consideration, respect and attention to individuals who may come into conflict with the institution itself and for whom the psychologist, whenever it is legitimate, must be their protector before institutional authorities.

If Dr. Gonzales was in Spain, she would not be in violation of Article 15 of this code. In fact, because she acted as a "protector" of the minority applicant by voting and speaking against what she believed to be a biased decision, and next, by filing a formal complaint against proceedings she deemed unjust, Dr. Gonzales has acted to uphold the intent and letter of this portion of Spanish code. Article 15 mandates that psychologists who provide services in institutions not exempt their duty toward individuals, which is to "give consideration . . . attention" to those who conflict with an institution in which a psychologist is working. Dr. Gonzales has upheld this portion of the Spanish code.

American Moral Values

1. How does Dr. Gonzales view her relationships with the board as accuser and defendant? Was her application to join the board hypocritical in light of her complaint, or did she wish to join precisely because of what she experienced during the oral examination, as well as her determination to attempt to change the process as a member of the board?
2. How will the board formally respond to this complaint? Will Dr. Gonzales have to recuse herself from contributing as a hearing examiner or as a witness? Will her decision depend upon whether a third party is called in to judge the complaint or serve as other

witnesses to the discriminatory behavior that was alleged to have occurred throughout the examinations?

3. Can Dr. Gonzales develop more skills at working efficaciously with racial bias by participating on the board than she could through filing and pursuing the complaint? Given the licensing board's larger role in writing laws and determining policy pertaining to psychologists, will this complaint undercut her future influence on such laws? Will the complaint erode trust among Dr. Gonzales and her colleagues? Should she explain her complaint to the rest of the board before they take it up formally, just to clear the air?

4. Does Dr. Gonzales's appointment to the board demonstrate a willingness to hear her perspectives on bias? If she fails to pursue the complaint, will she appear to have made it in order to join the board or at least obtain attention? Does she have to pursue it doggedly in order to maintain her integrity? Or will the prosecution of the complaint lead others to think she wants to oust current board members and put more members who may be on her side on the board? Will it look like a political ploy?

5. Should Dr. Gonzales fight against the specific denials of licensure delivered to the people of color she helped to interview? Or should she argue more generally against oral examinations, given how entrenched biases could skew their evaluation? Will that benefit candidates of color? Are there other considerations for oral exams that might prevent her from doing that?

Ethical Course of Action

Directive per APA Code

Standard 3.05 (c) requires that Dr. Gonzales clarify role expectations. Since the other board members are also psychologists, Standard 3.05 (c) also applies to them. Thus, Standard 3.05 (c) requires that everyone who is serving on the board clarify their role in relationship to the complaint and to Dr. Gonzales. Standard 3.05 (c) does not specify actions beyond clarification.

Dictates of One's Own Conscience

If you were either Dr. Gonzales or the department of licensing and found yourself in such an extraordinary circumstance, what do you think you would do?

1. As Dr. Gonzales:
    a. Consult with the state's attorney general's office for advice about how best to proceed.
    b. Recuse yourself from the proceedings in regards to the case in which you filed the complaint.
    c. Withdraw from membership on the board entirely.
2. As the state:
    a. Consult with the state's attorney general's office for advice about how best to proceed.
    b. Excuse Dr. Gonzales from involvement in the case except as a witness.
    c. Excuse all members who were sitting on the board at the time of the complaint so that the complaint can be fairly prosecuted.
    d. Ask Dr. Gonzales to withdraw from the board until the complaint is settled.
3. Do a combination of the previously listed actions.
4. Do something that is not previously listed.

If you were Dr. Gonzales serving in Spain, you would not face such a conflict since you have acted according to the Spanish code.

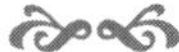

STANDARD 3.06: CONFLICT OF INTEREST

Psychologists refrain from taking on a professional role when personal, scientific, professional, legal, financial, or other interests or relationships could reasonably be expected to (1) impair their objectivity, competence, or effectiveness in performing their functions as psychologists or (2) expose the person or organization with whom the professional relationship exists to harm or exploitation.

A CASE FOR STANDARD 3.06: Uninvited Solicitations

Dr. Castillo specializes in treating anxiety, including phobias. She has successfully treated her client Jennifer, who worked as a cashier, for a phobia regarding handling money secondary to being robbed at gunpoint while at her workplace. Treatment is now progressing to other workplace anxieties. Jennifer appeared excited in session one day, asking Dr. Castillo to help prepare her to speak in public because through work she has been selected to be on a reality TV show that simulates and reenacts the robbery. The reenactment will be followed by interviews to discuss her recovery process, including her therapeutic work with Dr. Castillo.

Issues of Concern

Standard 3.06 would guide Dr. Castillo to refrain from taking on a dual professional–clinical role. Dr. Castillo is currently the treating psychologist for Jennifer. In this case, it appears that Dr. Castillo has unwittingly taken on the role of the treating psychologist for a reality TV show participant. If Jennifer performs well in the TV show, then the public perception of psychologists and treatment would be enhanced. If Jennifer specifically names Dr. Castillo, depending on Jennifer's performance, Dr. Castillo's stance and treatment with Jennifer will be affected regardless of whether Dr. Castillo accepts or declines being named as the treating psychologist for the show.

APA Ethics Code

Companion General Principle

Principle A: Beneficence and Nonmaleficence

> In their professional actions, psychologists seek to safeguard the welfare and rights of those with whom they interact professionally. . . Because psychologists' . . . professional judgments and actions may affect the lives of others, they are alert to and guard against personal, financial . . . factors that might lead to misuse of their influence.

Dr. Castillo, aspiring to the highest ideas of Principle A: Beneficence and Nonmaleficence, would be guided to help Jennifer examine the feasibility and advisability of entering into a reality TV show to reenact her traumatic robbery. Dr. Castillo is called upon to help Jennifer critically examine her options, regardless of the potential impact of Dr. Castillo's practice.

Principle B: Fidelity and Responsibility

> Psychologists . . . clarify their professional roles and obligations, accept appropriate responsibility for their behavior, and seek to manage conflicts of interest that could lead to exploitation or harm.

Principle B guides Dr. Castillo to clarify her role with Jennifer as they proceed into the journey of Jennifer appearing on a national reality TV show. Is Dr. Castillo, as the treating psychologist, guaranteed privacy? Is Dr. Castillo the consulting psychologist to a TV show, with understanding that confidentiality is not a privilege?

Principle E: Respect for People's Rights and Dignity

> Psychologists respect the . . . rights of individuals to . . . self-determination.

Regardless of what Dr. Castillo thinks of reality TV shows, or of the advisability of Jennifer's participation in such a venture, or of her own potential to gain, Principle E guides Dr. Castillo to respect whatever decision Jennifer ultimately makes in regards to her participation in the reality TV show.

Companion Ethical Standard(s)

Standard 5.05: Testimonials

> Psychologists do not solicit testimonials from current therapy clients.

Jennifer may feel exceptionally grateful to Dr. Castillo for having helped her through the traumatic recovery from being threatened at gunpoint. This state of gratitude makes Jennifer vulnerable to making positive public testimonials about Dr. Castillo. Given the circumstances of being on a national TV show talking about her trauma and recovery, it would be an easy step to suggest that Jennifer say only positive things about Dr. Castillo. Regardless of how Dr. Castillo makes the suggestion, encouraging Jennifer's participation may be regarded as a solicitation for a testimonial, thus violating the directive of Standard 5.05.

Standard 3.08: Exploitative Relationships

> Psychologists do not exploit persons over whom they have . . . authority such as clients.

Dr. Castillo may inadvertently exploit this relationship, thus violating Standard 3.08, if she reacts with excitement and encourages Jennifer to give a testimonial on TV about her positive experience in treatment with Dr. Castillo.

Standard 4.02: Discussing the Limits of Confidentiality

> (a) Psychologists discuss with . . . [those] they establish a . . . professional relationship (1) the relevant limits of

> confidentiality and (2) the foreseeable uses of the information generated through their psychological activities. (b) . . . the discussion of confidentiality occurs at the outset of the relationship and thereafter as new circumstances may warrant.

Standard 4.02 directs Dr. Castillo to now hold another conversation with Jennifer about confidentiality since "new circumstances" now warrant such a discussion.

Standard 2.01: Boundaries of Competence

> (a) Psychologists provide services . . . in areas only within the boundaries of their competence, based on their education, training, supervised experience, consultation, study, or professional experience. (c) Psychologists planning to provide services . . . new to them undertake relevant education, training, supervised experience, consultation, or study.

If Dr. Castillo is like most psychologists, she has not had special training or knowledge of how public media conducts business; thus the expected and foreseeable problems Jennifer will encounter are unknown. Combined with Principle A: Beneficence and Nonmaleficence, Dr. Castillo may not be competent to provide services to Jennifer as she prepares for reality TV. If both Jennifer and Dr. Castillo decide the therapeutic relationship should continue, Standard 2.01 (c) directs Dr. Castillo to undertake further study

Legal Issues 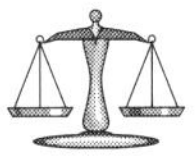

New York

> *N.Y. Comp. Codes R. & Regs. tit. 8, § 29.1 (2010). General provisions.*
>
> a. Unprofessional conduct shall be the conduct prohibited by this section . . .
>
> . . . 12. Advertising or soliciting for patronage that is not in the public interest: . . . iv. Testimonials, demonstrations, dramatizations, or other portrayals of professional practice are permissible provided that they otherwise comply with the rules of professional conduct and further provided that the following conditions are satisfied:
>
> a. the patient . . . expressly authorizes the portrayal in writing;
>
> b. appropriate disclosure is included to prevent any misleading information . . . as to the identity of the patient . . . ;
>
> c. reasonable disclaimers are included as to any statements made or results achieved in a particular matter.

Minnesota

> *Minn. R. 7200.4900 (2010). Client welfare.*
>
> *Subpart 7a. Exploitation of Client.* A psychologist must not exploit in any manner the professional relationship with a client for the psychologist's . . . financial . . . advantage or benefit.

The law of both jurisdictions focuses upon preventing exposure of the client to harm or exploitation due to circumstances in which the psychologist may become involved in conflicting roles. In New York, a specific prohibition exists against testimonials if misleading information may be disseminated. In Minnesota, a more general prohibition against client exploitation exists. In light of Dr. Castillo not being able to control the dissemination of information by the TV producers during the TV show, it is quite possible that if her client participates in the TV program, exploitation may occur.

Cultural Considerations

Global Discussion

Canadian Code of Ethics for Psychologists

> Principle III: Integrity in relationships.
>
> *Values statement.*
>
> As public trust in the discipline of psychology includes trusting that psychologists will act in the best interests of members of the public, situations that present real or potential conflicts of interest are of concern to psychologists. Conflict-of-interest situations are those that can lead to distorted judgment and can motivate psychologists to act in ways that meet their own . . . financial, or business interests at the expense of the best interests of members of the public.
>
> *Avoidance of conflict of interest.*
>
> III.34. Manage dual or multiple relationships that are unavoidable . . . in such a manner that . . . risk of exploitation are minimized. . .
>
> III.35. Inform all parties, if a . . . conflict of interest arises, of the need to resolve the situation in a manner that is consistent with Respect for the Dignity of Persons . . . and Responsible Caring . . . and take all reasonable steps to resolve the issue in such a manner.

If Dr. Castillo and Jennifer were in Canada, the code would require her to inform all parties of the potential conflict of interest. Being transparent about the potential impacts, both positive and negative, on her professional standing as a psychologist, including monetary gains if the outcomes are good, as well as discussing the changing dynamics of their relationship with her client seems indicated by this portion of the code. It can be argued that obtaining ongoing supervision or consultation from an uninterested third party for the duration of the multiple relationship would satisfy this dictate of the Canadian code.

American Moral Values

1. What are the different elements of Jennifer's request to Dr. Castillo? How does the task of helping Jennifer's anxiety for the sake of public speaking relate to the overall TV project and its representation of their therapy work together? How much influence should Dr. Castillo have in Jennifer's decision to appear on the TV show? Or is Dr. Castillo just responsible for not having their therapy work misrepresented?
2. How does this TV project fit into the work Jennifer has done in therapy? Does Dr. Castillo need to share with Jennifer possible concerns about the harm of reenactment? What does Dr. Castillo know about TV shows and their possible aftereffects for people who have done this type of reenactment?
3. How does Jennifer's career background and prospects play into Dr. Castillo's response? Could this be a way for Jennifer to start a career in media? Would this be a less dangerous, less potentially traumatic career choice than being a cashier? Is Jennifer trying to avoid working in a place where she was robbed?
4. Does Dr. Castillo know how Jennifer chose this project? Was she in need of money? Was she preyed upon by producers who convinced her it would be easier than it might be?
5. What will be the impact on other victims of similar trauma who watch Jennifer's profile? Will this be a good model for them? In particular, will it be a good model of resilience for women? Or will it be more exploitative, heightening the drama of violent crime and underscoring Jennifer's victim status?
6. What claims about therapy will be made on the TV program? Will this be a good representation of psychologists and the therapy they provide? Will it function as an advertisement for Dr. Castillo's services? Should she take advantage of that opportunity? Should she avoid any appearance of self-promotion?

Ethical Course of Action

Directive per APA Code

Standard 3.06 directs Dr. Castillo to refrain from taking on a professional role that could either impair objectivity and competence or expose Jennifer to harm or exploitation. Upholding Jennifer's right to self-determination, Principle E guides Dr. Castillo to work toward enabling Jennifer to make such a self-determining decision. One way to refrain from taking on an additional role is for Dr. Castillo to request that Jennifer not mention Dr. Castillo by name but only by her profession of psychologist.

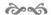

Dictates of One's Own Conscience

If you were in Dr. Castillo's position and someone handed you an opportunity for free publicity on national TV, but this seems to be in conflict with professional ethics, what would you do?

1. Focus solely on the therapeutic implications between you and Jennifer.
2. Focus solely on helping Jennifer make an informed decision about whether to participate in the reality TV show.
3. Tell Jennifer that her ability and desire to participate in such a reenactment is a sign of positive treatment outcome and could be seen as progress.
4. Tell Jennifer that you will work with her on this phobia as you have worked with her on other phobias in the past, and whether Jennifer mentions your name or not, it is her decision.
5. Jokingly say to Jennifer that you have always wondered about how psychologists are involved in consultations to such shows and would be willing to visit the set with Jennifer.
6. With Jennifer's permission, contact the producer of the TV show and introduce yourself as the treating psychologist.
7. Resign your license before the licensing board of your state can act on your behavior, go on the air, advertise yourself as the next Dr. Phil, make buckets of money, and retire quickly.
8. Do a combination of the previously listed actions.
9. Do something that is not previously listed.

If you were Dr. Castillo practicing in Canada, you would most likely proceed with Jennifer's treatment and engage in extra supervision to guard against exploitation of Jennifer in treatment.

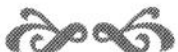

STANDARD 3.07: THIRD-PARTY REQUESTS FOR SERVICES

> When psychologists agree to provide services to a person or entity at the request of a third party, psychologists attempt to clarify at the outset of the service the nature of the relationship with all individuals or organizations involved. This clarification includes the role of the psychologist (e.g., therapist, consultant, diagnostician, or expert witness), an identification of who is the client, the probable uses of the services provided or the information obtained, and the fact that there may be limits to confidentiality.

A CASE FOR STANDARD 3.07: Welfare of Client Versus Welfare System

Ronald is a 32-year-old single white male living by himself with the financial support of his sister, Marilyn. At insistence from his sister, Ronald has applied for public assistance with the state. The state welfare office has referred Ronald to the office of Dr. Russell for a psychological evaluation to determine the nature and extent of Ronald's claim for assistance based on mental illness. The referral is accompanied by a release of information, a payment voucher, and stipulation that the psychological assessment report is sent directly to the welfare office.

Marilyn accompanied Ronald to the assessment sessions. At the beginning of the first appointment, Ronald requested that Marilyn come into the session with him. As the session started with Ronald, Marilyn, and Dr. Russell in the room, Dr. Russell informed Ronald of the fact that the report is requested by, paid for, and will be sent directly to the welfare office. Ronald responded with "OK" and signed all of the necessary consent and release forms.

After several days of extensive assessment, which includes a clinical interview, history, Minnesota Multiphasic Personality Inventory (MMPI), Wechsler Adult Intelligence Scale-IV (WAIS-IV), and the Rotter Incomplete Sentence Blank, Ronald was told again that the report would go to the welfare office. Upon hearing this, Ronald said he did not want the welfare office to know anything because "they are nosy and evil people who do whatever Marilyn says."

Dr. Russell informed Marilyn, who had transported Ronald to the sessions, and the welfare office that the assessment confirms the diagnosis of schizophrenia but that Ronald had rescinded his consent for release of the assessment report.

Issues of Concern

Standard 3.07 directs Dr. Russell to have clarified his role and the limits of confidentiality, which was indeed done. The conflict here is primarily focused on the identification of who is the client—whether it is Ronald or the state welfare office. It is doubtful that Dr. Russell would have proceeded with the assessment had Ronald not initially agreed and signed a release allowing the assessment report to be sent to the state welfare office. However, once the work is done and the state welfare office is the payor, how will Dr. Russell be reimbursed for his time and work if the report is not sent?

APA Ethics Code

Companion General Principle

Principle E: Respect for People's Rights and Dignity

> Psychologists respect . . . the rights of individuals to privacy, confidentiality, and self-determination. Psychologists are aware that special safeguards may be necessary to protect the rights and welfare of persons . . . whose vulnerabilities impair autonomous decision making.

Principle E affirms that psychologists believe in the right of self-determination for all people. The application of that right in the case of Ronald would be for Dr. Russell to affirm Ronald's right to give and then to rescind permission for release of assessment results. Principle E goes on to give guidance for those situations where, similarly to Ronald, the individual whose mental illness impairs their ability for autonomous decision making. If Ronald rescinds consent based on paranoid delusions, Principle E would guide Dr. Russell to enact safeguards to protect Ronald's welfare. Those safeguards may include affirming the signed documents and disregarding Ronald's verbal claim to rescind.

Principle B: Fidelity and Responsibility

> Psychologists . . . clarify their professional roles and obligations, accept appropriate responsibility for their behavior, and seek to manage conflicts of interest that could lead to exploitation or harm.

Principle B guides Dr. Russell to clarify his role in relationship to Ronald, Marilyn, and the state welfare office.

Companion Ethical Standard(s)

Standard 3.10: Informed Consent

> (a) When psychologists . . . provide assessment . . . they obtain the informed consent of the individual . . . except when conducting such activities without consent is mandated by law or governmental regulation or as otherwise provided in this Ethics Code.
>
> . . . (b) For persons who are legally incapable of giving informed consent, psychologists nevertheless . . .
>
> . . . (1) provide an appropriate explanation, . . . (2) seek the individual's assent, . . . (3) consider such persons' preferences and best interests, and (4) obtain appropriate permission from a legally authorized person, if such substitute consent is permitted or required by law.

Standard 3.10 defines the application of Principle E, where psychologists affirm people's right to self-determination through giving consent to engage in the assessment. At the beginning of the assessment, Dr. Russell followed the directives of Standard 3.10 (a). At the end of the assessment, once determined that Ronald may be paranoid, Standard 3.10 (b) may give guidance for Dr. Russell's response to Ronald rescinding permission for release of assessment results.

Standard 9.03: Informed Consent in Assessments

> (a) Psychologists obtain informed consent for assessments, . . . except when . . . (3) one purpose of the testing is to evaluate decisional capacity.
>
> . . . (b) Psychologists inform persons with questionable capacity to consent . . . about the nature and purpose of the proposed assessment services, using language that is reasonably understandable to the person being assessed.

As directed by Standard 9.03, Dr. Russell obtained informed consent as evidenced by Ronald's signature on the consent forms. However, as allowed by Standard 9.03 (a) (2) and 9.03 (a) (3), it is possible that Dr. Russell did not necessarily need Ronald's consent to conduct and release the assessment report.

Standard 4.01: Maintaining Confidentiality

> Psychologists have a primary obligation and take reasonable precautions to protect confidential information obtained through . . . any medium, recognizing that the extent and limits of confidentiality may be regulated by . . . professional . . . relationship.

Standard 4.01 directs Dr. Russell to be responsible for keeping all the information gathered in the assessment process confidential.

Standard 6.01: Documentation of Professional and Scientific Work and Maintenance of Records

> Psychologists . . . disseminate . . . records and data relating to their professional and scientific work in order to (1) facilitate provision of services . . . by other professionals.

Standard 6.01 directs Dr. Russell to be responsible for dissemination of the data and psychological report generated by his assessment of Ronald. Thus it is Dr. Russell's decision to make as to whether to release the assessment report to the state welfare office.

Standard 4.02: Discussing the Limits of Confidentiality

> (a) Psychologists discuss with persons (including, to the extent feasible, persons who are legally incapable of giving informed consent and their legal representatives) and organizations with whom they establish a . . . professional relationship. . .
>
> . . . (1) the relevant limits of confidentiality and . . . (2) the foreseeable uses of the information generated through their psychological activities.
>
> . . . (b) Unless it is not feasible or is contraindicated, the discussion of confidentiality occurs at the outset of the relationship and thereafter as new circumstances may warrant.

As directed in Standard 4.02 (a), Dr. Russell informed Ronald (considered the person who may be legally incapable of giving informed consent) in the presence of his sister Marilyn (considered the legal representative) of the limits of confidentiality. The discussion was done at the beginning of the assessment process as directed by Standard 4.02 (b).

Legal Issues 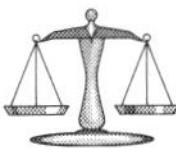

Florida

Fla. Admin. Code Ann. r. 64B19-19.006 (2010). Confidentiality.

. . . (2) In cases where an evaluation is performed upon a person by a psychologist for use by a third party, the psychologist must explain to the person being evaluated the limits of confidentiality in that specific situation, document that such information was explained and understood by the person being evaluated, and obtain written informed consent to all aspects of the testing and evaluative procedures.

Illinois

Ill. Admin. Code tit. 68, § 1400.80 (2010). Unethical, unauthorized, or unprofessional conduct.

The Department may . . . take . . . disciplinary action, based upon its finding of "unethical, unauthorized, or unprofessional conduct" . . . to include, but is not limited to, the following acts or practices:

. . . b) Revealing . . . information relating to a client . . . , except as allowed under Section 5 of the Act or under the Mental Health and Developmental Disabilities Confidentiality Act [740 ILCS 110]. The release of information "with the expressed consent of the client" as provided for in Section 6 of the Act is interpreted to mean that the psychologist, prior to the release of the information, obtained written consent and made certain that the client understood the possible uses or distributions of the information.

It appears that Florida law would permit the release of the evaluation results to the welfare office even though Ronald expressly revoked his consent to release the evaluation results. In Illinois, such an expressed revocation would preclude Dr Russell from releasing the results.

Cultural Global Considerations

Global Discussion

The Professional Board for Psychology Health Professions Council of South Africa: Ethical Code of Professional Conduct (April 2002)

2.6.1. Third-Party Requests for Service.

2.8.1. If there is a foreseeable risk of the psychologist's being called upon to perform conflicting roles because of the involvement of a third party, the psychologist shall clarify the nature and direction of her responsibilities, keep all parties appropriately informed as matters develop, and resolve the situation in accordance with the Code.

At play here are issues involving client autonomy, a client's right to refuse services, and the sister's right to avail herself and her brother of whatever resources can be legally and fairly qualified for by virtue of her brother's mental illness. Although Dr. Russell did clarify both role and limits of confidentiality at the outset of the relationship and again once the report had been completed, now that Ronald has rescinded his consent to the release of the report, Dr. Russell is in a conflicting role. Because Dr. Russell agreed to perform an evaluation requested by and paid for by the state, it is likely that they, the state, are the client, not Ronald; therefore, the psychologist could decide that the "nature and direction of his responsibilities" toward his client, the state, would require him to release the final report to them, as he had gained consent from Ronald at the outset of the evaluation.

American Moral Values

1. How does Dr. Russell judge Ronald's consent? How does Ronald's final objection relate to his previous agreement with the conditions of the evaluation? Does it deserve to be honored?

2. What is Dr. Russell's moral obligation to the welfare office? Do the disclosures for the evaluations include an obligation to report to this office? Does Dr. Russell believe the welfare office is part of a government institution that deserves respect? Does Dr. Russell fear repercussions to his own career from violating these conditions of serving in a subcontractor role with the welfare office? Does the office paying for the service change Dr. Russell's obligation? Should Dr. Russell refuse the payment voucher if he refuses to release the report?

3. Does Ronald's specific diagnosis of schizophrenia affect one's moral relationship to Ronald? Are Ronald's words more a symptom than a deliberate wish? Does one have a therapeutic responsibility to see Ronald's condition treated? How will that treatment relate to Ronald's welfare application?

4. Does Dr. Russell take confidentiality to be more important than third-party requests? Does Ronald's relationship as a client, no matter the conditions stated at the beginning, establish a right to confidentiality that can override those conditions? Is that based on

Ronald's wish or Dr. Russell's concern for what the welfare office might do with his diagnosis? Does Dr. Russell believe that acting against Ronald's wishes will threaten his ability to help Ronald?

Ethical Course of Action

Directive per APA Code

Standard 3.07 directs Dr. Russell to clarify who the client is. The state is the purchaser and consumer of the assessment report, and these conditions had been explained and agreed to by Ronald; therefore, Dr. Russell can consider the state his client. In terms of confidentiality, given that the assessment is being conducted for the purpose of applying for state welfare, per Standard 9.03 (a), consent to release information is implied. Thus, regardless of Ronald's rescinding permission to release the report, Dr. Russell does not violate ethical standards or aspirational principles if he chooses to send the report to the state welfare office.

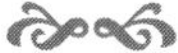

Dictates of One's Own Conscience

It is equally plausible that some psychologists would choose to uphold confidentiality and Ronald's right to self-determination by not releasing the assessment report to the state welfare office. If you were in Dr. Russell's position, what would you do?

1. Say that it is Ronald's right to rescind his permission to release the report, and tell Marilyn that you are sorry but cannot help her any further.
2. Contact the welfare office to say that Ronald has rescinded his permission to release confidential information and that no report will be filed; however, since time was spent by you, you will be cashing the payment voucher.
3. Remind Ronald that he acknowledged both orally and in writing that the report would be released to the welfare office.
4. Provide an oral recitation of the evaluation findings, and ask if Ronald knows of any other information that he would like included in the evaluation report by way of convincing him to reinstate his consent to release an evaluation report.
5. Withhold the report until you can ascertain further the reason for Ronald's refusal. (This is to assure yourself that Ronald is not acting out of the paranoid symptoms of his mental illness.)
6. Persuade Ronald that it is in his own (and his sister's) best interests to release the report to the state, because he has a qualifying diagnosis of schizophrenia and would be entitled to state benefits.
7. Release the results, knowing that the final outcome—hopefully Ronald's qualifying for services through the state—and relieving the financial burden on the sister, is a large enough "good" to justify what may be seen as a violation of Ronald's autonomy and rights to confidentiality.
8. Do a combination of the previously listed actions.
9. Do something that is not previously listed.

If you were Dr. Russell practicing in South Africa, nothing prohibits you from releasing the full report to the state welfare office.

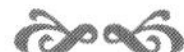

STANDARD 3.08: EXPLOITATIVE RELATIONSHIPS

Psychologists do not exploit persons over whom they have supervisory, evaluative, or other authority such as clients/patients, students, supervisees, research participants, and employees.

A CASE FOR STANDARD 3.08: The Seduction

Dr. Griffin works as clinical psychology faculty at a local university. One of his students, Brenda, is especially bright and promises to be an excellent clinical psychologist. Brenda is near the end of her studies and will be graduating very soon. Brenda already holds a license to practice as a mental health professional at the MA level. Dr. Griffin is opening a new office and Brenda accepted his invitation to sublease office space from him.

Brenda is having significant trouble in her marriage, which she discussed with Dr. Griffin. One day in the office, Brenda confessed that she has been attracted to Dr. Griffin since having him as her professor, and the reason for the failure of her marriage is that she, Brenda, has fallen in love with Dr. Griffin. Upon hearing this confession, Dr. Griffin is flattered. Several weeks later, the chair of the department called Dr. Griffin into her office; Brenda's husband had contacted the university to inquire about filing a formal complaint against Dr. Griffin, as his wife confessed her love for her professor and now current office mate. The husband wanted to know if it is against university policy for a faculty member to seduce a current or former student.

Issues of Concern

It is not unusual for new graduates to turn to their professors for professional networking and at times the sharing of an office suite. Depending on the nature of the invitation, Dr. Griffin could have taken advantage of his access to early career psychologists to obtain sublessees for his office, thus relieving him of the time consuming task of looking for sublessees. Though he is flattered, it is not clear that he has seduced or has thoughts of a romantic relationship with Brenda. Neither is it clear that he has not been subtly grooming Brenda for an affair.

Dr. Griffin needs to address two different audiences, one the university and the other an office sublessee. Standard 3.08 can direct Dr. Griffin's response to both audiences. If Dr. Griffin can demonstrate that he has not exploited Brenda, to both Brenda and her husband as well as to the university, then this incident can be considered one in which Dr. Griffin acted blamelessly.

APA Ethics Code

Companion General Principle

Principle A: Beneficence and Nonmaleficence

> Because psychologists'... actions may affect the lives of others, they are alert to and guard against personal, financial... factors that might lead to misuse of their influence...

Being omniscient regarding one's effects on other's lives is impossible. However, it is probably reasonable to expect Dr. Griffin to have had some inkling of Brenda's feelings for him and have thus predicted her husband's sense of betrayal by her professor.

Principle E: Respect for People's Rights and Dignity

> Psychologists are aware that special safeguards may be necessary to protect the rights and welfare of persons ... whose vulnerabilities impair autonomous decision making...

Aspiring to Principle E, not only are psychologists aware of the need to safeguard against undue influence over their patients but professors also must take special safeguards against the all-too-easy exploitation of their students. In this case, possibly being aware of his positive regard for Brenda or Brenda's positive regard for him, Dr. Griffin should be guided by Principle E to take special safeguards to protect against any semblance of exploitation.

Companion Ethical Standard(s)

Standard 3.05: Multiple Relationships

> (a) A multiple relationship occurs when a psychologist is in a professional role with a person and (1) at the same time is in another role with the same person...
>
> A psychologist refrains from entering into a multiple relationship if the multiple relationship could reasonably... [risk] exploitation or harm to the person with whom the professional relationship exists.
>
> Multiple relationships that would not reasonably be expected to cause impairment or risk exploitation or harm are not unethical.

Being a professor with evaluative authority over Brenda and being Brenda's landlord qualifies as a multiple relationship per Standard 3.05 (a) (1). Standard 3.05 (a) does not specify that multiple relationships are uniformly harmful and thus prohibited. Brenda's husband considered Dr. Griffin's relationship with his wife to have been harmful to him. The more pointed question is whether the relationship was harmful to Brenda and ultimately harmful to Dr. Griffin now that Brenda's husband has filed a complaint with the university.

Standard 3.06: Conflict of Interest

> Psychologists refrain from taking on a professional role when... financial... interests... could reasonably be expected to... (2) expose the person... with whom the professional relationship exists to harm or exploitation.

Standard 3.06 directs Dr. Griffin to have refrained from taking on Brenda as a sublessee, if it could have been reasonably foreseen that such an arrangement could have caused harm. Under most normal circumstances, unless there is something amiss about the office arrangement, such an arrangement would usually be seen as beneficial to the student since the student would be assisted in establishing a practice for him/herself.

Standard 7.07: Sexual Relationships
With Students and Supervisees

> Psychologists do not engage in sexual relationships with students . . . over whom psychologists have or are likely to have evaluative authority . . .

Standard 7.07 is a very clear prohibition against Dr. Griffin engaging in sexual relations with Brenda. At what point does a sexual relationship start? Dr. Griffin's response of being flattered could reasonably be considered as engaging in a romantic relationship with Brenda. Given the undue influence a professor has over a student, anything but a resounding rejection of the profession of love from a student would probably come across to the student as engaging in a romantic relationship.

Legal Issues 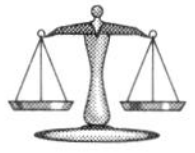

Washington

> *Wash. Admin. Code § 246-924-361 (2009). Exploiting supervisees and research subjects.*
>
> Psychologists shall not exploit persons over whom they have . . . evaluative, or other authority . . .

Pennsylvania

> *49 Pa. Code § 41.61 (2010). Code of ethics.*
>
> Principle 7. Professional Relationships.
>
> . . . (e) Psychologists do not exploit their professional relationships with . . . students. . . Psychologists do not condone or engage in sexual harassment. Sexual harassment is defined as deliberate or repeated comments, gestures or physical contacts of a sexual nature that are unwanted by the recipient.

The law of both jurisdictions precludes exploitation of students, including sexual relationships by their psychologist teachers. When Brenda professed her love for Dr. Griffin, Dr. Griffin must set an unequivocal boundary with Brenda and separate from any other association except the student–teacher relationship. It is quite likely that any other course of action would continue to suggest an appearance of exploitation to the ethics boards of both jurisdictions.

Cultural Considerations

Global Discussion

Code of Ethics for Psychology: Netherlands

> Principle III: Role integrity.
>
> III.1.3.4. Avoidance of mixing professional and non-professional roles.
>
> The psychologist avoids mixing professional and non-professional roles which may influence each other to such an extent that he is not able anymore to maintain his professional detachment towards those involved or that the interests of those involved may be harmed.
>
> III.1.3.5 Refraining from improper promoting of personal interests.
>
> In his professional activities the psychologist refrains from improper furthering of his personal . . . interests.
>
> III.1.3.7 No sexual behaviour towards the client.
>
> The psychologist refrains from sexual advances towards his client and does not comply with such advances from the client's side. He refrains from sexually tinted behaviour or from behaviour which could be seen as such in general.

In the Netherlands, Dr. Griffin would be prohibited from utilizing his students as a source of potential income (vis-à-vis sublessees) by using his professional role as faculty to further his own personal interests (III.1.3.5). Further, he would need to "not comply" with Brenda's sexual advances, although this portion of the code of the Netherlands (III.1.3.7) specifies clients, rather than former students. Dr. Griffin would be considered in violation of the Netherlands code by soliciting Brenda to be his office sublessee, as this clearly furthers his personal gains. Although it is unclear what "not complying" with sexual advances means specifically in this case, it can be argued that continuing to lease space to someone who has revealed romantic feelings and admitting being flattered by these admissions is also in violation of the Netherlands code.

American Moral Values

1. How does Dr. Griffin judge his current relationship with Brenda? Does Brenda's confession make it possible to have a collegial relationship while Brenda subleases space? Does that change how Dr. Griffin regards her acceptance of his invitation?

2. How should Dr. Griffin handle his own feelings of flattery about Brenda's confession? Has he confronted any feelings on his end that could complicate their professional relationship?

3. How does Dr. Griffin judge his past relationship with Brenda as her instructor? What was the nature of his invitation to Brenda? Was this just a chance to help an up-and-coming psychologist, one whose association with Dr. Griffin could help both of their careers? Did Brenda feel coerced to sublease for the sake of her career?

4. How will Dr. Griffin handle the husband's complaint? Will he share information that Brenda gave him in her "confession"?

Ethical Course of Action

Directive per APA Code

If Dr. Griffin had any inclinations of greater than normal positive regard for Brenda, Standard 3.08 directs him to have not invited her to sublease from him. Now that Brenda has professed her love for him, Standards 3.08 and 7.07 directs Dr. Griffin to disengage himself from Brenda. Dr. Griffin would do well to indicate such to the chair of his department at the university and proceed to enact the directive of Standards 3.08 and 7.07 by separating himself from Brenda.

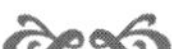

Dictates of One's Own Conscience

It is quite possible that Dr. Griffin may not wish to take such draconian measures in a reactionary response to Brenda's husband. Not knowing the nature of the marital discord, disengaging from Brenda so immediately and completely may cause excessive harm to Brenda. If you were in Dr. Griffin's position, what would you do?

1. Talk with the chair of the department to find out the exact nature of the complaint and then talk to Brenda.

2. Talk to an attorney to find out if the university has any right to concern themselves with Brenda's marital problems.

3. Invite Brenda to start looking for another office after explaining the complaint lodged by her husband against you with the university.

4. Among the numerous potential office mates available, you admit it was an obvious mistake to choose someone over whom you have academic authority and apologize to Brenda and her husband.

5. Sympathize with Brenda and consider that Brenda had good reason for a problematic marriage given that her husband's action regarding the complaint is ample evidence of his meanness by blaming you for his marital problems and then maliciously making trouble for you.

6. Tell the chair that the assertion by Brenda's husband is groundless and the ranting of a rejected husband.

7. Do a combination of the previously listed actions.

8. Do something that is not previously listed.

If you were Dr. Griffin teaching and practicing in the Netherlands, the Netherlands code would have you admit it was an obvious mistake to choose someone over whom you have academic authority, and invite Brenda to start looking for another office.

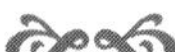

STANDARD 3.09: COOPERATION WITH OTHER PROFESSIONALS

When indicated and professionally appropriate, psychologists cooperate with other professionals in order to serve their clients/patients effectively and appropriately.

A CASE FOR STANDARD 3.09: Protecting the Public

Dr. Diaz returned a call left on her voice mail from Dr. Hayes, a psychologist who said she has a practice in a city on the East Coast. Upon contact, Dr. Hayes said to Dr. Diaz, "I gave your name and one other psychologist's name to a client of mine who moved to your city last week. I told him to give you, or the other psychologist, a call as soon as he arrives in town. I want you to know that he is a sexual predator. He ended treatment as soon as he told me he is afraid that he is attracted to and sexually aroused by little girls. He is extremely slippery, and for the sake of everyone, would you please contact me and discuss the case with me as you progress with treatment? His name is Chad ___."

A week after the conversation with Dr. Hayes, Dr. Diaz received a call from Chad requesting treatment.

Issues of Concern

Standard 3.09 directs Dr. Diaz to cooperate with Dr. Hayes in order to serve Chad. In the absence of a patient or a signed release of information, it appears that Dr. Hayes may have been overly eager to protect the public from a possible predator and has violated Chad's confidentiality. If Dr. Hayes has a signed release of information for both referred psychologists, would this allow Dr. Hayes to contact Dr. Diaz and disclose confidential information during the phone call but prior to Chad contacting Dr. Diaz?

Once Chad contacted Dr. Diaz, Standard 3.09's directive is for her to cooperate with Dr. Hayes. Standard 3.09 does not specify the nature of that cooperation. On one extreme, should Dr. Diaz contact Dr. Hayes to obtain further information and engage in peer consultation regarding the best course of treatment for Chad? On the other extreme, should Dr. Diaz's collaboration only extend to obtaining records with an appropriate signed release of information? Or, having received the relevant information already, might Dr. Diaz choose not to contact Dr. Hayes now?

Can Dr. Diaz provide services to this client (assuming she can remain unbiased and is competent to work with him) despite the unethical nature of the referral?

Did Dr. Hayes violate her patient's confidentiality by telling his name and issue to another therapist without his consent?

APA Ethics Code

Companion General Principle

Principle B: Fidelity and Responsibility

> Psychologists establish relationships of trust with those with whom they work. They are aware of their professional . . . responsibilities to society. . . They are concerned about the ethical compliance of their colleagues' . . . professional conduct.

Aspiring to the highest principle of responsibility, Dr. Hayes most probably acted as a responsible citizen with good reason to believe that a dangerous sexual predator will be entering into the city in which Dr. Diaz practices. To the extent that psychologists are members of a larger community, we have a responsibility to protect the public by ensuring that treatment focused on prevention of sexual abuse is provided to Chad. However, by contacting Dr. Diaz in the absence of a confirmed treatment relationship, Dr. Hayes may have violated Chad's privacy.

Aspiring to the highest principle of responsibility, Principle B guides Dr. Diaz to be concerned about Dr. Hayes's possible violation of privacy and confidentiality.

Principle E: Respect for People's Rights and Dignity

> Psychologists respect . . . the rights of individuals to privacy, confidentiality.

Principle E's guide for psychologists to respect Chad's privacy and confidentiality means that Dr. Hayes's contacting of Dr. Diaz in the absence of a confirmed treatment relationship between Dr. Diaz and Chad and without a signed release of confidential information is problematic. Respect for self-determination would guide Dr. Diaz to remember that it is up to Chad to decide whether to contact Dr. Diaz and to decide whether he wants Dr. Diaz to obtain information from Dr. Hayes.

Companion Ethical Standard(s)

Standard 1.04: Informal Resolution of Ethical Violations

> When psychologists believe that there may have been an ethical violation by another psychologist, they attempt to resolve the issue by bringing it to the attention of that individual . . .

Standard 1.04, which asks for the application of aspirational Principle B: Responsibility, directs Dr. Diaz to raise and address the fact that Dr. Hayes has broken confidentiality by giving Dr. Diaz private information without proper consent from the patient and in the absence of Chad having engaged Dr. Diaz to be his treating psychologist.

Standard 2.01: Boundaries of Competence

> (a) Psychologists provide services . . . with populations and in areas only within the boundaries of their competence. . .

Not knowing Dr. Diaz's areas of competency, it may be an inappropriate referral. Should Dr. Diaz not hold competence in treatment of sexual deviance, might Dr. Diaz decline taking Chad on as a patient based solely on information from Dr. Hayes without independent verification of the diagnosis?

Standard 4.01: Maintaining Confidentiality

> Psychologists have a primary obligation and take reasonable precautions to protect confidential information. . .

Standard 4.05: Disclosures

> (a) Psychologists may disclose confidential information with the appropriate consent of the . . . individual client.
>
> . . . b) Psychologists disclose confidential information without the consent of the individual only . . . where permitted by law for a valid purpose such as to . . . (1) provide needed professional services . . . (3) protect . . . others from harm . . .

Per Standard 4.05, in the absence of a confirmed appointment with a referral, discussion of confidential information is not necessary in that Dr. Diaz does not need to know anything about Chad if Chad is not a patient. Simply knowing about Chad's previous clinical history and his whereabouts in her city does not allow Dr. Diaz to affect Chad's behavior if he is not yet her client. Per Standard 4.01, Dr. Hayes has the responsibility to keep Chad's information confidential. And per Standard 4.05, in the absence of an executed release of information, Dr. Hayes could argue that she informed Dr. Diaz of Chad's diagnosis in order to protect Chad, Dr. Diaz, and the public from harm.

Standard 4.06: Consultations

> When consulting with colleagues, psychologists . . . (2) . . . disclose information only to the extent necessary to achieve the purposes of the consultation.

Standard 4.06 does not apply at the initial phone call since Dr. Diaz cannot engage in consultation regarding a patient she does not yet have. Once Dr. Diaz agrees to accept Chad as a patient and she contacts Dr. Hayes, then Standard 4.06 (a) directs both Dr. Diaz and Dr. Hayes to disclose only necessary information

Legal Issues 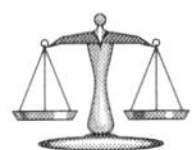

Georgia

> *Ga. Comp. R. & Regs. 510-5-.06 (2010). Welfare of clients and other professional relationships.*
>
> (1) Consultations and Referrals.
>
> (a) Psychologists arrange for appropriate consultations and referrals based principally on the best interests of their client/patients, with appropriate consent, and subject to other relevant considerations, including applicable law and contractual obligations.
>
> . . . (2) Continuity of Care.
>
> (b) Psychologists make reasonable efforts to plan for continuity of care in the event that psychological services are interrupted . . . by the client/patient's relocation . . .

New York

> *N.Y. Comp. Codes R. & Regs. tit. 8, § 29.1 (2010). General provisions.*
>
> . . . b. Unprofessional conduct in the practice of any profession licensed . . . shall include:
>
> . . . 8. revealing of personally identifiable . . . information obtained in a professional capacity without the prior consent of the patient . . . , except as authorized or required by law. . .

Both jurisdictions require Dr. Hayes to obtain appropriate consent from Chad before contacting Dr. Diaz to establish the referral. The law of neither jurisdiction permits violating the confidentiality of Chad in this manner to guard the public against harm.

Cultural Considerations

Global Discussion

Czech-Moravian Psychological Society Code of Ethics

> 4.6. Psychologists approach other psychologists in the spirit of principles of professional cooperativeness, with trust and will to cooperate; they do not diminish each other's professional competence.

A psychologist in Czech-Moravia could satisfy this portion of code by approaching another professional in a "spirit" of professional cooperativeness. If Dr. Diaz refuses Dr. Hayes's request, citing client confidentiality, it could be argued that this would violate this section of code, as it might "diminish" the professional competence of Dr. Hayes to be informed by a colleague that she, Dr. Hayes, has violated her clients' right to confidentiality. However, if Dr. Diaz approaches Dr. Hayes with a "spirit . . . of professional cooperativeness, with trust" one way to approach that would be for Dr. Diaz to assume that Dr. Hayes is correct in her professional assessment of Chad.

American Moral Issues

1. How does Dr. Diaz react to Dr. Hayes's breaking of Chad's confidentiality? Does she need to confront Dr. Hayes's decision before considering whether Chad will be a client?
2. Does Dr. Hayes's diagnosis affect whether Dr. Diaz will take Chad as a client? Does Chad require special therapeutic care with the breach of confidentiality needing to be sorted out later? What if he volunteers right away that he is a sexual predator and confirms Dr. Hayes's account? Does that affect what to do about Dr. Hayes's decision?
3. What if Chad asks Dr. Diaz if Dr. Hayes said anything about him and complains that he doesn't trust Dr. Hayes?
4. How does the case of a sexual predator require different evaluation and treatment than other diagnoses? Would the egregiousness of Chad's actions of sexual violence or the grievous harm done to victims of sexual violence justify Dr. Hayes's special handling of this case?

Ethical Course of Action

Directive per APA Code

Standard 3.09 directs Dr. Diaz to cooperate with Dr. Hayes in the treatment of Chad. In the first phone call when Dr. Diaz had no contact from Chad, it is not a violation of Standard 4.05 for Dr. Diaz to listen to Dr. Hayes. Standard 1.04 directs Dr. Diaz to address Dr. Hayes's breach of confidentiality. Other standards bracket the parameters of cooperation, such as Standard 4.05 to assure privacy and confidentiality and Standard 2.01 to assure that referral to Dr. Diaz was appropriate. It is unclear whether the danger feared by Dr. Hayes justifies setting aside privacy and confidentiality to guard the public against harm from Chad.

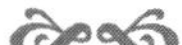

Dictates of One's Own Conscience

In the first phone call, you listen to Dr. Hayes and suggest that it may be more appropriate to hold this conversation if Chad contacts you and appropriate releases of information are signed. If and when you receive the phone call from Chad, what would you do?

1. Tell Chad that you are not taking on new clients at this point. You make this decision based on the fact that you are not competent to treat sexual predators.
2. Hold off making an appointment with Chad and send him an intake packet, including releases to all prior mental health professionals that he must fill out before scheduling the first session. Decide whether to schedule an appointment based upon whether Chad is forthcoming about his history and the identities of prior treatment providers.
3. Make an appointment with Chad and send him an intake packet with release of information for Dr. Hayes. Once the intake packet is received, regardless of whether it is before the appointment or not, then contact Dr. Hayes.
4. Make an appointment with Chad. During the first session, ask Chad whether he signed a release of information for Dr. Hayes to disclose confidential information to you.
5. Make an appointment with Chad. During the first session, tell Chad you have been contacted by Dr. Hayes and discuss the content of the conversation with Dr. Hayes.
6. Make an appointment with Chad, and proceed to conduct your own assessment without mention or regard for information from Dr. Hayes.
7. After you have arrived at the same clinical impression of sexual deviance, then contact Dr. Hayes for consultation.
8. Contact the licensing board in the state in which Dr. Hayes practices to report her breach of confidentiality.
9. Report Chad for child abuse based on the report from Dr. Hayes.
10. Do a combination of the previously listed actions.
11. Do something that is not previously listed.

If and when you receive the phone call from Chad and you were practicing in Czech-Moravia, know that Dr. Hayes contacted you with trust and will to cooperate. Based on Dr. Hayes's information, you take action as mandated by the laws of Czech-Moravia.

STANDARD 3.10: INFORMED CONSENT

(a) When psychologists conduct research or provide assessment, therapy, counseling, or consulting services in person or via electronic transmission or other forms of communication, they obtain the informed consent

> of the individual or individuals using language that is reasonably understandable to that person or persons except when conducting such activities without consent is mandated by law or governmental regulation or as otherwise provided in this Ethics Code.

A CASE FOR STANDARD 3.10 (A): Doing It My Way

Dr. Meyers was contacted by Mrs. Kathryn for family therapy. Mrs. Kathryn's initial contact indicated the family was having school attendance problems with their 12-year-old daughter, Jennifer. Dr. Meyers set up the first appointment with the parents and the two children, Elizabeth and Jennifer.

During the first session, Mrs. Kathryn and Jennifer confirmed that the reason Jennifer does not want to go to school is because she has missing facial hair because she has pulled out eye lashes from her right eye, half of her right eyebrow, and was starting to pull out hairs from the left side. Elizabeth thinks its "gross" that her sister pulls out her eyelashes and eyebrows.

Dr. Meyers informed the family that trichotillomania is a disorder that is not best treated with family therapy but with individual cognitive behavioral therapy (CBT) treatment. Dr. Meyers was very clear with the family that he is not competent to conduct CBT treatment for trichotillomania. Mrs. Kathryn said that CBT had been tried with no success. They had heard that Dr. Meyers is a child psychologist who can do family therapy and that Dr. Meyers has successfully treated the child of a close friend, and they want whatever kind of treatment Dr. Meyers does.

Issues of Concern

Standard 3.10 directs Dr. Meyers to obtain informed consent for treatment. In this case informed consent means that Dr. Meyers needs to inform the family of the recommended best course of treatment for Jennifer's diagnosis and to disclose to the family that he does not provide such treatment. As directed by Standard 3.10, Dr. Meyers informed the family of the standard treatment for trichotillomania and that he is not competent to provide such treatment. The parents are asking for family therapy, which Dr. Meyers *is* competent to provide. If the family acknowledges that the presenting problem is outside the competency area of the psychologist and consents to a modality that is within the competency of that psychologist, does this then constitute informed consent? In other words, has Dr. Meyers complied with the directive of Standard 3.10 and obtained the family's informed consent to proceed with treatment?

APA Ethics Code

Companion General Principle

Principle A: Beneficence and Nonmaleficence

> Psychologists strive to benefit those with whom they work and take care to do no harm.

Principle A guides psychologists to not only do no harm but also be of benefit.

It is likely that family therapy would not harm Jennifer in her management of the symptoms of trichotillomania, but it is unclear as to whether family therapy would benefit Jennifer in the treatment of trichotillomania.

Principle E: Respect for People's Rights and Dignity

> Psychologists respect . . . the rights of individuals to . . . self-determination.

Having been thus informed, Principle E would guide Dr. Meyers to respect the family's right to self-determination and decision regarding which treatment modality to engage for Jennifer. In the case of a minor and a family, Dr. Meyers would need to decide who has the right to self-determination. What if Mrs. Kathryn wishes to engage in family therapy but the daughters do not?

Principle C: Integrity

> Psychologists strive to keep their promises and to avoid unwise or unclear commitments.

Principle C: Integrity would guide Dr. Meyers to consider whether he can follow through with his commitment to provide treatment to this family should he accept the case. If Dr. Meyers accepts this case, is he making a commitment to treat the school truancy, the trichtotillimania, or the family discord? Principle C guides Dr. Meyers to be clear about his commitment to treat this family.

Companion Ethical Standard(s)

Standard 2.01: Boundaries of Competence

> (a) Psychologists provide services . . . in areas only within the boundaries of their competence. . .

Having clearly stated to the family that conducting CBT for the treatment of trichtotillimania is outside his boundary of competence, is Dr. Meyers within reasonable limits of the APA Ethics Code to offer family therapy instead, with which he can be considered competent?

Standard 3.04: Avoiding Harm

> Psychologists take reasonable steps to avoid harming their clients/patients . . . and to minimize harm where it is foreseeable and unavoidable.

Standard 3.04 is the enactment of Principle A. Standard 3.04 directs Dr. Meyers to consider whether proceeding or not proceeding with family therapy will harm the family and ultimately Jennifer.

Legal Issues 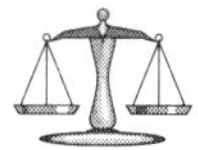

Illinois

> *Ill. Admin. Code tit. 68, § 1400.80 (2010). Unethical, unauthorized, or unprofessional conduct.*
>
> The Department may . . . take . . . disciplinary action, based upon its finding of "unethical, unauthorized, or unprofessional conduct" . . . to include, but is not limited to, the following acts or practices:
>
> . . . k) Pursuant to Section 15(7) of the Act, the Department hereby incorporates by reference the "Ethical Principles of Psychologists and Code of Conduct" American Psychological Association . . .

Maryland

> *Md. Code Ann., Health Occ. § 18-313 (LexisNexis 2009). License denial, suspension, or revocation.*
>
> . . . (20) Does an act that is inconsistent with generally accepted professional standards in the practice of psychology.
>
> *Md. Code Regs. 10.36.05.05 (2010). Representation of services and fees.*
>
> A. Public Statements and Advertising.
>
> (1) A psychologist shall: (a) Represent accurately and objectively the psychologist's professional qualifications, education, experience, and areas of competence;
>
> B. Informed consent.
>
> When conducting . . . psychotherapy, a psychologist shall:
>
> (1) In general.
>
> (a) Obtain informed consent using appropriate language understandable to the client;
>
> (b) Vary appropriate informed consent forms and procedures to ensure that the client:
>
> (i) Has the capacity to consent;
>
> (ii) Has been provided with information concerning participation in the activity that reasonably might affect the willingness to participate . . .
>
> (iii) Is aware of the voluntary nature of participation and has freely and without undue influence expressed consent; and
>
> (iv) Is given the opportunity to ask questions and receive answers regarding the activity;
>
> (3) In therapeutic relationships, explain to the client:
>
> (a) The clarification of reasonable expectations . . .

In both jurisdictions, by providing the family full disclosure about treatment focusing on Jennifer returning to school and further advising that Jennifer's symptoms of trichtotillomania would best be treated by CBT, sufficient disclosure was made. The family was provided the information necessary to select whether to proceed with treatment with Dr. Meyers. As long as Dr. Meyers practices within the boundaries of his competence, he would not engage in unethical behavior.

Cultural Considerations

Global Discussion

Code of Ethical Conduct
Psychologists of New South Wales

> A. Responsibilities to clients, students supervisees and research participants.
>
> 1. Nothing of a psychological nature should be done with, for or to clients . . . without obtaining proper informed and voluntary consent from them. This will involve being willing to explain the nature and purpose of therapy . . . , or any other intervention, the alternatives available. . . If the client does not have this capacity (for example, is a child, . . .) informed consent should be obtained from the person legally responsible for him or her. This could be a parent. . . Withdrawal of consent should always remain possible.

It seems as though this family is competent to provide consent—they understand what their daughter's condition is, they have tried other treatments that have so far proven unsuccessful, and are likely aware of other providers and other available options. It also seems that they are determined to have Dr. Meyers as their treating psychologist for family therapy, even though family therapy is usually not indicated for trichtotillomania. These clients have both the capacity and willingness to give informed consent, according to the New South Wales code.

Dr. Meyers has explained the nature and purpose of therapy, both family and the CBT recommended for the presenting problem; he has clearly stated the limits of his own competence, and the family is assumed to have understood. Therefore, it can be argued that Dr. Meyers has not violated the intent or letter of the New South Wales code. His clients have made a choice that Dr. Meyers does not likely agree with, but this in and of itself does not indicate that he, Dr. Meyers, has failed in his obligation to obtain informed consent.

American Moral Values

1. How does Dr. Meyers weigh the will of the family against the therapeutic needs of Jennifer? Could family therapy supplement CBT for Jennifer? Should Dr. Meyers only do family therapy if someone else treats with Jennifer with CBT? If the parents were to refuse CBT for Jennifer, must Dr. Meyers turn them away? Will Dr. Meyers be able to accept the family's decision to not receive any help at all?

2. How should Dr. Meyers help the parents make the best decision? Are they placing too much hope in Dr. Meyers based on a friend's recommendation? What is Dr. Meyers's obligation to ensure they have reasonable expectations about what family therapy can accomplish? Will the family therapy impede Jennifer's progress with CBT? Or will family therapy address ways for the parents to support Jennifer's struggles?

3. Dr. Meyers has explicitly informed the family about his expertise and his advice for Jennifer, and the family still wants to work in family therapy. At what point does Dr. Meyers need to respect the judgment of the family as he would other families seeking treatment? When is the parents' consent sufficient to proceed with treatment? Does Dr. Meyers expect the therapy to become about more than Jennifer anyway? Should that be made clear to the family?

Ethical Course of Action

Directive per APA Code

Standard 3.10 directs Dr. Meyers to provide his client with sufficient information for them to make an informed decision regarding the best course of action to reach the family's goal of having Jennifer attend school. Standard 2.01 directs Dr. Meyers to practice within the boundaries of his competence. Combining these two standards, with guidance based on Principle E, Dr. Meyers is ethically correct to proceed with family therapy for treatment of school truancy. In such a circumstance, Dr. Meyers would consider Jennifer's symptoms of trichtotillomania as any other difficulties experienced by a family member but not a focus of treatment.

Dictates of One's Own Conscience

Regardless of whether accepting the case for family therapy would be ethical, if you were in Dr. Meyers's situation, what would you do?

1. Be clear to the family that regardless of their wishes you know what they want will not work, thus you decline to accept the family for treatment. You then provide them with a few names of other psychologists for referral.

2. Accept the case, and proceed with family therapy per the request of the family.

3. Accept the case, and seek out consultation and education on treatment of trichotillomania as specified in Standard 2.01 (c), in combination with family therapy.

4. Request that the family sign a release of information for the previous psychologist who treated Jennifer with CBT for the symptoms of trichotillomania, and engage in other forms of behavioral activations than were used by the previous psychologist.

5. Tell the family that you will start a period of assessment that includes gathering of background information from school and previous treatment providers, and that after the assessment period, you would consult with them on the best course of treatment for Jennifer and may refer them to more a appropriate treatment provider at that point.

6. Do a combination of the previously listed actions.

7. Do something that is not previously listed.

If you were Dr. Meyers practicing in New South Wales, the previously listed options would still apply since the guideline for informed consent is not substantially different from those listed by the APA Ethics Code.

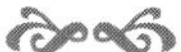

STANDARD 3.10: INFORMED CONSENT

> . . . (b) For persons who are legally incapable of giving informed consent, psychologists nevertheless (1) provide an appropriate explanation, (2) seek the individual's assent, (3) consider such persons' preferences and best interests, and (4) obtain appropriate permission from a legally authorized person, if such substitute consent is permitted or required by law. When consent by a legally authorized person is not permitted or required by law, psychologists take reasonable steps to protect the individual's rights and welfare.

A CASE FOR STANDARD 3.10 (B): The First Manic Episode

Mrs. Kathleen received a call from Jason, roommate of her son Matthew. Two years ago, Matthew left home to attend college in a large city on the East Coast. Last year, Matthew moved out of the college dormitory into an apartment with his friend Jason. Jason told Mrs. Kathleen that he is concerned about Matthew. Matthew had not paid this month's rent, was spending money on seemingly frivolous items, had been overly friendly to strangers, and now had started to stay up until all hours of the night. Soon after Jason's call, Mrs. Kathleen received a call from Matthew saying that everything is fabulous, that he is planning a big concert event that will earn him a lot of money, and he would like his mom to invest in this event. The next day, Mrs. Kathleen arrived at Matthew's apartment and asked Matthew to go with her. Matthew thought he was going to a lunch where his mother was going to invest in his concert event. Instead, Matthew was taken to the office of Dr. Ford, a clinical psychologist at an inpatient psychiatric hospital. Matthew was baffled and hurt that his mother would take him to see a clinical psychologist and, he reported that he has never felt better in his life and is not willing to give consent for treatment. Mrs. Kathleen reported that there is a history of bipolar illness in the family from the father's side, and she thinks Matthew is having his first manic episode.

Issues of Concern

Is a young man in the middle of a manic, possibly psychotic, episode capable of giving or withholding consent for treatment? Standard 3.10 specifies that should Matthew be considered "legally incapable" of giving consent then Mrs. Kathleen's consent should then be sought. Is it in the best interests of Matthew for Dr. Ford to proceed with the necessary steps to have Matthew deemed legally incapable of giving consent to treatment in order to assure that Matthew receives the needed treatment for a manic episode? Is it in the best interests of Matthew for Dr. Ford to advise Mrs. Kathleen on how best to protect herself and her son in the event that Matthew does not meet the criteria for involuntary hospitalization?

APA Ethics Code

Companion General Principle

Principle A: Beneficence and Nonmaleficence

> Psychologists strive to benefit those with whom they work and take care to do no harm.

Principle A guides psychologists to be of benefit. If in Dr. Ford's clinical judgment Matthew would benefit from treatment, does this professional opinion supersede an individual's right to refuse treatment?

Principle E: Respect for People's Rights and Dignity

> Psychologists respect . . . the rights of individuals to . . . self-determination. Psychologists are aware that special safeguards may be necessary to protect the rights and welfare of persons or communities whose vulnerabilities impair autonomous decision making.

Principle E guides psychologists to consider people's right to self-determination on equal footing with a psychologist's wish to be of benefit. The second sentence of Principle E guides psychologists to be sensitive to special considerations for the welfare of individuals who have vulnerabilities, such as when someone is mentally ill like Matthew or those whose ability to make decisions is impaired. Thus the principle of beneficence, in the case of someone whose decision making is impaired, may be of more importance than protecting people's rights for self-determination, such as by refusing treatment.

Companion Ethical Standard(s)

Standard 3.07: Third-Party Requests for Services

> When psychologists agree to provide services to a person . . . at the request of a third party, psychologists attempt to clarify at the outset of the service the nature of the relationship with all individuals . . . involved. This clarification includes the role of the psychologist (e.g., therapist, . . .), an identification of who is the client, the probable uses of the services provided or the information obtained, and the fact that there may be limits to confidentiality.

Although Dr. Ford has not spoken to Matthew but nonetheless has an appointment with Matthew and his mother it seems that Mrs. Kathleen made an appointment with Dr. Ford on Matthew's behalf. To the extent that Mrs. Kathleen is requesting services for Matthew, Dr. Ford has agreed to provide services to Matthew at the request of a third party. Standard 3.07 directs Dr. Ford to do four things: (1) clarify his role, which in this case is most likely the role of a consultant; (2) identify the client, which in this case is Matthew; (3) explain the uses of information provided, which in this case most likely will be used to proceed with involuntary treatment proceedings; and finally (4) clarify limits of confidentiality, which in this case (if Matthew is committed for involuntary treatment) there are no privileges of confidentiality.

Legal Issues 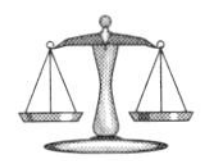

Florida

> *Fla. Admin. Code Ann. r. 64B19-19.006 (2010). Confidentiality*
>
> . . . (2) In cases where an evaluation is performed upon a person by a psychologist for use by a third party, the psychologist must explain to the person being evaluated the limits of confidentiality in that specific situation, document that such information was explained and understood by the person being evaluated, and obtain written informed consent to all aspects of the testing and evaluative procedures.
>
> (3) This rule recognizes that minors and legally incapacitated individuals cannot give informed consent under the law. Psychologists, nonetheless, owe a duty of confidentiality to minor and legally incapacitated service users consistent with the duty imposed by subsection (1) This does not mean that the psychologist may not impart the psychologist's own evaluation, assessment, analysis, diagnosis, or recommendations regarding the minor or legally incapacitated individual to the service user's guardian or to any court of law.

New Jersey

> *N.J. Admin. Code § 13:42-10.8 (2010). Professional interactions with clients.*
>
> (a) A licensee shall not abandon or neglect a client in need of professional care without making reasonable arrangements for the continuation of such care or offering to help the client find alternative sources of assistance.
>
> . . . (c) A licensee shall not willfully harass, abuse or intimidate a client regarding delivery of client services, either physically or verbally.
>
> . . . (e) A licensee shall terminate a clinical or consulting relationship when it is reasonably clear that the client is not benefiting from it. In such instances, the licensee shall offer to help the client find alternative sources of assistance.

In both jurisdictions, Matthew's refusal of treatment and the facts alleged by Matthew's mother may be sufficient to engage in an involuntary treatment evaluation. The due process protections of such a proceeding would protect Matthew but allow Dr. Ford shelter from violating either jurisdiction's ethical standards.

Cultural Considerations

Global Discussion

Code of Ethics: Netherlands

> I.5.3 Legally adult client, incapable of giving informed consent.
>
> If a client is a legal adult but is deemed incapable of adequately exercising his rights, the rights granted to him in terms of the Code will be exercised by his legal representative(s). . . If a representative of the latter kind has not been appointed, the client's rights will be exercised by his . . . parent, . . . unless the client objects to this or the psychologist deems this to be in conflict with the interests of the client. Regardless of the aforesaid, any adult client incapable of giving informed consent will be stimulated to seek full and active participation in decisions which affect them.
>
> I.5.4 Decisions in conflict with the clients' interests.
>
> The psychologist does not comply with any decision taken by the aforementioned representatives if he believes that, under the prevailing circumstances, this would undermine the interests of his client.

Does Matthew's mother have the right to make decisions for him because Matthew can be considered a legal but temporarily incompetent adult? Since Matthew has no legal representative that we are aware of, appointed or otherwise, and no partner, then his mother can "exercise the client's rights." However, the code of the Netherlands also states that if the client objects to this representation—or if the psychologist deems it to be "in conflict" with Matthew's interests—then this exercising of rights by Matthew's mother cannot occur. In that case, the psychologist here would be in violation of the Netherlands' code. However, this section of the code also states that adults found incapable of giving consent will still be included as full and active participants in decisions that affect them. If Dr. Ford decides that greater harm would come by respecting Matthew's wish to not enter treatment (spending money frivolously, having intimate contact with strangers, etc.) than by going against Matthew's wishes and treating him anyway, he would not be in violation of the code of the Netherlands.

American Moral Values

1. How does Dr. Ford relate bipolar illness to the notions of consent and reasoned judgment? If Matthew is indeed bipolar, is he stable enough for his wishes to be respected?
2. Is there a way to suggest to Matthew why treatment may be helpful for him if he does have bipolar symptoms? Or is reasoning with Matthew not an effective approach to bipolar illness?
3. How does Dr. Ford judge Mrs. Kathleen's behavior? Was her "intervention" appropriate for a person in Matthew's condition? Will Dr. Ford's relationship with Matthew be undermined if he is seen as endorsing her tactic? Can Dr. Ford criticize Mrs. Kathleen's "trick" while still suggesting to Matthew that therapy might address his symptoms?
4. What risks might Dr. Ford be taking by not treating an unwilling Matthew? Is his possible turn toward psychotic mania or clinical depression too much to risk?
5. Would Dr. Ford treat Matthew differently if the nature of the mental illness was different, say a manic episode induced by use of amphetamines?

Ethical Course of Action

Directive per APA Code

Standard 3.10 (b) directs Dr. Ford to first make a decision as to whether Matthew is legally capable of giving consent for treatment. If Dr. Ford decides that Matthew, despite his report of manic symptoms from his mother and roomate, is capable of giving consent, then Principle E guides and Standard 3.10 (a) directs Dr. Ford to respect Matthew's wish to not engage in treatment. However, if Dr. Ford decides that Matthew is not legally capable of autonomous decision making, then Standard 3.10 (b) directs Dr. Ford to explain the situation and try to obtain Matthew's agreement to enter treatment. Failing to obtain assent, Standard 3.10 (b) directs Dr. Ford to obtain permission from a legally authorized person, which in this case would not be Matthew's mother but the courts.

Dictates of One's Own Conscience

In the case of a first manic episode, if you were working for a psychiatric hospital, would you move to commit Matthew or try to persuade Mrs. Kathleen to attempt outpatient treatment?

1. Give Mrs. Kathleen referrals for other resources, and say that your hands are tied because Matthew has declined treatment.
2. Tell Matthew that he is mentally ill and should be in the hospital and should listen to his mother who has his best interests at heart.
3. Tell Matthew that he is experiencing a manic episode that has rendered him temporarily incompetent, and therefore he should be in treatment.
4. Reason that diagnostically Matthew meets many of the signs and symptoms of a manic episode diagnosis, and mania would certainly be expected to impair one's judgment and decision-making ability severely enough to render one incompetent; thus proceed to initiate involuntary commitment proceedings.
5. Reassure Matthew that he should trust his mother and would thank his mother for this intervention after treatment has been administered.
6. Fear that if Matthew remains untreated and presumably is having a manic episode, that he would next encounter either the legal or inpatient mental health system. In such an event you would be seen as negligent for not attempting to prevent this possible harm to Matthew by overriding his personal wishes and treating him anyway.

7. Perform a combination of the previously listed actions.
8. Do something that is not previously listed.

If you were Dr. Ford practicing in the Netherlands, you could proceed with treatment of Matthew based on the consent of his mother, Mrs. Kathleen.

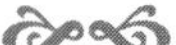

STANDARD 3.10: INFORMED CONSENT

> . . . (c) When psychological services are court ordered or otherwise mandated, psychologists inform the individual of the nature of the anticipated services, including whether the services are court ordered or mandated and any limits of confidentiality, before proceeding.

A CASE FOR STANDARD 3.10 (C): To Whom Does the Court Order Apply?

Rebecca presents for outpatient individual psychotherapy with Dr. Hamilton, a psychologist specializing in child/family problems. Rebecca reported she needs to improve her parenting skills. On intake, Dr. Hamilton found out that Rebecca has lost custody of her 2-year-old son to her ex-husband and is court ordered into treatment as a condition of her receiving visitations with her son. She thinks the court system is biased against her because she is a member of an indigenous tribe and biased in favor of her ex-husband because he is white, rich, and well connected. She does not want Dr. Hamilton to be in contact with the courts beyond providing verification that she is in treatment; nor does Rebecca want Dr. Hamilton to keep notes of what she talks about in session beyond the date and time of her appointments. Dr. Hamilton said to Rebecca, "The court has ordered you to provide information that would persuade the judge that you are a good parent. Just the fact that you come to treatment may or may not persuade a judge of your ability to parent. I can do what you want, but you may not meet the requirements of the court order."

Issues of Concern

Enacting that part of Principle E that respects people's rights to self-determination, Standard 3.10 (c) directs Dr. Hamilton to inform Rebecca of the following: first, "the nature of the anticipated services" or that his area of competence is in treatment of children. Second, he must inform her of "whether the services are court ordered or mandated" and talk to Rebecca about what the court has ordered. Third, he must inform Rebecca of "any limits of confidentiality, or that the courts could order him to discuss content of their sessions even if he does not provide them with chart notes."

The court order is directed at Rebecca, not at Dr. Hamilton. Dr. Hamilton is under no obligation to conform to the stipulations of the court's order. Dr. Hamilton is directed by the profession of psychology to comply with the directives of Standard 3.10 (c). If both Dr. Hamilton and Rebecca are clear about what kind of treatment Rebecca will obtain and what Dr. Hamilton will provide the courts, Dr. Hamilton has met the directives for Standard 3.10 (c).

Once Dr. Hamilton has satisfied the specifics as directed by Standard 3.10 and Rebecca persists with her request to limit his contact with the courts, is Dr. Hamilton in violation of Standard 3.10 (c) if he proceeds with treatment? By agreeing to the limits of confidentiality requested by Rebecca, does Dr. Hamilton knowingly harm Rebecca's chances of gaining visitation with her children?

APA Ethics Code

Companion General Principle

Principle A: Beneficence and Nonmaleficence

> Psychologists . . . take care to do no harm. In their professional actions, psychologists seek to safeguard the welfare and rights of those with whom they interact professionally and other affected persons. . .

Dr. Hamilton's application of Principle A would be a delicate balance between beneficence and nonmaleficence. Hopefully Dr. Hamilton's services, if done with cultural competence, would be of benefit to Rebecca. However, if Dr. Hamilton agrees to Rebecca's terms for treatment, Dr. Hamilton may knowingly harm Rebecca by providing service that does not comply with Rebecca's court-ordered treatment, thus violating the principle of nonmaleficence.

Principle B: Fidelity and Responsibility

> Psychologists establish relationships of trust with those with whom they work. Psychologists uphold professional

> standards of conduct, clarify their professional roles and obligations, accept appropriate responsibility for their behavior . . .

Standard 3.10 (c) is the enactment of the aspirational principle of fidelity. One condition for building trust between Dr. Hamilton and Rebecca is for Dr. Hamilton to be very clear as to his role in her legal affairs.

Principle E: Respect for People's Rights and Dignity

> Psychologists respect . . . the rights of individuals to privacy, confidentiality, and self-determination. . . Psychologists are aware of and respect cultural, individual, and role differences, including those based on . . . gender, . . . race, ethnicity, culture, . . . and consider these factors when working with members of such groups.
>
> Psychologists try to eliminate the effect on their work of biases based on those factors, and they do not knowingly participate in or condone activities of others based upon such prejudices.

Standard 3.10's directives for informed consent are the application of Principle E, with respect to people's rights to self-determination. For Dr. Hamilton to apply Principle E in his dealings with Rebecca requires that he be knowledgeable about the way that Rebecca's cultural history interacts with her attitude with the legal system.

Companion Ethical Standard(s)

> Guidelines on Multicultural Education, Training, Research, Practice, and Organizational Change for Psychologists (APA, 2003)
>
> **Guideline 5**
>
> Psychologists strive to apply culturally appropriate skills in clinical and other applied psychological practices.
>
> Client-in-context.
>
> Psychologists are also encouraged to be aware of the role that culture may play in the establishment and maintenance of a relationship between the client and therapist. Culture, ethnicity, race, and gender are among the factors that may play a role in the perception of, and expectations of therapy and the role the therapist plays. (pp. 47–48)

Rebecca is of a different culture from mainstream European American ancestry. Rebecca's request may be based on the cultural context of Native Americans' treatment by the U.S. court system. As guided by the previously cited guideline, Dr. Hamilton needs to consider the role of culture in his response to Rebecca's request and his subsequent interactions with the courts.

Standard 10.01: Informed Consent to Therapy

> (a) When obtaining informed consent to therapy . . . psychologists inform clients/patients as early as is feasible in the therapeutic relationship about . . . involvement of third parties, and limits of confidentiality and provide sufficient opportunity for the client/patient to ask questions and receive answers.

Standard 3.10 directs psychologists to obtain informed consent regardless of the services provided, be they research, organizational consultation, etc. In this situation, Dr. Hamilton is providing court-ordered treatment for Rebecca. Thus both Standard 3.10 (c) and Standard 10.01 apply.

Standard 4.01: Maintaining Confidentiality

> Psychologists have a primary obligation and take reasonable precautions to protect confidential information obtained through . . . any medium, recognizing that the extent and limits of confidentiality may be regulated by law.

Rebecca appears to be an individual who is able to give consent, thus Dr. Hamilton is directed by Standard 4.01 to protect Rebecca's privilege of confidentiality.

Standard 4.05: Disclosures

> (a) Psychologists may disclose confidential information with the appropriate consent of the . . . individual client/patient. . .
>
> . . . (b) Psychologists disclose confidential information without the consent of the individual only as mandated by law. . .

Standard 4.05 (a) allows for Dr. Hamilton to break confidentiality under the condition that Rebecca has given him permission. In this situation, Rebecca gave permission, or consent, for Dr. Hamilton to give information to a specific entity—the court, in a very specific area—when she came to treatment. Standard 4.05 (b) further specifies that Dr. Hamilton is allowed to disregard Rebecca's wishes if a court orders him to do so.

Legal Issues 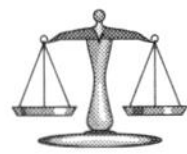

California

Cal. Bus.& Prof. Code § 2918 (West 2003). Confidential relations and communications; privilege; law governing.

The confidential relations and communications between psychologist and client shall be privileged . . .

Virginia

18 Va. Admin. Code § 125-20-150 (2010). Standards of practice.

A. . . . Psychologists respect the rights, dignity and worth of all people, and are mindful of individual differences.

B. Persons licensed by the board shall:

. . . 9. Keep confidential their professional relationships with patients . . . and disclose client records to others only with written consent except:

. . . (iii) as permitted by law for a valid purpose . . .

In both jurisdictions, Dr. Hamilton may not be able to protect the confidences of Rebecca even if a statute creates a psychologist/client privilege. In family law cases, the courts frequently issue orders that compel treating psychologists to report their observations and records of each session as fact witnesses rather than expert witnesses.

Cultural Considerations

Global Discussion

Canadian Code of Ethics for Psychologists

Principle I: Respect for the integrity of persons.

Freedom of consent.

I.27. Take all reasonable steps to ensure that consent is not given under conditions of coercion, undue pressure, or undue reward. (Also see Standard III.32)

I.29. Take all reasonable steps to confirm or re-establish freedom of consent, if consent for service is given under conditions of duress or conditions of extreme need.

I.30. Respect the right of persons to discontinue . . . service at any time,

Because Rebecca's treatment with Dr. Hamilton is court ordered, this could be an example of consent given under " . . . conditions of coercion, undue pressure." Dr. Hamilton's obligation under the Canadian code is to "re-establish freedom of consent." Therefore, informing Rebecca of the limits of confidentiality per the court-ordered confines of treatment would be a reasonable first step, as well as informing her of both the freedom and responsibility to discontinue treatment or withhold consent. If she continues treatment under the previously listed conditions or chooses to withdraw and risks the possibility of losing her custody case, either way, Dr. Hamilton's role here is to clearly communicate both options.

American Moral Values

1. How can Dr. Hamilton best address Rebecca's needs and interests? Does she understand what treatment might entail beyond just "parenting skills"? Should Dr. Hamilton promise not to tell the court what occurs in treatment? How will Dr. Hamilton's response relate to Rebecca's perception that her race and class are held against her by legal authorities? Would refusing her treatment reinforce her view?
2. What is Dr. Hamilton's responsibility to Rebecca's child? Would helping her with parenting justify not divulging confidences? Short of any mandatory reporting for abuse or neglect in Rebecca's parenting, is their any other behavior that would justify breaking confidentiality?
3. Can Dr. Hamilton help Rebecca's case by sharing information about her treatment with the court? How should Rebecca be included in that decision? Should Dr. Hamilton tell her from the beginning about this possibility?

Ethical Course of Action

Directive per APA Code

Standard 3.10 (c) directs Dr. Hamilton to make sure that Rebecca is clear about his services and that regardless of what Rebecca wishes or what Dr. Hamilton agrees to do that the courts could order him to discuss content of their sessions even if he does not provide them with chart notes.

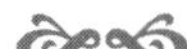

Dictates of One's Own Conscience

If you were Dr. Hamilton, having told Rebecca the courts may not look favorably on his refusal to provide the courts with details of her treatment at her request or that you may be ordered by the courts to give details of her treatment, what else might you do?

1. Decline to accept Rebecca as a client, and refer her to other psychologists.
2. Consider Rebecca's request for confidentiality in the face of a courts' order to be a central therapeutic topic for Rebecca and therefore focus on exploring the release of information as the first area of focus for treatment. Only after a full discussion of the implications for complying with Rebecca's request would you decide whether to continue treatment with Rebecca or to give her referrals for other psychologists.
3. Consider that you have not only complied with the letter but also the spirit of Standard 3.10 after providing Rebecca with an explanation of the limits of confidentiality and proceed with treatment.
4. Request to see a copy of the court order, and take time to fully examine the meaning of the specific order with Rebecca.
5. Discuss with Rebecca the possibility of her seeking treatment through services provided at the tribal center, as that course of action may cause the least harm.
6. Perform a combination of the previously listed actions.
7. Do something that is not previously listed.

If you were Dr. Hamilton practicing in Canada, you would discharge your obligations after assuring that Rebecca is aware of her options in relation to the court order.

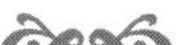

STANDARD 3.10: INFORMED CONSENT

> . . . (d) Psychologists appropriately document written or oral consent, permission, and assent.

A CASE FOR STANDARD 3.10 (D): But I Thought She Already Knew

Dr. Graham is the treating psychologist for Pamela, who is court ordered as a condition of her probation. Pamela presents for her first session somewhat disoriented to place and person. She was somewhat confused in reporting the circumstances of her court case and the reason for her court-ordered treatment. Pamela said that her probation officer would know "what needs to be done." For the next session, Pamela arrived to her session accompanied by Ms. Virginia, her probation officer. Pamela told Dr. Graham that Ms. Virginia knew "what needs to be done" and wanted Ms. Virginia to come into the session with them, to which Dr. Graham agreed. Dr. Graham asked Ms. Virginia the conditions of the probation.

Issues of Concern

Standard 3.10 (d) directs Dr. Graham to document Pamela's consent for treatment. It may be doubtful whether Pamela is capable of giving consent for treatment in her confused state. Under this circumstance, if Ms. Virginia is able to provide the legal mandate for treatment as a condition of Pamela's parole, can Dr. Graham take such legal mandate as consent for treatment?

Of secondary but equally important concern is the question of whether Pamela has given consent for release of information for Dr. Graham to converse with Ms. Virginia. It can reasonably be argued that though Pamela has not provided Dr. Graham with a written release of information, by physically being present when Dr. Graham and Ms. Virginia discuss the specifics of Pamela's situation, Pamela has given implied consent.

APA Ethics Code

Companion General Principle

Principle B: Fidelity and Responsibility

> Psychologists consult with, refer to, or cooperate with other professionals and institutions to the extent needed to serve the best interests of those with whom they work . . .

Principle B places psychologists in the context of a team of service providers who work collaboratively to assure the most benefit to a client. Aspiring to the highest principle of Responsibility, Dr. Graham would need to consult and work with Pamela's probation officer.

Principle E: Respect for People's Rights and Dignity

> Psychologists are aware that special safeguards may be necessary to protect the rights and welfare of persons . . . whose vulnerabilities impair autonomous decision making. . .

Recognizing Pamela's apparent confusion, Principle E guides Dr. Graham to adopt special safeguards to protect Pamela's rights to self-determination and confidentiality.

Companion Ethical Standard(s)

Standard 4.01: Maintaining Confidentiality

> Psychologists have a primary obligation and take reasonable precautions to protect confidential information obtained through or stored in any medium, recognizing that the extent and limits of confidentiality may be regulated by law . . .

Dr. Graham is directed by Standard 4.01 to protect Pamela's privilege of confidentiality.

Standard 4.05: Disclosures

> (a) Psychologists may disclose confidential information with the appropriate consent of the . . . individual client/patient. . .

Standard 4.05 (a) allows for Dr. Graham to break confidentiality under the condition that Pamela has given him permission. In this situation, it can be construed that Pamela has given implied consent to the release of her information.

Standard 3.10: Informed Consent

> . . . (c) When psychological services are court ordered or otherwise mandated, psychologists inform the individual of the nature of the anticipated services, including whether the services are court ordered or mandated and any limits of confidentiality, before proceeding.

Standard 3.10 (c) applies given that Pamela is seeking treatment as part of her probation.

Standard 3.10: Informed Consent

> . . . (b) For persons who are legally incapable of giving informed consent, psychologists nevertheless . . . (1) provide an appropriate explanation, . . . (2) seek the individual's assent, . . . (3) consider such persons' preferences and best interests, and . . . (4) obtain appropriate permission from a legally authorized person . . .

Standard 3.10 (b) may apply depending of the severity and length of Pamela's confusion.

Legal Issues 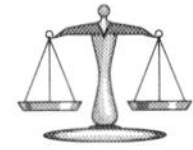

Ohio

> *Ohio Admin. Code 4732:17-01 (2010). General rules of professional conduct pursuant to section 4732.17 of the revised code.*
>
> (C) Welfare of the Client.
>
> . . . *(3) Informed Client.* A psychologist . . . shall give a truthful, understandable, and reasonably complete account of a client's condition to the client or to those responsible for the care of the client. The psychologist . . . shall keep the client fully informed as to the purpose and nature of any . . . procedures, and of the client's right to freedom of choice regarding services provided.

Washington

> *Wash. Admin. Code § 246-924-359 (2009). Client welfare.*
>
> *(1) Providing explanation of procedures.* The psychologist shall upon request give a truthful, understandable, and reasonably complete account of the client's condition to the client or to those responsible for the care of the client. The psychologist shall keep the client fully informed as to the purpose and nature of any . . . procedures, and of the client's right to freedom of choice regarding services. . .

In both jurisdictions, Dr. Graham would document Pamela's consent to treatment. In the event that such consent appears uncertain, Dr. Graham would assess whether Pamela has the capacity to provide informed consent to treatment and document the results of such an assessment. Ms. Virginia can provide collateral evidence about Pamela's capacity to provide consent. If Dr. Graham does decide to provide the court-ordered treatment as part of probation, he still must establish that Pamela has consented to treatment.

Cultural Considerations

Global Discussion

Canadian Code of Ethics for Psychologists

> Principle I: Respect for the dignity of persons.
>
> *Informed consent.*
>
> I.17. Recognize that informed consent is the result of a process of reaching an agreement to work collaboratively, rather than of simply having a consent form signed.
>
> I.18. Respect the expressed wishes of persons to involve others (e.g., family members, community members) in their decision making regarding informed consent. . .
>
> I.22. Accept and document oral consent, in situations in which signed consent forms are not acceptable culturally or in which there are other good reasons for not using them . . .

If Dr. Graham was practicing in Canada, he would be in violation of this part of the code, as it is unclear that Pamela made an "expressed wish" that her probation officer be privy to her court history and case details. However, according to the Canadian code, if written consent is not obtained, oral consent can be accepted and noted if there are "good reasons" for not using written forms. As Dr. Graham did not do either of these steps before beginning to discuss Pamela's private information in front of her probation officer, he needs to take immediate corrective action, as he is in violation of both the intent and letter of the Canadian code. Although an accompanying person's presence can be reasonably assumed to constitute a tacit, nonverbal consent, the Canadian code has specific guidelines for both oral and written consent, and neither of these mentions unspoken assumptions of the psychologist.

American Moral Values

1. What type of consent does Dr. Graham have from Pamela to talk with Ms. Virginia? Does bringing Ms. Virginia and saying she knows "what needs to be done" imply a consent for Ms. Virginia to inform Dr. Graham about the court order and receive information about Pamela's treatment?
2. Would pausing to gain explicit consent imply a lack of trust in Pamela? Would it convey to Pamela a sense that she might not know what she was doing in bringing Ms. Virginia to the meeting? How would these attributions affect Pamela's treatment by Dr. Graham?
3. Dr. Graham has also failed to check Ms. Virginia's credentials as Pamela's supposed probation officer. Would checking those at this point communicate a lack of trust in both Pamela and Ms. Virginia?
4. How does Dr. Graham value standards of confidentiality and authorization in the context of this court-ordered treatment? Is building trust and rapport with Pamela worth bending these rules in order to treat Pamela more effectively? Or could there be coercion of Pamela by the court and even Dr. Graham? Does part of her confusion come from being intimidated and self-conscious in the presence of Dr. Graham? Is she using Ms. Virginia just to avoid looking bad, rather than out of a genuine desire for help with her treatment? How can Dr. Graham be more certain that is not the case?

Ethical Course of Action

Directive per APA Code

To meet the directive of Standard 3.10 (d), Dr. Graham is to document Pamela's "consent, permission or assent" to treatment. It is unclear, due to Pamela's apparent disorientation, whether Pamela is capable of giving consent to treatment. Dr. Graham could take the court mandate for treatment to be permission to engage Pamela in treatment with Dr. Graham. If Dr. Graham does accept court-ordered treatment as part of probation, Standard 3.10 (d) directs that he so documents such a stance.

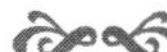

Dictates of One's Own Conscience

If you were Dr. Graham, sitting in the office with Pamela who is confused and a probation officer who could attest to treatment as condition of probation, would you deem such a condition as having obtained permission for treatment? Which would you do?

1. Ask Pamela to sign your consent to treatment form before proceeding.
2. Engage in clarification of the nature of treatment with Pamela in attempt to uphold Principle E.
3. Ask Ms. Virginia to obtain a specific court order for Pamela to be in treatment with Dr. Graham as a way to address the problem of Pamela's apparent inability to provide true informed consent to treatment.
4. Tell Ms. Virginia that you cannot provide treatment to Pamela because she is not in any mental condition to engage in treatment.
5. Refer Pamela for a medication evaluation on the grounds that she is not capable of giving consent at this point; and without consent to treatment, you cannot provide services.
6. Perform a combination of the previously listed actions.
7. Do something that is not previously listed.

If you were Dr. Graham practicing in Canada, you would not proceed to meet with anyone except Pamela but instead would proceed to further discuss and explore the concept of consent until such time you are assured that Pamela has understood and provided consent to treatment.

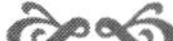

STANDARD 3.11: PSYCHOLOGICAL SERVICES DELIVERED TO OR THROUGH ORGANIZATIONS

> (a) Psychologists delivering services to or through organizations provide information beforehand to clients and, when appropriate, those directly affected by the services about (1) the nature and objectives of the services, (2) the intended recipients, (3) which of the individuals are clients, (4) the relationship the psychologist will have with each person and the organization, (5) the probable uses of services provided and information obtained, (6) who will have access to the information, and (7) limits of confidentiality. As soon as feasible, they provide information about the results and conclusions of such services to appropriate persons.
>
> (b) If psychologists will be precluded by law or by organizational roles from providing such information to particular individuals or groups, they so inform those individuals or groups at the outset of the service.

A CASE FOR STANDARD 3.11 (A) (1): Who Is My Client?

Dr. Sullivan had recently been admitted onto a managed care insurance panel that promises to increase her clientele substantially. To increase her visibility to the referral sources of this managed care panel, she agreed to take on the employee assistance program (EAP) cases of companies that directly contract with this managed care company. Thursday morning she received a call from the managed care company informing Dr. Sullivan there was an EAP case that was to be seen within the next 24 hours and asking whether she has an opening either Thursday or Friday. Dr. Sullivan said that she indeed has an opening at 2:00 pm that afternoon. The managed care company confirmed that a Mr. Gary will be informed of the appointment time and of the address of Dr. Sullivan's office. For background information, would Dr. Sullivan please call a Ms. Debra in the company's human resources (HR) department?

On contact, Ms. Debra informed Dr. Sullivan that Mr. Gary's supervisor had contacted the HR department reporting that Mr. Gary was unfit for work and could not return to work without a doctor's clearance. Would Dr. Sullivan please evaluate Mr. Gary this afternoon so that he would not be unnecessarily absent from work? The company would require that Dr. Sullivan provide a written evaluation addressed to the HR department with an opinion regarding Mr. Gary's ability to return to work.

Issues of Concern

Is Dr. Sullivan delivering service to Mr. Gary through the managed care company and/or through Mr. Gary's employer? Normally in a situation where an employee is self-referred, Dr. Sullivan would not be requested or required to write evaluations of an employee's mental status. Depending on the terms of the EAP contract, Dr. Sullivan may be considered a contract employee of the managed care company. As an employee of the managed care company, she would be delivering services to Mr. Gary through the organization of the managed care company. As such, Standard 3.11 applies. The specifics of Standard 3.11 direct Dr. Sullivan to inform Mr. Gary what HR has requested and how the information he shares with her will be used.

APA Ethics Code

Companion General Principle

Principle A: Beneficence and Nonmaleficence

> In their professional actions, psychologists seek to safeguard the welfare and rights of those with whom they interact professionally.

In this situation with Mr. Gary, the principle of focus here is nonmaleficence. Because it is easy to compromise Mr. Gary's privilege of confidentiality, Dr. Sullivan needs to attend to safeguarding his welfare. If she aspires to Principle A and if Dr. Sullivan thinks that given the situation with HR she may not be able to safeguard Mr. Gary's right to privacy then it behooves Dr. Sullivan to decline this referral.

Principle E: Respect for People's Right and Dignity

> Psychologists respect the . . . rights of individuals to privacy, confidentiality, and self-determination. Psychologists are aware that special safeguards may be necessary to protect the rights and welfare of persons or communities whose vulnerabilities impair autonomous decision making.

Principle E reiterates Principle A in that both guide psychologists to protect and respect individual's rights to self-determination. For Mr. Gary, this right to self-determination may come in the form of his right to refuse the conditions of the evaluation. Likewise for Dr. Sullivan, to safeguard Mr. Gary's rights she may need to modify or decline the terms of the referral.

Companion Ethical Standard(s)

Standard 3.07: Third-Party Requests for Services

> When psychologists agree to provide services to a person . . . at the request of a third party, psychologists attempt to clarify at the outset of the service the nature of the relationship with all individuals . . . involved. This clarification includes the role of the psychologist (e.g., . . . consultant . . .), an identification of who is the client, the probable uses of the services provided or the information obtained, and the fact that there may be limits to confidentiality.

Dr. Sullivan is delivering services through the managed care company (Standard 3.11) at the request of Mr. Gary's employer (Standard 3.07). When the managed care company agrees to provide services to Mr. Gary at the request of Mr. Gary's employer, per the directives of Standard 3.07, the HR department of Mr. Gary's employer needs to be informed of the parameters of the various relationships. And again, when Dr. Sullivan converses with Ms. Debra in HR, per Standard 3.07, Dr. Sullivan must clarify her role (contract employee of managed care company acting as an evaluator) and that of the client being Mr. Gary's employer.

Standard 3.05: Multiple Relationships

> (a) A multiple relationship occurs when a psychologist is in a professional role with a person and . . . (2) at the same time is in a relationship with a person closely associated with or related to the person with whom the psychologist has the professional relationship. . .
>
> A psychologist refrains from entering into a multiple relationship if the multiple relationship could reasonably be expected to impair the psychologist's . . . effectiveness in performing his or her functions as a psychologist. . .
>
> Multiple relationships that would not reasonably be expected to cause impairment or risk exploitation or harm are not unethical.

Because there are four entities involved in this situation, Standard 3.05 (a) (2) seems to apply. Dr. Sullivan will be the assessment psychologist for Mr. Gary, while at the same time she is a contract employee of the managed care company that is servicing Mr. Gary's employer. Situations like these probably have a low risk of affecting Dr. Sullivan's objectivity in her work with Mr. Gary, although there may be a chance that Dr. Sullivan may feel pressured to submit findings that are in agreement with or favor the employer.

Standard 2.01: Boundaries of Competence

> (a) Psychologists provide services . . . with populations and in areas only within the boundaries of their competence, based on their education, training, supervised experience, consultation, study, or professional experience.

As in any referral, regardless of whether services are delivered at the request of a third party or through an organization, Standard 2.01 directs Dr. Sullivan to only provide services in areas in which she is competent. Thus in Dr. Sullivan's conversation with Ms. Debra in the HR department sufficient information needs to be obtained for Dr. Sullivan to determine whether Mr. Gary's problems are within her area of competence.

Standard 4.01: Maintaining Confidentiality

> Psychologists have a primary obligation and take reasonable precautions to protect confidential information obtained through or stored in any medium, recognizing that the extent and limits of confidentiality may be regulated by . . . professional . . . relationship.

In this case, the limit of confidentiality is established by the professional contract Dr. Sullivan has with the managed care company and the contract that the managed care company has with Mr. Gary's employer. Dr. Sullivan needs to be aware of the stipulations regarding confidentiality by these two contracts.

Standard 9.03: Informed Consent in Assessments

> (a) Psychologists obtain informed consent for . . . evaluations, . . . except when . . . (2) informed consent is implied because testing is conducted as a routine . . . organizational activity (e.g., when participants voluntarily agree to assessment when applying for a job). . . Informed consent includes an explanation of the . . . limits of confidentiality and sufficient opportunity for the client/patient to ask questions and receive answers.

Standard 9.03 is the enactment of Principle E, respect for people's right to self-determination. It does not appear that the exceptions to informed consent as specified in Standard 9.03 apply to this situation.

Thus, per Standard 9.03, when Dr. Sullivan meets with Mr. Gary, she is to obtain consent from him for the evaluation after she explains the limits of confidentiality and her role in relationship to his employer.

Standard 4.05: Disclosures

> (a) Psychologists may disclose confidential information with the appropriate consent of the organizational client, the individual client/patient . . .

Standard 4.05 directs Dr. Sullivan to only provide information to Mr. Gary's employer after obtaining the informed consent for evaluation and signed release of information which names his employer.

Legal Issues 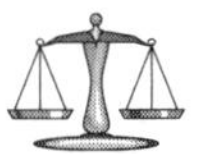

Pennsylvania

> *49 Pa. Code § 41.61 (2010). Code of ethics.*
>
> Principle 8. Utilization of Assessment.
>
> . . . (b) Persons examined at the request of or under the auspices of a sponsoring entity such as an employer . . . shall have, irrespective of who pays for the service, the same rights to information as set out in subsection (a), unless limitations are agreed upon in advance in writing among the psychologist, the person to be examined . . . and the sponsoring entity. The psychologist shall provide the examination results to the sponsoring entity only upon authorization in writing signed by the person to be examined. . . The psychologist shall ensure that the person to be examined . . . makes an informed decision . . . as to giving up one or more of the rights in subsection (a) and as to releasing information to the sponsoring entity.

Texas

> *22 Tex. Admin. Code § 465.11 (2010). Informed consent/ describing psychological services.*
>
> . . . (d) When a licensee agrees to provide services to a person . . . at the request of a third party, the licensee clarifies to all of the parties the nature of the relationship between the licensee and each party at the outset of the service and at any time during the services that the circumstances change. This clarification includes the role of the licensee with each party, the probable uses of the services and the results of the services, and all potential limits to the confidentiality between the recipient(s) of the services and the licensee.

Under both jurisdictions' laws, Dr. Sullivan must let Ms. Debra and Mr. Gary know that the company is her client. Before Dr. Sullivan evaluates Mr. Gary, Dr. Sullivan should inform Mr. Gary that all information provided by Mr. Gary to Dr. Sullivan can and probably will be forwarded to his employer and the information and her observations of Mr. Gary will lead to her providing a professional opinion about his fitness to work. Dr. Sullivan also should inform Mr. Gary that he has the right to refuse the conditions of the evaluation and that if he refuses the limits of confidentiality then evaluation will not proceed but Ms. Debra will be informed about his refusal to proceed.

Cultural Considerations

Global Discussion

Association of Greek Psychologists

> Ethical codes & guidelines.
>
> IV. Relationships with the institutions where the psychologist works.
>
> 1. During their professional practice in the areas of . . . industrial psychology, . . . psychologists preserve the confidentiality of information;
>
> 2. The psychologist should not criticize in public the department or organization where he works. Instead, he should directly announce his doubts or reservations to the organization, provided that this could lead to an amelioration of the working conditions and human relationships.
>
> 3. A psychologist who assumes responsibilities in an institution, informs his employer promptly on the restrictions and obligations defined by his code of ethics.

If this situation occurred in Greece, pursuant to 3, Dr. Sullivan is to state the limitations and "restrictions" of the code of ethics, including the obligation to preserve client confidentiality, and in that way attempt to safeguard Mr. Gary's privacy. However, if the company itself is seen as the client, then Dr. Sullivan must preserve both the confidentiality of that organization, and safeguard against making statements which could be construed as critical of that organization.

American Moral Values

1. How do the priorities of the managed care panel conflict or coincide with the values of the client–therapist relationship itself? Are the EAP cases beyond Sullivan's competence? If so, what justifies her work on this panel?

2. Under what terms should Dr. Sullivan agree to break confidentiality about Mr. Gary's treatment? Does determining his fitness for work merit breaking confidentiality to his employer? Does that serve Mr. Gary's interests as someone the company would want to retain, or is it wrong even to threaten his employment by discussing his case with the company?
3. If Mr. Gary does not want his information released for any reason, should Dr. Sullivan still evaluate him? What should her continuing role with the panel be?
4. Would leaving the panel change the way it works? Might Dr. Sullivan want to lend her skills to an imperfect system on the assumption that other therapists would not be as good as she is? Could she consider her work to be better for EAP case clients than if she left?

Ethical Course of Action

Directive per APA Code

Combining Standard 3.11: Psychological Services Delivered To or Through Organizations, Standard 3.07: Third-Party Request for Services, and Standard 9.03: Informed Consent in Assessments, Dr. Sullivan is to first let Ms. Debra know that she considers the company to be her client. After ascertaining that Mr. Gary's problem is within her area of competence, Dr. Sullivan would then agree to evaluate Mr. Gary. Dr. Sullivan sees Mr. Gary but prior to his revealing any information, Dr. Sullivan is to clarify with Mr. Gary that she is acting as a contract employee of the managed care company, whose client is his employer. Thus all information provided by Mr. Gary to Dr. Sullivan can and probably will be forwarded to his employer including her professional opinion of his fitness for work. Finally, Dr. Sullivan can inform Mr. Gary that he has the right to refuse the conditions of the evaluation, and that if he refuses the limits of confidentiality, then evaluation will not proceed.

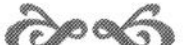

Dictates of One's Own Conscience

If you were in Dr. Sullivan's position and you decided that you are competent to provide the evaluation for Mr. Gary, regardless of the contracted terms of confidentiality, what would you do?

1. Conduct a full assessment, regardless of the length of time needed, in order to provide a sound basis for your opinion.
2. Conduct a clinical interview with mental status exam within the scheduled first appointment, inform Ms. Debra of your conclusions, and then schedule follow-up appointments per further EAP benefits.
3. Discuss with Mr. Gary your findings after an assessment, and give Mr. Gary an opportunity to reaffirm consent or rescind consent for you to send the report to his employer.
4. Tell Ms. Debra that you cannot conduct an evaluation because psychologists cannot predict the future, and thus you cannot say how Mr. Gary will function at work.
5. Advise Mr. Gary against consenting to the limits of confidentiality per contract with his employer and to seek out an independent evaluation.
6. Perform a combination of the previously listed actions.
7. Do something that is not previously listed.

If you were Dr. Sullivan working in Greece, you are to let Ms. Debra know that, per your professional ethics, information from Mr. Gary is confidential unless otherwise stated by Mr. Gary.

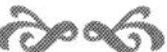

STANDARD 3.12: INTERRUPTION OF PSYCHOLOGICAL SERVICES

Unless otherwise covered by contract, psychologists make reasonable efforts to plan for facilitating services in the event that psychological services are interrupted by factors such as the psychologist's illness, death, unavailability, relocation, retirement, or by the client's/patient's relocation or financial limitations.

A CASE FOR STANDARD 3.12: But I Wasn't Available Anyway (Holding a Client Even During Absences)

Dr. Wallace is a postdoctoral intern working for a local community mental health clinic. One of his clients, Amanda, has a previous history of suicidality and substance abuse, although her current risk of relapse or suicidal acts is deemed to be low. Dr. Wallace decided to go out of town over the long Labor Day weekend. While he was away on vacation, he impulsively decided to spend one more day away since he had no regularly scheduled clients on that following Tuesday. He called the clinic to alert them of his updated plan. Since the clinic is closed over the weekend, he left a message on the front desk's voice mail saying he would not be in on Tuesday but would be available through his cell phone. Upon his return, he discovered a voice mail message from Amanda from the day before, indicating that she was in crisis and wanted to talk to Dr. Wallace right away. As Dr. Wallace was not going to miss any regularly scheduled therapy days, he did not inform Amanda that he would be out of town. When he queried the front desk as to whether anyone had called Amanda or why he had not been alerted about this situation, the receptionist replied that Dr. Wallace's message about extending his vacation was not received.

Issues of Concern

Standard 3.12 directs Dr. Wallace to make "reasonable efforts" for coverage in the event of his being unavailable. Would his calling in to the main switchboard of the clinic where he works be considered a reasonable effort? Leaving his cell phone number and being available for emergency calls during vacation would, by most measures, be considered more than adequate coverage. The system that failed is the clinic not picking up his message from the main voice mail box. Does Standard 3.12 direct Dr. Wallace to have planned for such an eventuality and placed his phone call to a specific person, perhaps his supervisor? Does the requirement of Standard 3.12 necessitate Dr. Wallace notifying every one of his clients of his absence over a long weekend?

APA Ethics Code

Companion General Principle

Principle B: Fidelity and Responsibility

> Psychologists establish relationships of trust with those with whom they work. They are aware of their professional and scientific responsibilities to society and to the specific communities in which they work. Psychologists uphold professional standards of conduct, clarify their professional roles and obligations, accept appropriate responsibility for their behavior, and seek to manage conflicts of interest that could lead to exploitation or harm.

Aspiring to Principle B: Fidelity and Responsibility, Dr. Wallace needed to uphold his professional obligations. Based on the directives of Standard 3.12, those professional obligations include making reasonable efforts for coverage should he be out of town. Does such an obligation extend to not making sudden unexpected changes like extending his vacation for one more day? Does such an obligation only extend to making sure that his patients are covered in the event he is unavailable? Does such an obligation require that Dr. Wallace ascertain the efficiency of the clinic administrative system and foresee such an occurrence as the possibility that his phone messages might not be received?

Companion Ethical Standard(s)

Standard 2.05: Delegation of Work to Others

> Psychologists who delegate work to employees . . . take reasonable steps to . . . (2) authorize only those responsibilities that such persons can be expected to perform competently on the basis of their education, training, or experience, either independently or with the level of supervision being provided; and (3) see that such persons perform these services competently.

Standard 2.05 requires that Dr. Wallace ascertain for himself that the front office staff and the voice mail system are functioning competently. If Dr. Wallace had any hints that the arrangements for coverage would not have been adequate, then calling the main number and leaving a message regarding how best to contact him would be in violation of Standard 2.05.

Legal Issues 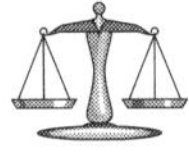

Michigan

> *Mich. Admin. Code r. 338.2515 (2010). Prohibited Conduct Rule 15.*
>
> Prohibited conduct includes, but is not limited to, the following acts or omissions by any individual covered by these rules:
>
> . . . (h) Willful or negligent failure to arrange for the continuity of necessary therapeutic service.

Georgia

> *Ga. Comp. R. & Regs. 510-5-.06 (2010). Welfare of clients and other professional relationships.*
>
> (2) Continuity of care.
>
> . . . (b) Psychologists make reasonable efforts to plan for continuity of care in the event that psychological services are interrupted by factors such as the psychologist's illness, death, unavailability or by the client/patient's relocation or financial limitations.

The laws of both jurisdictions direct Dr. Wallace to provide continuity of care by making reasonable efforts to extend coverage when he is unavailable. At the very least, Dr. Wallace should have advised his supervisor about his absence in light of a client on his caseload who has a history of suicidal behavior and alcohol relapse, even if such risks were viewed as low. The policy and procedure manual of the clinic would have defined reasonable efforts that Dr. Wallace should have followed and would be used to establish that he violated the ethical standards of the jurisdiction.

Cultural Considerations

Global Discussion

Canadian Code of Ethics for Psychologists

> Principle II: Responsible caring.
>
> *Minimize harm.*
>
> II.31. Give reasonable assistance to secure needed psychological services or activities, if personally unable to meet requests for needed psychological services or activities.
>
> II.34. Give reasonable notice and be reasonably assured that discontinuation will cause no harm to the client, before discontinuing services.

If Dr. Wallace were practicing in Canada, he would be seen as having made a mistake when he did not inform his clients of his upcoming absence. Barring the correct practice, which would have been to inform clients of any possible disruption of service in advance, provide several referral resources for emergencies, as well as updated schedules of availability on his own voice mail, Dr. Wallace is now in the unenviable position of having to address a preventable but potentially lethal disruption of services to his own client. Voice mail messages do become lost, or clinic front desks fail to check them; it is still the responsibility of the treating psychologist to prevent any foreseeable gaps in service, most especially to those clients deemed to be at high risk. As Dr. Wallace failed to give "reasonable notice" or any notice about his unavailability and was not successful in his attempts to communicate with the clinic staff, he is in violation of this portion of Canadian code. If he had informed his clients of his upcoming vacation and given at least one viable off-hours referral, he likely would not have been found in violation of this portion of Canadian code.

American Moral Values

1. What were Dr. Wallace's obligations to Amanda and the rest of the clients with respect to going on vacation? To his office staff? Was the chain of communication properly executed? Was Dr. Wallace obliged to notify a client like Amanda of plans for a long weekend?
2. Does Dr. Wallace need to provide an emergency line (e.g., mobile phone) to clients? Or is it sufficient to include on one's voice mail message a reminder to call 911 (or another colleague) if one needs emergency assistance? Can suicidal clients be expected to call those numbers, or will they insist on obtaining help solely from their own therapist?
3. What was the protocol for staff to call Dr. Wallace? Did the staff fail to uphold that protocol, or does there need to be a better plan for when calls like Amanda's come in on the weekend?

Ethical Course of Action

Directive per APA Code

Standard 3.12 directs Dr. Wallace is to make reasonable efforts for coverage in the event of his being unavailable. Regardless of whether he left a message in the general clinic voice mail box or not, reasonable efforts generally consist of a way to notify clients and/or supervisor directly of how best to contact Dr. Wallace if for any reason he is not in his office. In this case, the policy and procedure manual of the clinic would have defined reasonable efforts. Unless Dr. Wallace followed the procedure for contact while away on vacation, he is in violation of the directives of Standard 3.12

Dictates of One's Own Conscience

Presuming if you were Dr. Wallace that what was done was per the policy and procedure manual and you were dubious regarding the adequacy of such procedures, what would you do?

1. Leave a message on your own voice mail box as to how best to contact you when away.
2. Forward your work phone to another clinician so that clients are covered regardless of what happens in the general clinic.
3. Inform clients of your plan to be out of town, regardless of whether regularly scheduled appointments would have been missed.
4. Discuss any at-risk client with the clinician covering for the long weekend before leaving on holiday.
5. Call in on Tuesday to talk to a live person to make sure someone had your cell phone number to contact you for emergencies.
6. Check your voice mail from out of town, and take care of any client emergencies without relying on clinic backup.
7. Think better of it, and come back to town as previously scheduled.
8. Do a combination of the previously listed actions.
9. Do something that is not previously listed.

If you were Dr. Wallace and this occurred in Canada, you would have been better served to arrange for off-hours coverage while you were away and communicate clearly with all clients the matter of your absence.

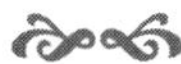

CHAPTER 4

Privacy and Confidentiality

Ethical Standard 4

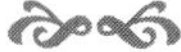

CHAPTER OUTLINE

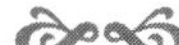

STANDARD 4.01: MAINTAINING CONFIDENTIALITY

Psychologists have a primary obligation and take reasonable precautions to protect confidential information obtained through or stored in any medium, recognizing that the extent and limits of confidentiality may be regulated by law or established by institutional rules or professional or scientific relationship.

A CASE FOR STANDARD 4.01: Confidentiality and Age of Majority

Last year Dr. Brooks treated Stephanie, a 12-year-old girl, for depression. Although Stephanie's mother drove her to the sessions, she had expressed at the beginning of the first session that she did not want to be involved in her daughter's treatment because the daughter did not want her to know what was said to the psychologist. Dr. Brooks conducted regular weekly sessions with Stephanie for 3 to 4 months. In the course of treatment, Stephanie reported that she was pregnant. Dr. Brooks inquired about whether Stephanie had seen a doctor to confirm the pregnancy, and she said she had it confirmed at a local clinic. Dr. Brooks discussed options with

Stephanie, including the possibility of telling her parents. She was very afraid of this option given that her parents are fundamentalist Christians. After the session in which Dr. Brooks discussed talking to the parents, Stephanie did not show for her next appointment. Stephanie said she wanted to "quit" therapy when Dr. Brooks made a follow-up call to find out why Stephanie missed the appointment. Dr. Brooks recommended against termination to both Stephanie and her parents, but Stephanie terminated anyway with her parents' agreement. Four months later, Stephanie is now 13 years old. Dr. Brooks receives a phone message from Stephanie's parents. Her parents are irate and demand that copies of records be sent to them.

Issues of Concern

What age of the client does your jurisdiction consider necessary to provide consent to treatment and retain the right to confidentiality? At what age does your jurisdiction consider participation in sexual intercourse a crime against a minor, regardless of whether the minor consented? Can the fact that Stephanie's mother only drove her to therapy and did not interact with Dr. Brooks except to tell Dr. Brooks that at her daughter's request she was not going to be part of treatment constitute implied consent to secure the privilege of confidentiality regardless of the law of the jurisdiction?

APA Ethics Code

Companion General Principle

Principle A: Beneficence and Nonmaleficence

> Psychologists strive to benefit those with whom they work and take care to do no harm.

To abide by the principle of nonmaleficence, Dr. Brooks needs to consider whether predictable harm might arise if Stephanie's parents gain knowledge of the content of treatment records.

Principle B: Fidelity and Responsibility

> Psychologists establish relationships of trust with those with whom they work.

To abide by the principle of fidelity, Dr. Brooks would retain the trust of the client by keeping to the confidentiality agreement established at the beginning of the treatment. This attests to the importance of the confidentiality portion of informed consent to treatment.

Principle E: Respect for People's Rights and Dignity

> Psychologists respect the dignity and worth of all people, and the rights of individuals to privacy, confidentiality, and self-determination.

To abide by the various elements of Principle E, Dr. Brooks needs to determine who has the right to access information obtained from Stephanie in session; to ensure confidentiality, Dr. Brooks needs to determine whether Stephanie holds the privilege of confidentiality. With regard to self-determination, Dr. Brooks needs to decide who has consented to treatment for Stephanie: her parents or Stephanie.

Companion Ethical Standard(s)

Standard 3.10: Informed Consent

> . . . (b) For persons who are legally incapable of giving informed consent, psychologists nevertheless . . . (4) Obtain appropriate permission from a legally authorized person . . . (d) Psychologists appropriately document written or oral consent, permission, and assent.

The application of self-determination, Standard 3.10 (b), directs Dr. Brooks to obtain consent from Stephanie's mother for Stephanie to be in treatment if Stephanie is considered a minor in your state. Additionally, Standard 3.10 (d) directs Dr. Brooks to have that consent documented.

Standard 10.01: Informed Consent to Therapy

> (a) When obtaining informed consent to therapy . . . , psychologists inform clients . . . as early as is feasible in the therapeutic relationship about the . . . limits of confidentiality. . .

Standard 10.01 (a) directs Dr. Brooks to have had a conversation about who has access to information obtained from Stephanie in session. A verbal statement from Stephanie's mother that she does not wish to have access to treatment information indicates that such a conversation occurred, thus Dr. Brooks is in compliance with Standard 10.01 (a).

Standard 10.02: Therapy Involving Couples or Families

> (a) When psychologists agree to provide services to several persons who have a relationship (such as . . . parents and children), they take reasonable steps to clarify at the outset. . .
>
> . . . (1) which of the individuals are clients/patients and . . . (2) the relationship the psychologist will have with each person. This clarification includes the psychologist's role and the probable uses of the services provided or the information obtained.

Unless indications existed at the beginning of psychological services that the parents wanted to be involved in the services, this section does not apply to the vignette.

Standard 6.02: Maintenance, Dissemination, and Disposal of Confidential Records of Professional and Scientific Work

> (a) Psychologists maintain confidentiality in . . . accessing . . . records under their control . . .

Regardless of who has legal right to Stephanie's records, it is Dr. Brooks's responsibility to keep those records confidential. A necessary element to assure compliance with Standard 6.02 (a) is for Dr. Brooks to determine who has legal rights to Stephanie's records before releasing the records.

Legal Issues 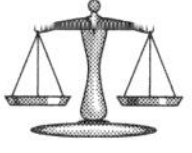

Florida

> *Florida Statute § 394.4784 (2010). Minors; access to outpatient crisis intervention services and treatment.*
>
> For the purposes of this section, the disability of nonage is removed for any minor age 13 years or older to access services. . .

California

> *Cal. Fam. Code § 6920 (West 2004).*
>
> . . . A minor may consent to the matters provided in this chapter, and the consent of the minor's parent or guardian is not necessary. . .
>
> *Cal. Fam. Code § 6924(b)(2)(d) (West 2004).*
>
> The mental health treatment . . . of a minor . . . shall include involvement of the minor's parent . . . unless, in the opinion of the professional person who is treating . . . the minor, the involvement would be inappropriate. The professional person who is treating . . . the minor shall state in the client record whether and when the person attempted to contact the minor's parent or guardian, and whether the attempt to contact was successful or unsuccessful, or the reason why, in the professional person's opinion, it would be inappropriate to contact the minor's parent or guardian.

For Florida, the age of consent for the purpose of mental health treatment is 13. If Dr. Brooks was practicing in Florida State and Stephanie's mother had consented to treatment for her, the parents would have held the authority for releasing confidential information at the time of treatment. If the parents requested Stephanie's records at that point, the psychologist legally could release the information and records. However, at the time of the request for records, Stephanie had turned 13 and thus gained authority concerning her records and the release of confidential information. Unless Stephanie provided a release of information, Dr. Brooks may not release the records as requested by the client's parents.

If Dr. Brooks was practicing in California, the age of consent, for the purpose of mental health treatment depends upon the circumstances of the case. Stephanie would hold the authority for releasing confidential information at the time of treatment as well as at the time of request for records. Dr. Brooks may not release the records as requested by the client's parents.

In both jurisdictions, Dr. Brooks would make a report to Child Protective Services (CPS) because reasonable suspicion of child abuse had arisen.

Cultural Considerations

Global Discussion

Code of Ethics for Psychologists: Netherlands

> 1.5.1 Representation of clients; legally minor client.
>
> If the client is a legal minor . . . , the rights granted to him in terms of the Code are exercised by his legal representative(s), unless the psychologist has reason to believe that their participation in the professional relationship would seriously undermine the interests of the client. The client aged 16 years and over is in all cases deemed to have reached the age of discretion, unless he is deemed incapable of adequately exercising his rights. The client aged 12 years and over will be stimulated to

seek full and active participation in decisions which effect him, regardless of the claims of his legal representative(s).

Given that this situation involves a client between the ages of 12 and 16, a psychologist practicing in the Netherlands would need to discuss the parent's request for release of records with the client before any action is taken.

American Moral Values

1. Does Dr. Brooks attach a special moral status to pregnancy (as opposed to, say, drug abuse)? If she considers being pregnant an especially private and personal matter (having to do with one's own body, one's sexuality, one's own child being considered), does she keep the client's confidentiality? Or does she view pregnancy as too important not to involve other family members for support and moral guidance, especially given the client's age?
2. What if Dr. Brooks considers it impossible that pregnancy at age 12 could be consensual, even if the 12-year-old claims that it was not child abuse? If Dr. Brooks has an abhorrence of child abuse and/or statutory rape, will that lead her to release the records to Stephanie's parents?
3. Does Dr. Brooks believe that the mother's earlier statement that she did not wish to be "involved" was a promise to keep the treatment confidential? Was the treatment based on that understanding, in which case informing the parents would violate Dr. Brooks's own implicit promise to the client?
4. How does Dr. Brooks view her responsibility to protect her client from further harm? Does she anticipate harm coming to Stephanie from her parents gaining knowledge of her pregnancy? What is Dr. Brooks's assessment of Stephanie's family and their ability to be supportive?

Ethical Course of Action

Directive per APA Code

Standard 4.01, in conjunction with Standards 6.02, directs Dr. Brooks to protect the information contained in Dr. Brooks's record of Stephanie's sessions. Standard 4.01 directs Dr. Brooks to enact the directive of Standard 6.02 by keeping the records confidential. In addition to Standard 4.01, Dr. Brooks needs to act within limitations established by law. If Dr. Brooks was practicing in California or Florida, she would not release the records to Stephanie's parents. She would make a CPS report as a mandatory reporter.

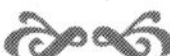

Dictates of One's Own Conscience

If you were Dr. Brooks and you did not know the situation with Stephanie after a 4-month interval, you would not be able to determine whether it might be harmful or beneficial to Stephanie to release records. Aspiring to the highest principle of beneficence and nonmaleficence, what might you do?

1. Respond with a letter that references the age of consent in your state, with enclosed records if your state law deems Stephanie to be a minor.
2. Respond with a letter that references the age of consent in your state, and do not enclose records if your state law deems Stephanie to be the age of majority for the purpose of mental health treatment.
3. Discuss the issue with Stephanie to ascertain the realistic impact and potential harm of releasing the records.
4. Remind the client as to the extent of her confidentiality protections regarding the records.
5. Make it clear to Stephanie that records would not be sent to her parents without her permission.
6. If Stephanie agrees to the release of information, request that Stephanie be present during the disclosures.
7. If Stephanie agrees to the disclosure of confidential information, insist that Stephanie be present so that you can help with the processing of the parental reactions.
8. Instead of release of records, ask that the parents and Stephanie come in to discuss the release of records in person. Tell the parents that Stephanie is the client, and that to avoid a multiple or dual relationship, Stephanie and you will discuss the records and the therapy with them as collaterals to the psychotherapy. You reason that you will be more likely able to support Stephanie in such sessions.
9. Do a combination of the previously listed actions.
10. Do something that is not previously listed.

If you were Dr. Brooks practicing in the Netherlands, the previously listed options would still apply since the age of majority for the purpose of mental health treatment is not substantially different from those listed for Florida or California.

STANDARD 4.02: DISCUSSING THE LIMITS OF CONFIDENTIALITY

> (a) Psychologists discuss with persons (including, to the extent feasible, persons who are legally incapable of giving informed consent and their legal representatives) and organizations with whom they establish a scientific or professional relationship; (1) the relevant limits of psychological activities.

A CASE FOR STANDARD 4.02 (A): At Wit's End

Carolyn, a 29-year-old single mother, has been in treatment for the past 9 months with Dr. Woods for generalized anxiety. Carolyn is a former methamphetamine and alcohol abuser. She has sustained recovery for 1.5 years and is doing well (no cravings). She has been seeing her Alcoholic Anonymous (AA) sponsor and attending AA meetings regularly. She lives with her new boyfriend whom she's known for 6 months and is currently receiving food stamps. Lately, she's been having trouble with her 5-year-old daughter who refuses to eat any of the food that Carolyn prepares at home. Her daughter will only eat McDonald's fast food. Carolyn has to drive 2 miles each way to the nearest McDonald's. Carolyn reports feeling stressed, worried about money, and feeling exhausted. This week in session Carolyn reported that her stress level had risen to the point where she could not sleep. Feeling exhausted, sleep deprived, and at her wit's end, Carolyn lost her temper with her 5-year-old daughter. Last week, with no extra money for gas or McDonald's food, she told Dr. Woods, she found herself shaking her daughter and calling her a selfish, uncaring brat at the top of her lungs.

Issues of Concern

Standard 4.02 directs Dr. Woods to have discussed, presumably at intake, the limits of confidentiality. In most states and provinces, psychologists are mandatory reporters for child abuse. Should Dr. Woods have informed Carolyn at the onset of treatment that authorities would be contacted should anything occur during the course of treatment that indicates child abuse may or has occurred? If so, would Carolyn expect Dr. Woods to report the incident to an agency such as CPS? Even if Dr. Woods had provided Carolyn with an office policy document that explicated the conditions under which psychologists are mandated to report in the state, it does not mean that Carolyn understood that one of the foreseeable uses of the information might be a report to the state against her.

Dr. Woods has the choice of reporting Carolyn to CPS, which may come as a surprise to Carolyn since this may be one of the unforeseen uses of treatment information. If Dr. Woods believes that reasonable suspicion of child abuse has not arisen, another option would be to discuss with Carolyn that they need to immediately develop a plan to avoid any other such situations where Carolyn may abuse her children. Such an intervention would constitute a reminder to the client of the possible foreseeable use of confidential information.

APA Ethics Code

Companion General Principle

Principle A: Beneficence and Nonmaleficence

> Psychologists seek to safeguard the welfare and rights of those with whom they interact professionally and other affected persons. . .

Principle A guides Dr. Woods to safeguard Carolyn's welfare as the person with whom the interaction is occurring. Principle A additionally guides Dr. Woods to safeguard the welfare of "other affected persons," which would include the 5-year-old daughter.

Principle B: Fidelity and Responsibility

> Psychologists establish relationships of trust with those with whom they work. They are aware of their professional . . . responsibilities to society. . .

Dr. Woods, aspiring to the principle of fidelity, would try to uphold his client's trust by keeping his client's confidences. In some cases, as in mandatory reporting situations, psychologists are pulled between the opposing needs of therapeutic necessity of confidentiality and the social responsibility of reporting child abuse.

Companion Ethical Standard(s)

Standard 4.05: Disclosures

> Psychologists disclose confidential information without the consent of the individual only as mandated by law . . . for a valid purpose such as to . . . protect the client/patient, . . . or others from harm.

In most states, psychologists are mandatory reporters of child abuse. If Dr. Woods was practicing in such a state, he would be obligated to report Carolyn to the state for having committed an abusive act, that of shaking a 5-year-old child.

Legal Issues 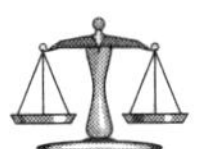

Alabama

> *Ala. Admin. Code 750-X-6-.02 (2009).*
>
> American Psychological Association Ethical Principles Of Psychologists And Code Of Conduct, 2002 Edition (Appendix II) . . . Adopt By Reference: . . . Filed May 13, 2003; effective June 17, 2003.
>
> *Ala. Admin. Code § 26-14-3 (2009). Mandatory reporting.*
>
> (a) All . . . mental health professionals . . . called upon to render aid . . . to any child, when the child is known or suspected to be a victim of child abuse or neglect, shall be required to report, or cause a report to be made of the same, orally, either by telephone or direct communication immediately, followed by a written report, to a duly constituted authority.

Alaska

> *Alaska Stat. § 08.86.200 (2008). Confidentiality of communication.*
>
> (a) A psychologist . . . may not reveal to another person a communication made to the psychologist . . . by a client about a matter concerning which the client has employed the psychologist . . . in a professional capacity. . .
>
> (b) Notwithstanding (a) of this section, a psychologist . . . shall report to the appropriate authority incidents of child abuse or neglect . . .

In both jurisdictions, Dr. Woods is a mandatory reporter who must make a report to CPS. In Arkansas, the report must be made orally and in writing. In Alaska, an oral report is likely to be sufficient.

Cultural Considerations

Global Discussion

Code of Ethics: Netherlands

> III.2.4 . Confidentiality.
>
> III.2.4.3. Breach of confidence.
>
> The psychologist is not obliged to observe confidentiality if he has legitimate reason to believe that a breach of confidence is the sole remaining measure that can prevent clear and imminent danger to any individual, or if they are required by law to disclose confidential information.
>
> III.2.4.4. Information about breach of confidence.
>
> If circumstances of this kind are likely to arise, the psychologist informs, if possible, those involved that a breach of confidence may prove inevitable at some point in time.
>
> III.2.4.5. Range of breach of confidence.
>
> If the psychologist decides to disclose confidential information, then he . . . shall inform those involved of his decision to do so.

If Dr. Woods was practicing in the Netherlands, it would have been sufficient to inform Carolyn at the outset of the treatment relationship of the limits to confidentiality, including imminent harm to others, and to have informed Carolyn, "if possible," prior to contacting authorities to report possible child endangerment. It is ideal, but it is not mandated nor obligated for Dr. Woods to discuss this with Carolyn in advance of a report. He would be within the letter and intent of this code if he reported to Carolyn after-the-fact what actions he had taken.

American Moral Values

1. How does Dr. Woods weigh the need to protect children from abuse against the confidentiality of the client and, more importantly, the prospects of helping a client become a better parent? Will informing CPS threaten Dr. Woods's relationship with Carolyn, and will that be in the best interests of the child? Or will neglecting to tell CPS be dangerous for Carolyn's child, since Dr. Woods alone cannot necessarily protect the daughter from future harm?

2. How does Carolyn's status as a recovering addict alter Dr. Woods's moral view? Is the struggle of recovery, when added to the stress of parenting,

more likely to send Carolyn over the edge? Is this further reason to tell CPS, or is this a reason why maintaining Carolyn's trust through engaging in the report together paramount?

3. How does Dr. Woods consider his own abilities as a therapist in this situation? Can treatment succeed in helping Carolyn adapt better to parental stress fast enough that a CPS report can be made and a voluntary service plan be entered into so that Carolyn does not lose her child to foster care?

4. Has Dr. Woods given Carolyn enough information about confidentiality at the outset? If not, will that affect how Dr. Woods feels about CPS? How can that best be remedied? Will Carolyn feel betrayed if he suddenly explains its limits as a prelude to informing CPS about her behavior?

Ethical Course of Action

Directive per APA Code

Standard 4.05 directs Dr. Woods to report Carolyn should he live in a state that mandates psychologists to report child abuse. Dr. Woods, following the directive of Standard 4.02 (a), would now have another conversation with Carolyn about how some confidences must be disclosed under the law. He can engage in the principle of fidelity by reporting Carolyn's behavior to CPS with Carolyn present.

Dictates of One's Own Conscience

For most clients, the act of disclosing confidential information to the state without a client's consent is experienced as an act of betrayal that usually results in clients terminating treatment. Ever aware of such a possibility, if you were Dr. Woods, what additional intervention might you consider in addition to informing Carolyn of your legal responsibility?

1. Tell Carolyn you will be reporting the incident to CPS but reassure her that in most cases where a mother is in treatment, CPS will not investigate.
2. Tell Carolyn, as you told her at the beginning of therapy, that should you find out child abuse is occurring, you will report the incident for the ultimate protection of her children.
3. As soon as Carolyn started to say anything that hinted at child abuse, remind her about the limits of confidentiality and guard her against saying anything that might incriminate herself. Explore the details of the situation more with Carolyn, discussing what she did and the impact that it had on her daughter.
4. Convince Carolyn that a CPS report and doctor's visit is best for her daughter, to make sure that she is OK.
5. Jointly, with Carolyn on a conference call, report the incident to CPS.
6. Have Carolyn make the CPS call with you in the room for support.
7. Do a combination of the previously listed actions.
8. Do something that is not previously listed.

If you were Dr. Woods practicing in the Netherlands, you would have discharged your ethical obligation by informing Carolyn you had made a CPS report after such a report was entered with the proper authorities.

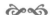

STANDARD 4.02: DISCUSSING THE LIMITS OF CONFIDENTIALITY

> . . . (b) Unless it is not feasible or is contraindicated, the discussion of confidentiality occurs at the outset of the relationship and thereafter as new circumstances may warrant.

A CASE FOR STANDARD 4.02 (B): Taking Sides

Dr. Sanders was providing couples therapy to Christine and Russell. Christine was concurrently in individual treatment with Dr. Cole, who is Dr. Sanders's office mate in the same group practice. At the onset of treatment with Dr. Sanders, Christine had signed a release of information for Dr. Cole and Dr. Sanders to exchange information. As treatment progressed, both Christine and Russell said it was fine for Dr. Sanders to discuss the content of the couple's session with Dr. Cole, but no release of information had yet been signed.

During a peer consultation session in the office with Dr. Cole present, Dr. Sanders discussed witnessing an interaction between Christine and Russell where Christine's behavior toward Russell was indicative of contempt, blame, character assassination, and overall emotional abuse, because it seemed unwarranted and excessive. During the next session, Christine said, "I know you side with Russell. You have now put in his head that I have been abusing him. Not only that, but I know you have turned my therapist (Dr. Cole) against me. Now both of you are out to get me. Well, I'll get you first. I never signed that piece of paper for you to talk to Dr. Cole about Russell. I don't want you as my therapist anymore. I want the name and telephone number of your direct supervisor, and I am going to report you."

Issues of Concern

As directed by Standard 4.02 (a) and (b), Dr. Sanders discussed and obtained written consent for an exchange of information between appropriately engaged service providers. As seen in this situation, it is often not sufficient that the discussion of limits of confidentiality be relegated to the outset of the therapeutic relationship. Information that is revealed as treatment unfolds gives clients a very different perspective and willingness to release privilege of confidentiality. Was it sufficient to have previously obtained verbal release of information to discuss this case with Dr. Cole if such a verbal release was documented in the chart notes?

APA Ethics Code

Companion General Principle

Principle B: Fidelity and Responsibility

> . . . Psychologists consult . . . with other professionals . . . to the extent needed to serve the best interests of those with whom they work.

Within the context of respecting client confidentiality, psychologists do not work in isolation. When appropriate, psychologists consult for collaboration and for peer consultation. Dr. Sanders, to assure best service to her clients, consults with fellow psychologists for peer consultation and collaboration with Dr. Cole to coordinate treatment.

Companion Ethical Standard(s)

Standard 4.01: Maintaining Confidentiality

> Psychologists have a primary obligation and take reasonable precautions to protect confidential information obtained through . . . any medium, recognizing that the extent and limits of confidentiality may be regulated by law . . .

Standard 4.01 clearly places the burden of keeping information confidential in Dr. Sanders's domain.

Standard 3.09: Cooperation With Other Professionals

> When indicated and professionally appropriate, psychologists cooperate with other professionals in order to serve their client/patients effectively and appropriately.

Standard 3.09 directs Dr. Sanders to work with Dr. Cole in order to serve their mutual client in such a way that both Christine and Russell are effectively and appropriately served. In this case, it can be argued that sharing information between Drs. Sanders and Cole assures the most effective service.

Standard 4.05: Disclosures

> . . . (b) Psychologists disclose confidential information without the consent of the individual . . . where permitted by law for a valid purpose such as to . . . (2) obtain appropriate professional consultations . . .

From time to time, all psychologists are encouraged to engage in supervision and/or peer consultation to ensure the provision of ethical and efficacious service to clients. As permitted by Standard 4.05 (b) (2), Dr. Sanders's office consultation is within the ethical behavior of psychologists.

Standard 4.06: Consultations

> When consulting with colleagues, (1) psychologists do not disclose confidential information that reasonably could lead to the identification of a client/patient, . . . unless they have obtained the prior consent of the person . . . and (2) they disclose information only to the extent necessary to achieve the purposes of the consultation.

If Dr. Sanders did disclose information only to the extent necessary, such as not using Christine's and Russell's names during consultation, such consultation would be within the directives of Standard 4.06 as well as the boundaries of the verbal consent provided by Christine and Russell.

Standard 10.01: Informed Consent to Therapy

> (a) When obtaining informed consent to therapy . . . psychologists inform clients/patients as early as is feasible

> in the therapeutic relationship about the . . . limits of confidentiality and provide sufficient opportunity for the client/patient to ask questions and receive answers.

As directed by Standard 10.01 (a), at the onset of treatment Dr. Sanders should have informed her clients of her peer consultation situation. Thus, even without a signed written release of information from Christine and Russell, Dr. Sanders's consultations with Dr. Cole were within the ethical directives of Standard 10.01, 4.05, and 4.01.

Standard 10.02: Therapy Involving Couples or Families

> (a) When psychologists agree to provide services to several persons who have a relationship (such as spouses . . .), they take reasonable steps to clarify at the outset (1) which of the individuals are clients/patients and (2) the relationship the psychologist will have with each person. This clarification includes the psychologist's role and the probable uses of the . . . information obtained.

Standard 10.02 (a) is applicable in this situation with Dr. Sanders providing couples therapy. As directed by Standard 10.02 (a), Dr. Sanders should have clarified the difference between individual therapists, as is the role of Dr. Cole and a couples therapist. Part of that clarification of roles would include an explanation of exactly the issues that Christine is concerned mean that Dr. Sanders has "taken sides."

Standard 10.04: Providing Therapy to Those Served by Others

> In deciding whether to . . . provide services to those already receiving mental health services elsewhere, psychologists carefully consider the treatment issues and the potential client's/patient's welfare. Psychologists discuss these issues with the client/patient . . . in order to minimize the risk of confusion and conflict, consult with the other service providers when appropriate, and proceed with caution and sensitivity to the therapeutic issues.

Dr. Sanders is providing couples psychotherapy to Christine, who is also being served by Dr. Cole. Thus Standard 10.04 is applicable to this situation. The risk of confusion and conflict is evident in Christine's reaction to Dr. Sanders and Dr. Cole's coordination, as directed by Standard 3.09 and Standard 4.06.

Legal Issues

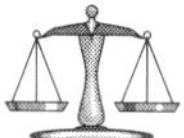

Arkansas

> *074-00-1 Ark. Code R. § 16 (2010). Code of ethics.*
>
> The Arkansas Psychology Board adopts the Ethical Principles of Psychologists and Code of Conduct of the American Psychological Association as part of these Rules and Regulations. The principles shall constitute one standard by which appropriate professional practices are determined.

Colorado

> *Colo. Rev. Stat. Ann. § 12-43-218 (West 2010). Disclosure of confidential communications.*
>
> (1) A licensee . . . shall not disclose, without the consent of the client, any confidential communications made by the client, . . . without the consent of the person to whom the knowledge relates.

In both jurisdictions, Christine would have no legitimate complaint against Dr. Sanders for engaging in consultation with Dr. Cole. Christine had provided consent to the consultation and coordination of services when asked. Both clinicians relied upon that verbal consent, and it was not revoked throughout the pendency of the couples and individual psychotherapy.

Cultural Considerations

Global Discussion

Canadian Code of Ethics for Psychologists

> Principle I: Respect for dignity of persons.
>
> *Informed consent.*
>
> I.24. Ensure, in the process of obtaining informed consent, that at least the following points are understood[:] . . . confidentiality protections and limitations . . .
>
> I.25. Provide new information in a timely manner, whenever such information becomes available and is significant enough that it reasonably could be seen as relevant to the original or ongoing informed consent.

Dr. Sanders has not violated the Canadian code as she has obtained a release of information to talk to Dr. Cole about Russell and Christine. The Canadian code calls for Dr. Sanders to explain to both Christine and Russell the significance and relevance of the information that she wants to share with Dr. Cole; what the benefits and risks to such disclosures might be; and modify the original consent, whether by documentation or by documenting the oral conversation. One original consent form or process does not cover every circumstance and as new information becomes relevant to share outside of Dr. Sanders's treatment room, the Canadian code demands that the original consent be modified.

American Moral Values

1. Should Dr. Sanders have mentioned Christine and Russell's case in a peer review consultation session? What is the benefit of that sharing compared to Christine's eventual move to end treatment and report her?
2. Should Dr. Sanders have continued treatment and the consultation without obtaining a written release confirming the verbal agreement about the consultation? Would that have jeopardized the rapport Dr. Sanders had with the couple?
3. Even if Dr. Sanders received Christine's written approval for an exchange of information at the beginning of her work with Dr. Cole, what is the best way to treat Christine given what she feels now? Will citing her signed paperwork put her in a corner? Is there any way to preserve the relationship without citing legal documents? Can Dr. Sanders explain more clearly why Christine's stated endorsement of the exchange opened the door to the consultations?

Ethical Course of Action

Directive per APA Code

Standard 4.02 (b) directs Dr. Sanders to have discussed the sharing of information between herself and Dr. Cole, which she did. Standard 4.02 (b) also directs Dr. Sanders to repeat this conversation throughout treatment as "new circumstances may warrant." Christine's reaction to an individual session appears to warrant another discussion from Dr. Sanders on the limits of confidentiality, the benefit of professional consultation and collaboration, and the meaning of her prior verbal consent.

Dictates of One's Own Conscience

In addition to all of the steps taken by Dr. Sanders, with perhaps the addition of making sure the written release of information was signed when the verbal release was given, what would you do to help the couple and possibly avoid an ethics complaint?

1. Review your chart notes and those of the consultant, the individual psychotherapist, to make sure that the verbal release was documented.
2. Argue back to the clients that what you did was within legal directives and that they have no grounds for a complaint.
3. Inform the couple that coordination between health care personnel is necessary to assure the best care for them.
4. Inform the couple that their name was not used in consultation, that you had not had a chance to discuss the case with Dr. Cole, so what Dr. Cole figured out about Christine had nothing to do with the couples treatment.
5. Ask Christine what action she would like you to take to rectify the situation.
6. Explore and use the conflict between you and Christine as a therapeutic intervention.
7. Ask if both of them wish to end treatment.
8. Do a combination of the previously listed actions.
9. Do something that is not previously listed.

If you were Dr. Sanders practicing in Canada, in addition to all of the steps already taken in the vignette, with perhaps the addition of making sure the written release of information was signed when the verbal release was given, what would you do to help the couple and possibly avoid an ethics complaint?

1. Apologize to Christine for surprising her regarding the content of professional consultation and the exact nature of the verbal release of confidential information with Dr. Cole.
2. Offer to discuss the content of consultation with Dr. Cole before the consultation next time.
3. Explore with Christine the reasons why she thought the opinion shared with Dr. Cole was inaccurate, regardless of whether she liked it or not.

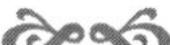

STANDARD 4.02: DISCUSSING THE LIMITS OF CONFIDENTIALITY

> . . . (c) Psychologists who offer services, products, or information via electronic transmission inform clients/patients of the risks to privacy and limits of confidentiality.

A CASE FOR STANDARD 4.02 (C): A Suicide in Progress

Larry is a psychology graduate student who has chosen to conduct a study of individuals who are gay/lesbian identified and who, in their youth, had attempted suicide. With permission from the institutional review board (IRB) and the chair of his Dissertation Committee, Larry posted a solicitation notice for research subjects on Craigslist with an e-mail address, webpage address, and phone number to contact for further information on the study. The webpage contact information was to Larry's professional page, which clearly outlines the other services Larry offers, including psychotherapy under his master's degree licensure and consultation for sexual minorities. One of the resources listed under Information on the website's home page discusses the Top Ten Warning Signs That Someone You Love Is Suicidal.

The day after the solicitation posting, Larry received an e-mail from Jeffrey. Jeffrey sent the e-mail detailing his difficult life as a gay-questioning 18-year-old who is constantly demeaned by his father for his nonmasculine ways. Jeffrey indicated that as he was typing he had a cord of rope on his lap and was ready to go to the garage to hang himself sometime before his family came home from a long weekend. Larry noticed that the e-mail was sent yesterday, with 2 days left before the ending of the long weekend.

Issues of Concern

What did Larry put into his solicitation invitation that was posted on Craigslist? If Larry were offering services, products, or information, then Standard 4.02 would guide Larry to have included information about limits of confidentiality in the solicitation, including Larry's duty to protect should a mandated reporting situation arise. Solicitation to participate in a research study would not generally be considered in the realm of services, products, or information. However, because the posting contained his professional webpage, which did contain information regarding services, Standard 4.02 does apply.

Since the message from Jeffrey was electronic, there is no way to verify the veracity of the claim that Jeffrey is indeed who he says he is and undergoing a suicide in progress. This could be some sort of attack from someone else using Jeffrey as an alias. On the other hand, it could be a real request for assistance. Has a client/psychotherapist relationship been established? Has a duty of confidentiality arisen in light of a unilateral contact?

Would Larry be obligated to reply to Jeffrey's e-mail with a response email? If Jeffrey had included any types of identifier in his email, would Larry be mandated to break confidentiality to make a report? Is it ethical for Larry to take any actions about the possible suicide attempt of a person with whom he has no prior personal or professional relationship?

APA Ethics Code

Companion General Principle

Principle B: Fidelity and Responsibility

> Psychologists uphold professional standards of conduct, clarify their professional roles and obligations, accept appropriate responsibility for their behavior, and seek to manage conflicts of interest that could lead to exploitation or harm.

Larry posted an ad on Craigslist with a webpage address and by doing so may have established himself as an expert in Jeffrey's mind. While Larry has not officially begun a professional relationship with Jeffrey, he has nonetheless become aware of a potentially dangerous situation. To accept appropriate responsibility for the resultant e-mail from his advertisement on Craigslist may entail Larry responding in some fashion that is of benefit to Jeffrey while upholding the professional role of a researcher.

Principle C: Integrity

> Psychologists strive to keep their promises and to avoid unwise or unclear commitments.

Larry may not have been clear in his intentions, expectations, or limitations within his advertisement. Even if the Craigslist solicitation has been clearly confined to the study, the webpage contained information about providing treatment services. The content of the webpage could have lead to confusion regarding the limited extent of Larry's intent in the Craigslist solicitation.

Companion Ethical Standard(s)

Standard 3.10: Informed Consent

> (a) When psychologists conduct research . . . via electronic transmission . . . they obtain the informed consent of the

> individual . . . using language that is reasonably understandable to that person. . .

Presumably Larry would have obtained consent from individuals who contacted him to participate in his research. The situation with Jeffrey is one in which Larry has not made contact with him thus has not had an opportunity to discuss consent or any other relevant issues pertaining to the research project. In the absence of informed consent, as specified in Standard 3.10, does Larry have any professional obligations to Jeffrey?

Standard 4.05: Disclosures

> . . . (b) Psychologists disclose confidential information without the consent of the individual only as mandated by law. . .

Chances are there was some mention of confidentiality in the solicitation for a research subject. It is doubtful whether the limit of confidentiality was specified in the solicitation. There is higher probability of a confidentiality clause mentioned on Larry's webpage. Even if Larry did include limit of confidentiality, it is doubtful if Jeffrey fully understood its implications. Even if Larry wished to alert some authority of Jeffrey's imminent danger to himself, it may not be possible to give law enforcement enough information to locate Jeffrey. Given all of these conditions, should Larry attempt to intervene in what appears to be a suicide in progress by contacting law enforcement authorities?

Standard 7.01: Design of Education and Training Programs

> Psychologists responsible for education and training programs take reasonable steps to ensure that the programs are designed to provide the appropriate knowledge and proper experiences, . . . for which claims are made by the program.

Larry's status as a graduate student means that his research activities are guided under the supervision of a faculty. The structure of the supervision for Larry's work, as specified under Standard 7.01, is incorporated into the design of the training program. Regardless of whether it should have been foreseen, does the program provide Larry with access to his professors for guidance in handling this situation as suggested by Standard 7.01?

Legal Issues 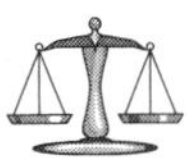

Florida

Fla. Admin. Code Ann. r. 64B19-19.002 (2010). Definitions.

A "client", . . . is that individual who, by virtue of private consultation with the psychologist, has reason to expect that the individual's communication with the psychologist during that private consultation will remain confidential, regardless of who pays for the services of the psychologist.

Fla. Admin. Code Ann. r. 64B19-11.005 (2010). Supervised experience requirements.

(1) Definitions. Within the context of this rule, the following definitions apply:

. . . (b) "Psychology Resident or Post-Doctoral Fellow." A psychology resident or post-doctoral fellow is a person who has met Florida's educational requirements for licensure and intends from the outset of the supervised experience to meet that part of the supervised experience requirement for licensure which is not part of the person's internship.

. . . (e) The psychology resident or post-doctoral fellow shall inform all service users of her or his supervised status and provide the name of the supervising psychologist. . .

Fla. Admin. Code Ann. r. 64B19-19.006 (2010). Confidentiality.

(1) One of the primary obligations of psychologists is to respect the confidentiality of information entrusted to them by service users . . .

Florida Statute 490.0147 (2010). Confidentiality and privileged communications.

Any communication between any person licensed under this chapter and . . . his . . . client shall be confidential. This privilege may be waived under the following conditions:

. . . (3) When there is a clear and immediate probability of physical harm to the . . . client, . . . and the person licensed under this chapter communicates the information only to the . . . appropriate family member, or law enforcement or other appropriate authorities.

Hawaii

Haw. Code R. § 16-98-4 (2010). Direction of an individual [psychology trainee].

Only a licensed psychologist in the State shall be considered eligible to direct the services of an individual and only if the licensed psychologist meets the following requirements:

> ...(3) Is responsible for the direct and continuing administrative and professional direction of the person being directed;
>
> ...(8) Establishes and maintains a level of supervisory contact consistent with establish professional standards, and be fully accountable in the event that professional, ethical, or legal issues are raised.

Haw. Code R. § 16-98-34 (2010). Unethical practice of psychology.

> ...(d) Safeguarding information about an individual that has been obtained by the psychologist in the course of...investigation is a primary obligation of the psychologist. Such information shall not be communicated to others unless certain important conditions are met:
>
> (1) Information received in confidence may be revealed only after careful deliberation and where there is a clear and imminent danger to an individual...and then only to appropriate professional workers or public authorities.

In Florida and Hawaii, the law requires Larry to disclose that he is in training and the name of his supervisor. The law in Florida also suggests that Jeffrey would not be viewed as having entered into a professional relationship because no interaction had occurred between Larry and Jeffrey. In Hawaii, the law remains silent on whether the type of contact Jeffrey engaged in is sufficient to establish a professional relationship with the resulting duties. If Jeffrey's e-mail was viewed by the Florida and Hawaii licensing boards as having established the expectation of a professional relationship, Larry could disclose all information from the record created by Jeffrey to protect Jeffrey from harm, and not violate the confidentiality laws.

Cultural Considerations

Global Discussion

The Professional Board for Psychology Health Professions Council of South Africa:
Ethical Code of Professional Conduct (April 2002)

> 3.1. Discussing the limits of confidentiality.
>
> 3.2.2. When engaging in electronically transmitted services psychologists shall ensure that confidentiality and privacy are ensured and shall inform clients of the measures undertaken to guarantee confidentiality.

In order to comply with South Africa's code, Larry would inform all potential visitors to his website about confidentiality, privacy, and the possible exceptions to confidentiality. Further, Larry is obligated to inform prospective clients about the measures to safeguard confidential information. The code remains unclear about whether Jeffrey can be considered a potential client when he was rerouted from the Craigslist ad to Larry's website, rather than directly seeking out the website himself. South Africa's code is one of the only other extant psychological codes of ethics to address electronic services.

American Moral Values

1. What is Larry's responsibility to the e-mailer, who appears to be on the verge of attempting suicide? Does a suicide threat in an exchange of e-mails permit the release of the details provided in order to obtain the e-mailer's identity/whereabouts?
2. What if Jeffrey is not the author of the e-mails? What are the possible effects of taking action on "Jeffrey's" suicide? Would it unwittingly "out" the real Jeffrey? Or would it be an empty pursuit that distracts Larry from his research?
3. Does Larry find communication over e-mail or other online forms to lead to personal accountability for the people interacting with this medium? Does e-mail justify as high a sense of accountability to others' sufferings as does a face-to-face or even phone contact?
4. What is Larry's and his supervisor's responsibility for recruiting people in the way that he did? Was it not fairly predictable that teens who struggle with their sexual identity and once considered suicide might call in with a "crisis" question? Should Larry's supervisor foresee the real possibility of such a scenario from a Craigslist advertisement? As a psychology graduate student, should Larry have included the identity of his supervising psychologist in the Craigslist solicitation?

Ethical Course of Action

Directive per APA Code

Under the umbrella of Standard 4.02 (a), relationships include those scientific or professional in nature. Jeffrey's relationship to Larry is both scientific, as part of a research project, and professional, as part of Larry's professional activities. Standard 4.02 (c) does name relevant activities to include only services, products, or information. Though Larry's research activities may not fall under services, products, or information, it does fall under scientific or professional as referenced in Standard 4.02 (a). In addition, the reference to a webpage that advertises treatment services links Larry's research activities with his treatment services. Standard 4.02 (a) dictates that Larry's electronic transmissions include information on the limits of confidentiality.

If Larry was conducting his research in the state of Florida and Larry does not respond to Jeffrey's e-mail, then no further obligation is incurred and Larry does not need to report this suicide incident. However, this does not preclude Larry choosing to respond to Jeffrey or to notify police of a possible suicide in progress.

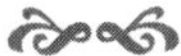

Dictates of One's Own Conscience

If you were Larry attending graduate school in Florida and received the e-mail from Jeffrey in response to your solicitation for research subjects, what would you do?

1. Reply by e-mail to Jeffrey, tell him that you are concerned and care about his safety, and ask him if he would like to talk about this further.
2. Provide him with your number as well as that of any local suicide prevention resources and/or crisis lines and encourage him to call.
3. Leave it up to him to decide his next step without any intervention.
4. Acting as a mandated reporter, contact the police and provide them with the e-mail address and the information that suggests the possibility of a suicide in progress.
5. Modify your Craigslist recruitment tool with the notations about the fact that you are in training and your supervisor's name.
6. Modify your Craigslist recruitment tool further by adding a number to a teen suicide prevention hotline.
7. Do a combination of the previously listed actions.
8. Do something that is not previously listed.

If you were Larry attending graduate school in South Africa and received the e-mail from Jeffrey in response to your solicitation for research subjects, what would you do?

1. Respond to the e-mail from Jeffrey as follows:
   a. With information about the limit of confidentiality
   b. With information about the research project
2. Do not release Jeffrey's information without his consent.

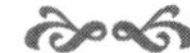

STANDARD 4.03: RECORDING

> Before recording the voices or images of individuals to whom they provide services, psychologists obtain permission from all such persons or their legal representatives.

A CASE FOR STANDARD 4.03: Retroactive Destruction of Records

Eric, a psychology graduate student, is meeting his first client. Both the school clinic staff and Eric have explained to the client that all treatment sessions will be video recorded for the purpose of providing Eric with supervision. Authorization is obtained both verbally and in writing before the first treatment session. The client, Stephen, works as a contract carpenter in the city. Treatment progressed smoothly until the fifth session when Stephen refused to enter the treatment room. Standing in the hallway, and speaking in a half-whisper, Stephen said that he had just run into an ex-girlfriend of his, who, to his alarm, was attending school here and was in a counseling program. Stephen thought his ex-girlfriend could gain access to his treatment videos and did not want to enter into the treatment room until the recording device was turned off and all previous videos were destroyed. He also would not engage in any further video recordings of the future sessions.

Issues of Concern

Eric and the clinic have faithfully followed the directives of Standard 4.03, which clearly directs Eric not to make further recordings of sessions. Stephen has essentially revoked his permission for recordings. Can the earlier records be altered? In requesting the deletion of video recordings, Stephen is asking for alteration of his records, not for disposal of the record. Video recording is typically only part of a file that is created for a client. Can a client retroactively rescind permission for creation of a part of the treatment record? Would destruction of the previous recordings be considered as an alteration of records and a violation of the law?

APA Ethics Code

Companion General Principle

Principle B: Fidelity and Responsibility

> Psychologists establish relationships of trust with those with whom they work... Psychologists ... clarify their professional roles and obligations ... and seek to manage conflicts of interest that could lead to ... harm.

Stephen is asking Eric to keep to the principle of fidelity. Stephen needs to trust that the content of the treatment sessions are confidential with no possibility of access by anyone he knows. To ensure trust from clients, Eric is guided to make sure that the training clinic's policies and procedures are in place to ensure file security. Might Eric be caught between meeting the client's request versus his role as a student, which entails obtaining supervision with video recording?

Principle E: Respect for People's Rights and Dignity

> Psychologists respect ... the rights of individuals to privacy, confidentiality, and self-determination.

Aspiring to make certain Stephen's rights to privacy and confidentiality are upheld, Eric first needs to be assured himself that Stephen's ex-girlfriend has no access to Stephen's video or written records. Should Stephen not be adequately assured of his privacy and choose to end treatment, Principle E guides Eric to respect Stephen's right to make such a decision as part of Stephen's right to self-determination.

Companion Ethical Standard(s)

Standard 6.01: Documentation of Professional and Scientific Work and Maintenance of Records

> Psychologists create, and to the extent records are under their control, maintain ... records and data relating to their professional ... work in order to ... (1) facilitate provision of services later by them or by other professionals ... [and] (3) meet institutional requirements.

Standard 6.01 stipulates that "to the extent" that the video and the written record are under Eric's control, he is to manage the files.

Standard 6.02: Maintenance, Dissemination, and Disposal of Confidential Records of Professional and Scientific Work

> (a) Psychologists maintain confidentiality in creating, storing, accessing, transferring, and disposing of records under their control, whether these are written, automated, or in any other medium.

Does Standard 6.01 and 6.02 absolve Eric of the responsibility for Stephen's privacy given that Eric does not have control of records, whether it is a video recording or a written file, except for the creation of the information? Are records the clinic's to control? Standard 6.01 directs psychologists to assure confidentiality is kept, even in the disposal of records. The standards are silent as to whether records are to be altered once created. Thus the question becomes whether Eric and the clinic can comply with Stephen's request for alteration of records.

Standard 4.07: Use of Confidential Information for Didactic or Other Purposes

> Psychologists do not disclose ... confidential, personally identifiable information concerning their clients/patients ... that they obtained during the course of their work, unless ... (1) they take reasonable steps to disguise the person ..., [and] (2) the person ... has consented in writing.

Standard 4.07 does not pertain to Eric since he is using the information for supervision. However, except for the purpose of supervision, Standard 4.07 directs Eric's supervisor to keep all information about Stephen confidential and disguise all involved should the material be used in any other way besides supervision of Eric.

Standard 7.06: Assessing Student and Supervisee Performance

> ... (b) Psychologists evaluate students and supervisees on the basis of their actual performance on relevant and established program requirements.

With the removal of the video recordings, Eric's supervisor would no longer be able to access Eric's actual performance. When Eric's supervisor conducts an evaluation of Eric's work, he/she would be in violation of Standard 7.06 unless the supervisor had access to other video recordings of Eric's work.

Legal Issues 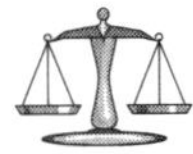

Idaho

Idaho Code Ann. § 54-2309 (2007). Nonissuance and revocation of license.

No license may be issued, and a license previously issued may be revoked, suspended, restricted or otherwise disciplined if the person applying, or the person licensed be:

. . . (5) Found by the board to have been unethical as detailed by the current, and future amended, ethical standards of the American Psychological Association.

Iowa

Iowa Admin. Code r. 645-240.9 (2010). Psychologists' supervision of unlicensed persons in a practice setting.

The supervising psychologist shall:

1. Be vested with administrative control over the functioning of assistants in order to maintain ultimate responsibility for the welfare of every client . . .

2. Have sufficient knowledge of all clients, . . . in order to plan effective service delivery procedures. The progress of the work shall be monitored through such means as will ensure that full legal and professional responsibility can be accepted by the supervisor for all services rendered . . .

. . . 9. Establish and maintain a level of supervisory contact consistent with established professional standards, and be fully accountable in the event that professional, ethical or legal issues are raised.

Iowa Admin. Code r. 645-242.2 (2010). Grounds for discipline.

(1) Failure to comply with the Ethical Principles of Psychologists and Code of Conduct of the American Psychological Association, as published in the December 2002 edition of American Psychologist, hereby adopted by reference.

. . . (9) Falsification, alteration or destruction of client or patient records with the intent to deceive.

In both jurisdictions, Eric would stop video recording of the psychotherapy because of Stephen's revocation of consent. Under Iowa law, the prior videotapes could be erased, as no intention of deception is present. If Eric's supervisor believed that appropriate supervision could not be conducted without video recording, Eric would need to either find another supervisor who could work within the demands of the context or withdraw from the case, in order to not violate the law of either jurisdiction.

Cultural Considerations

Global Discussion

British Psychological Society Code of Ethics

4: Confidentiality.

Specifically they shall:

4.5. Only make video recordings of recipients of services . . . with the expressed agreement of those being recorded both to the recording being made and to the subsequent conditions of access to it . . .

Any video or audio recording of a service recipient is the property of that recipient, not the psychologist or the clinic in which they practice. The client must agree to the recording itself and the "subsequent conditions of access" to those recordings.

American Moral Values

1. How does Eric weigh possible problems between Stephen and his ex-girlfriend and his therapeutic agenda with Stephen? Why is the preservation of the previous week's tapes so important to Eric's project? Is Stephen's wish not to be seen important enough to threaten the pedagogical use of his own sessions?
2. Does Eric's position as the person evaluated with those tapes complicate his appeal to Stephen? Does it not appear as if Eric is looking out for his own job rather than Stephen's process of healing?
3. What would be the impact of showing the tapes on the relationship between Stephen and Eric? Would this erode trust between them? Is that cost too high for Eric?
4. Does Stephen's socioeconomic or cultural background make a difference in how Eric views this issue? Would his girlfriend use her knowledge of his therapy to discredit him in the eyes of his family

or community, especially if they regard therapy as disloyal or selfish? Or would this stay confined to his relationship with his girlfriend?

Ethical Course of Action

Directive per APA Code

Standard 4.03 directs Eric to have obtained permission before making recordings of sessions with Stephen. Eric was in compliance with the directives of Standard 4.03 at the beginning of treatment. Following the directives of Standard 4.03, Eric is now not to video record sessions with Stephen because permission for such recording no longer exists. Standard 6: Recordkeeping and Fees is silent on redaction of records. Therefore, Eric and his supervisor would need to address the possible violation of Standard 7.06 (b) by not having an ability to evaluate Eric's performance based on direct access to actual performance.

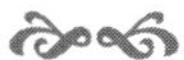

Dictates of One's Own Conscience

It is clear from the directive of Standard 4.03 that no further video recording of Stephen is permissible. If you were Eric and needed the video recording to obtain supervision, what might you do? In addition, if you were Eric's supervisor and/or the clinic director, on the receiving end of a request for alteration of records, what would you do?

1. As the student therapist, you would do as follows:
   a. Turn off the video recording device and then proceed with the session.
   b. Turn off the video recording device and proceed with the content of the hallway conversation but not proceed with any other topic.
   c. Reschedule the session with Stephen.
   d. Stay in the hallway to finish the conversation before deciding to either proceed with the treatment session or to reschedule.
   e. Ask Stephen the name of his ex-girlfriend in order to find out whether she is a student in the program and thus has access to the recordings.
   f. Ask the clinic staff to find out if Stephen's ex-girlfriend is a student in the same program, and proceed with the session without recording.
   g. Explore the nature of Stephen's reluctance in session and use this situation for a therapeutic intervention.
   h. Discuss the possibility of referral to another clinic.
2. As the supervisor, you would do as follows:
   a. Tell Eric that you cannot provide supervision without some way to access the interactions of the session.
   b. Tell Eric sessions with Stephen need to be terminated because supervision cannot proceed.
   c. Tell Eric that records cannot be altered, and Stephen has to wait for the routine cycle of video deletion in the clinic.
3. As the clinic manager, you would do as follows:
   a. Assure Eric that only he and the supervisor can access video recordings.
   b. Tell Eric that policy is for destruction of video recording at the end of the semester and no earlier.
   c. Tell Eric he needs to obtain the request in writing from the client and authorization from the supervisor before records can be redacted.
4. Do a combination of the previously listed actions.
5. Do something that is not previously listed.

If Eric was practicing in England and Stephen made a decision to deny access to video by asking for their cessation or destruction, Eric would be obligated to comply. In England, you would stop recording and redact all previously recorded treatment sessions.

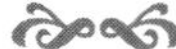

STANDARD 4.04: MINIMIZING INTRUSIONS ON PRIVACY

(a) Psychologists include in written and oral reports and consultation only information germane to the purpose for which the communication is made.

A CASE FOR STANDARD 4.04 (A): In the Closet

Ann entered into treatment with Dr. Price for depression. As the sessions progressed, it was clear that Ann was subjected to sexual harassment at her work from her boss and that she was struggling with her sexual identity. Under

Dr. Price's care, Ann realized that in order to decrease her depression she had to find some way to stop the constant sexual harassment. Ann decided to apply for other jobs and in the meantime had filed a sexual harassment complaint against her boss. As the complaint proceeded, the employer requested Dr. Price's records. Ann's attorney thought Dr. Price's records could support her claim of pain and suffering from work. Dr. Price witnessed and recorded the poignancy of the sexual harassment in the context of Ann's sexual identity. Ann was in agreement with her attorney about releasing the treatment record. However, Ann was not open about her homosexuality and did not want information pertaining to her sexual identity revealed.

Issues of Concern

Standard 4.04 directs Dr. Price to include germane information in Ann's report. This means that Dr. Price only needs to include information pertaining to the sexual harassment in the released record and/or in any reports from him. The request from Ann is not to destroy or to alter the record. Ann is giving Dr. Price permission to release only certain parts of the record.

The dilemma is twofold. The first is a practical question of whether it is advisable to redact the information if the records are written in such a way that it is not possible to retain any semblance of coherence once redacted. The other issue is not one that relates to possible conflict within professional ethics as much as with the definition of the word *germane*. Dr. Price may deem Ann's homosexuality clinically germane to her situation regarding sexual harassment.

APA Ethics Code

Companion General Principle

Principle A: Beneficence and Nonmaleficence

> Psychologists strive to benefit those with whom they work and take care to do no harm. . .

Aspiring to Principle A of beneficence, Dr. Price might wish to release the record without substantially redacting parts of the record. It may be Dr. Price's clinical opinion that it is of utmost benefit for Ann to win the sexual harassment case. And the pain and suffering portion of her grievance is even more poignant within the context of her homosexuality, particularly if the person alleged to have engaged in the sexual harassment suspected Ann's sexual identity and engaged in behavior that egregiously attempted to exploit her sexual identity. Both Ann's attorney and Dr. Price may be of the opinion that releasing the whole record without redacting any portion of the record may be significantly more beneficial to Ann.

Principle B: Fidelity and Responsibility

> Psychologists establish relationships of trust with those with whom they work. . .

Principle B guides Dr. Price to proceed with the awareness that whatever he says to Ann or does with the records, he needs to proceed with a focus on maintaining Ann's trust.

Principle E: Respect for People's Rights and Dignity

> Psychologists respect the . . . rights of individuals to privacy, confidentiality, and self-determination. . .

Principle E guides Dr. Price to respect Ann's right to self-determination, which in this case means Dr. Price is to respect Ann's request that the records be redacted. In addition, respecting Ann's right to privacy means Dr. Price is not to release any part of her record without Ann's explicit consent.

Companion Ethical Standard(s)

Standard 6.02: Maintenance, Dissemination, and Disposal of Confidential Records of Professional and Scientific Work

> (a) Psychologists maintain confidentiality in creating, storing, accessing, transferring, and disposing of records under their control, whether these are written, automated, or in any other medium.

Standard 6.02 directs Dr. Price to maintain confidentiality in accessing Ann's records.

Standard 4.05: Disclosures

> (a) Psychologists may disclose confidential information with the appropriate consent of . . . the individual client. . .

Standard 4.05 directs Dr. Price to only release records with Ann's "appropriate consent." Appropriate consent in this case most probably calls for a signed release for Dr. Price to provide Ann's attorney with parts of the record that address her sexual harassment.

Standard 3.05: Multiple Relationships

> (a) A multiple relationship occurs when a psychologist is in a professional role with a person and . . . (1) at the same time is in another role with the same person. . . A psychologist refrains from entering into a multiple relationship if the multiple relationship could reasonably be expected to impair the psychologist's objectivity, competence, or effectiveness in performing his or her functions as a psychologist, or otherwise risks exploitation or harm to the person with whom the professional relationship exists. Multiple relationships that would not reasonably be expected to cause impairment or risk exploitation or harm are not unethical.

Inherent in the deliberation as to whether or not to redact the record may be Dr. Price's opinion regarding the extent of harm sustained by Ann. Implied in the deliberation is whether Dr. Price takes on the role of an expert witness. As an expert witness, Dr. Price is called upon to render an opinion regarding the merit of Ann's case. However, in assuming the role of an expert witness, Dr. Price enters into a multiple relationship, both in the role of a treating psychologist, which is a fact witness, and additionally taking on the role of an expert witness. Assuming both roles puts Dr. Price in a multiple relationship situation with Ann. While Standard 3.05 does not prohibit such multiple relationships, it does caution against it.

Legal Issues 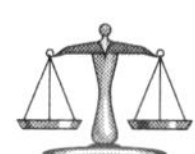

Indiana

> *Ind. Code Ann. § 16-39-1-1 (LexisNexis Supp. 2010). Right of access; written requests; effective duration.*
>
> Sec. 1.
>
> . . . (d) On a patient's written request and reasonable notice, a provider shall furnish to the patient or the patient's designee the following:
>
> . . . (2) At the option of the patient, the pertinent part of the patient's health record relating to a specific condition, as requested by the patient.
>
> *868 Ind. Admin. Code 1.1-11-4.1 (2010). Relationships within professional practice.*
>
> Sec. 4.1.
>
> (a) A psychologist shall not enter into a dual relationship with a . . . client if such relationship could impair professional judgment. . .
>
> . . . (h) In areas beyond the scope of the psychologist's competence, the psychologist shall refer to a professional who is competent in that area of practice.

Kansas

> *Kan. Admin. Regs. § 102-1-10a (2010). Unprofessional conduct.*
>
> Each of the following shall be considered unprofessional conduct:
>
> . . . (f) ignoring client welfare, which shall include the following acts:
>
> (1) Failing to provide copies of . . . records . . . unless the release of that information is restricted . . .

If Dr. Price was practicing in Kansas, his equivocation about which part of the record to release may be deemed unprofessional conduct. In Indiana, it may be deemed as denial of client's right to access her records. In both jurisdictions, Dr. Price should release those portions of the records indicated in the client's request for release of records.

Cultural Considerations

Global Discussion

Canadian Code of Ethics for Psychologists

> Principle I: Respect for the dignity of persons.
>
> *Privacy.*
>
> I.38. Take care not to infringe, in . . . service activities, on the . . . culturally defined private space of individuals[,] . . . unless clear permission is granted to do so.
>
> *When principles conflict.*
>
> Principle II: Responsible caring.
>
> This principle generally should be given the second highest weight. Responsible caring requires competence and should be carried out only in ways that respect the dignity of persons . . .

In this instance, Dr. Price would be infringing on the "culturally defined private space" of Ann by revealing her sexual identity as part of a sexual harassment lawsuit. For someone to disclose personal information in a workplace setting is potentially harmful to one's privacy. For someone who is a sexual minority and is also in an antagonistic position with her employer, harm could easily come to Ann if Dr. Price's records were revealed. Dr. Price would have to have "clear permission" to infringe on Ann's private space, which he does not. In that case, no matter how sound his argument or passionate his feelings about the necessity of Ann's revealing her sexual identity, if he were to do so in Canada, he would be considered in violation of this portion of code.

If there are conflicting principles, respect for the dignity of persons has a higher weight and moral value than responsible caring. Therefore, if one undergoes the process of weighing conflicting principles in this situation, Ann's right to privacy of her information has the highest value, above the psychologist trying to conform to the principle of responsible caring by including the information about her sexual identity. Therefore, after weighing conflicting principles, the psychologist must respect Ann's position, autonomy, and right to be treated with individual dignity.

American Moral Values

1. How can Dr. Price balance the need to share Ann's struggles with sexual harassment against the limits Ann wants to set on his testimony, specifically its discussion of sexual orientation? Does Dr. Price implicitly believe Ann's need not to be harassed trumps her desire not to be "outed," or is it vice versa? Are there basic principles or priorities for life that make sense of that conflict, and can they help Dr. Price adhere to his client's request? How is the freedom to work weighed in relation to sexual/personal privacy?
2. Has Dr. Price fully disclosed that a competent cross-examining lawyer will likely investigate any personal issues that could undermine Ann's claim of sexual harassment?
3. Does the "poignancy" of Ann's struggles with sexual identity justify including it in testimony against Ann's will? Is Ann even willing to win the case if that confidentiality about her sexual identity is broken?
4. How would breaking confidentiality affect Ann's subsequent struggle with her sexual identity? Is this taking power out of her hands when she needs it most? Or does helping her resist her boss's harassment ultimately signify a greater victory? Is this a decision that Dr. Price should make without Ann's input?

Ethical Course of Action

Directive per APA Code

Standard 4.04 directs Dr. Price to only release portions of the record that are "germane" to the dictates of the sexual harassment grievance. Similar to the reasoning behind the Canadian code, regardless of what Dr. Price might think best for Ann, Standard 4.04 in combination with Standard 4.05 directs Dr. Price to act in accordance within the limits set by Ann in releasing her records.

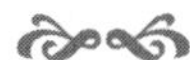

Dictates of One's Own Conscience

If you were Dr. Price, in consultation with Ann's attorney, thinking that the greatest benefit to both the grievance case and Ann's mental health is to release the whole record and knowing the directives of Standard 4.04 and 4.05, what might you do?

1. Reassure Ann that no matter what you think, you will only release that portion of the record that Ann has specified.
2. Review the records in session with Ann to determine what part Ann does not want released.
3. Explore with Ann the cost and possible repercussions of releasing the whole record or portions of the record.
4. Discuss with Ann the likelihood of your being questioned by the opposing attorney and specifying how you must not engage in perjury if the opposing attorney raises questions about Ann's sexual identity.
5. Inform Ann that you must be very careful to adhere to the role of a fact witness because in such legal matters rarely will opposing lawyers permit the limited release of any such record; therefore, Ann's sexual identity may be revealed regardless of wishes.
6. Decide that you are not competent to weigh in on the matter of records, so you decide to consult with a forensic psychologist who will prepare you to perform competently as a fact witness and to provide sufficient clarification to your client so that she is prepared for the likely disclosure about all of the facts revealed during psychotherapy.
7. Do a combination of the previously listed actions.
8. Do something that is not previously listed.

If you were Dr. Price and Ann was your client in Canada, which would you do?

1. Attempt to persuade Ann that being open about her sexuality is of benefit not only to her harassment case but to her overall mental well-being.
2. Agree to limit the release of Ann's records in accordance with her wishes.

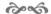

STANDARD 4.04: MINIMIZING INTRUSIONS ON PRIVACY

> ... (b) Psychologists discuss confidential information obtained in their work only for appropriate scientific or professional purposes and only with persons clearly concerned with such matters.

A CASE FOR STANDARD 4.04 (B): What Do You Do For a Living?

Dr. Bennett, who has lived in his urban neighborhood for several years, now finds himself living in the same block as another psychologist, Dr. Wood. Dr. Wood had purchased the house five doors down from Dr. Bennett. At the annual block party, the conversation turned to self-introductions and work. The neighbors all found out that both Drs. Bennett and Wood are clinical psychologists. The neighbors were curious and asked them to talk about their work. Dr. Wood proceeded to regale the party with funny stories about her client's activities.

Issues of Concern

Standard 4.04 (b) directs Drs. Bennett and Wood to limit their discussion of their clients only with "persons clearly concerned with such matters." It is clear that neighbors at a party do not constitute people who are "clearly concerned" with their clients. If Dr. Wood has disguised the identity of her clients to the extent that no identity could be derived, would it not be possible for her to share her work experience? Does Dr. Bennett have a professional obligation to have a conversation with Dr. Wood about the impression of malfeasance she may have left with her audience when discussing her practice in such a cavalier manner?

APA Ethics Code

Companion General Principle

Principle A: Beneficence and Nonmaleficence

> Psychologists strive to benefit those with whom they work and take care to do no harm...

It is doubtful that Dr. Wood's clients would not feel embarrassed or betrayed by Dr. Wood's exhibitionistic display of their struggles. Dr. Wood may well have benefited her clients with the treatment she has provided, but she risks harming them now if they were to become aware of her behavior. She also may have left an impression with her neighbors that psychologists are cavalier with the confidences of their clients.

Principle B: Fidelity and Responsibility

> Psychologists establish relationships of trust with those whom they work. They are aware of their professional ... responsibilities to society and to the specific communities in which they work. Psychologists uphold professional standards of conduct ... [and] clarify their professional roles and obligations... They are concerned about the ethical compliance of their colleagues' ... professional conduct.

Hearing a psychologist like Dr. Wood discuss the emotional pain of a person does not convey a level of respect owed to people's struggles nor does it instill a sense of trust should one of the neighbors be in therapy with a psychologist or in contemplation of beginning treatment with a psychologist. By her behavior, Dr. Wood does not uphold the value of fidelity stated in Principle B. Aspiring to enact the highest level of professional responsibility as stated in Principle B, Dr. Bennett is placed in an ethically awkward position with regard to the ethical compliance of Dr. Wood's professional conduct.

Companion Ethical Standard(s)

Standard 3.04: Avoiding Harm

> Psychologists take reasonable steps to avoid harming their clients/patients...

Harm can be done if any one of Dr. Wood's clients comes to think that she has made his/her emotional pain into a laughable matter at a party. Standard 3.04 directs Dr. Wood to guard against such harm. One way to avoid such harm is to abide by the directives of standard 4.04 (b).

Standard 1.04: Informal Resolution of Ethical Violations

> When psychologists believe that there may have been an ethical violation by another psychologist, they attempt to resolve the issue by bringing it to the attention of that individual, if an informal resolution appears appropriate and the intervention does not violate any confidentiality rights that may be involved.

No specific client is involved, thus Standard 1.04 directs Dr. Bennett to talk with Dr. Wood about her inappropriate use of client information, in violation of Standard 4.04.

Legal Issues 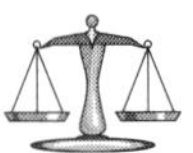

Kentucky

> *Ky. Rev. Stat. Ann. § 319.082 (West 2002). Disciplinary actions against license and certificate holders.*
>
> (1) The board may suspend, revoke, or refuse to issue or renew a license . . . upon proof that the credential holder has:
>
> . . . (p) Improperly divulged confidential information.

Maine

> *Me. Rev. Stat. Ann. tit. 32, § 3816 (1999). Code of ethics.*
>
> The board shall adopt rules establishing a code of ethics in keeping with those standards established by the American Psychological Association or its successor or other organization approved by the board to govern appropriate practices or behavior as referred to in this chapter.

In both jurisdictions, psychologists would violate the ethical standards by divulging client confidences in such a manner. Kentucky has no reporting law that Dr. Bennett must follow. In Maine, Dr. Bennett would engage in an informal resolution process with Dr. Wood.

Cultural Considerations

Global Discussion

Singapore Psychological Society: Code of Professional Ethics

> Specific principles.
>
> Principle 1. Responsibility.
>
> . . . 3. As a practitioner, the psychologist knows that a heavy social responsibility is borne because the work may touch intimately the lives of others.
>
> Principle 6. Confidentiality.
>
> Safeguarding information about an individual that has been obtained by the psychologist in the course of . . . practice . . . is a primary obligation of the psychologist. Such information is not communicated to others unless certain important conditions are met.
>
> . . . 2. Information obtained in clinical . . . relationships . . . are discussed only for professional purposes and only with persons clearly concerned with the case . . . [and] every effort should be made to avoid undue invasion of privacy.

Socializing at a party does not meet Singapore's standard of "important conditions" under which confidential information about clients may be shared. Neither Drs. Bennett nor Wood have any idea if the information being casually revealed will somehow cause harm to any of the partygoers, their overall impression about the trustworthiness of psychologists in general, and the possibility that confidentiality can be temporarily suspended for the amusement of party guests by otherwise well-meaning psychologists. It is clear that Singapore's code holds psychologists responsible for the "heavy social burden" we have undertaken along with our professional roles and privilege and that our work deeply touches the intimate lives of others in many ways.

American Moral Values

1. Do Dr. Wood's stories, without names being divulged, violate the confidentiality and privacy her patients deserve? Is there a chance people will figure out the subject of some of the stories, based on context, personal characteristics, the size of the town, the nature of gossip, etc.? Or is Dr. Wood just venting about "the office," thus deflating the caricature of an arrogant, smug therapist? Would saying, "I can't talk about clients" be off-putting and hurt the image of psychologist in partygoers' minds?
2. How will Dr. Bennett's action relate to the larger community's impression of psychologists? Does Dr. Bennett need to intervene if people at the party implicitly take away the wrong ideas from Dr. Wood's stories—about confidentiality, what psychologists "really" think about their patients, etc.? Will Dr. Bennett discussing Dr. Wood's behavior at the

party possibly backfire if she feels humiliated? Should Dr. Bennett wait to talk in an office setting? Or should Dr. Bennett openly contest Dr. Wood's actions at the party, to send a message that such stories do not meet professional standards for "good" psychologists?

3. Are there appropriate contexts for laughing about clients with friends or strangers who are curious about what it is like to be a psychologist? How is this similar or different from those contexts? What is the difference between laughing to oneself and laughing with others in terms of how that client is truly regarded by the therapist and how that attitude relates to treatment? Could the attitude itself be more problematic than the sharing? If so, then should Dr. Bennett talk to Dr. Wood not just about confidentiality but about her attitude toward her clients as well?

Ethical Course of Action

Directive per APA Code

Dr. Wood has violated the directives of Standard 4.04. Even if she does disguise all identifiers, such general intrusions into privacy of clients were witnessed by all of her neighbors. Standard 1.04 directs Dr. Bennett to contact Dr. Wood to informally resolve his concerns about her misconduct.

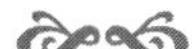

Dictate's of One's Own Conscience

Besides contacting Dr. Wood to request that she not use confidential information for the party entertainment regardless of the fact that no names and other identifiers were used, if you were Dr. Bennett, what might you do to further mitigate the possible harm done by Dr. Wood?

1. Educate your neighbors (briefly) about psychologists' need to protect their clients' privacy.
2. Do not mention the embarrassment about Dr. Wood's behavior with the neighbors.
3. Avoid contact with Dr. Wood and any of the other neighbors and ignore the matter entirely.
4. Engage in informal resolution with Dr. Wood about the impression she may have created by disclosing client information in such a disrespectfully cavalier manner.
5. File a formal complaint with the licensing board.
6. Do a combination of the previously listed actions.
7. Do something that is not previously listed.

If you were Dr. Bennett attending the party in Singapore, which would you do?

1. Engage in an informal conversation with Dr. Wood about her behavior and lapse of judgment in discussing her clients in such a manner.
2. File a formal complaint with the licensing body of Singapore.

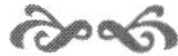

STANDARD 4.05: DISCLOSURES

(a) Psychologists may disclose confidential information with the appropriate consent of the organizational client, the individual client/patient, or another legally authorized person on behalf of the client/patient unless prohibited by law.

A CASE FOR STANDARD 4.05 (A): Mother's Rights

Dr. Barnes provides family therapy to a family that consists of the father, Jerry; the mother, Joyce; the 10-year-old son, Gregory; and the 12-year-old son, Joshua. The family had recently separated, and Jerry sought treatment for his two sons. On the night of the separation, Jerry came home to find Joyce somewhat intoxicated and screaming at the children. Jerry tried to intercede on behalf of the children when Joyce turned on him, accused Jerry of having an affair, and proceeded to throw objects at him. Joshua called the police when Joyce started throwing knives at Jerry. Upon arrival, the police escorted Joyce out of the house, and the next day Jerry applied for and received a duly executed restraining order against Joyce, barring her from having any contact with Jerry or the kids.

Gregory said that he wants to go live with his mom because his brother, Joshua, is beating him and otherwise mistreating him after school before father comes home. Joshua denies these charges, saying that he tells Gregory to do his chores before his father comes home and tells Gregory not to talk to mom when dad is not home.

Then Dr. Barnes received a call from Joyce, requesting information about her children and demanding to be part of the treatment of her children.

Issues of Concern

Standard 4.05 (a) directs Dr. Barnes to disclose information with client's consent unless prohibited by law. Both Gregory and Joshua are minors. It appears that custody has not yet been determined. Thus Joyce has rights as a parent to treatment information from Dr. Barnes. However, does the presence of a restraining order constitute legal prohibition against Dr. Barnes responding to Joyce's request to be part of the family therapy? Does the restraining order extend to prohibiting Joyce access to treatment information? In addition, does Gregory's claim of abuse cause Dr. Barnes to act in such a way as to ensure his safety?

APA Ethics Code

Companion General Principle

Principle B: Fidelity and Responsibility

> . . . Psychologists uphold professional standards of conduct, clarify their professional roles and obligations, accept appropriate responsibility for their behavior, and seek to manage conflicts of interest that could lead to exploitation or harm. . .

Principle B guides Dr. Barnes to consider her responsibilities to society, which in this case may involve the legal mandate to report child abuse. Principle B also encourages psychologists to be knowledgeable about the legal definition of child abuse and stipulations of when child abuse needs to be reported.

Principle B also guides Dr. Barnes to clarify her role to each member of the family. In this situation, role clarification needs to include the influence of the restraining order and its impact on Joyce's involvement in treatment as well as Dr. Barnes's role as a mandated reporter of child abuse.

Companion Ethical Standard(s)

Standard 6.02: Maintenance, Dissemination, and Disposal of Confidential Records of Professional and Scientific Work

> (a) Psychologists maintain confidentiality in . . . accessing . . . records under their control. . .

Standard 6.02 places the responsibility of deciding whether Joyce is to have access to treatment information upon Dr. Barnes, as the psychologist.

Standard 4.05: Disclosures

> . . . (b) Psychologists disclose confidential information without the consent of the individual only as mandated by law. . .

Psychologists are mandated by law to report child abuse in many states. If Gregory's claim that Joshua is beating him constitutes child abuse, then Standard 4.05 allows for Dr. Barnes to break confidentiality without the consent of the client to file a report of child abuse.

Standard 10.02: Therapy Involving Couples or Families

> (a) When psychologists agree to provide services to several persons who have a relationship (such as . . . parents and children), they take reasonable steps to clarify at the outset (1) which of the individuals are clients/patients and (2) the relationship the psychologist will have with each person. This clarification includes the psychologist's role and the probable uses of the services provided or the information obtained.
>
> . . . (b) If it becomes apparent that psychologists may be called on to perform potentially conflicting roles (such as family therapist and then witness for one party in divorce proceedings), psychologists take reasonable steps to clarify and modify, or withdraw from, roles appropriately.

Standard 10.02 and enacting elements of Principle B: Fidelity and Responsibility directs Dr. Barnes to clarify her role in relationship to each at each step of the legal process until injunctive relief provides more information.

Section (b) of Standard 10.02 further specifies that Dr. Barnes's clarification of her role is to include who, including attorney and courts, has access to what information from Dr. Barnes at what point in treatment and the court proceedings. Where there is an ongoing legal proceeding, Dr. Barnes might wish to consider the option of negotiating an agreement with the family that specifically prohibits her from entering into any interactions with the legal system.

Legal Issues 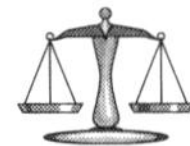

Louisiana

> *La Admin. Code tit. 46, § 1301 (2009). Ethical principles and code of conduct.*
>
> A. The Board of Examiners of Psychologists incorporates by reference and maintains that Psychologists

shall follow the APA Ethical Principles of Psychologists and Code of Conduct as adopted by the American Psychological Association's Council of Representatives during its meeting, August 21, 2002, and made effective beginning June 1, 2003.

Nebraska

172 Neb. Admin. Code § 156-006 (2010). Regulations defining unprofessional conduct by a psychologist.

Confidentiality. A psychologist shall hold in confidence information obtained from a client, except in those unusual circumstances in which to do so would result in clear danger to the person or to others or where otherwise required by law. Failure to do so shall constitute unprofessional conduct.

In both jurisdictions, the protective order creates a barrier to releasing further information to the person restrained. Dr. Barnes would not be able to discuss any information about the family therapy with Joyce before the restraining order was lifted. Dr. Barnes must file a report of the brother's behavior with children's protective services as a mandatory reporter in both jurisdictions.

Cultural Considerations

Global Discussion

The Professional Board for Psychology Health Professions Council of South Africa:
Ethical Code of Professional Conduct (April 2002)

3.3 Disclosures.

3.3.1. Psychologists may disclose confidential information only with the permission of the individual or as mandated by law, or when permitted by law for a valid purpose, such as . . . to protect the client or others from harm . . .

The restraining order against the mother means that she no longer has parental rights over her children, and Dr. Barnes would be prohibited from providing treatment information without permission from the father. However, if the possibility of abuse occurring to one of the children meets the criteria of "protecting clients or others from harm," Dr. Barnes would disclose this information, although information disclosed would be limited to the minimum necessary to safeguard the welfare of the minor children.

American Moral Values

1. What relationships take priority in this situation? Is protecting the children the first priority? What actions help to protect them the best? How is Gregory's safety best protected?
2. How does Dr. Barnes view the restraining order in the context of the family relationships at hand? Is Joyce setting up the psychologist to violate the privacy between Jerry and his children?
3. What value does Joyce's relationship with her sons carry when thinking about her request for information? Does motherhood elicit different value judgments than fatherhood when it comes to confidentiality and the law?
4. What value does Dr. Barnes place on the family staying together? Does it seem especially troubling to consider splitting Joshua and Gregory between the parents?
5. How does the restraining order pertain to future treatment of the family? Is it about Joyce and Jerry rather than the two of them with the children? Does Joyce present a threat to the children as well? What clarification does Dr. Barnes need from the court in order to proceed with family therapy?

Ethical Course of Action

Directive per APA Code

Standard 4.05 directs Dr. Barnes not to disclose confidential information in response to the restraining order. This means Dr. Barnes may not tell Joyce the time and location of the therapy appointments because such knowledge may allow Joyce physical access to the children. This also means Joyce may not join in the family therapy sessions. Depending on the specifics of the restraining order, Dr. Barnes may discuss the case and possibly the specifics of the abuse alleged by Gregory with Joshua.

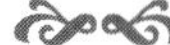

Dictates of One's Own Conscience

As permitted by Standard 4.05 and directed by the restraining order, Dr. Barnes may not allow for Joyce to be in contact with the children or father while the restraining order is in effect. However, Joyce is an interested parent, and at some point the restraining order will lapse.

In preparation for the day that the restraining order is no longer in effect, what would you do if you were Dr. Barnes?

1. Recommend that Joyce obtain some type of alcohol treatment.
2. Explore with the family how they wish to move forward after the restraining order ends.
3. Advise that Joyce enter into individual therapy with another provider until the restraining order ends.
4. Have no contact with Joyce until such time the restraining order ends, then request that she join the family sessions.
5. Have no contact with Joyce until such time the restraining order ends, then request that she join the family sessions with the children separately from Jerry and the children.
6. Once the restraining order ends and treatment resumes with all members of the family, ask that Joyce and Jerry review with their attorneys a stipulation prepared by you and sign the stipulation that precludes your taking part or your records being disclosed in any future litigation.
7. Seek to influence the restraining order given the report of sibling abuse by writing a report to the courts.
8. Seek to disentangle yourself from their court proceedings by requesting the family refrain from using any part of treatment in any court proceedings, and proceed with family therapy with the boys.
9. Do a combination of the previously listed actions.
10. Do something that is not previously listed.

If you were Dr. Barnes working with Joyce and Jerry in South Africa, which would you do?

1. Explain to Joyce that until the restraining order lapses or Jerry gives permission, you cannot release any information to her about the treatment of her children.
2. Decide that the issue of potential abuse of one of the sons is serious enough to warrant notification of both parents; notify both Jerry and Joyce of possible abuse of the one son, but limit disclosures of information to only that topic when discussing treatment with Joyce.

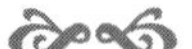

STANDARD 4.05: DISCLOSURES

> . . . (b) Psychologists disclose confidential information without the consent of the individual only as mandated by law, or where permitted by law for a valid purpose such as to (1) **provide needed professional services;** (2) obtain appropriate professional consultations; (3) protect the client/patient, psychologist, or others from harm; or (4) obtain payment for services from a client/patient, in which instance disclosure is limited to the minimum that is necessary to achieve the purpose.

A CASE FOR STANDARD 4.05 (B) (1): To Report or Not to Report?

Diane is in treatment with Dr. Ross for severe depression. Diane reported that she has been having difficulties with her husband, Jack, for some time in the area of sexual partnership. Jack is bisexual and wants a polyamorous arrangement where a male partner joins the relationship. Diane knows that Jack has engaged in homosexual relationships and is actively seeking a partner who is open to a polyamorous relationship. Lately Diane has reported feeling like she has had the flu for weeks on end. One day Diane came into the session extremely distressed at having received a positive result on an HIV/AIDS lab test, which she administered to herself at home anonymously and sent to the mail-order lab that supplied the test. She had called in for the results that morning.

Issues of Concern

In many states, psychologists are mandated reporters for communicable diseases, like HIV/AIDS. This usually entails a report to the state public health department. Like child abuse mandates, psychologists are not required to affirm the positive presence of a communicable disease but just to have good professional reasons for believing that the client is ill with a communicable disease. Standard 4.05(b), under the phrase "as mandated by law," would direct Dr. Ross to file a communicable disease report.

APA Ethics Code

Companion General Principle

Principle A: Beneficence and Nonmaleficence

> Psychologists strive to . . . take care to do no harm. In their professional actions, psychologists seek to safeguard

> the welfare and rights of those with whom they interact professionally and other affected persons . . .

Aspiring to the highest level of Principle A of nonmaleficence, Dr. Ross would take into consideration the harm that may come to Diane should she make a report to the health department.

Principle B: Fidelity and Responsibility

> . . . They are aware of their professional and scientific responsibilities to society and to the specific communities in which they work.

Principle B directs Dr. Ross's attention to her professional responsibility to society in the form of making known a situation of possible danger to the public health. Not reporting a communicable disease to the state health department would place the public at risk, thus violating the intent of Principle B. Balancing the harm to Diane, as stated in Principle A, is Dr. Ross's responsibility to society as mandated by state law.

Principle E: Respect for People's Rights and Dignity

> Psychologists respect the dignity and worth of all people, and the rights of individuals to privacy, confidentiality, and self-determination.

Principle E guides Dr. Ross to respect Diane's right to privacy and confidentiality. Regarding the value of self-determination, perhaps Dr. Ross might best enact the highest level of Principles A, B, and E by assisting Diane in exploring the details of such a report to the health department.

Companion Ethical Standard(s)

Standard 4.01: Maintaining Confidentiality

> Psychologists have a primary obligation and take reasonable precautions to protect confidential information obtained through . . . any medium, recognizing that the extent and limits of confidentiality may be regulated by law. . .

Standard 4.01 recognizes that client confidentiality is not absolute, and in some circumstances the law establishes that disclosures to public health authorities or other public agencies are mandatory. Standard 4.01 allows Dr. Ross to adhere to the mandates of law should the state stipulate that psychologists are mandated reporters of communicable diseases.

Standard 4.02: Discussing the Limits of Confidentiality

> . . . (b) Unless it is not feasible or is contraindicated, the discussion of confidentiality occurs at the outset of the relationship and thereafter as new circumstances may warrant. . .

Standard 4.02 directs Dr. Ross to discuss again the requirement of reporting communicable diseases as new circumstances have occurred and this occasion warrants such a discussion.

Legal Issues 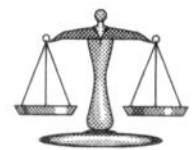

Minnesota

> *Minn. Stat. Ann. § 214.18 (West 2009). Definitions.*
>
> . . . *SUBD. 5.* REGULATED PERSON.
>
> "Regulated person" means a licensed dental hygienist, dentist, physician, nurse who is currently registered as a registered nurse or licensed practical nurse, podiatrist, a registered dental assistant, a physician's assistant, and for purposes of sections 214.19, subdivisions 4 and 5 . . .
>
> *Minn. Stat. Ann. § 214.19 (West 2009). Reporting obligations.*
>
> . . . *SUBD. 3.* MANDATORY REPORTING.
>
> A person . . . required to report HIV, HBV, or HCV status to the commissioner . . . shall . . . notify the commissioner if the person or institution knows that the reported person is a regulated person.
>
> . . . *SUBD. 4.* INFECTION CONTROL REPORTING.
>
> A regulated person shall, within ten days, report to the appropriate board personal knowledge of a . . . failure . . . by another regulated person to comply with accepted and prevailing infection control procedures related to the prevention of HIV, HBV, and HCV transmission. . .

Washington

> *Wash. Admin. Code § 246-101-010 (2009). Definitions within the notifiable conditions regulations.*
>
> . . . (15) "Health care provider" means any person having direct or supervisory responsibility for the delivery of health care who is:
>
> (a) Licensed or certified in this state under Title 18 RCW [the law of this title includes licensed psychologists].
>
> *Wash. Admin. Code § 246-101-105 (2009). Duties of the health care provider.*

> Health care providers shall:
>
> (1) Notify the local health department where the patient resides (in the event that patient residence cannot be determined, notify the local health department where the health care providers practice) . . . regarding: (a) Cases . . . of notifiable conditions specified as notifiable to local health departments in Table HC-1 [including Human immunodeficiency virus (HIV) infection within three days of knowledge, *see* Wash. Admin. Code § 246-101-101 (2009)].

The law in both jurisdictions permits disclosure of the HIV health condition. In Minnesota, however, psychologists are not one of the regulated professionals under this statute. In Washington, it is a mandatory reporting duty. In Washington, the psychologist must file the report, although the law does not preclude the psychologist's client from engaging in the reporting process with the psychologist.

Cultural Considerations

Global Discussion

Code of Ethics for the Psychologist: Spain

> ***Article 40.*** All information gathered by psychologists in the practice of their profession . . . is subject to the duties and rights for professional secrecy, from which they can only be relieved with the client's express consent. Psychologists must keep awake to ensure that any colleagues abide by this professional secret.

If Dr. Ross was practicing in Spain, she would be unable to reveal any information about Diane's HIV positive status without Diane's "express consent." Moreover, Dr. Ross would need to safeguard Diane's confidential information from being revealed by other professionals and colleagues.

American Moral Values

1. What are the public health concerns that Dr. Ross would have to consider before notifying the board of health of Diane's test result in a jurisdiction that does not have a mandatory duty to report? Is her monogamy with Jack a sufficient reason to consider her a small risk for spreading the virus? Does her presumed sexual fidelity make her more "deserving" of privacy?
2. How does Jack's sexual behavior factor into Dr. Ross's decision? Is notifying the board of health a way of making Jack more accountable? Would his having affairs solely with women change Dr. Ross's perspective on the need to break confidentiality?
3. Is Diane's home test dependable enough to proceed as if she did have HIV/AIDS? Is waiting to say anything too much of a gamble?

Ethical Course of Action

Directive per APA Code

Standard 4.05 (b) allows for Dr. Ross to disclose Diane's confidential information should there be a legal mandate to do so. Dr. Ross needs to be certain that such a legal mandate exists for psychologists to report communicable diseases in the state that both Dr. Ross and Diane reside in and where Dr. Ross practices.

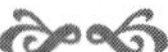

Dictates of One's Own Conscience

Presuming that such a legal mandate does exist in the state in which your clients live and you practice, knowing the harm to Diane from breaking confidentiality as well as the certainty that no one is in danger of contracting HIV/AIDS from Diane, what would you do?

1. Do not report this situation to the state department of health, reasoning that since Diane is not sexually active with anyone else except her husband, she is of no danger to the community.
2. Do not report this situation to the state department of health, reasoning that the disclosure might have adverse effects in her workplace and possibly with her health insurance.
3. Do not report this situation to the state department of health, reasoning that such a report implicates her husband as the possible carrier/spreader of the disease, which could easily result in his discrimination, almost regardless of what profession he's in.
4. Tell Diane that she needs to seek diagnostic confirmation from her physician immediately, also warning her of the possibility that primary care physicians are mandated reporters of communicable diseases.
5. Report this situation to the state department of health, reasoning that such a report implicates her husband as the possible carrier/spreader of the disease, and his behavior already has established that he has acted irresponsibly.

6. Remind Diane that, as already discussed at intake, you are a mandatory reporter and proceed with the report. Process with Diane how the report can be conducted with her present and participating in a manner that would best preserve the therapeutic alliance.
7. Recommend that Jack join in the next therapy session to discuss this situation within a certain time that permits the 72-hour limit of the law to be satisfied.
8. Encourage Diane to make the report herself either through her primary care physician or directly to the health department.
9. Do a combination of the previously listed actions.
10. Do something that is not previously listed.

If you were Dr. Ross, treating Diane in Spain, which would you do?

1. Refuse to file a report about her possible HIV condition to the health department, citing the need for her "express consent."
2. Attempt to get express consent from Diane to release her health status information to the health department, reasoning that protection of public welfare is important.
3. Assure Diane that you will not report her health status, nor will you attempt to persuade her to do so, and moreover, you will attempt to keep her information away from other health professionals.

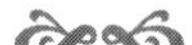

STANDARD 4.05: DISCLOSURES

> . . . (b) Psychologists disclose confidential information without the consent of the individual only as mandated by law, or where permitted by law for a valid purpose such as to (1) provide needed professional services; (2) obtain appropriate professional consultations; **(3) protect the client/patient, psychologist, or others from harm;** or (4) obtain payment for services from a client/patient, in which instance disclosure is limited to the minimum that is necessary to achieve the purpose.

A CASE FOR STANDARD 4.05 (B) (3): An Uncomfortable Marriage

Mr. Raymond is a man in his early 40s who has been in therapy with Dr. Henderson for about eight sessions. Raymond's initial complaints included stress at work and in his marriage. At intake, he mentioned his wife had told him she had been sexually molested by one of her uncles when she was 10 years old. However, Mr. Raymond reported his marriage was primarily satisfactory, but his work situation was significantly more distressing, so therapy began with work-related issues. Mr. Raymond had come to every appointment and made good progress.

One day at the end of a session, Mr. Raymond indicated his wife and 10-year-old daughter would be going to visit her family in another state in a few weeks. Mr. Raymond noted that the uncle who molested his wife would be at the gathering. Dr. Henderson stated they should discuss this topic further in the next session.

Issues of Concern

Since neither the child, the wife, nor the uncle is a client of Dr. Henderson's, this is not a situation in which Dr. Henderson is mandated by law to break confidentiality. However, Standard 4.05 (b) (3) permits Dr. Henderson to report the possibility of sexual abuse to protect Mr. Raymond's daughter from harm. Should Dr. Henderson enact permission as indicated in Standard 4.05 (b) (3) and make contact with the state authorities? What harm might such a report have on Mr. Raymond's marriage? What harm might *not* reporting have on Mr. Raymond's daughter?

APA Ethics Code

Companion General Principle

Principle A: Benevolence and Nonmaleficence

> In their professional actions, psychologists seek to safeguard the welfare and rights of those with whom they interact professionally and other affected persons . . .

Aspiring to the highest level stated in the second sentence of Principle A, Dr. Henderson should seek to protect the welfare of "other affected persons," which in this case is Mr. Raymond's daughter.

Principle B: Fidelity and Responsibility

> . . . They are aware of their professional and scientific responsibilities to society and to the specific communities in which they work . . .

Principle B guides Dr. Henderson to consider her professional responsibility not only to her client and/or his daughter but to society in general. By reporting the possible danger to Mr. Raymond's daughter, might Dr. Henderson be protecting the many other preadolescent girls this uncle has contact with and access to?

Companion Ethical Standard(s)

Standard 4.02: Discussing the Limits of Confidentiality

> . . . (b) Unless it is not feasible or is contraindicated, the discussion of confidentiality occurs at the outset of the relationship and thereafter as new circumstances may warrant . . .

Standard 4.02 directs Dr. Henderson to discuss again the limits of confidentiality and to consider with Mr. Raymond whether a report to CPS would be in Mr. Raymond's best interest or his daughter's best interest.

Legal Issues 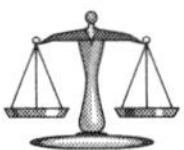

Nevada

> *Nev. Admin. Code § 641.224 (2010). Confidential information.*
>
> . . . 3. A psychologist may disclose confidential information without the informed written consent of a patient if the psychologist believes that disclosure of the information is necessary to protect against a clear and substantial risk of imminent serious harm . . . to . . . another person and:
>
> (a) The disclosure is limited to such persons and information as are consistent with the standards of the profession of psychology in addressing such problems. . .
>
> 4. A psychologist may disclose confidential information without the informed written consent of a patient if:
>
> . . . (b) Disclosure is required by a state . . . law . . . , including a law . . . that requires a psychologist to report the abuse of a child . . .

New Hampshire

> *N.H. Admin. Rules, Mental Health Practice 501.02 (2010). Code of ethics.*
>
> (a) A licensee shall adhere to the ethical principles of the profession in which they are licensed, as adopted by the following entities: (1) For "psychologists" the American Psychological Association . . .

In both Nevada and New Hampshire, the law mandates that psychologists report child abuse. In Nevada, Dr. Henderson cannot disclose the possibility that child abuse may have occurred without a release from her client, unless a clear and substantial risk of imminent serious harm exists. In New Hampshire, it appears that Dr. Henderson could make the report to protect Mr. Raymond's daughter from potential abuse.

Cultural Considerations

Global Discussion

Singapore Psychological Society:
Code of Professional Ethics

> Principle 6. Confidentiality.
>
> Safeguarding information about an individual that has been obtained by the psychologist in the course of . . . practice . . . is a primary obligation of the psychologist. Such information is not communicated to others unless certain important conditions are met.
>
> 1. Information received in confidence is revealed only after most careful deliberation and when there is clear and imminent danger to an individual or to society, and then only to appropriate professional workers or public authorities.

If Dr. Henderson was in Singapore, she would undergo "careful deliberation" before revealing confidential information and then only do so to appropriate professionals. The safety of the public, and particularly of identifiable, vulnerable others, is a greater good to protect than the confidentiality of one's client or that client's information.

American Moral Values

1. In light of the reported problems with the marriage, can Dr. Henderson trust the secondhand report of Mr. Raymond about his wife's alleged sexual molestation from her uncle?
2. Can Dr. Henderson assess Mr. Raymond's wife? Has Mr. Raymond misunderstood his wife's statements or reported them inaccurately? Is Mr. Raymond's wife a parental protector who will look out for her daughter? Does she have a parental or personal authority to deal with her uncle in the way she sees fit or believes to be best? Does her experience in the family make her a better judge of how that protection can work?

3. Does Mr. Raymond's daughter need protection of the external authorities? Does his wife have a better way of protecting her daughter from her own alleged assailant? Or does her alleged traumatic experience make her an unreliable protector?
4. What can Dr. Henderson assess about Mr. Raymond's wife? Is she thought of as a parental protector who will look out for her daughter? Does she have a parental or personal authority to deal with her uncle in the way she sees fit or believes to be best? Does her experience in the family make her a better judge of how that protection can work?
5. How will Mr. Raymond's family be confronted if Dr. Henderson breaks confidentiality? Could this kind of intervention threaten the functioning of this larger family? To what degree should Dr. Henderson consider what Mr. and Mrs. Raymond stand to lose by Dr. Henderson's informing the authorities about Mrs. Raymond's uncle? Does Dr. Henderson need to account for what Mr. Raymond's family thinks about therapy in general?
6. How will breaking confidentiality affect Mr. Raymond's relationship to Dr. Henderson? Might Mr. Raymond feel pushed to the side in Dr. Henderson's attempt to protect his daughter? How does Dr. Henderson cultivate Mr. Raymond's ability to understand his wife's abuse and support her, in addition to looking out for his daughter?

Ethical Course of Action

Directive per APA Code

Standard 4.05 (b) (3) permits Dr. Henderson to make such a report to CPS should she deem it appropriate. Different states may prohibit such disclosure. If Dr. Henderson lived in a state that permitted a report to CPS, then clinical judgment and the specifics of the situation, as hinted at in the Moral Values section, are the best guides for Dr. Henderson at this point.

Dictates of One's Own Conscience

If you were in Dr. Henderson's situation and you had serious concerns for the safety of Mr. Raymond's daughter, what might you do?

1. Consider that the secondhand report of your client may have been made for strategic purposes in light of the marital problems that were reported. Inquire more about whether your client's marital problems still exist, the nature of those problems, and whether your client is considering whether to engage in any legal action.
2. Explore with Mr. Raymond the nature and extent of the danger, as in whether the extended family is aware of the uncle's proclivity to sexual abuse.
3. Explore with Mr. Raymond the level of alarm expressed by his wife about the possibility of harm to their daughter.
4. Suggest that Mr. Raymond invite his wife into the next session to discuss the need to protect their daughter and whether arrangements can be made to protect their daughter sufficiently.
5. Suggest to Mr. Raymond that he accompany his wife and daughter on the family trip, taking care not to leave his daughter alone at any time.
6. With consent of Mr. Raymond, contact the state CPS of the other jurisdiction.
7. Do a combination of the previously listed actions.
8. Do something that is not previously listed.

If you were practicing in Singapore and Mr. Raymond was your client, which would you do?

1. Stress the importance of making a report to authorities in order to protect Mr. Raymond's daughter.
2. State to Mr. Raymond that regardless of his agreement or not you will report the possibility of imminent harm to Mr. Raymond's daughter to the authorities.

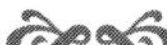

STANDARD 4.06: CONSULTATIONS

When consulting with colleagues, (1) psychologists do not disclose confidential information that reasonably could lead to the identification of a client/patient, research participant, or other person or organization with whom they have a confidential relationship unless they have obtained the prior consent of the person or organization or the disclosure cannot be avoided, and (2) they disclose information only to the extent necessary to achieve the purposes of the consultation.

A CASE FOR STANDARD 4.06: Six Degrees of Separation

Dr. Coleman is a newly licensed psychologist working in a behavioral health practice. Dr. Coleman specializes in couples' work, using a variety of techniques, including videotaping client sessions so that the couple can review and reflect on their body language, posture, expressions, etc., in between sessions. Dr. Coleman shares a group practice with several colleagues, and as part of the informed consent process, couples' clients are informed that short segments of their videos may be used for consultation among the practice partners. All clinic treatment is video recorded for consultation and is also analyzed and coded by trained psychologists who specialize in body language. One of Dr. Coleman's newest colleagues is Dr. Jenkins, a visiting practice member filling in for a psychologist who is away on maternity leave. Dr. Coleman has previously discussed this couples' case in consultation without identifiers. This day Dr. Coleman was scheduled to conduct the full presentation of his clinic case, with video recording. Dr. Coleman went the extra step of obtaining special permission from his clients to show a specific 10-minute video clip to his consultation group, although he did not reveal the name of his newest colleague, Dr. Jenkins, to his couples' client. As soon as the video clip appeared on the screen, Dr. Jenkins instantly recognized the face on the screen as her neighbor's daughter, who has been babysitting her young children.

Issues of Concern

Despite all precautions, there is always the possibility of clients being recognized from nonclinic contexts and thus unintentional breaches of confidentiality. With all precautions taken as directed in Standard 4.06, Dr. Jenkins and Dr. Coleman now find themselves in an awkward position. Standard 4.06 (2) directs Dr. Coleman to disclose information only to the extent necessary to achieve the purpose of the consultation. In this situation, was it necessary to obtain the level of consultation available through video recording without the possibility of this awkward circumstance? Was such a situation foreseeable, and could the clinic have provided the technical fix of showing the video with the client's face blurred?

What should Dr. Jenkins do now that she is aware that the video being shown during a consultation is actually her neighbor who babysits her daughter?

APA Ethics Code

Companion General Principle

Principle A: Beneficence and Nonmaleficence

> When conflicts occur among psychologists' obligations or concerns, they attempt to resolve these conflicts in a responsible fashion that avoids or minimizes harm.

Clearly a conflict has occurred. Principle A directs Dr. Coleman and Dr. Jenkins to resolve this conflict in such a way as to avoid harm.

Companion Ethical Standard(s)

Standard 4.01: Maintaining Confidentiality

> Psychologists have a primary obligation and take reasonable precautions to protect confidential information obtained through or stored in any medium, . . .

Standard 4.01 places the primary responsibility to maintain client confidentiality on Dr. Coleman, the treating psychologist.

Standard 4.02: Discussing the Limits of Confidentiality

> (a) Psychologists discuss with persons . . . with whom they establish a . . . professional relationship (1) the relevant limits of confidentiality and (2) the foreseeable uses of the information generated through their psychological activities.

If there is going to be any possible breach of confidentiality, Standard 4.02 directs psychologists to obtain client consent. In this case, Dr. Coleman followed the directives of both Standard 4.02 and Standard 4.06.

Standard 2.05: Delegation of Work to Others

> Psychologists who delegate . . . take reasonable steps to . . . (1) avoid delegating such work to persons who have a multiple relationship with those being served that would likely lead to exploitation or loss of objectivity; . . . (2) authorize only those responsibilities that such persons can be expected to perform competently on the basis of their education, training, or experience . . .

The consult group members appeared to be appropriately qualified to engage in the work of peer consultation. To the extent the group members are qualified, Dr. Coleman ensured that he only delegated the work of consultation to those persons who can be expected to perform competently on the basis of their education, training, and experience.

Legal Issues 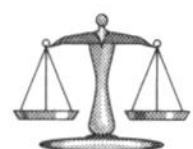

New Mexico

> *N.M. Code R. § 16.22.2.12 (2010).*
>
> Protecting Confidentiality
>
> A. Safeguarding confidential information. The psychologist shall safeguard confidential information obtained in the course of practice... The psychologist shall disclose confidential information to others only with the written informed consent of the patient or client...
>
> ... I. Discussion of client information among professionals. When ... interacting with other appropriate professionals concerning the welfare of the client, the psychologist may share confidential information about the client provided the psychologist ensures that all persons receiving the information are informed about the confidential nature of the information and abide by the rules of confidentiality.
>
> ... K. Observation and electronic recording. The psychologist shall ensure that diagnostic interviews or therapeutic sessions with a patient are ... electronically recorded only with the informed written consent of the patient...

Oregon

> *Or. Admin. R. 858-010-0075 (2010).*
>
> Code of Professional Conduct.
>
> The Board adopts for the code of professional conduct of psychologists in Oregon the American Psychological Association's "Ethical Principles of Psychologists and Code of Conduct" effective June 1, 2002.

In both jurisdictions, once the informed consent of the client occurred, the videotape could be used for consultation among the psychologists within the office. The new consulting psychologist would maintain confidentiality under the law even when she became aware that she knows the family from a personal context.

Cultural Considerations

Global Discussion

The Professional Board for Psychology Health Professions Council of South Africa:
Ethical Code of Professional Conduct (April 2002)

> 3.9. Professional consultations.
>
> ... 3.9.2. When consulting with colleagues (1) psychologists shall not disclose confidential information that reasonably could lead to identification of a client, ... unless they have obtained the prior consent of the person ..., and (2) they disclose information only to the extent necessary to achieve the purposes of the consultation.

Dr. Coleman is in violation because when the couples' client gave consent at the beginning of their treatment, it did not account for the inclusion of Dr. Jenkins. To be in compliance with South Africa's code, he would have needed to either alter the identity of his couples' client to such a degree that their faces and voices are not recognizable or have modified his consent with the client to alert his couple that a new colleague had temporarily joined the practice and would be viewing their session tapes.

American Moral Values

1. What is the professional purpose of the consultation? What are Dr. Jenkins's obligations as a participant? Can she treat this case with her full analytical abilities intact? Will it serve the consultation's purpose best to declare she knows one of the subjects? Would it be best to excuse herself, given how that awareness might affect her colleagues' discussion of the case? Or would that disrupt her colleagues' ability to help with Dr. Coleman's case?
2. What is the balance to be struck between using video to gain insight on body language and risking a patient's privacy and anonymity? Are there sufficient resources to blur the faces on future videos? Or are facial expressions too important to lose for the edification of the therapists?
3. Does Dr. Jenkins's status as a visiting professor influence her decision? Does she feel like the faculty would not appreciate a visitor advising on videotaping practice?
4. What is the effect on Dr. Jenkins and her babysitter, assuming that the employer/employee relationship

continues? Should she tell her babysitter about the video? Can Dr. Jenkins keep her on as a caregiver if she goes ahead and watches it? Will it even help if she does not watch, knowing that her babysitter may have a serious mental health issue?

Ethical Course of Action

Directive per APA Code

Dr. Coleman followed all relevant directives to ensure confidentiality and to ensure appropriate ongoing consultation for his work. Both the APA (American Psychological Association) Ethics Code and the reviewed state laws are silent on what Dr. Jenkins should do once she recognized the identity of Dr. Coleman's client. Presumably Standard 4.01 binds Dr. Jenkins to confidentiality. Thus, cognizant of her professional obligation of client confidentiality, she would keep her knowledge of Dr. Coleman's client confined to the professional setting and not reveal her knowledge to her neighbor or her babysitter.

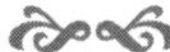

Dictates of One's Own Conscience

If you were Dr. Jenkins, what would you do?

1. Keep the information about Dr. Coleman's client being your babysitter confidential and never reveal the knowledge to anyone, then proceed with the consultation.
2. Instantly inform the consultation group of the relationship between yourself and Dr. Coleman's client. Then ask the consultation group for a discussion on the best course of action.
3. Instantly inform the consultation group of the relationship between yourself and Dr. Coleman's client. Recuse yourself and leave the consultation room immediately.
4. Instantly inform the consultation group of a conflict of interest with the subject matter without revealing the relationship between yourself and Dr. Coleman's client. Request that the consultation not proceed with Dr. Coleman's client.
5. Instantly inform the consultation group of a conflict of interest with the subject matter without revealing the relationship between yourself and Dr. Coleman's client. Request that you be excused from the consultation for the week.
6. Do a combination of the previously listed actions.
7. Do something that is not previously listed.

If you were Dr. Jenkins and this situation had occurred in South Africa, which would you do?

1. Abide by the limits of confidentiality, not reveal the relationship of Dr. Coleman's client and yourself, and proceed with the consultation.
2. Immediately reveal that a breach of confidentiality has occurred, and discuss with Dr. Coleman the necessity of updating or revising his informed consent process as new circumstances, such as new visiting psychologists, arise.

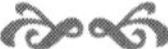

STANDARD 4.07: USE OF CONFIDENTIAL INFORMATION FOR DIDACTIC OR OTHER PURPOSES

Psychologists do not disclose in their writings, lectures, or other public media, confidential, personally identifiable information concerning their clients/patients, students, research participants, organizational clients, or other recipients of their services that they obtained during the course of their work, unless (1) they take reasonable steps to disguise the person or organization, (2) the person or organization has consented in writing, or (3) there is legal authorization for doing so.

A CASE FOR STANDARD 4.07: But I Didn't Reveal His Identity, Did I?

Dr. Perry, in her first job after graduation, was teaching psychopathology. To illustrate what paranoid schizophrenia looks like, Dr. Perry utilized some of her work with a client she calls "John Doe." As part of the background, she gave a disguised version of an actual case but retained distinguishing details of a suicide attempt. After the class, one of Dr. Perry's students approached and said, "I think you talked about my older brother. John, my brother, is the guy who tried to kill himself and has schizophrenia. I don't think he would be very happy about his information being shared in front of people he doesn't know."

Issues of Concern

Presumably Dr. Perry did not obtain written consent from John to use his information for educational purposes. In the absence of such written consent, Standard 4.07 directs psychologists not to disclose personally identifiable information. Dr. Perry had not identified her previous client by name, occupation, age, or other common features of identifiable information. Were the details of a suicide attempt sufficiently identifiable to have violated Standard 4.07? How disguised does the situation need to be in order to be deemed in compliance with Standard 4.07? In this situation, was there any way for Dr. Perry to have avoided violating Standard 4.07 if the illustration of the psychopathology necessitated providing some details of a suicide attempt? Or is it possible there will always be someone in the audience who knows someone who fits enough of the distinguishing features in a case illustration that Dr. Perry will often find herself being accused of violating confidentiality, regardless of how much she alters the details of a case?

APA Ethics Code

Companion General Principle

Principle E: Respect for People's Rights and Dignity

> Psychologists respect the dignity and worth of all people, and the rights of individuals to privacy. . .

One activity in enacting Principle E is safeguarding the client's privacy. In most situations, privacy means protecting John Doe's identity. In this situation, Dr. Perry is not to reveal specific information that may identify John Doe.

Companion Ethical Standard(s)

Standard 3.04: Minimizing Harm

> Psychologists take reasonable steps to avoid harming their clients. . .

Not protecting the client's privacy is a way Dr. Perry could have harmed her client. Even if John Doe was not the student's brother, the belief that Dr. Perry was talking about her brother might have harmed the student. The student may take information back to the family regarding treatment of someone whom she believed to be her brother, thus inadvertently spreading erroneous information about her brother.

Standard 4.01: Maintaining Confidentiality

> Psychologists have a primary obligation . . . to protect confidential information obtained through . . . any medium . . .

Standard 4.05: Disclosures

> (a) Psychologists may disclose confidential information with the appropriate consent of . . . the individual client . . .

Standard 4.01, in combination with Standard 4.05, dictates that Dr. Perry needs to ensure confidentiality unless John Doe signed a consent form for his information to be used for educational purposes. If Dr. Perry had a written consent from John Doe, then discussing the diagnosis with specific details of a suicide attempt would not be a breach of confidentiality.

Legal Issues 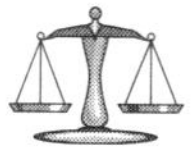

South Carolina

> *S.C. Code Ann. Regs.100-4 (2010). Code of ethics.*
>
> G. Protecting confidentiality of clients.
>
> (1) In general. The psychologist shall safeguard the confidential information obtained in the course of practice. . . With the exceptions set forth below, the psychologist shall disclose confidential information to others only with the informed written consent of the client.
>
> . . . (10) Disguising confidential information. When case reports or other clinical materials are used as the basis of teaching, . . . the psychologist shall exercise reasonable care to insure that the reported material is appropriately disguised to prevent client identification.

South Dakota

> *S.D. Admin. R. 20:60:07:01 (2010). Code of ethics.*
>
> The code of ethics for psychologists licensed in this state is the "ASPPB Code of Conduct," 2005.

. . . III. Rules of Conduct

. . . F. Protecting Confidentiality of Clients

1. In general. The psychologist shall safeguard the confidential information obtained in the course of practice. . . With the exceptions set forth below . . . the psychologist shall disclose confidential information to others only with the informed written consent of the client.

. . . 10. Disguising confidential information. When . . . confidential information is used as the basis of teaching, . . . the psychologist shall exercise reasonable care to insure that the reported material is appropriately disguised to prevent client identification.

If Dr. Perry was teaching in South Carolina or South Dakota, the use of client related confidential information would be permitted if the information were appropriately disguised. Neither state defines what would entail an *appropriate disguise* of the facts, thus it is unclear whether Dr. Perry has violated state law.

Cultural Considerations

Global Discussion

Code of Ethics: Netherlands

III.2.6. Disclosure of information.

III.2.6.5. Use of information for purposes of scientific publications or education, supervision, etc. . .

The psychologist is entitled to use for the purposes of . . . education . . . only information in which a client is not personally identifiable. The combination of personal data and described circumstances should not enable third parties to identify the client in question.

Dr. Perry would likely be in violation of the Netherlands Code if she failed to disguise her client enough that he would not be identifiable to any "third party"—that is, gave actual diagnostic information and specific details of a suicide attempt, if that information could reasonably be used to identify her client. Acquaintances, friends, coworkers, or family members may feel as though they are hearing information about someone they know that should better be kept confidential, but in this case, Dr. Perry's decision to reveal the actual details of the suicide attempt is likely to violate the client's confidentiality.

American Moral Values

1. How does Dr. Perry assess the effectiveness of her vignette? What makes it good enough to risk someone recognizing its source, however much she disguises the person by race, gender, etc.? Does she owe it to her students to give them the most instructive example for their training in the field? To what degree is an instructor responsible for speculation that might go on among students about the real-life person behind the vignette?
2. What does Dr. Perry owe to John's brother and the rest of his family? Did the brother have an unusually perceptive guess, piecing together details no one else could have? What if the brother was the only one to recognize John in the story? Is one person enough to scrap the vignette, or can Dr. Perry argue that John's life will be impossible to detect by students?
3. How should Dr. Perry discuss the issue with John's sister? What role would his own embarrassment about his brother's suicide attempt play in his objection? Can she try to convince him that with additional tweaking no one will know the case? Would it be morally permissible to deny to John's brother that the vignette was about John, given how she changed it?
4. Does Dr. Perry need to discuss her vignette with John himself? Is John's approval sufficient to continue using the vignette? What if one of John's younger relatives or friends encounters this story as a student? Could Dr. Perry seem exploitative regardless of John's attitude?

Ethical Course of Action

Directive per APA Code

Per Standard 4.05 (a) and Standard 4.07 (2), if Dr. Perry had obtained written consent from John Doe, then no violation of privacy has occurred, regardless of whether a student in the class thinks John Doe is his brother. However, if Dr. Perry does not have written consent from John Doe, Standard 4.07 still allows for use of client information for didactic purposes if steps were taken to disguise the client. Disguising the identity of a client for the purpose of teaching goes beyond changing a person's status such as sex, age, social/economic status (SES), etc. To disguise an identity requires that any disclosed information does not include sufficient details that are unique and recognizable enough that an acquaintance of the client would be able to guess that person's identity. Similarly, if Dr. Perry was practicing in the Netherlands, her decision to reveal the actual details of the suicide attempt places her at risk of violating her client's confidentiality.

Dictates of One's Own Conscience

If you were Dr. Perry, hopefully you would not have furnished revealing details of such specificity that could identify your client. However, if the student was correct and indeed John Doe was her brother, which would you do?

1. Assure the student that John Doe was not his/her brother, but the details of such a suicide attempt are common for clients diagnosed with schizophrenia.
2. Apologize to the student, and vow not to use the vignette in the future.
3. Reason that the use of clinical information for didactic purposes is allowed and can be particularly useful in teaching situations; decide you will be more vigilant when creating clinical vignettes based on actual client cases.
4. Do a combination of the previously listed actions.
5. Do something that is not previously listed.

If you were Dr. Perry, teaching in the Netherlands, which would you do?

1. Immediately alter the vignette for future use; combine it with others to make a composite vignette, and alter other similar vignettes.
2. Assure your student that the client you spoke of was not his/her brother but allow for the possibility that hearing about such a similar case may be distressing for your student.
3. Apologize to your student, explain that many clients with schizophrenia attempt suicide, and although it is likely not about his/her brother, assure the student you will no longer use that particular vignette.

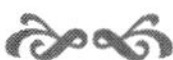

CHAPTER 5

Advertising and Other Public Statements

Ethical Standard 5

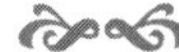

CHAPTER OUTLINE

- Standard 5.01: Avoidance of False or Deceptive Statements
- Standard 5.02: Statements by Others
- Standard 5.03: Descriptions of Workshops and Non-Degree-Granting Educational Programs
- Standard 5.04: Media Presentations
- Standard 5.05: Testimonials
- Standard 5.06: In-Person Solicitation

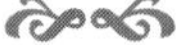

STANDARD 5.01: AVOIDANCE OF FALSE OR DECEPTIVE STATEMENTS

(a) Public statements include but are not limited to paid or unpaid advertising, product endorsements, grant applications, licensing applications, other credentialing applications, brochures, printed matter, directory listings, personal resumes or curricula vitae, or comments for use in media such as print or electronic transmission, statements in legal proceedings, lectures and public oral presentations, and published materials. Psychologists do not knowingly make public statements that are false, deceptive, or fraudulent concerning their research, practice, or other work activities or those of persons or organizations with which they are affiliated.

A CASE FOR STANDARD 5.01(A): Inadvertent Grandiosity

Dr. Black is a licensed psychologist in private practice. Taking the marketing advice from various professional publications, she has decided to join the town's chamber of commerce. A standard joining practice is for the chamber of commerce to ask for a sample of goods or services provided by new members. To fulfill this requirement for membership, Dr. Black was asked to provide an example of her services through a donation to the chamber of commerce's annual charity auction. The suggestion, to which Dr. Black had agreed, was for Dr. Black to "donate a psychological evaluation" to the auction. The auction bid sheet has Dr. Black listed as a psychologist and the psychological evaluation as "testing to answer questions you have about yourself or your family members."

Issues of Concern

Standard 5.01 (a) addresses public statements. The bid sheet for the silent auction is a document that is open for the public to read. On the auction bid sheet is a statement about Dr. Black's practice, which involves provision of psychological evaluations. Standard 5.01 (a) directs Dr. Black not to "knowingly" make "false, deceptive, or fraudulent" statements regarding her practice. The statement about "testing to answer questions you have about yourself or your family members" is misleading at best and may be fraudulent because it implies that Dr. Black can conduct testing for any type of concern. It is doubtful that Dr. Black has been trained and is competent to use any type of diagnostic assessment and/or for any type of diagnosable mental condition. If Dr. Black did not create the auction bid sheet, she has not "knowingly" made a deceptive or fraudulent statement about her practice. Is Dr. Black still in violation of Standard 5.01 (a)?

APA Ethics Code

Companion General Principle

Principle E: Respect for People's Rights and Dignity

> Psychologists respect the dignity and worth of all people, and the rights of individuals to privacy, confidentiality, and self-determination.

Respecting right to privacy, Principle E guides Dr. Black to ensure that each step of acquiring her services is kept as confidential as possible. Respecting right to self-determination, each step of the referral process must hold no element of coercion. The process of public auction does not engender privacy or self-determination. If the person who purchased the service did so with the intention of using it for someone else, Dr. Black has not established a referral process that is focused on self-determination but contributed to a process which may result in collusion with coercive behavior.

Principle B: Fidelity and Responsibility

> Psychologists uphold professional standards of conduct, clarify their professional roles and obligations, accept appropriate responsibility for their behavior, and seek to manage conflicts of interest that could lead to exploitation or harm. . .

Dr. Black holds some responsibility toward the people who end up coming to her office through purchasing the auction item. If the person who won the bid for psychological evaluation purchased it for a spouse but the spouse thinks the first partner is blaming him or her for all of their marital problems and does not want to be evaluated, Dr. Black cannot proceed with the assessment because the second partner has not consented to an evaluation. Also, if the purchase is not used, what responsibility does Dr. Black hold for the cost of the purchased service?

Companion Ethical Standard(s)

Standard 5.02: Statements By Others

> Psychologists who engage others to create or place public statements . . . retain responsibility for such statements.

Standard 5.02 places the responsibility for the professional integrity of public statements made by others in the hands of the psychologist. It was with Dr. Black's knowledge and consent that the chamber of commerce included her in the silent auction. Thus Dr. Black "engaged" others in the chamber of commerce to create a public statement in the form of the auction bid sheet.

Standard 2.01: Boundaries of Competence

> (a) Psychologists provide services . . . with populations and in areas only within the boundaries of their competence . . .

It is not within Dr. Black's control as to who enters or wins the bid for the psychological evaluation. The referral questions could involve a multitude of issues from child ADHD to traumatic brain injury, for example, depending upon who wins the silent auction bid and what their individual concerns or questions may be. It is not possible for any psychologist to be competent to conduct evaluations for any and all situations. The potential for violation of Standard 2.01 is tremendous in this situation.

Standard 3.05: Multiple Relationships

> . . . (b) If a psychologist finds that . . . a potentially harmful multiple relationship has arisen, the psychologist takes reasonable steps to resolve it with due regard for the best interests of the affected person and maximal compliance with the Ethics Code.

The unforeseen circumstances related to the outcome of the auction leaves Dr. Black at risk. It is within the realm of possibility that the person who shows up to claim the psychological evaluation is known to Dr. Black or is known to someone close to her.

Standard 1.01: Misuse of Psychologists' Work

> If psychologists learn of . . . misrepresentation of their work, they take reasonable steps to correct or minimize the . . . misrepresentation.

Now that Dr. Black has learned of this public statement associated with her psychology practice, Standard 1.01 directs her to "take reasonable steps" for correction of the situation.

Legal Issues 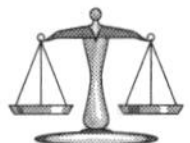

Tennessee

> *Tenn. Comp. R. & Regs. 1180-01-.15 (2010). Advertising and other public statements.*
>
> (1) Definition of public statements. Public statements include but are not limited to paid or unpaid . . . printed matter . . . and published materials.
>
> (2) Statements by others.
>
> (a) Licensees . . . holders who engage others to create or place public statements that promote their professional . . . activities retain professional responsibility for such statements.
>
> (b) In addition, licensees or certificate holders make reasonable efforts to prevent others whom they do not control (such as . . . sponsors . . .) from making deceptive statements concerning licensees' . . . practice . . . activities.
>
> (c) If licensees . . . learn of deceptive statements about their work made by others, licensees . . . make reasonable efforts to correct such statements.

Utah

> *Utah Admin. Code 156-61-502 (2010). Unprofessional conduct.*
>
> "Unprofessional conduct" includes:
>
> (1) violation of any provision of the "Ethical Principles of Psychologists and Code of Conduct" of the American Psychological Association (APA) as adopted by the APA, August 2002 edition, which is adopted and incorporated by reference . . .

In both jurisdictions, the auction statement is overly broad and could be viewed as deceptive. To meet the standards of the law, the psychologist should narrow the statement by delineating her area of evaluative competence and limiting the evaluation to the person bidding upon the service at auction.

Cultural Consideration

Global Discussion

Hong Kong Psychological Society: Professional Code of Practice

> Chapter 11: Public statements.
>
> 11.1. Promotional activities of Members serve the purpose of helping the public make informed judgments and choices. Members shall represent accurately and objectively their professional qualifications, affiliations, and functions, as well as those of their institutions or organizations.
>
> 11.2. Public statements include, but are not limited to . . . circular . . . directory and business card. . . Public statements made by Members in announcing or advertising the availability of psychological . . . services, shall not contain: a. any statement which is . . . misleading . . . or likely to mislead or deceive; . . .

To auction off a psychological evaluation is a violation of Hong Kong's Code, as it interferes with the ability of the public to "make informed judgments and choices" regarding the purpose and intent of a psychological evaluation, as well being "misleading or . . . likely to mislead or deceive." Because Dr. Black cannot predict who will win or undergo such an evaluation and what possible presenting problems or mitigating circumstances will enter her office with that person, she cannot accurately write a disclaimer for all of the likely (and preventable) harms caused by her decision. Finally, depending on what other items are in the auction bid sheet, Dr. Black may have lessened the value or impact of psychological evaluations and services in the minds of those attending the auction—actions that could be seen as a violation of 11.1: " . . . helping the public make informed judgments and choices."

American Moral Values

1. In what respects does Dr. Black consider her work a product to be sold? Does belonging to a chamber of commerce compromise the standards of a psychologist as a care provider? Or is it just this auction and its promotion that is objectionable? Does the need

to gain clients and make a living have limits in the context of providing mental health care?

2. Does the auction bid promise too much in implying Dr. Black will "answer questions" about a person's life, mental health, etc.? Is asking about family members, for example, even an appropriate topic for an assessment or therapy?
3. What is Dr. Black's responsibility as a representative practitioner of psychology? Will this auction harm the way that psychology is viewed in the community? Or does this represent a largely harmless form of outreach to community members who might otherwise go untreated? Is this way of publicizing her work meeting the community where they are?
4. Is this auction a unique demand made by the chamber of commerce, or will Dr. Black have to meet additional requirements as part of her membership? Will her membership entail being collegial with other chamber members? Will it entail an understood reciprocity between her and the other members in terms of access, services provided, etc.?

Ethical Course of Action

Directive per APA Code

The auction bid sheet is a public statement and thus falls under the directive of Standard 5.01. She did not knowingly make a deceptive public statement, thus is not in violation of Standard 5.01. But regardless of whether Dr. Black knowingly made deceptive public statements or not, Standard 5.02 does not absolve Dr. Black of responsibility for the public statement. Standard 1.01 directs Dr. Black to now engage in corrective behavior to resolve the misunderstanding.

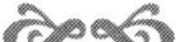

Dictates of One's Own Conscience

If you were Dr. Black, knowing that you are clearly responsible for corrective action, what would you do?

1. Speak to the auction organizer and ask to have the auction item removed immediately.
2. Insert a qualifier in the auction bid sheet to have bidders consult with you before making a bid to assure the appropriateness of the referral not only about type of service but also about who could be evaluated.
3. Post your qualifications on the auction bid sheet with a request that only those who want an evaluation within your area of competence should bid for the evaluation.
4. Do a combination of the previously listed actions.
5. Do something that is not previously listed.

If you were Dr. Black and this situation occurred in Hong Kong, which would you do?

1. Consider submitting an addendum to the auction bid sheet, explaining the nature, limitations, and conditions under which you can perform a psychological evaluation for the winner of the bid.
2. Explain to the person in charge at the chamber of commerce that although you wish to join, it would be unethical for you to perform a psychological evaluation that is so open-ended and undefined.
3. Go ahead with the evaluation on whoever wins the bid, after clearly explaining your limitations and areas of competence; resolve to limit your affiliation with the chamber in the future.

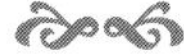

STANDARD 5.01: AVOIDANCE OF FALSE OR DECEPTIVE STATEMENTS

> . . . (b) Psychologists do not make false, deceptive, or fraudulent statements concerning (1) their training, experience, or competence; (2) their academic degrees; (3) their credentials; (4) their institutional or association affiliations; (5) their services; (6) the scientific or clinical basis for, or results or degree of success of, their services; (7) their fees; or (8) their publications or research findings.

A CASE FOR STANDARD 5.01 (B): Are We There Yet?

Patrick is a certified public accountant (CPA). After some years of practicing as an accountant, Patrick decided to return to graduate school in psychology. Patrick's dissertation defense is scheduled in late May, with his anticipated graduation with his doctorate occurring in June. Being a devoted father and active in his community, Patrick had been persuaded to run for the local school board. The public statement pamphlet is developed in May and distributed in August, a few weeks before the primaries in his state. At the time of submission for the pamphlet Patrick had every reason to believe he would graduate and hold his doctorate in psychology by summer. Thus the short biographic statement in the pamphlet lists Patrick as "Dr. Patrick__, CPA, PhD."

Unplanned and unanticipated by all, Dr. Palmer, the chair of Patrick's dissertation committee, suffered a heart attack the day before Patrick's scheduled defense. With Dr. Palmer in the hospital and no time to make any other arrangements, his defense was canceled and could not be rescheduled until Dr. Palmer was medically released to return to work. By the time Dr. Palmer was given medical clearance to return to work, other faculty members on the dissertation committee had already begun their summer traveling schedules. Thus, Patrick's dissertation defense was rescheduled for mid-August when faculty were all due to return to campus before the start of the fall semester.

In last-minute campaign moves, Patrick's opponent publicly charged Patrick with making false claims about his educational achievements. When the local newspaper and radio station contacted the university, the statement from the university's registrar's office confirmed that Patrick has not yet received his doctorate.

Issues of Concern

The voter's pamphlet contains a statement that references his academic credentials, regardless of whether the publication is intended for use in the professional arena or in some aspect of the psychologist's private life activities, such as running for the local school board. Patrick did not *knowingly* make a false public statement. Does it matter that he had every expectation of graduating by August? As it turns out, he did make a false statement concerning his training and credentials and is now in violation of Standard 5.01 (b) (3).

APA Ethics Code

Companion General Principle

Introduction and Applicability

> The Ethics Code applies only to psychologists' activities that are part of their scientific, educational, or professional roles as psychologists. Areas covered include but are not limited to the clinical, counseling, and school practice of psychology; research; teaching; supervision of trainees; public service; policy development; social intervention; development of assessment instruments; conducting assessments; educational counseling; organizational consulting; forensic activities; program design and evaluation; and administration. The Ethics Code applies to these activities across a variety of contexts, such as in person, by post, telephone, internet, and other electronic transmissions. Such activities are distinguished from the purely private conduct of psychologists, which is not within the purview of the Ethics Code.

The Ethical Principles and Code of Conduct apply to psychologists in their " . . . role as a psychologist . . . distinguished from the purely private conduct of psychologists, which is not within the purview of the Ethics Code." Therefore, the published material, because it is not within the domain of Patrick's professional activities in his role as a psychologist, is not within the purview of any principle or standards of the code.

Principle B: Fidelity and Responsibility

> . . . They are aware of their professional and scientific responsibilities to society and to the specific communities in which they work. Psychologists uphold professional standards of conduct, clarify their professional roles and obligations, accept appropriate responsibility for their behavior, and seek to manage conflicts of interest that could lead to exploitation or harm.

The political system in the United States seems to consider all aspects of a person's life to be available for scrutiny if the person is running for or serving in public office. To the extent that Patrick has voluntarily entered into an arena where all aspects of his life, including his profession as a psychologist, are open for examination, he should expect to be measured against the standards of the profession of psychology. As such, regardless of whether psychology considers his private life to be within the domain of psychology, the public considers his profession of both roles as an accountant and psychologist to be within the public domain. Thus Principle B, which guides Patrick to be "aware of . . . professional . . . responsibilities to . . . the specific communities in which they work," hopes Patrick is cognizant of the fact that he has a responsibility to uphold the honor of psychology in the public eye.

Principle C: Integrity

> Psychologists seek to promote accuracy, honesty and truthfulness in . . . psychology. In these activities psychologists do not . . . engage in . . . intentional misrepresentation of fact . . .

Principle C is the companion value that corresponds to the directives of Standard 5.01. Hopefully we all aspire to honesty and truthfulness in every aspect of our professional and private lives.

Companion Ethical Standard(s)

Standard 5.02: Statements by Others

> Psychologists who engage others to create or place public statements. . . retain responsibility for such statements.

Even presuming Patrick had campaign staff that developed the content of the pamphlet for him, Patrick is still responsible for everything printed in the pamphlet.

Standard 1.01: Misuse of Psychologists' Work

> If psychologists learn of . . . misrepresentation of their work, they take reasonable steps to correct or minimize the . . . misrepresentation.

Claiming a degree that has not yet been earned is misrepresentation of work. Standard 1.01 directs Patrick to "take reasonable steps to correct" the mistake.

Legal Issues 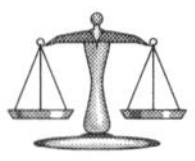

Vermont

> *20-4-1600 Vt. Code R. § 5.01 (2010). Avoidance of false or deceptive statements.*
>
> . . . (b) Psychologists do not make false . . . statements concerning . . . (2) their academic degrees . . .

Virginia

> *18 Va. Admin. Code § 125-20-150 (2010). Standards of practice.*
>
> . . . B. Persons licensed by the board shall:
>
> . . . 2. When making public statements regarding credentials . . . , ensure that such statements are neither fraudulent nor misleading.

In both jurisdictions, representing that a doctorate had been obtained before it was conferred is unethical. As the doctoral student's representation was published in the public statement pamphlet, reasonable steps must be taken to address the misleading impression left with all potential voters. Even then, it is likely Patrick's act was unethical.

Cultural Considerations

Global Discussion

Code of Ethics: Netherlands

> Basic principles worked out in guidelines.
>
> III. 2 Honesty.
>
> III.1.2.1. Avoidance of deception.
>
> The psychologist refrains from any form of deception in his professional conduct.
>
> III.1.2.3. Representation of education, qualifications, experience, competence and titles.
>
> The psychologist represents his academic background . . . accurately. This representation will be done only when this is strictly relevant.

Although Patrick's "deception in his professional conduct" was unintentional, nonetheless, he has publicly laid claim to credentials he had not yet earned. Running for a local school board is not relevant to the practice of psychology, nor is a doctorate in psychology particularly relevant to political office or campaigning for the school board. Using a credential that one has not earned in an attempt to be more credible, qualified, or somehow a better choice as a political candidate violates both the intent and the letter of this portion of the Netherlands code. Doing so before the credential has actually been earned, no matter how well-intentioned, is also a significant violation.

American Moral Values

1. Patrick has published an incorrect claim on a campaign flyer, despite his reasonable anticipation of having the PhD by the time the pamphlet was to be used. Is that anticipation enough to justify making a claim that may not be true at that later time? Is there an academic standard or law or protocol that conflicts with standards for campaign literature and the media? Is the former standard something Patrick would identify with and defend in a public discussion of the issue?

2. What are Patrick's views about the public and its use of information? Does he basically believe they buy negative campaigning, diversionary tactics, and made-up scandals? Or does he sympathize with the views of an average voter, who might wonder why someone is claiming a degree they haven't earned yet? Is his incorrect pamphlet an example of not being strictly accountable to the voters? Does he owe voters just an explanation, or does he owe them an apology as well? Is his action serious enough to quit the campaign?

3. Claiming a CPA and PhD is itself a politically and culturally loaded act for a candidate, involving associations with accountants and psychologists, among others. Does Patrick anticipate extra resentment for his misstatement because of the degrees involved? Should he challenge that resentment as part of defending academic institutions and fields he believes in?

4. Was the inclusion of the PhD a standard part of any resume he would have sent out at the time? Has Patrick considered whether he was using that degree for political legitimacy in his campaign? What does Patrick owe the university for bringing its name into this political attack? What does he owe his colleagues in the psychology department?

Ethical Course of Action

Directive per APA Code

Even if the psychology ethics code is not intended to apply to the situation described, the public has an expectation that they will be protected from errant behavior of psychologists based on the psychology ethics code. Although Patrick has not violated the directives of Standard 5.01 (a) because he did not intentionally make a false statement about his academic credentials, if he were living in Vermont or Virginia, he would be in violation of the law. In addition, he is in violation of Standard 5.01 (b) because he did technically make a false statement concerning his academic degree. Following the directive of Standard 1.01, Patrick now needs to take reasonable steps to rectify the situation.

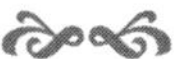

Dictates of One's Own Conscience

If you are of the opinion that the ethics code does apply in this situation and that something does need to be done to correct the misrepresentation, if you were Patrick, what would you do?

1. Avoid possible misconduct by publishing the pamphlet with "Dr. Patrick __, CPA, PhD candidate" instead of the CPA, PhD.
2. Make a public statement in May to the fact that your anticipated graduation date has been moved to August.
3. Make a public statement about the specifics about Dr. Palmer's health and why the degree was not awarded in May as originally expected.
4. Make a public apology with a statement that you should have known better than to claim a degree not yet awarded.
5. Do a combination of the previously listed actions.
6. Do something that is not previously listed.

If you were Patrick, running for local office in the Netherlands, would you have avoided the entire situation by not adding your academic credentials to the public pamphlet, reasoning that a degree in psychology is not relevant to candidacy for the school board?

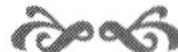

STANDARD 5.01: AVOIDANCE OF FALSE OR DECEPTIVE STATEMENTS

> . . . (c) Psychologists claim degrees as credentials for their health services only if those degrees (1) were earned from a regionally accredited educational institution or (2) were the basis for psychology licensure by the state in which they practice.

A CASE FOR STANDARD 5.01 (C): Crossing Professions

Heather came to her graduate program in clinical psychology with a license as a massage therapist. To keep up with her bills, Heather has continued working at a private massage clinic on a part-time basis. The massage clinic is owned by Dr. Mills, a naturopathic physician. Other employees of Dr. Mills's clinic include an acupuncturist, a nutritionist, and two massage therapists, one of whom is Heather. One and half years after entering the graduate program with her comprehensive examinations successfully completed, Heather was now looking for ways to increase her clinical training hours to be more competitive for internship applications. In casual office conversation, Heather updated Dr. Mills on her progress and mentioned that she had now learned how to give "all of these psychological assessments, like screening for eating disorders." Dr. Mills asked Heather if she would informally give tests to clients that he refers for massage, especially women who may possibly be developing or hiding eating disorders.

Seeing a good opportunity, Heather agreed and created all of the appropriate disclosure and consent notices informing clients that her assessments are informal and information will go to Dr. Mills. Everything seems to be progressing smoothly. Heather engaged in practicing administering several assessments, Dr. Mills provided information about possible eating disorder symptomology, and clients received appropriate consultation from the nutritionist in the office.

At the end of the first month, Heather noticed that the clinic has billed a client's insurance for the exam performed by Dr. Mills, the massage therapy performed by Heather, and additional charges for psychological assessment performed by Heather under her massage therapy license.

Issues of Concern

Heather does hold a massage therapy license duly granted by the state in which she is now practicing. The services submitted to the insurance company were claimed under her massage therapy license. The difficulty is regarding what type of service is specified under which license. Should Heather provide psychological assessment under the auspices of her massage therapy license? Has Dr. Mills's office violated Standard 5.01 (c) by billing for psychological services under Heather's massage therapy license? As Heather provided the services, is it most appropriate that the services be billed under Heather's name?

APA Ethics Code

Companion General Principle

Principle D: Justice

> Psychologists recognize that fairness and justice entitle all persons to access to and benefit from the contributions of psychology and to equal quality in the processes, procedures, and services being conducted by psychologists.

Presuming that Heathers and Dr. Millss clients are appropriately referred and would benefit from the eating disorder assessment, does Principle D guide Heather to provide such services? Since Heather is not yet a licensed psychologist, should the assessment be conducted free of charge?

Principle C: Integrity

> Psychologists seek to promote accuracy, honesty, and truthfulness in the . . . practice of psychology. In these activities psychologists do not . . . engage in fraud . . . or intentional misrepresentation of fact. . .

Principle C guides Heather to bill accurately for psychological services. Billing for eating disorder assessments under her massage therapist license appears to be either fraudulent or at the least an intentional misrepresentation about the scope of her practice.

Companion Ethical Standard(s)

Introduction and Applicability

> Membership in the APA commits . . . student affiliates to comply with the standards of the APA Ethics Code . . .

Heather, being a student in a psychology program, is in the category of "student affiliates" regardless of whether she has applied for American Psychological Association (APA) membership as long as the graduate program is accredited by the APA Commission on Accreditation. Heather's professional activities in the realm of psychology are under the purview of this ethics code. Thus, the eating disorder assessment is under the domain of psychology, not her massage therapy license.

Standard 2.01: Boundaries of Competence

> (a) Psychologists provide services . . . only within the boundaries of their competence, based on their . . . supervised experience . . .

Standard 2.01 directs Heather, being a student affiliate, to practice only within her area of competence. Since students are not licensed for independent practice, Standard 2.01 directs Heather to stay within her area of competence based on supervision. Dr. Mills is acting outside of the scope of his practice and is an inappropriate person to provide oversight or supervision since he is not a psychologist. Practicing under inappropriate supervision likely will lead to administration errors or inaccurate interpretation of tests which may lead to inappropriate or unnecessary medical treatments.

Standard 9.07: Assessment by Unqualified Persons

> Psychologists do not promote the use of psychological assessment techniques by unqualified persons, except when such use is conducted for training purposes with appropriate supervision.

Was Heather qualified, as a student, to conduct assessments and provide results without appropriate supervision? Here we assume that supervision by a naturopathic physician is not appropriate for administration of psychological assessments.

Standard 6.04: Fees and Financial Arrangements

> . . . (b) Psychologists' fee practices are consistent with law.
> (c) Psychologists do not misrepresent their fees.

Massage therapy does not encompass psychological assessments for eating disorders, and it is illegal to submit bills for psychological services under a massage therapy license. At the very least, it is a misrepresentation to bill for psychological assessments under a massage therapy licensure.

Standard 6.06: Accuracy in Reports to Payors and Funding Sources

> In their reports to payers for services . . . psychologists take reasonable steps to ensure the accurate reporting of the nature of the service provided[,] . . . the fees, charges, . . . and where applicable, the identity of the provider, the findings, and the diagnosis.

Standard 6.06 directs Heather to ensure accurate reporting to the insurance company. Specifically Standard 6.06 tells Heather to "take reasonable steps" to ensure accuracy. Since billing is not under Heather's control, what would be considered "reasonable steps" for Heather to take in this situation?

Standard 1.03: Conflicts Between Ethics and Organizational Demands

> If the demands of an organization . . . for whom they are working conflict with this Ethics Code, psychologists clarify the nature of the conflict, make known their commitment to the Ethics Code, and to the extent feasible, resolve the conflict in a way that permits adherence to the Ethics Code.

Dr. Mills's office is considered the organization in Standard 1.03 that is implicitly demanding that Heather bill for all of her services, massage and psychological assessments. In accordance with Standard 6.04, Heather should not bill for assessments under her massage therapy license. As Dr. Mills' office submitted the bill and Dr. Mills is Heather's employer, Heather is caught between Standard 6.04 and the implicit demand of Dr. Mills's office. Standard 1.03 directs Heather to talk to whoever made the decision to submit the insurance bill, whether it is Dr. Mills, the billing clerk, or the office manager, in order to make known that such misleading and fraudulent billing to the insurance companies should not occur. Standard 1.03 does not direct Heather to necessarily take further action but simply to resolve the conflict to whatever extent feasible.

Legal Issues 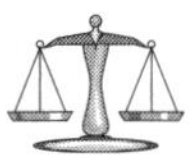

West Virginia

> *W. Va. Code R. § 17-3-6 (2010). Professional ethics.*
>
> The Board hereby adopts the Ethical Principles of Psychologists and Code of Conduct of the American Psychological Association . . . , and all provisions of this Code of Ethics have the same effect as if they were specifically promulgated rules of the Board.

Alaska

> *Alaska Stat. § 08.86.170 (2008). Use of title.*
>
> (a) Unless licensed under this chapter, a person may not use . . . a . . . device indicating or tending to indicate that the person is a psychologist or practices psychology.
>
> *Alaska Admin. Code tit. 12, § 60.185 (2010). Ethics and standards.*
>
> (a) The ethics to be adhered to by . . . licensed psychological associates are the Ethical Principles of Psychologists and Code of Conduct (June 2003), of the American Psychological Association, Inc. Ethical Principles of Psychologists and Code of Conduct is incorporated by reference in this section.
>
> *Alaska Admin. Code tit. 12, § 60.190 (2010). Misrepresentation.*
>
> A licensed . . . psychological associate may not misrepresent or permit the misrepresentation of the licensee's professional . . . products or services with which the licensee is associated.

In both jurisdictions, the psychological testing should not occur without competent supervision being provided to the doctoral student. Nor should the service be charged under another license where the scope of practice does not include psychological testing.

Cultural Considerations

Global Discussion

Singapore Psychological Society: Code of Professional Ethics

> Principle 4. Misrepresentation.
>
> The psychologist avoids misrepresentation of professional qualifications . . . and those of the . . . organizations with which the psychologist is associated.

1. A psychologist does not claim . . . professional qualifications that differ from actual qualifications. . . Psychologists are responsible for correcting others who misrepresent their professional qualifications or affiliations.

Heather is claiming "... by implication professional qualifications that differ from actual qualifications," because she has been performing psychological assessments under a massage therapy license, and they are being billed to the insurance company as such. Heather is obligated to correct Dr. Mills, the naturopathic physician; the clinic office manager who performed the billing; and the insurance companies themselves. Further, it would seem that Heather must also correct the misleading impression that her massage therapy license somehow qualifies her to perform psychological assessments with her patients.

American Moral Values

1. Can Heather justify billing a patient for a non-massage assessment? Should she permit the clinic to correct the billing this time and then redefine her assessments with the clinic going forward? Should they be presented to clients as part of Heather's training, implying that they might not be qualified assessments? Or should they just be presented as unbilled services that help with the overall treatment of the patient by the whole clinic? In other words, does making the assessments free remove the moral obligation to warn clients of Heather's status as trainee?
2. If Heather sees the billing as wrong, should she reassess her relationship with the clinic? Was this a one-time mistake, or should she be wary about how the clinic operates? Has Heather explained exactly how the assessments will serve to build experience hours and who should supervise her experience hours, or is the clinic just interested in her ability to identify eating disorders?
3. As a psychologist-in-training, should Heather seek supervision by a psychologist qualified to perform these kinds of assessments? How does practicing at the clinic help her if she does not have that source of instruction? Is she putting clients at risk by practicing without in-house supervision or any qualified supervision?
4. What value does Heather attach to spotting symptoms of eating disorders? Has this been neglected by mainstream medicine? If so, is it important enough to risk inaccuracies in order to help the clinic treat clients whose problem would otherwise go unnoticed? Would quitting the clinic damage how effective they could be in treating women with such eating disorders?

Ethical Course of Action

Directive per APA Code

Standard 5.01 (c) directs Heather to be appropriately credentialed for the health services provided. This means Heather should hold a psychology license in order to provide and to bill for psychological assessment, unless appropriately supervised (Standard 9.07). Standard 5.01 (c) combined with the directives of Standard 9.07 dictate that Heather's assessment for eating disorders should not be billed to insurance companies under her massage therapy license. Nor would it be ethical for the services to be provided without charge. To be in compliance with Standard 9.07, the services still must be supervised by a competent psychologist. Also, standard 1.03 demands that Heather make known to Dr. Mills's office personnel the problems associated with billing for assessments under her massage therapy license.

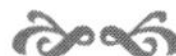

Dictates of One's Own Conscience

Violations of 5.01 (c) and 9.07 compel Heather to acknowledge the inappropriateness of the billing practice for her assessments. After making your objections known, per Standard 1.03, if you were Heather, what might you do?

1. Tell Dr. Mills that on second thought you really cannot perform clinical assessments, and to ask him to stop giving you referrals.
2. Tell the office manager to call the insurance company to obtain instructions about how to bill for the assessments under someone else's scope of practice.
3. Tell Dr. Mills that since the assessments were done under his supervision, the insurance claims need to go under his license instead of your massage therapy license.
4. Tell Dr. Mills that if the office wants to charge insurance companies for psychological assessment, they need to purchase supervision for you so that insurance can be charged under your psychology supervisor's name if in fact such a charge is permitted under the various insurance policies of the clinic's clients.
5. Contact the insurance company to redact the charge.

6. Obtain your own supervision from your professional psychology program to continue administering and interpreting assessments or hire an independent competent supervisor.
7. Do a combination of the previously listed actions.
8. Do something that is not previously listed.

If you were Heather, working in Singapore, which would you do?

1. Immediately have a conversation with Dr. Mills, the office manager, and the insurance companies about the problems and violations stemming from billing for psychological evaluations under a massage therapy license.
2. Ask Dr. Mills to stop giving you referrals until you have supervision from a licensed psychologist.

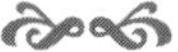

STANDARD 5.02: STATEMENTS BY OTHERS

(a) Psychologists who engage others to create or place public statements that promote their professional practice, products, or activities retain professional responsibility for such statements.

A CASE FOR STANDARD 5.02 (A): A PROFESSORSHIP

Dr. Nichols is a newly licensed psychologist opening her first private practice office. As part of the marketing work, Dr. Nichols has hired a web designer to create an electronic presence for herself. Douglas, the web designer, comes highly recommended as someone who is knowledgeable about health practices. Dr. Nichols gave Douglas her curriculum vitae and some digital pictures of herself, with the instruction to design something that best highlights her expertise and downplays the newness of her licensure. She is pleased with the mock-up but a little uneasy that the design prominently shows her "professor" status. The "professor" title refers to her having taught one course as an adjunct instructor in her final year of graduate school. Douglas said that the information on the webpage is accurate and is best designed to attract the kind of clients Dr. Nichols wants in her practice.

Issues of Concern

Standard 5.02 (a) states that Dr. Nichols retains responsibility for public statements, regardless of who designs the webpage. Douglas has expertise in the area of marketing and web design. Dr. Nichols pays for and wants value from the advice of the expert. However, the reference to her teaching appears inaccurate. Is the claim of academic experience after teaching only one class deceptive and misleading? Standard 5.02 (a) does not absolve Dr. Nichols of responsibility for contents of the webpage. Dr. Nichols needs to come to terms with her uneasiness.

APA Ethics Code

Companion General Principle

Principle C: Integrity

> Psychologists seek to promote accuracy, honesty, and truthfulness in the . . . practice of psychology. In these activities psychologists do not . . . engage in . . . intentional misrepresentation of fact.

Dr. Nichols's "uneasiness" about the inclusion of the title of "professor" on the website gives reference to a conflict with Principle C: Integrity.

Companion Ethical Standard(s)

Standard 5.01: Avoidance of False or Deceptive Statements

> Psychologists do not knowingly make public statements that are . . . deceptive . . . concerning their . . . work activities . . .

If the webpage is published with the reference to her "professor" status, Dr. Nichols would be in violation of Standard 5.01 because she would be "knowingly" making public statements that are deceptive.

Legal Issues 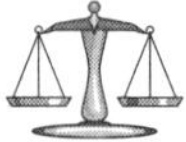

California

> *Cal. Bus. & Prof. Code § 17500 (West 2003). False or misleading statements; penalty.*
>
> It is unlawful for any person . . . to . . . cause to be made or disseminated . . . in any . . . advertising device, . . . including over the Internet, any statement, . . . concerning any circumstance or matter of fact . . . , which is . . . misleading, and which is known . . . to be . . . misleading. . . . Any violation of the provisions of this section is a misdemeanor . . .

Wisconsin

> *Wis. Stat. Ann. § 455.08 (West 2006). Code of Ethics.*
>
> The examining board shall adopt such rules as are necessary under this chapter and shall, by rule, establish a reasonable code of ethics governing the professional conduct of psychologists, using as its model the "Ethical Standards of Psychologists" established by the American Psychological Association.

In both jurisdictions, making or knowing that false statements or misrepresentations had been made about the psychologist's background would be unethical. The differences between instructor and professor within the field are considerable, and to allow the misleading characterization to be published would be actionable.

Cultural Considerations

Global Discussion

Singapore Psychological Society:
Code of Professional Ethics

> Principle 5: Public statements.
>
> Psychologists who supply information to the public . . . are expected to show due regard for the limits of present knowledge and exercise modesty and scientific caution in all such statements.

Dr. Nichols has not shown "due regard for the limits of present knowledge," namely, that claiming professorship status after teaching only one course is deceptive and misleading. The dictate to "exercise modesty" is violated by overstating or inflating her credentials on her webpage, even if she did not design it herself.

American Moral Values

1. How does Dr. Nichols view her relationship with Douglas? Can she defer to his standards of accuracy as the hired advertiser for her services? Is he fulfilling his stated mission of attracting the kind of clients she wants? Should she consider whether other service providers are advertising themselves along the same lines as Douglas is proposing? Is she violating an unspoken protocol among therapists who advertise? Or is Douglas's way just "how it's done"?
2. What exactly is Dr. Nichols's reservation about the term *professor*? What does her feeling of uneasiness represent as a moral objection? Does she feel it is a misrepresentation of her teaching position, misleading clients about her status as a psychologist? How much of her objection is embarrassment over being called "professor," a hesitancy to assume the aura of authority accorded to that term?
3. If the professor designation is technically accurate, how does Dr. Nichols view its practical effect on prospective clients? Is it not reasonable to assume they will put more stock in her experience and expertise, without necessarily digging into her resume to find out what made her a "professor"? What would she say to clients who cite that title as part of the reason they chose her? Does she consider those clients illegitimately recruited, or does she feel like her subsequent work with clients will vindicate that stretching of the truth?

Ethical Course of Action

Directive per APA Code

Aspiring to the highest value of integrity, Dr. Nichols would make no public statements that are not accurate without being misleading. Standard 5.02 (a), in combination with Standard 5.01 directs Dr. Nichols not to publish references to her "professor" claim.

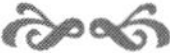

Dictates of One's Own Conscience

If you were Dr. Nichols, probably overwhelmed with graduate school debt, spending money on expert advice on starting a private practice, what would you do?

1. Pay Douglas only when the webpage is published.
2. Ask Douglas to go back to the drawing board and come up with another design that does not show the "professor" status so prominently on the webpage.
3. Change the academic status from "professor" to "instructor," and go with the rest of the design.
4. Thank Douglas for his mock-up and say that you have decided not to use his services.
5. Explain to Douglas the ethical violation of claiming the title of "professor," and ask that he design something that is within the ethical limits of psychologists.
6. Do a combination of the previously listed actions.
7. Do something that is not previously listed.

If you were Dr. Nichols, opening a practice in Singapore, your options would be similar as to the ones previously listed, as both Singapore's and the U.S. codes of ethics are similar on this point.

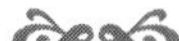

STANDARD 5.02: STATEMENTS BY OTHERS

> . . . (b) Psychologists do not compensate employees of press, radio, television, or other communication media in return for publicity in a news item.

A CASE FOR STANDARD 5.02 (B): The Business Lunch

Dr. Grant is a forensic psychologist who specializes in determining competency to stand trial. An old high school buddy, Carl, who is a reporter for the local newspaper, contacted Dr. Grant. Carl is writing a news article on the death penalty and doing research on the use of psychological evaluations in the sentencing phase of the court proceedings. Carl wanted to know if Dr. Grant was willing to talk to him about this topic. Dr. Grant said, "I'm on my way to try out that new golf course in town. You can come as my guest, and I'll pay for 18 holes of golf. I'll talk to you about psych evaluations only if you are going to use my information positively and give me proper credit. But I am not going to take the time to do this interview if you cannot guarantee that you'll use the information or properly credit me for this information. If you can't guarantee me that, we can still play a round and just talk about our old times in high school."

Issues of Concern

Standard 5.02 (b) prohibits psychologists from paying reporters for publicity. Does Dr. Grant's offer to pay for a round of golf if the reporter will give him press coverage violate the directive of Standard 5.02 (b)?

APA Ethics Code

Companion General Principle

Principle B: Fidelity and Responsibility

> Psychologists . . . cooperate with other professionals . . . to the extent needed to serve the best interests of those with whom they work. . .

Principle B guides Dr. Grant to cooperate with Carl in order to serve the best interests of his client. It is certainly of benefit to the public and society in general to be accurately informed of the beneficial use of psychological assessments. Aspiring to act responsibly on behalf of his clients, Dr. Grant would be guided to give Carl an interview.

Principle A: Beneficience and Nonmaleficence

> Because psychologists' . . . judgments and actions may affect the lives of others, they are alert to and guard against personal, financial . . . factors that might lead to misuse of their influence.

In the aspiration to the principle of beneficence, the psychologist guards against actions that are self-serving. Offering to pay for a round of golf does not seem on the surface, at least, related to talking about business in exchange for press coverage. Dr. Grant's offer does not seem to be primarily driven by wanting to increase publicity for his practice.

Companion Ethical Standard(s)

Standard 3.09: Cooperation With Other Professionals

> When indicated and professionally appropriate, psychologists cooperate with other professionals in order to serve their clients/patients effectively and appropriately.

The reporter did the solicitation for the interview. As the recipient of a request from another professional, in this case a reporter, Standard 3.09 directs Dr. Grant to cooperate with Carl "in order to serve his clients effectively and appropriately." Does giving an interview to a reporter on the general topic of psychological evaluations "serve his clients effectively and appropriately"?

Standard 3.05: Multiple Relationships

> (a) A multiple relationship occurs when a psychologist is in a professional role with a person and . . . (1) at the same time is in another role with the same person. . . . A psychologist refrains from entering into a multiple relationship if the multiple relationship could reasonably be expected to impair the psychologist's objectivity . . . in performing his or her functions as a psychologist. . . . Multiple relationships that would not reasonably be expected to cause impairment . . . are not unethical.

Dr. Grant and Carl were high school friends. With the interview, Dr. Grant now enters into a professional relationship with Carl. Per Standard 3.05 (a), a situation of multiple relationships now exists. The cautionary note in Standard 3.05 is for Dr. Grant to avoid such a situation if it could impair his objectivity. Could the prospect of press coverage with his name attached be expected to influence, and possibly impair his objectivity? Might Dr. Grant be unduly influenced to tell Carl what Carl wants to hear in order for Dr. Grant to receive positive press coverage?

Legal Issues 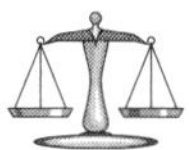

Hawaii

Haw. Code R. § 16-98-34 (2010). Unethical practice of psychology.

. . . (f) (3) The psychologist shall not enter into a professional relationship with . . . intimate friends . . . whose welfare might be jeopardized by such a dual relationship.

. . . (h) The psychologist shall act with integrity in regards to colleagues . . . in other professions.

(i) Financial arrangements in professional practice shall be in accord with professional standards that safeguard the best interest of the . . . profession.

Illinois

225 Ill. Comp. Stat. Ann. 15/15 (West 2007).

. . . (7) Unethical, unauthorized or unprofessional conduct as defined by rule. In establishing those rules, the Department shall consider . . . the ethical standards for psychologists promulgated by recognized national psychology associations.

Ill. Admin. Code tit. 68, § 1400.80 (2010). Unethical, unauthorized, or unprofessional conduct.

The Department may suspend or revoke a license, refuse to issue or renew a license or take other disciplinary action, based upon its finding of "unethical, unauthorized, or unprofessional conduct" . . . to include, but is not limited to, the following acts or practices:

. . . f) Directly or indirectly giving to . . . any person . . . any . . . form of compensation for any professional services not actually rendered.

It appears that in both jurisdictions even the *de minimus* "form of compensation" of a round of golf at a private golf course probably would be viewed as an unethical act. The context becomes even more plagued as a preexisting friendship exists between the psychologist and the reporter. It is likely that the preexisting personal relationship may affect the integrity of the professional relationship.

Cultural Considerations

Global Discussion

Singapore Psychological Society:
Code of Professional Ethics

Principle 5: Public statements.

3. A psychologist who engages in radio or television activities does not participate in commercial announcements recommending purchase or use of a product.

Singapore's code is one of the only ones that discuss the limitations placed on psychologists who do either radio or television "activities." Singapore's code is silent on whether it would be problematic to compensate other media professionals for free publicity. Therefore, as long as Dr. Grant does not attempt to sell a particular product on the radio or television, he is adhering to Singapore's code.

American Moral Values

1. What does this exchange mean for the relationship between Carl and Dr. Grant? Has Dr. Grant placed obtaining business above professional integrity? Could he have asked Carl to mention his practice as a matter of policy (such as a professor's university being mentioned)? Does the offer of a golf round for publicity suggest that Dr. Grant has no such policy, that instead this is an informal bargain?
2. How will Carl work with Dr. Grant going forward? Will Carl limit his psychologist consultations to Dr. Grant in order to receive more free rounds of golf? Will Carl adjust his reporting to make Dr. Grant look good, especially in cases where Dr. Grant testifies? Could this have repercussions for defendants who may or may not be fit for trial?
3. How will Dr. Grant regard Carl's work in the future? Will Dr. Grant consider Carl's need for a story before giving his opinion?
4. What will other golf club members think about their relationship if they see them playing together? Does golf, when played by two professionals or "successful" men, have cultural validity—that is, no necessary associations of a quid pro quo? Would it be different if Dr. Grant were a woman?

Ethical Course of Action

Directive per APA Code

Standard 5.02 (b) clearly directs Dr. Grant not to engage in "compensation" that may affect the integrity of a professional relationship. By offering to pay for a round of golf and giving Carl an interview in exchange for a guarantee of positive press coverage, Dr. Grant violates Standard 5.02 (b).

Dictates of One's Own Conscience

If you were Dr. Grant, approached by a high school buddy on your way to a relaxing afternoon before a game of golf, and you wish to do a good turn for your old high school buddy, what would you do?

1. Tell Carl that you would like to become reacquainted, and he could join you in a round of golf but no interview will be given.
2. Tell Carl he should schedule the interview with another forensic psychologist who does not have a preexisting friendship.
3. Tell Carl to schedule the interview during your normal workday and proceed with your golf game.
4. Tell Carl he can come along for the golf game and some conversation but that Carl would have to pay his own way.
5. Tell Carl that you will talk to him if you can trust an old high school buddy to report accurately what you say, regardless of whether information is attributed to you or not.
6. Tell Carl that you don't give interviews because of potential for misquotes, but you could direct him to some published research on the topic.
7. Do a combination of the previously listed actions.
8. Do something that is not previously listed.

If you were Dr. Grant and this situation occurred in Singapore, which would you do?

1. Readily agree to a round of golf with your old friend, and pay his way, hoping for positive publicity from him in return, reasoning that these are the ways in which business is done and information traded.
2. Readily agree to a round of golf with your old friend, and pay his way, reasoning that publicity and positive press for psychology benefits other psychologists and potential clients.

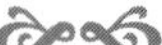

STANDARD 5.02: STATEMENTS BY OTHERS

> . . . (c) A paid advertisement relating to psychologists' activities must be identified or clearly recognizable as such.

A CASE FOR STANDARD 5.02 (C): Top of the Heap

Dr. Knight has recently purchased a condominium inside the city. With all her children out of the house, Dr. Knight was planning to sell her suburban home and move both her professional and private life to the city. She has subleased a private practice office close to her condo. Dr. Knight is contacted by the town newspaper, who is selling ads for their annual edition of "Top Doctors in Town." This year, the publication is adding a new section for psychologists, and they wished to know if Dr. Knight would like to be listed. In addition to simply being listed, the paper would like to know whether Dr. Knight is interested in purchasing a larger ad space. Dr. Knight decided to purchase an ad for this issue, with copy that reads: "You'll find Top Docs at our clinic!" with a prominent picture of herself attached. In small print at the bottom is a statement to the fact that this is an advertisement paid for by Dr. Knight. Dr. Knight asked that her ad be placed on the page opposite from a listing of top psychologists of the year named by the state psychological association.

Issues of Concern

Standard 5.02 (c) directs Dr. Knight to design and affirm that her advertisement is paid for by her. Even if the advertisement made a statement that it is paid for by Dr. Knight, does the positioning of the ad violate the spirit of Standard 5.02 (c)?

APA Ethics Code

Companion General Principle

Principle C: Integrity

> Psychologists seek to promote accuracy . . . in . . . psychology. In these activities psychologists do not . . . engage in . . . intentional misrepresentation of fact.

Standard C guides Dr. Knight to be accurate. Has Dr. Knight intentionally misrepresented herself with her request for positioning of the advertisement?

Companion Ethical Standard(s)

Standard 5.01: Avoidance of False or Deceptive Statements

> (a) . . . Psychologists do not knowingly make public statements that are . . . deceptive . . . concerning their . . . practice. . .

Standard 5.01 is the operationalization of Principle C: Integrity. Assuming that Dr. Knight is accurate with the contents of her ad, the request for the positioning of her ad seems to be intentionally deceptive and self-serving.

Legal Issues 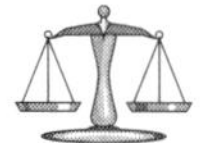

Indiana

> *868 Ind. Admin. Code 1.1-11-1 (2010). Relationship with the public.*
>
> . . . (d) Advertisements for professional services and other public statements:
>
> (1) must not contain . . . misleading, or deceptive information;
>
> (2) must not misinterpret . . . statements; and
>
> (3) must fully disclose all relevant information.
>
> . . . (g) A psychologist may not suggest or imply sponsorship of . . . his or her activities by professional associations or organizational affiliations.

Kentucky

> *201 Ky. Admin. Regs. 26:145 (2010). Code of conduct.*
>
> . . . Section 8. Representation of Services.
>
> . . . (3) Misrepresentation of affiliations. The credential holder shall not misrepresent directly or by implication his or her affiliations, or the . . . characteristics of institutions and organizations with which the credential holder is associated.
>
> (4) False or misleading information. The credential holder shall not include . . . misleading information in a public statement concerning professional services offered.

In both jurisdictions, the psychologist probably would be viewed as violating the laws by strategically placing her ad adjacent to the listings of top psychologists of the year named by the state psychological association. Such a placement is misleading even though it is identified as an advertisement. The psychologist's behavior was intended to be misleading: the labeling of the ad as paid was small; and the printing of the ad occurred on the day of, and adjacent to, the listing of top psychologists of the year named by the state psychological association.

Cultural Considerations

Global Discussion

The Professional Board for Psychology Health Professions Council of South Africa:
Ethical Code of Professional Conduct (April 2002)

> 8.2. Statements by others.
>
> 8.2.1. A paid advertisement relating to psychologists' activities must be identified or clearly recognisable as such, unless it is already apparent from the context of the advertisement.

If the annual "Top Doctors in Town" supplement can be commonly understood to be an advertisement or should be understood from context to be an advertisement, Dr. Knight would not be in violation of South Africa's code, particularly if she undergoes the additional step of noting the paid advertisement somewhere on her text. South Africa's Code does not describe how clearly or prominently a psychologist must make clear the nature of the advertisement.

American Moral Values

1. Is Dr. Knight misleading prospective clients with her ad? How does Dr. Knight judge an ad to be misleading? Does she believe it is the audience's responsibility to read ads carefully? Does technical accuracy fulfill her moral duties as a service provider placing an ad?
2. Why does Dr. Knight ask to put her ad where she does? Does she believe a listing of top psychologists who are endorsed by the state psychological association is where readers would naturally look to find psychological services? Or is she capitalizing on her position opposite that listing to make a subconscious visual linkage? Is that beneath an advertiser, or is that how the rules of advertising go? Should a psychologist play by those rules, or is a higher standard for aiding patient decision making expected of such a professional?
3. The use of "Top Docs" seems to be a near quote of "Top Doctors in Town" opposite Dr. Knight's ad. Should Dr. Knight have concluded that readers will

assume some of those top doctors will be in her clinic? Does that cross the line of false advertising?

4. What does Dr. Knight think about the state psychological association? Does she believe that their rankings are arbitrary and that her top docs are at least as good as the psychologists listed? Or is she just making a claim to drum up business because such an endorsement by the state psychological association is a great honor?

Ethical Course of Action

Directive per APA Code

Standard 5.02 (c) directs Dr. Knight to identify her ad as a paid advertisement. Most likely, Dr. Knight's ad does identify itself as a paid advertisement. However, her request for the positioning of the ad appears to be intentionally deceptive and is thus in violation of Standard 5.01 (a).

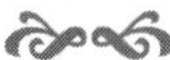

Dictates of One's Own Conscience

If you were Dr. Knight, wanting to obtain the most out of a very expensive advertisement, what would you do to ensure good visibility?

1. Call the newspaper back to say that you changed your mind about where the ad is to be placed and that you now have no specific request, so they can place the ad anywhere they think it best suits the publication.
2. Change the language of the ad so that it does not mirror the title of the special issue.
3. Decide not to take out an ad but spend your marketing funds for more personal contacts like lunches with referral sources.
4. Decide not to take out an ad, and spend the funds on printing brochures and business cards.
5. Do a combination of the previously listed actions.
6. Do something that is not previously listed.

If you were Dr. Knight, practicing in South Africa, you could keep the ad as it currently is, with the same placement, ensuring that the disclaimer of "paid advertisement" appears clearly on the ad itself.

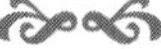

STANDARD 5.03: DESCRIPTIONS OF WORKSHOPS AND NON-DEGREE-GRANTING EDUCATIONAL PROGRAMS

To the degree to which they exercise control, psychologists responsible for announcements, catalogs, brochures, or advertisements describing workshops, seminars, or other non-degree-granting educational programs ensure that they accurately describe the audience for which the program is intended, the educational objectives, the presenters, and the fees involved.

A CASE FOR STANDARD 5.03: The Renowned Expert

Dr. Ferguson's office is located in a medical professional building located next to the local hospital. The hospital is opening a new women's health clinic. Gloria, the director of the women's health clinic, contacted the practicing health-related professionals in the building to invite doctors to conduct workshops at the clinic as part of a series of activities to celebrate the clinic's opening. The clinic would provide the site and pay for all advertisements; in trade, the doctors would obtain exposure. Gloria was persuasive in her argument that the doctor's time would be amply repaid with a significant increase of clients, usually self-referrals, who come in after attending such workshops. Dr. Ferguson signed up for an early November workshop time slot to provide a 1.5-hour workshop called "Depression and the Holidays." When the program brochure was published, Dr. Ferguson's workshop is billed as "Depression Busters—Guaranteed Ways to Ward Off Holiday Depression" with nationally renowned expert Dr. Ferguson. The women's health clinic is charging participants a fee of $25 for the workshop.

Issues of Concern

Ideally, organizations that publish flyers to advertise their events check with presenters before publication to ensure accuracy. However, many organizations do not double-check with their presenters. Standard 5.03 directs psychologists to ensure accuracy "to the degree to which they exercise control" regarding four items. The four items are (1) intended audience, (2) objective of the workshop, (3) presenters, and (4) fees. The brochure does meet Standard 5.03's directives. The brochure does state the fee of $25, does describe the presenter as Dr. Ferguson, does state the objective as warding off holiday season depression, and does implicitly describe the intended audience as those who are interested in avoiding holiday depression. Dr. Ferguson is not remiss in her participation with the workshop series. Nor has Dr. Ferguson been remiss or in violation of Standard 5.03 for her part in the oversight of the advertisement for the workshops because she did not have control over the advertisement nor the workshop fees.

At the same time, participants will be paying money to have Dr. Ferguson tell them how to avoid depression over the holidays. Is it misleading for Dr. Ferguson to participate in something that describes her as a nationally renowned expert and guarantees prevention of depression? Is it false to make such a claim if Dr. Ferguson is not nationally known in this specialty area and no research has demonstrated a guaranteed prevention for seasonal depression? Even if Dr. Ferguson was nationally renowned, is her area of expertise in seasonal depression?

APA Ethics Code

Companion General Principle

Principle C: Integrity

> Psychologists seek to promote accuracy, honesty, and truthfulness in the . . . practice of psychology. In these activities psychologists do not . . . engage in . . . intentional misrepresentation of fact.

The advertisement that claims Dr. Ferguson as nationally renowned and guarantees prevention of seasonal depression misrepresents the facts. Though Dr. Ferguson is not the person who made the claim, her silence regarding these claims violates the intent of Principle C: Integrity.

Principle B: Fidelity and Responsibility

> Psychologists uphold professional standards of conduct, clarify their . . . obligations . . . and seek to manage conflicts of interest that could lead to exploitation or harm. Psychologists consult with . . . or cooperate with other . . . institutions to the extent needed to serve the best interests of those with whom they work.

Principle B guides Dr. Ferguson to clarify her obligation to the workshop participants, cooperate with the women's health clinic, and seek to manage the ensuing conflicts over wording of the brochure.

Companion Ethical Standard(s)

Standard 2.01: Boundaries of Competence

> (a) Psychologists provide services . . . with populations and in areas only within the boundaries of their competence.

One could safely presume that Dr. Ferguson is competent to present a workshop about depression and the holiday season based on her having voluntarily signed up for the topic.

Standard 5.01: Avoidance of False or Deceptive Statements

> . . . (b) Psychologists do not make false . . . statements concerning (1) their . . . experience . . . or competence . . . [,] (6) the scientific or clinical basis for, or results or degree of success of, their services . . .

If Dr. Ferguson is not a nationally renowned expert in seasonal depression, then the brochure has violated Standard 5.01 (b) (1) by claiming to guarantee that a 1.5-hour workshop will ward off holiday depression, which is deceptive at best and fraudulent at worst.

Standard 2.04: Bases for Scientific and Professional Judgments

> Psychologists' work is based upon established scientific and professional knowledge of the discipline. . .

There is no "established scientific and professional knowledge" that can guarantee a person will not experience depression, thus the claim of the brochure that guarantees avoidance of depression violates Standard 2.04.

Standard 1.01: Misuse of Psychologists' Work.

> If psychologists learn of . . . misrepresentation of their work, they take reasonable steps to correct or minimize the . . . misrepresentation.

Standard 1.01 directs Dr. Ferguson to take responsibility for correcting the misinformation and exaggerated claims of the brochure.

Legal Issues 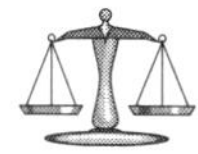

Kansas

> *Kan. Admin. Regs. § 102-1-10a (2010). Unprofessional conduct.*

. . . (h) misrepresenting the services offered or provided, which shall include the following acts:

. . . (2) making claims of professional superiority that cannot be substantiated;

(3) guaranteeing that satisfaction or a cure will result from the performance of professional services;

(4) knowingly engaging in . . . misleading advertising . . .

Maryland

Md. Code Ann., Health Occ. § 18-313 (2010). Denials, reprimands, suspensions, and revocations—grounds.

. . . (20) Does an act that is inconsistent with generally accepted professional standards in the practice of psychology.

Md. Code Regs. 10.36.05.05 (2010). Representation of services and fees.

(A)(2) A psychologist may not:

. . . (c) Make public statements that contain:

(i) False, fraudulent, misleading, or deceptive statements;

(ii) Partial disclosures of relevant facts that misrepresent, mislead, or deceive; or

(iii) Statements that create false or unjustified expectations of favorable results . . .

In both jurisdictions, Dr. Ferguson would likely be viewed as acting unethically unless she corrected the misrepresentations in the brochure about the guarantee to ward off holiday season depression and that she is nationally renowned. Neither jurisdiction's law provides specific direction about how to correct the misleading information.

Cultural Considerations

Global Discussion

The Professional Board for Psychology Health Professions Council of South Africa:
Ethical Code of Professional Conduct (April 2002)

8.4. Description of workshops and educational programmes.

Psychologists associated with . . . flyers . . . describing workshops . . . shall ensure that they accurately describe the audience for which the programme is intended, the educational objectives, the presenters, the fees involved, and the restrictions on practice, and shall not create any expectation that such activities will lead to registration or licensing.

Dr. Ferguson has allowed misleading information regarding the educational objectives, the presenter (herself), and the restrictions on practice. Dr. Ferguson has violated 8.4 by not ensuring the flyer had accurately described these elements.

American Moral Values

1. If Dr. Ferguson is not in fact a "nationally known expert," is she responsible for correcting a misleading ad? Could participants pay to attend based on that description?
2. Is the use of "guaranteed" to describe Dr. Ferguson's approaches promising too much? Is this usage a less informal, everyday way of saying the approaches work (e.g., tools, cleaning supplies)? Should that usage apply to therapy, or does therapy, as a form of health care, demand a higher standard for accuracy and fairness?
3. What are Dr. Ferguson's personal and professional commitments to the women's health clinic? Does she believe that the cause of women's health is important enough not to embarrass or undercut it by pulling out of the seminar? Would she not want to cause trouble for its staff by challenging its advertisement? Does she believe the new clinic's clients could benefit by being referred to her? Or is she mostly considering the business her practice could bring in?
4. In light of the participants being charged, in addition to their time loss, should a refund be offered because of the false advertising?
5. How does this promotion relate to Dr. Ferguson's practice? Does Dr. Ferguson believe this type of event is useful, or does this line of advertising lead her to question her involvement in it? Does she have a duty to the hospital to make sure they know what is being done in their name through this promotion?
6. How will Dr. Ferguson's actions affect larger relationships between health providers and the community? Will this promotion threaten perceptions about psychologists in general? Will readers decide not to attend based on what they feel is an overhyped ad?
7. Considering what has been implicitly promised, should Dr. Ferguson offer a different seminar altogether, one that will have no promises attached to it?

Ethical Course of Action

Directive per APA Code

Dr. Ferguson has not violated the directives of Standard 5.03. The brochure published by the women's health clinic did cover all of the necessary elements enumerated in Standard 5.03. However, the brochure's claim about Dr. Ferguson's credentials and reputation is probably misleading at best and does violate Standard 5.01 (b). The brochure's claim about the promised effects of the workshop violates Standard 2.04. Standard 1.01 directs Dr. Ferguson to take reasonable steps to correct the misrepresentation.

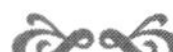

Dictates of One's Own Conscience

Unlike the vignette described under Standard 1.01, there is a presumption that there are no cross-cultural complications. If you were Dr. Ferguson, being concerned about the misleading statements in the brochure, what would you do? And what moral principle guides you to choose your course of action?

1. Let Gloria know your concerns.
2. Tell Gloria that although you would like to donate your time by running a workshop for the women's health clinic, you would not be able to do so until more accurate information was provided to the public.
3. Inform participants that corrective information could not be provided in a timely manner and then on the day of the workshop return the participant's fees with a statement that you could not guarantee they will not experience holiday depression.
4. Even if corrective information could be provided, reiterate your credentials and state you cannot guarantee remission or cure of depression.
5. Tell the workshop participants that based on the misleading information provided you are offering a refund of their fees. However, because you do not receive any money and their fees go to support the nonprofit women's health clinic, you ask that they voluntarily donate their workshop fees to the nonprofit organization as a tax write-off.
6. Make it a practice to negotiate prior approval of advertising information before it is published or made public with any organization.
7. Do a combination of the previously listed actions.
8. Do something that is not previously listed.

If you were Dr. Ferguson and this situation occurred in South Africa, which would you do?

1. Speak to Gloria about the inaccuracies of the workshop's claims, and ask her to release an addendum to the workshop advertisements.
2. Contact each participant for your upcoming workshop, and give them clear information about depression, treatment for depression, as well as your own experience and credentials.

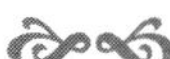

STANDARD 5.04: MEDIA PRESENTATIONS

When psychologists provide public advice or comment via print, internet, or other electronic transmission, they take precautions to ensure that statements (1) are based on their professional knowledge, training, or experience in accord with appropriate psychological literature and practice; (2) are otherwise consistent with this Ethics Code; and (3) do not indicate that a professional relationship has been established with the recipient.

A CASE FOR STANDARD 5.04: DEAR DR. STONE

Dr. Stone is writing a psychology advice column in her small town newspaper. Cheryl sent an e-mail request for advice about her weight problem. Cheryl gave a long history of her struggles with food. She wants to avoid gaining weight over the holidays. She read somewhere that a good way to enjoy the holidays and not gain weight is to eat small portions of food and spit them out. Dr. Stone's response in the newspaper advice column is that to eat and spit is an eating disorder that requires professional treatment. As it happens, Dr. Stone is the only psychologist in town who treats eating disorders.

Issues of Concern

Standard 5.04 applies in that Dr. Stone is doing an advice column in print media. It appears that she is careful to follow the directive enumerated in Standard 5.04. Her advice is based on professional knowledge and experience (5.04 (1)) since she is competent to treat eating disorder problems. The advice for Cheryl to seek professional treatment seems to be benign on the surface. However, if this advice is viewed in conjunction with Standard 5.06: In-Person Solicitation, could a reader in this small community infer that Dr. Stone is using her advice column to solicit clients, especially if it is generally known she is the only psychologist in the area who treats eating disorders? In addition, when Cheryl discovers that Dr. Stone is the only professional in town who would be competent to treat her problem, might Cheryl consider Dr. Stone's advice as a solicitation? Conversely, might Cheryl think a professional relationship has already been established between Dr. Stone and herself because of the extensive history of the eating disorder Cheryl has already told to Dr. Stone in her e-mail? At what point has a professional relationship been established?

APA Ethics Code

Companion General Principle

Principle B: Fidelity and Responsibility

> Psychologists establish relationships of trust with those with whom they work. They are aware of their professional and scientific responsibilities to society and to the specific communities in which they work...

Publication of a psychology advice column in a small town may be tantamount to taking on the responsibility of primary intervention for the mental health of the whole community. The relationship she is seeking to establish is one of trust with the townspeople who are the readers of the town newspaper. If the community concludes that Dr. Stone's advice column is somehow self-serving by soliciting patients for her practice, might she have broken trust with the community? Might this specific response to Cheryl accordingly be viewed as solicitation?

Companion Ethical Standard(s)

Standard 5.06: In-Person Solicitation

> Psychologists do not engage . . . in uninvited in-person solicitation of business from . . . potential therapy clients... However, this prohibition does not preclude . . . (2) providing . . . community outreach services.

If Dr. Stone were writing her Dear Dr. Stone column in a large city where there is a multitude of services providers who are competent to treat eating disorders, then any psychologist giving the advice for someone to seek professional treatment would not be construed as self-serving or as an act of solicitation. Given the nature of rural communities with very limited access to treatment with psychologists, such advice could easily be perceived as self-serving and thus be in violation of Standard 5.06. Standard 5.06 (2) provides an exception of community outreach services. Does writing a psychology advice column in a small rural newspaper constitute community outreach service? Would writing the column be seen as less self-serving if Dr. Stone did this as pro-bono work?

Standard 3.10: Informed Consent

> (a) When psychologists conduct . . . consulting services . . . they obtain the informed consent of the individual . . .

An advice column in a newspaper would fall under consulting services. As directed by Standard 3.10 (a), Dr. Stone would need to obtain informed consent from Cheryl. Does the very act of knowing one is writing in to a published advice column constitute informed consent, or does Dr. Stone need to take the extra step of contacting Cheryl for a signed consent form to have parts of Cheryl's email be published in the newspaper?

Standard 4.01: Maintaining Confidentiality

> Psychologists have a primary obligation and take reasonable precautions to protect confidential information obtained through . . . any medium, recognizing that the extent and limits of confidentiality may be . . . established by institutional rules . . .

Dr. Stone cannot protect Cheryl's privacy because of the public nature of an advice column. Is Dr. Stone responsible for keeping confidential all identifying information transmitted by Cheryl in the e-mail? Or is the nature of an advice column such that those who write to Dr. Stone would not expect any confidentiality?

Standard 6.02: Maintenance, Dissemination, and Disposal of Confidential Records of Professional and Scientific Work

> (a) Psychologists maintain confidentiality in creating, storing, accessing, transferring, and disposing of records under their control, whether these are written, automated, or in any other medium.

Dr. Stone is now holding information from Cheryl. Should the e-mail from Cheryl be treated in the same manner or equivalent to confidential treatment records by the newspaper? Should Dr. Stone create a secure file, either electronically or in hard copy, at the newspaper for all the correspondences received by the Dear Dr. Stone advice column?

Standard 3.05: Multiple Relationships

> (a) A multiple relationship occurs when a psychologist is in a professional role with a person and . . .
>
> . . . (3) promises to enter into another relationship in the future with the person. . . A psychologist refrains from entering into a multiple relationship if the multiple relationship could reasonably be expected to impair the psychologist's . . . effectiveness in performing his or her functions as a psychologist. . . Multiple relationships that would not reasonably be expected to cause impairment or risk exploitation . . . are not unethical.

How might the prior interaction between Dr. Stone and Cheryl affect Cheryl if Cheryl decides to seek treatment with Dr. Stone? Does Dr. Stone's advice for Cheryl to seek treatment in the context of a rural setting constitute multiple relationships as defined in Standard 3.05 (a) (3), where Dr. Stone implies a promise to enter into a treatment relationship in the future with Cheryl? Standard 3.05 does not prohibit such multiple relationships if such a relationship would not be expected to cause harm in some way.

Legal Issues 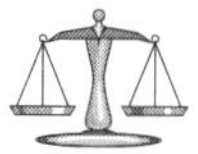

Colorado

> *Colo. Rev. Stat. Ann. § 12-43-222 (West 2010). Prohibited activities—related provisions.*
>
> . . . (j) Has exercised undue influence . . . , including the promotion of the sale of services . . . in such a manner as to exploit the client for the financial gain of the practitioner . . .

Maryland

> *Md. Code Regs. 10.36.05.05 (2010). Representation of services and fees.*
>
> (2) A psychologist may not:
>
> . . . (d) Solicit, either in person or through others, business . . .from clients who are vulnerable to undue influence.

If Dr. Stone were writing this advice column in either rural Maryland or rural Colorado, she would be in violation of the laws of both jurisdictions if her advice column came to be seen as a form of solicitation for her private practice. Cheryl, and other consumers similar to her, may be fearful about her eating habits and vulnerable to suggestions from a local advice column about eating disorders.

Cultural Considerations

Global Discussion

Hong Kong Psychological Society:
Professional Code of Practice

> Chapter 11: Public statements.
>
> 11.2. Public statements include, but are not limited to communication by means of . . . circular. . . Public statements made by Members in announcing or advertising the availability of psychological . . . services, shall not contain:
>
> d. Any statement intended or likely to appeal to a client's fears, anxieties or emotions concerning the possible results of failure to obtain the offered services;
>
> 11.5. Members shall provide individual diagnostic . . . services in the context of professional psychological relationships only, and not by means of . . . newspaper . . . publicity directed at unknown individuals.

By indicating to Cheryl in a newspaper article that she needs professional assistance for her possible eating disorder, Dr. Stone has violated 11.2 d. Hong Kong's code specifies in 11.5 that psychologists shall provide diagnostic services only in the context of a professional relationship, not by means of "newspaper." By "diagnosing" Cheryl with an eating disorder severe enough to warrant therapeutic intervention, Dr. Stone has assumed a professional relationship with Cheryl.

American Moral Values

1. What kind of confidentiality does Dr. Stone owe Cheryl? Is "Cheryl" a pseudonym? Does Cheryl's e-mail contain any other identifying detail that Dr. Stone would feel responsible for editing? Should Dr. Stone make sure Cheryl understands the risks of her letter being published in a small community newspaper? Does Cheryl understand that an advice column response does not entail the beginning of a client–therapist relationship?
2. What will Cheryl think about Dr. Stone's advice if she finds out Dr. Stone is the only psychologist in town who treats eating disorders? Will this create mistrust in Cheryl's mind? Will this prevent her from seeking treatment from Dr. Stone or anybody else? Will other readers, fairly or not, take Dr. Stone to be giving herself business by advising that Cheryl obtain treatment?

Would they suspect that even if Dr. Stone were not the only one who treated eating disorders in the area? Could public mistrust threaten Dr. Stone's practice?

3. Assuming Dr. Stone does not want her column to convey promotion, how does she weigh the possible social benefits of addressing these kinds of issues in an advice column? How important does Dr. Stone take it to counter false rumors and media buzz on issues like eating disorders and weight loss? Does the benefit of giving advice to a communal readership outweigh the possible conflict of interest of being the only therapist in the area to take on an issue? Should one's unique expertise, instead of being a cause for disqualification, instead serve as the most appropriate way to offer her expertise to as wide an audience as possible? What would be the detriment to the community if such information were not passed on?

4. If Dr. Stone's expertise is something of a "public good" for the community, should Dr. Stone have said more about "eat and spit" and why it would not be a good idea to try it? Does referring Cheryl to treatment cut the answer too short, at least in terms of a public health effort? How can Dr. Stone draw the line between implying professional treatment, or a promise of treatment, while providing as much useful information as possible for the public?

5. How does Dr. Stone view the newspaper's role in the community and beyond? Could the identification of eat and spit as an eating disorder cause a small community to gossip about who was considering it? How far beyond the community's subscribers could the advice reach? If the paper is available on the Internet, should Dr. Stone consider how her advice will function in a much wider public domain (e.g., appearing in Google searches for eat and spit)?

6. Could Dr. Stone have written back to Cheryl with her advice without publishing it? Should she tell Cheryl that she is the only one in the area treating eating disorders, by way of full disclosure?

7. Does Dr. Stone have a moral objection to society's general approach to the topic of eating disorders and the media-facilitated exchange of suggestions like eat and spit? Is there a particular urgency Dr. Stone ascribes to tackling such issues with a general readership?

8. Could she have written in her column that eat and spit is "generally thought to need professional treatment," distancing herself from a direct instruction to seek treatment? What does the demand to sell newspapers do to a psychologist's style in an advice column? Who chooses the e-mails? How much say does Dr. Stone have over this selection?

Ethical Course of Action

Directive per APA Code

On the surface of it, it appears that Dr. Stone has met the directives as specified in Standard 5.04. The only complication appears to be the rural context given the limited number of psychologists or health care providers who are competent to treat an eating disorder. Given the numerous possible pitfalls of straightforward advice to seek treatment, Dr. Stone might consider printing some type of disclaimer in the advice column.

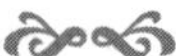

Dictates of One's Own Conscience

If you were Dr. Stone receiving this e-mail, what might you do between the time the e-mail was received from Cheryl and the time the advice column was published with Cheryl's situation?

1. Make sure that the e-mail is kept confidential from the rest of newspaper staff.
2. E-mail Cheryl with notice that her correspondence has been received.
3. Provide Cheryl with a full and detailed explanation regarding the nonconfidential nature of an advice column and the fact that a professional treatment relationship has not been established despite the fact that Dr. Stone will be providing advice.
4. Send the e-mail in #3, and request that Cheryl send a response that explicitly acknowledges consent for use of her information for publication in the advice column.
5. Do a combination of the previously listed actions.
6. Do something that is not previously listed.

If you were Dr. Stone, writing such a column in Hong Kong, which would you do?

1. Not be in this situation because there would have been a large disclaimer at the top of your column that read the following: "Advice is not intended for professional treatment use but for public education. This column is not intended to replace consultation with a physician or mental health services provider."
2. Contact Cheryl privately, and tell her that rather than publish her question in your column you feel she

would benefit from a professional consultation with you or another provider in a different city.

3. Contact Cheryl privately and suggest that a diagnosis or treatment recommendation cannot come via a public forum. Recommend Cheryl seek consultation from a psychologist in another city and if appropriate return to Dr. Stone for therapy.

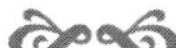

STANDARD 5.05: TESTIMONIALS

> Psychologists do not solicit testimonials from current therapy clients/patients or other persons who because of their particular circumstances are vulnerable to undue influence.

A CASE FOR STANDARD 5.05: Collateral Contact

Dr. Hawkins's wife received a job offer with a salary that the family could not turn down. Dr. Hawkins notified the clients in his clinic that he will be leaving in a month's time. Mildred, the mother of a current client, has been quite pleased with the treatment Dr. Hawkins has been providing to her daughter. On discovering that Dr. Hawkins is moving, Mildred expressed disappointment. Mildred also heard that Dr. Hawkins is moving to the town in which she grew up and still has many connections. Dr. Hawkins expressed his concern about difficulties with starting up a new practice in an unfamiliar town. Mildred assured Dr. Hawkins that she would tell her friends in her hometown about him the next time she goes home to visit and recommend him highly. Dr. Hawkins asked if Mildred would be willing to write a letter of introduction and give him several names he might be able to contact for referrals.

Issues of Concern

Does Dr. Hawkins's innocent inquiry violate Standard 5.05? Even though he does not solicit testimonials, does a letter of introduction pull for a testimonial-like statement from Mildred? Does Dr. Hawkins violate Standard 5.05 in that Mildred is not a client? Would Mildred's refusal of assistance to Dr. Hawkins lead to the daughter's treatment being adversely influenced? Dr. Hawkins must consider whether potential references from Mildred will be accurate and will not unduly influence new clients who come to his practice at her recommendation.

APA Ethics Code

Companion General Principle

Principle A: Beneficence and Nonmaleficence

> In their professional actions, psychologists seek to safeguard the welfare . . . of those with whom they interact professionally and other affected persons . . .

In his urge to maximize his chances of establishing a practice in a new town, Dr. Hawkins may have overlooked the welfare of Mildred and his future clients based on references from Mildred. Placing Mildred in the position of providing a testimonial affects her peace of mind about both the possibility that she might offend Dr. Hawkins, thus negatively impact her daughter's treatment, and the possibility that friends may not find Dr. Hawkins to be a good treatment provider, thus affecting her friendships.

Principle E: Respect for People's Rights and Dignity

> Psychologists are aware that special safeguards may be necessary to protect the . . . welfare of persons . . . whose vulnerabilities impair autonomous decision making. . .

In his request for letters of referral, Dr. Hawkins failed to recognize Mildred's vulnerabilities that impair her autonomous decision making. Mildred may feel compelled to provide a good letter of reference to ensure positive closure to Dr. Hawkins's treatment of her daughter.

Principle B: Fidelity and Responsibility

> Psychologists . . . seek to manage conflicts of interest that could lead to . . . harm. . .

Imagine the possibility that a close friend of Mildred is a radio talk show host. Based on this letter of referral from Mildred, this friend invites Dr. Hawkins for a live on-air interview. Such a chance for press coverage is something that Dr. Hawkins would be hard-pressed to refuse. Before the interview, Dr. Hawkins and this friend go for a cup of coffee to prepare for the show. During this time, the friend solicits information from Dr. Hawkins about Mildred. Dr. Hawkins is now in a position to either risk having a difficult show should he offend his interviewer or violating Mildred's confidentiality. Dr. Hawkins would not be in such a conflict of interest had he not used a letter of introduction from Mildred.

Companion Ethical Standard(s)

Standard 3.05: Multiple Relationships

> (a) A multiple relationship occurs when a psychologist is in a professional role with a person and . . .
>
> . . . (2) at the same time is in a relationship with a person closely associated with or related to the person with whom the psychologist has the professional relationship, or . . . (3) promises to enter into another relationship in the future with the person or a person closely associated with or related to the person. A psychologist refrains from entering into a multiple relationship if the multiple relationships could reasonably be expected to impair the psychologist's objectivity . . . in performing his or her functions as a psychologist, or otherwise risks . . . harm to the person with whom the professional relationship exists. Multiple relationships that would not reasonably be expected to cause impairment or risk exploitation or harm are not unethical.

Dr. Hawkins is the treating psychologist for Mildred's daughter (Standard 3.05 (a) (2)) and at the same time may develop relationships with friends of Mildred (Standard 3.05 (a) (3)).Though Standard 3.05 does not categorically prohibit multiple relationships per se, Dr. Hawkins is cautioned to refrain from knowingly entering into such situations.

Standard 3.08: Exploitative Relationships

> Psychologists do not exploit persons over whom they have . . . authority such as clients/patients. . .

Standard 3.08 implements aspects of both Principle A and Principle B by directing psychologists not to use their influence to exploit clients. Dr. Hawkins appears to be exploiting his relationship with Mildred to gain potentially valuable referral sources and possible personal relationships in his new town.

Standard 5.06: In-Person Solicitation

> Psychologists do not engage . . . in uninvited in-person solicitation of business from actual . . . therapy clients . . . or other persons who because of their particular circumstances are vulnerable to undue influence.

By asking for a letter of introduction from Mildred, Dr. Hawkins has engaged in solicitation of actual therapy clients for future business, and thus violates Standard 5.06.

Legal Issues 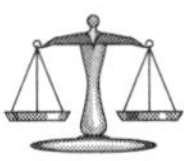

Michigan

> *Mich. Admin. Code r. 338.2515 (2010). Prohibited conduct.*
>
> . . . Rule 15. Prohibited conduct includes, but is not limited to, the following acts or omissions by any individual covered by these rules:
>
> . . . (d) Taking advantage of any professional relationship . . . to further the licensee's . . . financial interests, including inducing a patient . . . to solicit business on behalf of the licensee.

Minnesota

> *Minn. R. 7200.4900 (2010). Client welfare.*
>
> . . . I. to be free from exploitation for the benefit or advantage of the psychologist.
>
> Subp. 7a. Exploitation of client. A psychologist must not exploit in any manner the professional relationship with a client for the psychologist's . . . financial . . . benefit.

In both jurisdictions, Dr. Hawkins's request for a testimonial and introduction to Mildred's friends would be viewed as an exploitation to further his business or financial interests. Although the laws appear to apply to clients, the licensing boards would likely take a dim view of Dr. Hawkins's approach to Mildred, the mother of one of his clients.

Cultural Considerations

Global Discussion

Singapore Psychological Society:
Code of Professional Ethics

> 5. The use in a brochure of "testimonials from satisfied users" is unacceptable.

Does a letter of introduction count as a brochure? Singapore's code appears to focus more on testimonials as unacceptable. As such, Dr. Hawkins would be in violation of Singapore's code.

American Moral Values

1. What exactly is the relationship between Dr. Hawkins and Mildred? Does a relationship with the parent of a client carry with it the same principles and values

of staying within professional confines and avoiding coercion? How can a problem in this relationship lead to a problem with Dr. Hawkins's treatment of Mildred's daughter?

2. Does this move signify an end to Dr. Hawkins's relationship with Mildred's daughter, thus freeing his relationship to Mildred from professional considerations? Or could that relationship continue by other means (e.g., phone, e-mail), including Dr. Hawkins moving back in the future?
3. Dr. Hawkins would presumably wish to avoid coercing Mildred into helping him adjust to a new town, given the implication that he would not treat her daughter unless she helped him. Could a request for a letter of introduction be coercive to Mildred? What about complaining that Mildred's hometown is "unfamiliar?" Is that an indirect cue that Mildred might be in a position to help him? Would even mentioning where he was moving, if he knew Mildred was from there, be manipulating a client–therapist relationship?
4. What will be the effect of Mildred's interventions on her own hometown relationships? Will this request put her in an awkward position? Will it put her daughter in a position of losing confidentiality?
5. Is it appropriate for Mildred to talk to her hometown friends about Dr. Hawkins without his involvement? Could Dr. Hawkins have allowed this kind of "good word" to occur, for example telling her where he was moving if she asked?

Ethical Course of Action

Directive per APA Code

By requesting a letter of reference from Mildred, Dr. Hawkins entered into a multiple relationship against the cautionary note of Standard 3.05 and violated Standard 5.06 by engaging in direct solicitation. Dr. Hawkins has violated Standard 5.05 through his request to Mildred to write a letter of reference on his behalf.

Dictates of One's Own Conscience

If you were Dr. Hawkins, what might you do now? And what moral principle guides you to choose your course of action?

1. Rescind your request for a letter of reference from Mildred.
2. Ask Mildred if she would be willing to have a 15-minute conversation, without charge, for her to tell you what she knows of the town, such as where attorneys and physicians have their offices, culture of the town, neighborhoods, etc.
3. Thank Mildred for her offer of telling her friends about you and say that such good word-of-mouth advertisement is more than sufficient support for your new endeavors.
4. Do a combination of the previously listed actions.
5. Do something that is not previously listed.

If you were Dr. Hawkins, faced with this situation in Singapore, would you contact Mildred again, explain to her that you cannot seek out her help in directly acquiring new clients, and withdraw your request for a letter of introduction?

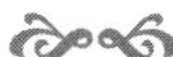

STANDARD 5.06: IN-PERSON SOLICITATION

> Psychologists do not engage, directly or through agents, in uninvited in-person solicitation of business from actual or potential therapy clients/patients or other persons who because of their particular circumstances are vulnerable to undue influence. However, this prohibition does not preclude (1) attempting to implement appropriate collateral contacts for the purpose of benefiting an already engaged therapy client/patient or (2) providing disaster or community outreach services.

A CASE FOR STANDARD 5.06: Saying Goodbye

Roger is in the last month of his internship. He has done his internship at an interdisciplinary medical and social services agency that provides treatment and support for persons suffering from life-threatening illness. Roger applied and has been invited to join a local group practice after his internship and graduation. In anticipation of his starting with the group practice, Roger has developed a letter of introduction, business cards, and a new brochure that includes his name and credentials. All of the advertisement materials cite Roger's specialty in "grief/loss, serious illness, and health psychology." As Roger terminated things with his individual and group patients, he handed out his new business card and brochure, saying to his treatment patients, "Stay in touch. I would really like to know how you are doing."

Issues of Concern

It is natural for Roger to let people know where he is going after his internship. If Roger were to move away from the area to another part of the country and in saying goodbye hands out his new business card, brochure, and says, "Stay in touch," it is doubtful that such actions would or could be construed as a realistic expectation for continued relationships. However, when Roger is relocating to somewhere the patients could easily access, an implicit expectation of a continued therapeutic relationship because of geographic proximity may arise. This implicit expectation may suggest an uninvited in-person solicitation for business.

APA Ethics Code

Companion General Principle

Principle A: Beneficence and Nonmaleficence

> In their professional actions, psychologists seek to safeguard the . . . rights of those with whom they interact professionally. . .

Roger is to safeguard the right of his internship clinic. Presumably the welfare of the clinic rests on their clientele. Seeking to take away their clients does not safeguard the welfare of the clinic. However, if one considers "those with whom they interact professionally" to be the clients Roger has been treating, then Roger's communication may be intended to safeguard the welfare of the clients through noninterruption of treatment.

Principle B: Fidelity and Responsibility

> Psychologists establish relationships of trust with those with whom they work. . .
>
> Psychologists uphold professional standards of conduct, clarify their professional roles . . . and seek to manage conflicts of interest that could lead to exploitation or harm. . .

In return for the training, supervision, and support provided to Roger, the clinic would expect a certain degree of fidelity from Roger. The clinic would expect that Roger not betray its trust by taking away the clinic's clients.

On the other hand, clients might trust that Roger has their best welfare in mind by giving these clients the choice of continued treatment with Roger. However, this perspective is offset by the expectation, as explicated in Principle B, that Roger would have explained his role as an intern and thus his leaving the clinic does not surprise clients, nor hopefully leave them ill-prepared to adjust to Roger's pending absence.

Companion Ethical Standard(s)

Standard 3.08: Exploitative Relationships

> Psychologists do not exploit persons over whom they have . . . authority such as clients. . .

Standard 3.08 enacts both Principle A and Principle B by directing psychologists not to exploit their influence over clients. Roger may be exploiting his relationship with his clients by implicitly inviting them to transfer care to his private practice.

Standard 7.01: Design of Education and Training Programs

> Psychologists responsible for education and training programs take reasonable steps to ensure that the programs are designed to provide the appropriate . . . experiences. . .

Since Roger's situation is one of ending his educational experience, the expectation is that his training program would have complied with the directives of Standard 7.01. Knowing that a normal part of internships is the short-term nature of the commitment, the training program would have ensured that the internship site has provision for orderly termination of Roger's placement and an organized process of transition for his professional relationships.

Standard 10.09: Interruption of Therapy

> When entering into . . . contractual relationships, psychologists make reasonable efforts to provide for orderly and appropriate resolution of responsibility for client/patient care in the event that the . . . contractual relationship ends, with paramount consideration given to the welfare of the client/patient.

A student entering into internship is deemed to hold a contractual relationship with the internship site. Standard 10.09 directs Roger and his training program to ensure that the clinic has provisions for transfer of patient care when Roger leaves. By giving clients the option to continue treatment without disruption, has Roger upheld the spirit of Standard 10.09?

Standard 10.10: Terminating Therapy

> ...(c) Except where precluded by the actions of... third-party payors, prior to termination psychologists provide pre-termination counseling and suggest alternative service providers as appropriate.

Meeting with his clients for pretermination sessions is expected of Roger, per the directives of Standard 10.10. Also per the directives of Standard 10.10, Roger is to suggest alternative service providers. Is it appropriate for Roger to have suggested himself in his private practice setting as an alternative service provider? Or is it more appropriate for Roger to have referred his clients to transfer therapists at his internship site?

Legal Issues 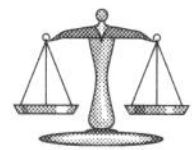

Montana

> *Mont. Admin. R. 24.189.2301 (2009). Representation of self and services.*
>
> (1) In representation of self or services, a licensee:
>
> ...(3)(f) shall not engage, directly...in uninvited in-person solicitation of business from actual... clients... are vulnerable to undue influence...

Nebraska

> *172 Neb. Admin. Code §§ 156-005, -007 (2010). Regulations defining unprofessional conduct by a psychologist.*
>
> ...005 PUBLIC STATEMENTS... Unprofessional conduct includes but is not limited to:
>
> 005.01 Advertising of psychological... services which contain:
>
> ...F) a statement of direct solicitation of individual clients.
>
> ...007 PROFESSIONAL RELATIONSHIPS. A psychologist shall safeguard the welfare of clients and maintain appropriate professional relationships with clients... Unprofessional conduct includes but is not limited to:
>
> 007.01 Using skills of the psychologist to exploit clients.

In Montana, Roger's acts would likely be viewed as engaging in an uninvited in-person solicitation of business from actual clients. None of the Nebraska laws seem to preclude informing his clients of the agency. His statements to "stay in touch" or providing them material about his new practice do not appear to be exploitive of the clients.

Cultural Considerations

Global Discussion

Singapore Psychological Society:
Code of Professional Ethics

> Principle 10: Announcement of services.
>
> A psychologist adheres to professional rather than commercial standards in making known the availability of professional services.
>
> 1. A psychologist does not directly solicit clients for individual diagnosis or therapy.

Roger, by virtue of handing out material advertising his new practice location and making requests for his clients to "keep in touch," can be seen as directly soliciting clients, regardless of circumstance. If Roger had been asked by clients where he was going after the end of his internship and if it was permissible for clients to voluntarily seek him out and see him professionally in his new location, then his actions would likely not constitute solicitation under Singapore's code. However, handing out advertising materials and asking clients to keep in touch likely violates both the letter and intent of Singapore's code on this issue.

American Moral Values

1. Does Roger solicit his clients by handing out a business card and brochure? Do these documents include an element of advertisement and promotion? Or is Roger celebrating his graduation and job with people he feels close to? Given that he is staying in town, is there an implied invitation to continue treatment with him?
2. What constitutes "staying in touch" with his clients? Is the brochure necessary for clients wishing to contact him in the future? What about the business card? Could he have referred clients to the agency's receptionist to pass on his personal information? Would that have been an impersonal way to deal with his clients? Were the business card and brochure necessary to maintain a personal connection with his clients?
3. What is contained within the statement "I want to know how you are doing"? Is that a basic friendly wish or a therapeutically loaded intention to continue service?
4. What significance does the life-threatening nature of his clients' illness have for Roger's behavior? Does this make it more justifiable to share information about his next job, for fear they might feel abandoned as

they confront life and death issues? Does Roger feel his treatment is better than what they could receive at the clinic after he leaves?

5. Roger is now moving on from his internship with the agency to graduate and take a job. Does he think of the agency as a support for his career, where people would be proud of his advancement? Does he think of them as "family" who would not mind him passing out business literature—a rite of passage of sorts? Or is he betraying an institution that trained and nurtured him by soliciting on their premises?

Ethical Course of Action

Directive per APA Code

Standard 5.06 directs Roger not to solicit his current clients for business in his private practice, whether that solicitation is explicit or implicit. The uninvited nature of the solicitation violates the standard.

Dictates of One's Own Conscience

It is unclear as to whether it benefits the clients to terminate treatment with Roger. If you were in Roger's situation and think that clients are best served when treatment is continued with the same person until treatment is no longer needed, what would you do? And what moral principle guides you to choose your course of action?

1. Talk with the clinic to allow your clients the option of continued treatment with you by transferring to your private practice.
2. Negotiate with the clinic for a continued relationship through a contractual arrangement that will allow you to continue with current clients until they are no longer in need of psychological treatment.
3. Make it explicitly clear to your clients that the invitation to stay in touch is not a suggestion that they transfer care to your private practice.
4. Make it explicitly clear to your clients that your contract prohibits direct transfer of them to you for treatment but does not prohibit their right to choose their treatment providers. Or explain what the clinic actually does, which is to keep business cards and referral information on file from all former interns still in the area for those who call in directly seeking therapy resources.
5. Do a combination of the previously listed actions.
6. Do something that is not previously listed.

If you were Roger, as an intern about to graduate in Singapore, which would you do?

1. Refrain from saying anything to your clients about your new private practice, instead discussing your impending absence as a termination/transfer issue relevant to therapy.
2. Ensure that all of your clinic clients had ample time and preparation to transfer to new intern therapists at the clinic, and leave your contact information behind at the clinic in case anyone directly asks to contact you.

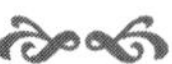

CHAPTER 6

Record Keeping and Fees

Ethical Standard 6

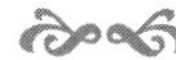

CHAPTER OUTLINE

- Standard 6.01: Documentation of Professional and Scientific Work and Maintenance of Records
- Standard 6.02: Maintenance, Dissemination, and Disposal of Confidential Records of Professional and Scientific Work
- Standard 6.03: Withholding Records for Nonpayment
- Standard 6.04: Fees and Financial Arrangements
- Standard 6.05: Barter With Clients/Patients
- Standard 6.06: Accuracy in Reports to Payors and Funding Sources
- Standard 6.07: Referrals and Fees

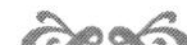

STANDARD 6.01: DOCUMENTATION OF PROFESSIONAL AND SCIENTIFIC WORK AND MAINTENANCE OF RECORDS

Psychologists create, and to the extent the records are under their control, maintain, disseminate, store, retain, and dispose of records and data relating to their professional and scientific work in order to **(1) facilitate provision of services later by them or by other professionals,** (2) allow for replication of research design and analyses, (3) meet institutional requirements, (4) ensure accuracy of billing and payments, and (5) ensure compliance with law.

A CASE FOR STANDARD 6.01 (1): A Grieving Son

Mr. Joe, a wealthy elderly male client, has been in treatment with Dr. West for about 3 months. Mr. Joe's presenting complaint was feelings of depression. During the course of treatment, Joe has discussed his many life regrets, including taking a hands-off approach in the upbringing of his only son, Craig. He berated himself for allowing his wife to spoil his son. Now his wife is long-deceased, and his son has run wild and accomplished nothing with his life. Uncharacteristically, one day Joe did not show up for his scheduled appointment. Dr. West called Joe's home phone, leaving a voice mail message regarding the missed appointment. Two days later, Dr. West received a voice mail from Craig, Joe's son, requesting a callback at Joe's home phone number.

On return call and conversation, Craig told Dr. West that Joe was found dead in his home by the house cleaner. Further, Joe died of an apparent overdose and the authorities were not certain whether the death was a suicide or an accident. Craig is tearful, saying that he and his family would like to know what was going on with his father because it might help them cope with his death to know the truth. He would like copies of Dr. West's treatment records. He also states that his lawyer needs copies of the records within a day or two.

Issues of Concern

Standard 6.01 speaks to the creation and dissemination of records for specific purposes. Standard 6.01 directs psychologists to only put into records information that would (1) comply with the law, (2) help Dr. West to remember what had been done, and (3) help other medical providers to figure out what kind of treatment had been conducted. Once the record is created, Standard 6.01 places some responsibility for deciding whether and to whom and when to release Dr. West's records of Joe. Items for Dr. West to consider in responding to Craig's request are as follows: Would the content of the records be harmful to Craig? What is the intent of Craig having an attorney review the record? Who now holds privilege of confidentiality since Joe is deceased?

APA Ethics Code

Companion General Principle

Principle E: Respect for People's Rights and Dignity

> Psychologists respect the . . . rights of individuals to privacy. . . Psychologists are aware that special safeguards may be necessary to protect the rights . . . of persons . . . whose vulnerabilities impair autonomous decision making.

Principle E guides Dr. West to respect Joe's rights to privacy and confidentiality. It is silent on whether or not Joe's right extends beyond death. In most normal circumstances, a person's rights are transferred to their designated heir. Does Principle E focus a psychologist's attention on the need to protect Joe's rights because of Joe's vulnerability, in this case Joe's death, which prohibits Joe from making any decisions?

Principle A: Beneficence and Nonmaleficence

> Psychologists strive to benefit those with whom they work and take care to do no harm. In their professional actions, psychologists seek to safeguard the welfare . . . of . . . other affected persons . . .

Principle A calls for simultaneous attention to the joint idea of benefiting clients and not doing clients any harm. Aiming for the highest ideal of Principle A, Dr. West's responsibility may now be to not harm "other affected persons," which in this case would be Craig.

Companion Ethical Standard(s)

Standard 4.01: Maintaining Confidentiality

> Psychologists have a primary obligation and take reasonable precautions to protect confidential information obtained through or stored in any medium . . .

Standard 4.01 directs Dr. West to protect Joe's information stored in Dr. West's records of professional work.

Standard 4.05: Disclosures

> . . . (b) Psychologists disclose confidential information without the consent of the individual only as mandated by law, or where permitted by law for a valid purpose such as to . . .
>
> . . . (1) provide needed professional services; . . . (2) obtain appropriate professional consultations; . . . (3) protect the client/patient, psychologist, or others from harm; or . . . (4) obtain payment for services from a client/patient, in which instance disclosure is limited to the minimum that is necessary to achieve the purpose.

Given that Joe is now deceased, any release of records by Dr. West would fall under directives of Standard 4.05 (b), which addresses disclosures without consent of the individual. Standard 4.05 (b) directs Dr. West to release confidential information as mandated by law. The state law may mandate that all rights are transferred to Craig. If so, then Standard 4.05 (b) allows Dr. West to release the information in Joe's confidential record to Craig.

If state law does not transfer right of privacy to legal executor of the estate once deceased, then Dr. West can release confidential information only for the four purposes listed in Standard 4.05 (b). Since the condition under which Craig is requesting records does not fit into any of the categories listed in Standard 4.05 (b), Dr. West cannot release Joe's confidential information to Craig.

Standard 4.04: Minimizing Intrusions on Privacy

> (a) Psychologists include in written . . . reports . . . only information germane to the purpose for which the communication is made.
>
> . . . (b) Psychologists discuss confidential information obtained in their work only for appropriate . . . professional purposes and only with persons clearly concerned with such matters.

Standard 4.04 (a) directs Dr. West to selectively release information from Joe's record to Craig. And Standard 4.04 (b) likewise directs Dr. West to selectively release information to the attorney. To follow the directives of Standard 4.04 (a) and (b), Dr. West would necessarily need to know the purpose for which the information will be used.

Legal Issues 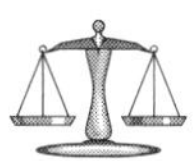

Nevada

> *Nev. Admin. Code § 641.215 (2010). Disclosure to patient or legal representative.*
>
> . . . 3. Shall not perform any professional service that has not been authorized by the patient or his legal representative.
>
> *Nev. Admin. Code § 641.224 (2010). Confidential information.*
>
> . . . 2. During the course of a professional relationship with a patient and after the relationship is terminated, a psychologist shall protect all confidential information obtained in the course of his practice. . .
>
> . . . 4. A psychologist may disclose confidential information without the informed written consent of a patient if:
>
> . . . administrator to whom authority has been lawfully delegated, orders the disclosure . . .

New Jersey

> *N.J. Admin. Code § 13:42-8.3 (2010). Access to copy of client record.*
>
> (a) For purposes of this section, "authorized representative" means, . . . a person designated by the client or a court to exercise rights under this section. An authorized representative may be client's attorney. . .
>
> (b) . . . No later than 30 days from receipt of a request from a client or duly authorized representative, the licensee shall provide a copy of the client record . . . Limitations on this requirement are set forth in (e) below. . .
>
> (c) The licensee may elect to provide a summary of the record, as long as the summary adequately reflects the client's history and treatment, unless otherwise required by law.
>
> . . . (e) A licensee may withhold information contained in the client record from . . . the client's guardian if . . . the licensee believes release of such information would adversely affect the client's . . . welfare.
>
> 1. That record or the summary, with an accompanying explanation of the reasons for the original refusal, shall nevertheless be provided upon request of and directly to:
>
> i. The client's attorney; . . .
>
> (f) Records maintained as confidential pursuant to N.J.A.C. 13:42-8.1 (c) shall be released:
>
> 2. Pursuant to an order of a court of competent jurisdiction.

In both Nevada and New Jersey, Dr. West can release information from Joe's confidential records to Craig only if Craig is a legally recognized representative of Joe's estate. In either state, Dr. West should require legal documentation that establishes who is the duly authorized representative that can provide a signed release for the records and discussions about any confidences.

Cultural Considerations

Global Discussion

Code of Ethics for the Psychologist: Spain

> Principle V: Gathering and use of information.
>
> ***Article 49.*** The death of the client . . . does not free the Psychologist from the obligations of professional secrecy.

Regardless of whether a client is known to be deceased, the psychologist is still obligated to maintain confidentiality. This article of Spain's code applies to both public and private institutions. Therefore, Craig should be denied access to Joe's treatment records by Dr. West.

American Moral Values

1. How does Dr. West view his relationship to Craig? What commitment does he have to a client's relative? Does he owe Craig any type of explanation, given that Craig might not know anything about why his father committed suicide?
2. Does Dr. West believe Craig just wants to "know the truth"? Is his lawyer's involvement an indication of hostility? Should Dr. West consider contacting a different representative of Joe's family to exchange information?
3. Is Dr. West guilty about Joe's suicide? Is there regret about the treatment he gave Joe? Would this lead Dr. West to be more obliged to help the family with their grieving?
4. Do Joe's complaints about Craig play a role in how he reacts to the request for records? Is Craig going to use them responsibly? What will be the result of Craig finding out about his father's opinion of him? Does Dr. West have an obligation to protect Craig from knowing this information? What purpose would it serve now? Can Dr. West claim that the information could be permanently damaging to Craig?
5. When someone dies, the heir to the estate typically takes a client's legal rights. Is Craig Joe's heir? Has Dr. West seen a will or death certificate declaring him so? If he is the heir, can Dr. West preserve the confidentiality of Joe's records? Does Joe deserve to have that confidentiality respected, even at the cost of Craig not getting access to his records?
6. Does Dr. West believe that Joe's death is a suicide? Could Craig be trying to shift blame to Dr. West? How suspicious should Dr. West be about that possibility? How can Dr. West be sure to protect his own career and reputation?

Ethical Course of Action

Directive per APA Code

Standard 4.01 directs Dr. West to protect Joe's information stored in Dr. West's records of professional work unless a proper release is provided. In this case, no executor has provided a release and no judicial officer has provided a court order.

Standard 6.01 provides Dr. West directives on what information should be placed in the client records. If Dr. West has followed directives of Standard 6.01, then only information that Dr. West needs to "facilitate provision of services later" would be included. Did Dr. West need to document the details of Joe's conversation about Craig in the records to facilitate services?

When releasing Joe's records, Dr. West should presume that Craig's attorney will provide a copy of the records to Craig. Principle A calls Dr. West's attention to the necessity of not causing harm to Craig while releasing the records. Standards 4.04 (a) and (b) direct Dr. West to release "only information germane to the purpose for which the communication is made."

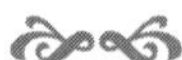

Dictates of One's Own Conscience

If you were Dr. West and you were following the directives of standards previously stated in this vignette, what would you do?

1. Write a letter to Craig requesting legal documentation from the executor or personal representative of Joe that provides access to Joe's private and confidential records.
2. Inform Craig's attorney that the executor or personal representative of Joe must provide a release.
3. Wait for the attorney to contact you, and request a copy of legal authority for confidential records.
4. Review your records on Joe to see what was recorded about Craig.
5. Explain to the executor or personal representative of Joe that you are concerned about the effect of Craig finding out information from his father, and invite the executor or personal representative of Joe to rescind his request for records.
6. Ask the executor or personal representative of Joe why Joe's records are being requested so that you know what to write in a treatment summary.
7. After the executor or personal representative of Joe provides a release, extend an invitation to the executor or personal representative of Joe and Craig to review the records in your office.
8. Release to the executor or personal representative of Joe the record with accompanying fee for copying and mailing.
9. Do a combination of the previously listed actions.
10. Do something that is not previously listed.

If you were Dr. West working in Spain with a request from Craig for copy of Joe's records, would you inform

Craig of your obligation to protect Joe's right to privacy and decline to release information from Joe's records?

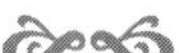

STANDARD 6.01: DOCUMENTATION OF PROFESSIONAL AND SCIENTIFIC WORK AND MAINTENANCE OF RECORDS

> Psychologists create, and to the extent the records are under their control, maintain, disseminate, store, retain, and dispose of records and data relating to their professional and scientific work in order to (1) facilitate provision of services later by them or by other professionals, **(2) allow for replication of research design and analyses,** (3) meet institutional requirements, (4) ensure accuracy of billing and payments, and (5) ensure compliance with law.

A CASE FOR STANDARD 6.01 (2): Moments of Panic

Joshua is nearing the end of his graduate career with only his dissertation to finish before graduation. He has finished the first draft of his dissertation. He sent this first write-up to Dr. Owens, the chair of his dissertation committee. Dr. Owens asked Joshua to bring all of his raw data and any hard copy items related to the data to their next meeting. In readiness for this meeting, Joshua has included the subject's signed consent forms, the institutional review board (IRB) approval, and the thumb drive onto which he has loaded all other relevant items. During the meeting with Dr. Owens, Joshua produced the signed consent forms to verify the number of participants. When it became time to review his analysis, Joshua could not find his thumb drive. Somewhere between his home and Dr. Owens's office Joshua had lost track of his thumb drive with all of the information. Included on this drive was the list of subject's names, their identifying information, and the data identifier numbers.

Issues of Concern

Standard 6.01 directs psychologists engaged in research to keep records of their scientific work. Presumably one of the primary purposes of such records is to allow for outside verification of findings as well as future replication. If Joshua had followed the directive of Standard 6.01, then Dr. Owens's request would have come as no surprise and the information would have been easy to produce. And indeed, Joshua appeared to have had no anxiety about producing the necessary information to allow for replication and to meet institutional requirements. However, Joshua was not able to produce such information at the time and place required by the chair of his dissertation committee.

APA Ethics Code

Companion General Principle

Principle E: Respect for People's Rights and Dignity

> Psychologists respect . . . the rights of individuals to privacy, confidentiality, and self-determination. . .

In research, the aspiration of Principle E is for psychologists to protect subjects' rights to participation and privacy. The right to self-determination is usually done through signed consent to research participation. The right to privacy is accomplished by Joshua keeping confidential all individually identifiable subject information.

Principle C: Integrity

> Psychologists seek to promote accuracy, honesty, and truthfulness in the science . . . of psychology. In these activities psychologists do not . . . engage in fraud. . . Psychologists strive to keep their promises and to avoid unwise or unclear commitments.

Based on the perspective of Dr. Owens, Joshua was unable to produce the records. Depending on the reason Dr. Owens requested review of all data, the "loss" of the thumb drive might have been a very unfortunate incident that could have happened to anyone, or Joshua might have lied about his research and now cannot satisfy the scrutiny of Dr. Owens's review of his records.

Principle C persuades psychologists to keep their promises. Joshua is to keep whatever promises were made to his subjects. If he promised to keep subjects' information confidential and to keep their participation anonymous, then the loss of the thumb drive may compromise his ability to fulfill the aspirations of Principle C.

Companion Ethical Standard(s)

Standard 8.10: Reporting Research Results

> (a) Psychologists do not fabricate data...

Standard 8.10 (a) is one of the implementations of Principle C., Joshua is in a position to provide evidence to Dr. Owens that the data reported in his dissertation is accurate.

Standard 3.10: Informed Consent

> (a) When psychologists conduct research..., they obtain the informed consent of the ... individuals...

Standard 3.10 is one of the implementations of Principle E. Standard 3.10 (a) directs Joshua to get informed consent from his subjects. Presumably the subject's consent was evidenced by subject's signed consent forms. Depending on the specifics outlined on the consent form, and whether the data were secured by a password on the thumb drive, Joshua may have violated the conditions of the research by the loss of the thumb drive.

Standard 8.02: Informed Consent to Research

> (a) When obtaining informed consent ... psychologists inform participants about ... (6) limits of confidentiality...

Standard 8.02 directs Joshua to have specified the nature of the research project and the extent of anonymity and confidentiality. If the consent form called for Joshua to promise anonymity and confidentiality as part of the research participation, then his loss of the thumb drive is of consequence to the research participants if the drive was not protected by a password.

Legal Issues 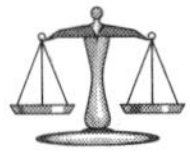

New Mexico

> *N.M. Code R. § 16.22.2.10 (2010). Patient welfare.*
>
> ... J. Avoiding harm. Psychologists take reasonable steps to avoid harming their ... research Participants ... and minimize harm where it is foreseeable and unavoidable.
>
> *N.M. Code R. § 16.22.2.12 (2010). Protecting confidentiality.*
>
> A. Safeguarding confidential information. The psychologist shall safeguard confidential information obtained in the course of ... research...
>
> ... M. Confidentiality of electronic transmission. The psychologist shall ensure that confidential information is not transmitted in any way that compromises confidentiality.

New York

> *N.Y. Comp. Codes R. & Regs. tit. 8, § 29.1 (2010). General provisions.*
>
> Unprofessional conduct shall be the conduct prohibited by this section...
>
> ... 5. Conduct in the practice of a profession which evidences moral unfitness to practice the profession; ...
>
> ... 8. Revealing of personally identifiable facts, data or information obtained in a professional capacity without the prior consent of the patient or client, except as authorized or required by law.

In both jurisdictions, even if the loss of the thumb drive was accidental, then Joshua would be in violation of confidentiality laws. The licensing boards of New York and New Mexico would likely expect Joshua to have protected the data on the thumb drive in a manner to protect it from being accessed by anyone except for authorized personnel. If, however, the loss of the thumb drive is a fabricated excuse to hide any variety of possible problems with the data, then such evidence would be viewed by the licensing boards as Joshua being unfit to practice in the profession of psychology.

Cultural Considerations

Global Discussion

New South Wales Code of Ethical Conduct

> Responsibilities to clients, students, supervisees and research participants.
>
> 1. Nothing of a psychological nature should be done with, for or to ... research participants without obtaining proper informed and voluntary consent from them...
>
> 2. Unless required by law, ... psychologists, even in supervision, must not release information about them unless the clients specifically authorizes the release, preferably in writing. Even under these circumstances, psychologists should be aware of the need to preserve

> as much confidentiality as possible... Computerised data bases should also be secured by the psychologists responsible.

The code of New South Wales, Article 2, specifies that psychologists are responsible for securing confidential material on computerized databases. Joshua is in violation of this portion of the code if information on his thumb drive was not password protected. It is the inherent responsibility of the psychologist to inform research participants of any possible breaches of confidentiality for that participant as part of the informed consent process. In this particular case, although unintentional, Joshua is in violation of New South Wales code.

American Moral Values

1. Does Dr. Owens judge Joshua's loss as unprofessional or just part of common academic absentmindedness? Could it be that Joshua actually never had the required data?
2. Should the subjects be contacted to announce the loss of data? In deciding whether to do so, does it matter what the experiment is about (e.g., pedophilia)? What is owed to those subjects in terms of the time and energy they gave to the project?
3. Given the need for documentation in the dissertation, should any more action be taken until Joshua has exhausted all possibilities of recovering the data? What can Dr. Owens do to move the dissertation forward (e.g., edits, analysis) while that is being determined?
4. What are the experimental ethics behind insisting that the documentation be present? Is it that the work needs to be replicated by other scholars? Or is it more about transparency about the content gained from subjects?
5. What are the larger effects of not enforcing these standards of documentation? Will Joshua become less of a scholar? Will the field be harmed? Could there be a subsequent problem if a subject or other interested party wants to see documentation?

Ethical Course of Action

Directive per APA Code

Standard 6.01 directs that psychologists who engage in research keep records of their scientific work. The institution now calls upon Joshua to produce the necessary information that would allow for examination of his professional and scientific work. Joshua was not able to produce such information at the time and place required by the chair of his dissertation committee. If the loss of the thumb drive were an unfortunate incident, Joshua and Dr. Owens would decide what steps to take, if any, to protect the confidentiality of the research subjects. If there is reason to believe the loss of the thumb drive was a convenient excuse, then Dr. Owens would need to take a different course of action.

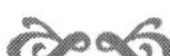

Dictates of One's Own Conscience

If you were Dr. Owens and were faced with a student who was not able to produce the research data as requested, what might you do?

1. Believe that it was an unfortunate incident that could have happened to anyone.
   a. Give comfort to Joshua and reschedule the appointment.
   b. Decide what steps to take, if any, to protect the confidentiality of the research subjects.
2. Direct Joshua to notify the participants that a breach of security has occurred.
3. Reprimand Joshua for this breach of research protocol by transporting confidential data in a nonsecure manner.
4. Request that he go home and get another set of data within the hour.
5. Believe that Joshua was unable to produce the information because some dishonest behavior has occurred.
6. Tell Joshua that you do not believe that he conveniently lost the thumb drive and will be calling for a full review from the faculty.
7. Do a combination of the previously listed actions.
8. Do something that is not previously listed.

If you were Dr. Owens working in New South Wales, faced with a student who was not able to produce the research data as requested, what might you do?

1. Ask Joshua about the layers of encryption for his research data on the thumb drive.

2. If password protected, then request that he go home and get another set of data within the hour.
3. If not protected, then initiate procedures for reprimand for violation of the ethics code and request that he go home and get another set of data within the hour.

STANDARD 6.01: DOCUMENTATION OF PROFESSIONAL AND SCIENTIFIC WORK AND MAINTENANCE OF RECORDS

> Psychologists create, and to the extent the records are under their control, maintain, disseminate, store, retain, and dispose of records and data relating to their professional and scientific work in order to (1) facilitate provision of services later by them or by other professionals, (2) allow for replication of research design and analyses, **(3) meet institutional requirements,** (4) ensure accuracy of billing and payments, and (5) ensure compliance with law.

A CASE FOR STANDARD 6.01 (3): The Evidence Box

Ms. Reynolds, a psychology intern, is doing a rotation in an outpatient treatment clinic. The clinic policy requires that Ms. Reynolds enter chart notes in a patient's file for each and every interaction with the patient. In addition, all information on clinic patients becomes part of the clinic records. Joan is referred to treatment by her primary care physician, who has signed for a 1-month medical leave of absence from work due to emotional stress. Joan works as a security guard for a private agency who contracts with businesses to provide security. Joan is the only female security guard in the agency. Joan reported that her stress has come primarily from her fellow security guards who, being all male, have multiple pictures of nude women in the guard's communal office space. Joan has tolerated the nude calendars because she knows it's "normal" for males. But in the months before her leave, there seemed to have been a shift in that the rude sexual jokes and sexually explicit remarks were directed more personally at Joan. As an example of this, Joan pulled out a Polaroid picture of a penis. Joan explained that this picture was left on her desk the last day she was at work. Joan handed over the picture to Ms. Reynolds and said, "I don't want it around me, but my friends tell me not to throw it away because it will be evidence of harassment. Will you keep it for me?"

Issues of Concern

Standard 6.01 (3) charges psychologists with the creation and care of patient records for the purpose of meeting "institutional requirements." To the extent that information generated from treatment sessions is part of the patient record, the Polaroid picture is now a part of Joan's medical records. As with most clinics, client records are usually kept in one central location, not in the individual staff's office. To the extent that Ms. Reynolds is working in a large institution, the Polaroid picture is now part of the patient record. As part of the record, the Polaroid picture should not remain in Ms. Reynolds's office. However, the reality of a pornographic picture traveling throughout the records office and other parts of the facility poses an institutional dilemma. If the clinic decides that this picture should be kept in a separate file in Ms. Reynolds's office, what responsibility does Ms. Reynolds have in regard to this portion of the patient's file when her rotation ends?

APA Ethics Code

Companion General Principle

Principle C: Integrity

> Psychologists seek to promote accuracy, honesty, and truthfulness in the . . . practice of psychology.

Joan is counting on the fact that Ms. Reynolds ascribes to Principle C: Integrity. Keeping to the highest ideals of integrity, Ms. Reynolds would embody "accuracy, honesty, and truthfulness." If Ms. Reynolds does behave with "accuracy, honesty, and truthfulness" then she would be a credible witness in court regarding the circumstances in which the Polaroid picture came into her possession.

Companion Ethical Standard(s)

Standard 4.01: Maintaining Confidentiality

> Psychologists have a primary obligation and take reasonable precautions to protect confidential information

> obtained through or stored in any medium, recognizing that the extent and limits of confidentiality may be . . . established by institutional rules . . .

Standard 6.02: Maintenance, Dissemination, and Disposal of Confidential Records of Professional and Scientific Work

> (a) Psychologists maintain confidentiality in creating, storing, accessing, transferring, and disposing of records under their control, whether these are . . . in any other medium.

Standard 4.01 and 6.02 (a) combined direct Ms. Reynolds and the clinic to keep the Polaroid picture confidential within the clinic. The question for the clinic is how best to protect the confidentiality of the record, the Polaroid picture being part of the record, and at the same time protect the clinic staff from exposure to pornography.

Standard 6.02: Maintenance, Dissemination, and Disposal of Confidential Records of Professional and Scientific Work

> . . . (c) Psychologists make plans in advance . . . to protect the confidentiality of records and data in the event of psychologists' withdrawal from positions or practice. . .

Standard 6.02 (c) directs Ms. Reynolds and the clinic to make plans for the care of the Polaroid picture when Ms. Reynolds moves on to her next rotation.

Standard 4.02: Discussing the Limits of Confidentiality

> (a) Psychologists discuss with persons . . . with whom they establish a . . . professional relationship . . . (1) the relevant limits of confidentiality and . . . (2) the foreseeable uses of the information generated through their psychological activities.

Since Joan is requesting that certain material be entered into her confidential file, it is most appropriate for Ms. Reynolds to take a moment to reiterate the directives of Standard 4.02.

Standard 4.05: Disclosures

> (a) Psychologists may disclose confidential information with the appropriate consent of . . . the individual client/patient. . .

As directed by Standard 4.05, once entered into the confidential record, Joan can access the Polaroid picture only with an appropriately signed release of information requesting review of the record, copying of the record, or release of record to another entity like her attorney or the courts.

Legal Issues

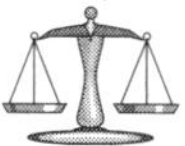

Ohio

> *Ohio Admin. Code 4732:17-01 (2010). General rules of professional conduct pursuant to section 4732.17 of the revised code.*
>
> (B) Negligence:
>
> . . . (6) Maintenance and retention of records.
>
> . . . (c) A psychologist . . . shall store and dispose of . . . records of clients in such a manner as to ensure their confidentiality. Licensees shall make plans in advance . . . to protect the confidentiality of records in the event of the psychologist's . . . withdrawal from positions or practice.
>
> (C) Welfare of the client:
>
> (1) Conflict of interest. When there is a conflict of interest between the client and a psychologist's . . . employing institution, the psychologist . . . shall clarify the nature and direction of his/her loyalties and responsibilities and keep all parties concerned informed of his/her commitments.

New Jersey

> *N.J. Admin. Code § 13:42-8.1 (2010). Preparation and maintenance of client records.*
>
> (a) A licensee shall prepare and maintain separately for each client a permanent client record which accurately reflects the client contact with the licensee . . .
>
> . . . (h) The licensee shall establish procedures for maintaining the confidentiality of client records in the event of the licensee's . . . separation from a . . . practice, and shall establish reasonable procedures to assure the preservation of client records which shall include at a minimum:
>
> 1. Establishment of a procedure by which patients can obtain treatment records or acquiesce in the transfer of those records to another licensee or health care professional who is assuming the responsibilities of that practice.
>
> *N.J. Admin. Code § 13:42-8.3 (2010). Confidentiality.*

> (a) A licensee shall preserve the confidentiality of information obtained from a client in the course of the licensee's . . . practice. . .

In both Ohio and New Jersey, the responsibility for confidential records is placed on Ms. Reynolds. She must be sure that the facility at which she works has a maintenance process for the records she creates that complies with the laws of the jurisdiction in which she practices. Her disclosure statement that is provided to the clients at the advent of services should specify how client records can be obtained. In this manner, Ms. Reynolds's clients would have notice about how to obtain their records even after she is transferred to another rotation. If the facility in which Ms. Reynolds works does not want to maintain the record of the photograph in Ohio, Ms. Reynolds should clarify the nature and direction of her loyalties and responsibilities and keep all parties concerned informed about her commitment to maintaining the record. In both jurisdictions, after informing the client and the facility in which she works, she should offer to maintain the record separately, along with a set of copies of the other parts of the record.

Cultural Considerations

Global Discussion

Association of Greek Psychologists Ethical Code and Guidelines

> IV. Relationships with the institutions where the psychologist works.
>
> 1. During their professional practice in the areas of . . . clinical . . . psychology[,] . . . psychologists preserve the confidentiality of information; this confidentiality concerns both individuals and issues relevant to these environments.

Greece's code mandates psychologists to hold as confidential all information pertinent to an individual or an institutional environment. However, it does not specify how such confidentiality is to be maintained, nor does it outline who should have access to such confidential information within an institutional environment such as a clinic. In Greece, the Polaroid is held to be part of a confidential treatment record and must be treated as part of the individual records because the Polaroid is individually clinically relevant. The Greek code's reference to "different environments" pertains to one, the clinic, and two, the security agency. The part that belongs to the clinic has to be kept confidential from other nonclinical parts of the agency. Should this case become litigated, the Greek code recognized that a different environment has arisen. In such an event, the Polaroid cannot be treated solely as individual clinical information.

American Moral Values

1. How do these pictures fit into the client–therapist relationship? Does Ms. Reynolds's role extend past talking about Joan's issues? How does keeping the picture change the client–therapist relationship? Is Ms. Reynolds more of a confederate now? Is this move of Joan's a way of transferring responsibility to Ms. Reynolds? Does this absolve Joan of her responsibility to represent herself?
2. What is the significance of this being evidence of sexual harassment? Would Ms. Reynolds mind keeping a picture of a gun as evidence of a death threat? How about a picture Joan believes is proof of theft? What makes this situation and its alleged offense a case where Ms. Reynolds should keep the picture?
3. If Ms. Reynolds does consider keeping the pictures, should she and Joan have a formal understanding of how it is to be kept? Can Ms. Reynolds have a private file expressly for this purpose? What responsibility is Ms. Reynolds willing to accept by keeping it? What recourse will Joan have if Ms. Reynolds loses it?
4. What will be the result of refusing Joan's request? Will this represent a loss of trust? Will Joan view this as rejection or disgust with her situation? Will she view it as an unwillingness to stick up for someone being sexually harassed?

Ethical Course of Action

Directive per APA Code

Standard 6.01 (3) directs Ms. Reynolds to accept the Polaroid picture as part of Joan's clinic records. Standards 4.01 and 6.02 (a) direct Ms. Reynolds and the clinic to keep the picture confidential. Due to the offensiveness of the picture, the clinic might need to develop a different strategy for keeping that part of the record more secure than normal. This may be accomplished by the creation of a separate file that does not travel throughout the clinic. Per Standard 6.02 (c), the clinic needs to develop a strategy for handling of the picture when Ms. Reynolds leaves this rotation.

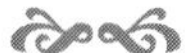

Dictates of One's Own Conscience

If you were Ms. Reynolds or the administrator at the clinic, besides endorsing permission for Ms. Reynolds to accept the Polaroid picture as part of Joan's record, what might you do to address the other problems?

1. Suggest that she keep the picture in a bank security box instead of giving the picture to you.
2. Accept the picture, and review the limits of confidentiality.
3. Reiterate the steps she needs to take should she want access to the picture again, then ask Joan whether she still wants to give you the picture.
4. Consult with your supervisor as to whether to accept the picture for Joan's records, and if the picture is to be kept, how the picture should be kept.
5. Ask that the agency create a "nontraveling" confidential file in the clinic's records office, and place the picture in that locked file cabinet.
6. Explain to Joan that you are an intern and are scheduled to leave the clinic in the next few months, and detail the arrangements about how the "nontraveling" file will be accessed by the new clinician who will replace Ms. Reynolds.
7. Do a combination of the previously listed actions.
8. Do something that is not previously listed.

If you were Ms. Reynolds or the administrator at the clinic in Greece, you might separate the Polaroid from the clinic file; create a separate confidential file for Joan that is within the clinic file system.

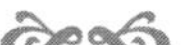

STANDARD 6.01: DOCUMENTATION OF PROFESSIONAL AND SCIENTIFIC WORK AND MAINTENANCE OF RECORDS

> Psychologists create, and to the extent the records are under their control, maintain, disseminate, store, retain, and dispose of records and data relating to their professional and scientific work in order to (1) facilitate provision of services later by them or by other professionals, (2) allow for replication of research design and analyses, (3) meet institutional requirements, **(4) ensure accuracy of billing and payments,** and (5) ensure compliance with law.

A CASE FOR STANDARD 6.01 (4): Confidentiality or Secrecy?

Dr. Ward practices out of his home office. He usually schedules new patient appointments immediately after lunch for 1.5 hours per appointment. This day he went to the waiting room for a Ms. Rose. Dr. Ward did not find a Ms. Rose but instead found the mayor of the town sitting in the waiting room. The mayor said that part of the reason Dr. Ward was chosen was because of the very private setting of his office. The mayor requested for the appointment book that Dr. Ward continue to use the name of Ms. Rose instead of his real name. In addition, the mayor asked that Dr. Ward keep no records of his treatment in any form, including financial ledgers. Instead, "Ms. Rose" would pay cash at the beginning of each session.

Issues of Concern

Standard 6.01 (4) directs psychologists to document professional work to "ensure accuracy of billing and payment." If the mayor is to pay cash out of pocket and does not request fee statements for insurance or tax purposes, does Standard 6.01 (4) allow for no documentation of any kind? What types of documentation are necessary for professional work, as directed in Standard 6.01 (1), or required by state law? Is it possible for treatment to occur without having any trace of the interaction be evident in records?

APA Ethics Code

Companion General Principle

Principle E: Respect for People's Rights and Dignity

> Psychologists respect the . . . rights of individuals to privacy, confidentiality, and self-determination. Psychologists are aware that special safeguards may be necessary to protect the rights and welfare of persons . . . whose vulnerabilities impair autonomous decision

> making. Psychologists are aware of and respect cultural, individual, and role differences, including those based on . . . culture . . . and consider these factors when working with members of such groups.

As applied to this vignette, Principle E is multifaceted. In aspiring to the highest ethical ideas to assure people's right to privacy, Dr. Ward should acknowledge the mayor's request for privacy by not keeping any form of documentation for services rendered. Principle E calls Dr. Ward's attention to the needs of special populations with whom he works. Dr. Ward may need to respect the way American culture deals with elected officials and take special safeguards to protect their rights of privacy and confidentiality. If Dr. Ward should not be able to comply with the mayor's request, he should respect the mayor's right to self-determination by not engaging in treatment with Dr. Ward.

Principle C: Integrity

> Psychologists seek to promote accuracy, honesty, and truthfulness in the . . . practice of psychology. In these activities psychologists do not . . . engage in fraud, subterfuge, or intentional misrepresentation of fact. Psychologists strive to keep their promises and to avoid unwise or unclear commitments. In situations in which deception may be ethically justifiable to maximize benefits and minimize harm, psychologists have a serious obligation to consider the need for, the possible consequences of, and their responsibility to correct any resulting mistrust or other harmful effects that arise from the use of such techniques.

Aspiring to the ideals of Principle C, Dr. Ward would ideally be truthful in his records and any other documentation of his work. Does agreeing to keep no records and enter the mayor as Ms. Rose in his appointment book constitute fraud, subterfuge, or intentional misrepresentation of the facts? Does the current situation justify deception to maximize treatment for the mayor and minimize harm should others be seeking ways to damage the mayor's reputation or violate his privacy?

Companion Ethical Standard(s)

Standard 3.10: Informed Consent

> (a) When psychologists . . . provide . . . therapy . . . in person, . . . they obtain the informed consent of the individual. . . (d) Psychologists appropriately document written or oral consent, permission, and assent.

Standard 3.10 (d) requires that Dr. Ward document the fact that the mayor has consented to treatment. If Dr. Ward knowingly allows for Ms. Rose to sign such a consent document, has Dr. Ward knowingly lied on the documentation? If Dr. Ward consents to not keeping records, including written documentation of consent to treatment, has Dr. Ward violated the directives of Standard 3.10 (a)?

Standard 4.02: Discussing the Limits of Confidentiality

> (a) Psychologists discuss with persons . . . with whom they establish a . . . professional relationship (1) the relevant limits of confidentiality. . .

It appears that the mayor has started the treatment relationship by engaging in a discussion of confidentiality. Standard 4.02 directs Dr. Ward to likewise engage with the mayor on this topic. The exact content of such a discussion regarding the limits of confidentiality depends on the state Dr. Ward practices in.

Standard 4.05: Disclosures

> . . . (b) Psychologists disclose confidential information without the consent of the individual only as mandated by law. . .

Following the directive of Standard 4.02 (a) (1), part of such a discussion should include the conditions under which Dr. Ward will disclose confidential information without the mayor's expressed consent for release of information as allowed by Standard 4.05 (b). This would include letting the mayor know that regardless of written documentation, what Dr. Ward knows—even if the information is not documented—may be accessed if a situation occurred where Dr. Ward were mandated by law to disclose what Dr. Ward knows about the mayor. Thus, even if Dr. Ward agrees to forgo all written documentation, total confidentiality cannot be assured.

Standard 3.04: Avoiding Harm

> Psychologists take reasonable steps to avoid harming their clients/patients . . . and to minimize harm where it is foreseeable and unavoidable.

Standard 3.04 directs Dr. Ward to engage in practices that would avoid harming the mayor. The mayor foresees harm to himself. Should knowledge of his seeking treatment be known, he is exposed to greater harm if the contents of the treatment sessions are accessible to anyone. The mayor's fears may be justified given the political culture in the United States.

Legal Issues 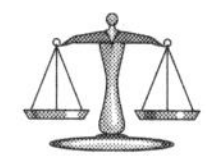

Pennsylvania

49 Pa. Code § 41.57 (2010). Professional records.

(a) This section sets out the Board's minimum requirements for the maintenance of professional records by psychologists. These requirements express the Board's belief that a psychologist's commitment to the welfare of a client/patient includes the duty to record accurately that person's progress through the evaluation and intervention process.

(b) A psychologist shall maintain a legible record for each client/patient which includes, at a minimum:

(1) The name and address of the client...

(2) The presenting problem or purpose or diagnosis.

(3) The fee arrangement.

(4) The date and substance of each service contact.

49 Pa. Code § 41.61 (2010). Code of ethics.

Principle 3. Moral and legal standards.

... (d) In their professional roles, psychologists avoid action that will violate or diminish the legal and civil rights of clients...

Principle 5. Confidentiality.

(a) Psychologists shall safeguard the confidentiality of information about an individual that has been obtained in the course ... practice... Psychologists may not, without the written consent of their clients ... be examined in a civil or criminal action as to information acquired in the course of their professional service on behalf of the client.

(2) Information obtained in clinical ... relationships ... are discussed only for professional purposes and only with persons clearly concerned with the case[;] ... every effort should be made to avoid undue invasion of privacy.

... (4) Confidentiality of professional communications about individuals is maintained. Only when the originator and other persons involved give their express written permission is a confidential professional communication shown to the individual concerned. The psychologist is responsible for informing the client of the limits of the confidentiality...

South Carolina

S.C. Code Ann. Regs.100-4 (2010). Code of ethics.

... I. Fees and statements.

... (3) Itemized fee statement. The psychologist shall itemize fees for all services for which the client ... is billed and ensure that the itemized statement is available to the client. The statement shall identify the date on which the service was performed, the nature of the service, the name of the individual providing the service and the name of the individual who is professionally responsible for the service.

Both Pennsylvania and South Carolina explicitly specify that records of clinical relationships must be kept. Not only do both states require records but each specifies that identifying information must be contained in the record. Neither state law provides a procedure under which Dr. Ward may dispense with keeping records. If she were to comply with the mayor's request, Dr. Ward would be in violation of law in both states.

Cultural Considerations

Global Discussion

Code of Ethics: Netherlands

III.1.2 Honesty.

III.1.2.1 Avoidance of deception.

The psychologist refrains from any form of deception in his professional conduct.

III.2.5 Record.

III.2.5.1 Restriction of the record to relevant information.

When compiling records, the psychologist only collects and retains information which is germane to and serves the purposes of the professional relationship.

III.2.5.8 Revision, supplementation or elimination of data in the record.

On the client's request, the psychologist ... eliminates those data in the record, of which the client demonstrates that they are ... irrelevant in view of the purpose of the record, and insofar they concern the client. The request to ... [eliminate] data will be presented in writing or, if necessary, formulated on paper by the psychologist in consultation with the client.

The Netherlands code forbids deception in any area of a psychologist's work. Dr. Ward would violate both III.1.2 and III.2.5 if he agrees to keep no records and to disguise the client's identity as Ms. Rose in his appointment book. Further, the Netherlands code states that a client may seek to have information removed from the record. The code is silent on a request not to keep any such records or change or alter the identity of the patient from the outset of the treatment relationship. While requesting the removal of irrelevant information from a treatment record is certainly reasonable, the Netherlands code specifies that such requests must be made in writing and kept as part of the record by the psychologist. Dr. Ward will need to decide whether or not the real identity of his client is "relevant" to treatment or what the relevance might be of the requests by the mayor.

American Moral Values

1. What moral importance does Dr. Ward ascribe to record keeping? Are records for the sake of a client's treatment? Are they a duty as part of upholding the legal system and the protection of citizens? How does the proper role of the media relate to the social function of record keeping? Under what circumstances should the public have a right to these records?
2. How does Dr. Ward view the relationship between media and politicians? Does he believe the media have gone too far if they prevent a public official from receiving mental health support? Or is the mayor trying to secure special privilege in his position as mayor? How would Dr. Ward handle another kind of celebrity who did not want the media to find out about their treatment?
3. Does it help or hurt the public's relationship to therapy and psychologists to keep this type of treatment private? Would it be better for the public to see that a figure like the mayor receives treatment? Or would it make therapy subject to crass political attacks and distortion?
4. Would Dr. Ward's view of confidentiality change in light of what the mayor shared in sessions? What if the mayor confessed to grafting, or allowing police brutality, or worse?
5. Would the mayor's treatment be adversely affected by the code name and lack of files he is requesting? Would Dr. Ward be able to remember details for their sessions? Would this compromise his professional standards?
6. How might treating the mayor impact how Dr. Ward's office runs? Would other clients be affected by media stakeouts, protests, etc.?

Ethical Course of Action

Directive per APA Code

Standard 6.01 directs psychologists to document professional work. Section (4) of Standard 6.01 requires Dr. Ward to create a record to "ensure accuracy of billing and payment." Principle E and Standard 3.04 allow Dr. Ward to not create a written document in order to protect the mayor's privacy. It appears that the answer to this dilemma lies in the state law for documentation.

Dictates of One's Own Conscience

If you were Dr. Ward and practicing in Pennsylvania or South Carolina, what would you do?

1. Be clear with the mayor that treatment cannot occur under the conditions requested of fraudulent and absent records.

If you were Dr. Ward and *not* practicing in Pennsylvania or South Carolina, what would you do?

1. Psychologists try to minimize harm. The psychologist here might weigh the possibility of harm that could arise both in honoring the mayor's request and in disregarding the mayor's request.
2. If the psychologist takes the mayor as a client, the relationship should be based on trust. If the mayor cannot trust the psychologist, or the psychologist feels that he cannot be honest about his obligations for record keeping, he might need to refer the client to another provider.
3. Whatever the psychologist does to remedy the situation, he should be honest about the decision he has made—that is, he should inform the client of his decision, and he should accurately document whatever decision is made.
4. The mayor has the right to psychological services if he and the psychologist agree on the terms of treatment. If the psychologist does not treat the client, it cannot be because of discrimination but because they could not agree on the terms of treatment, which includes

the records that will be kept and the manner in which they will be kept.

5. Do a combination of the previously listed actions.
6. Do something that is not previously listed.

If you were Dr. Ward and practicing in the Netherlands, would you tell the mayor that he needs to sign a document that attests to such a request and includes the statement that the record, in the mayor's opinion, is irrelevant for the purpose of his treatment?

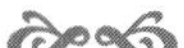

STANDARD 6.01: DOCUMENTATION OF PROFESSIONAL AND SCIENTIFIC WORK AND MAINTENANCE OF RECORDS

> Psychologists create, and to the extent the records are under their control, maintain, disseminate, store, retain, and dispose of records and data relating to their professional and scientific work in order to (1) facilitate provision of services later by them or by other professionals, (2) allow for replication of research design and analyses, (3) meet institutional requirements, (4) ensure accuracy of billing and payments, and **(5) ensure compliance with law.**

A CASE FOR STANDARD 6.01 (5): An Untimely Death

Dr. Torres has been treating Ashley, a 7-year-old who lives with her father, Jerry. Ashley has been having nightmares of her father dying in a variety of horrible ways. Ashley's father reported that these nightmares seem to have started around the time he had to travel for a 3-day conference a few months ago. On inquiry, Ashley says that she can't remember her mother because her mother died when she was 4 years old. One day, Dr. Torres picked up a voice mail from someone who claimed to be Elizabeth, Ashley's mother. Elizabeth would like a copy of Dr. Torres's treatment records for Ashley.

Dr. Torres spoke to Ashley's father at the next appointment and found out that, indeed, Ashley's mother is not deceased. Elizabeth was very dissatisfied with her life and walked out on the family 3 years ago. Jerry has allowed the belief of her death to continue because he thinks it is better to let Ashley think that her mother is dead than that her mother deserted them. He also never engaged in any legal process to end Elizabeth's parental rights.

A week after the phone call, Dr. Torres received a certified letter from Elizabeth requesting a copy of Ashley's treatment record. In the letter, Elizabeth stated that she remains Ashley's parent and has legal right to the treatment records of her daughter.

Issues of Concern

"Ensure compliance with the law" is one of the purposes stated in Standard 6.01 for keeping documentation of one's professional work. This means that Dr. Torres's record would show that he was in compliance with the law at the time treatment occurred. Thus one would expect to find in his intake records documentation that Dr. Torres believed Jerry to be the only person who could give legal consent to treatment as minors do not hold right to consent to treatment nor privilege of confidentiality in most states. The right to consent to treatment and privilege of confidentiality is usually vested in the parent(s) or legal guardian(s). Since there was no reason to believe that Jerry did not have sole custody of Ashley at the beginning of treatment, there was no reason to contact any other persons for legal permission to treat Ashley, a minor. Once contacted by Elizabeth, the documentation requirements change due to the mandate set forth in Standard 6.01 (5). Since Jerry and Elizabeth never divorced and since she never relinquished custody, by law Elizabeth has full access to Ashley's treatment records. Dr. Torres needs to somehow document that he is engaged in treatment with Ashley in due compliance with the law of his state.

APA Ethics Code

Companion General Principle

Principle A: Beneficence and Nonmaleficence

> Psychologists strive to benefit those with whom they work and take care to do no harm. In their professional actions, psychologists seek to safeguard the welfare and rights of those with whom they interact professionally and other affected persons... When conflicts

> occur among psychologists' obligations or concerns, they attempt to resolve these conflicts in a responsible fashion that avoids or minimizes harm.

Principle A inspires Dr. Torres to act in such a way as to benefit those with whom he works, which would be Ashley, Jerry, and Elizabeth. As Elizabeth reenters Ashley's life, conflict is bound to occur for all parties involved, including Dr. Torres.

Principle B: Fidelity and Responsibility

> Psychologists establish relationships of trust with those with whom they work... Psychologists uphold professional standards of conduct, clarify their professional roles and obligations [and] accept appropriate responsibility for their behavior.

With the unfolding of a new situation, Dr. Torres's professional role within Ashley's family also changes. Principle B asks that Dr. Torres would clarify his role as the situation evolves. The values espoused in Principle B would hopefully give a general basis for his decisions regarding contact with Elizabeth. The values reflected in Principle B include being trustworthy to Ashley, abiding by the law regarding rights of parents, and taking responsibility for not having asked for a certificate of the mother's death.

Principle E: Respect For People's Rights and Dignity

> ... Psychologists are aware that special safeguards may be necessary to protect the rights and welfare of persons ... whose vulnerabilities impair autonomous decision making ...

Principle E calls upon Dr. Torres to take special care in safeguarding Ashley's rights and welfare. Ashley, being a minor, is certainly included in the category of "persons whose vulnerabilities impair autonomous decision making."

Companion Ethical Standard(s)

Standard 3.10: Informed Consent

> ... (b) For persons who are legally incapable of giving informed consent, psychologists ... (4) obtain appropriate permission from a legally authorized person, if such substitute consent is ... required by law. (d) Psychologists appropriately document written or oral consent, permission, and assent.

Standard 3.10 (b) directs Dr. Torres to have obtained consent to treatment for Ashley from her legally authorized guardian and to have documented such consent. To guard against the later charge of not having complied with the directives of Standard 3.10 (b), should Dr. Torres have documented a certificate attesting to the mother's death before accepting only her father's signature for consent to treatment? Conversely, now that Elizabeth has reappeared, does Dr. Torres require a signed consent to treatment from her to "ensure compliance with the law" as directed in Standard 6.01 (5)?

Standard 4.04: Minimizing Intrusions on Privacy

> ... (b) Psychologists discuss confidential information obtained in their work only for appropriate ... professional purposes and only with persons clearly concerned with such matters.

A request has been made both verbally and in writing for Dr. Torres to release confidential information documented in his records. Standard 4.04 (b) directs Dr. Torres to determine whether releasing his records to Elizabeth is appropriate. If appropriate, such release is for the professional purpose of providing treatment to his client Ashley. Presumably, Elizabeth is a person who is concerned with Ashley's treatment.

Standard 3.04: Avoiding Harm

> Psychologists take reasonable steps to avoid harming their clients/patients ... and to minimize harm where it is foreseeable and unavoidable.

Standard 3.04 directs Dr. Torres to engage in practices that would primarily avoid harming his client, Ashley, and secondarily avoid harming Jerry or Elizabeth. In this situation, it is difficult to see how harm could be avoided with regard to all concerns, thus Dr. Torres is directed to minimize the harm. This means Dr. Torres should chart a course of action that primarily has the welfare of Ashley in mind. To this end, Dr. Torres may need to discover Jerry and Elizabeth's motives for renewed contact and orchestrate the mother's reintegration into Ashley's life.

Standard 10.02: Therapy Involving Couples or Families

> (a) When psychologists agree to provide services to several persons who have a relationship (such as ... parents and children), they take reasonable steps to clarify at the outset ...

> . . . (1) which of the individuals are clients/patients and . . . (2) the relationship the psychologist will have with each person. This clarification includes the psychologist's role and the probable uses of the services provided or the information obtained.
>
> . . . (b) If it becomes apparent that psychologists may be called on to perform potentially conflicting roles (such as family therapist and then witness for one party in divorce proceedings), psychologists take reasonable steps to clarify and modify, or withdraw from, roles appropriately.

Based on the vignette, it appears that Ashley is clearly identified as the client, thus Standard 10.02 (a) (1) has been satisfied. Presumably Dr. Torres discussed his role with both Ashley and Jerry at the onset of treatment, satisfying the dictates of Standard 10.02 (a) (2). With the phone call from an allegedly deceased mother, Dr. Torres now needs to satisfy the directive on Standard 10.02 (2) and redefine his role with all involved.

Legal Issues

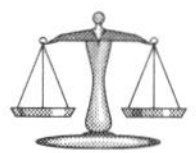

Texas

> *22 Tex. Admin. Code § 465.12 (2010). Privacy and confidentiality.*
>
> . . . (c) Licensees keep patients and clients informed of all changes in circumstances affecting confidentiality as they arise.
>
> *22 Tex. Admin. Code § 465.14 (2010). Misuse of licensee services.*
>
> . . . (b) If licensees become aware of misuse . . . of their services or the results of their services, they take reasonable steps to correct or minimize the misuse. . .
>
> *22 Tex. Admin. Code § 465.22 (2010). Psychological records . . .*
>
> . . . (b) Maintenance and Control of Records . . .
>
> . . . (8) No later than 15 days after receiving a written request from a patient to examine . . . all or part of the patient's mental health records, a psychologist shall:
>
> (A) make the information available for examination during regular business hours and provide a copy to the patient, if requested; or
>
> . . . (C) provide the patient with a signed and dated statement that having access to the mental health records would be harmful to the patient's . . . mental or emotional health. The written statement must specify the portion of the record being withheld, the reason for denial and the duration of the denial.

Washington

> *Wash. Admin. Code § 246-924-363 (2009). Protecting confidentiality of clients.*
>
> . . . (3) Services involving more than one interested party. In a situation in which more than one party has a legally recognized interest in the professional services rendered by the psychologist to a recipient, the psychologist . . . will act in the minor's best interests in deciding whether to disclose confidential information to the legal guardians without the minor's consent.

In Texas, Dr. Torres may decide after talking with Jerry that services were being misused. In which case, he must take reasonable steps to rectify the misuse of his services. It could include keeping Jerry and Elizabeth informed of the evolving nature of the situation and perhaps making the record available to Elizabeth if a misuse of the services is determined. In either state, Dr. Torres may move to deny Elizabeth access to Ashley's records on the grounds that the release of information may be harmful to Ashley.

Cultural Considerations

Global Discussion

Code of Ethics: Netherlands

> Principle 1. 5. Representation of clients.
>
> 1.5.2 Information issued to both parents.
>
> If one of the parents has legal custody of a legally minor client, any information concerning the client issued to the custodian by the psychologist, shall also be issued to the other parent upon request, unless this undermines the interests of the legally minor client.
>
> III.2.4 Confidentiality.
>
> III.2.4.3 Breach of confidence.
>
> The psychologist is not obliged to observe confidentiality . . . if they are required by law to disclose confidential information.
>
> III.2.4.4 Information about breach of confidence.
>
> If circumstances of this kind are likely to arise, . . . the psychologist informs . . . those involved that a breach of confidence may prove inevitable at some point in time.
>
> III.2.4.5 Range of breach of confidence.
>
> If the psychologist decides to disclose confidential information, then he shall disclose no more than the prevailing

circumstances demand and shall inform those involved of his decision to do so.

III.2.4.6 Appeal for exemption.

The psychologist is obliged to appeal for exemption before judicial bodies if his evidence or answers to specific questions conflict with his pledge of confidentiality.

The Netherlands code specifies information on minor children must be given to both parents unless to do so would "undermine" the interests of the minor child. Dr. Torres may breach confidentiality as required by law to give both parents treatment information about Ashley. Further, Dr. Torres must tell Jerry and Ashley that he is about to talk to Elizabeth if Elizabeth produces evidence of her legal status as mother.

If, however, Dr. Torres decides that Ashley's interests would be undermined by providing confidential treatment information to Elizabeth, he could decide not to as supported by Article III 2.4.6. If Dr. Torres deemed it was potential harm to Ashley even if Elizabeth provided evidence of parenthood, he could appeal for an exemption in order not to reveal confidential information to Elizabeth.

American Moral Values

1. How does Dr. Torres view Elizabeth's status with respect to his work with Ashley? Does Dr. Torres disregard her wishes and concerns about Ashley until Jerry says otherwise? As Jerry's legal spouse and Ashley's parent, how can Elizabeth be excluded from Ashley's treatment?
2. Is this person the real Elizabeth, Ashley's real mother? What kind of relationship does she want with Ashley? Will she use these files to attack Jerry or to gain sole custody? Did Jerry tell the truth about why and how she left? Does there need to be a meeting between Jerry and Elizabeth to sort out how her wishes will be treated? Should Dr. Torres offer to facilitate that discussion in a counseling capacity?
3. What will be the consequences of Ashley realizing her mother is alive? Is Jerry's "noble lie" still worth maintaining? On what terms? What if Elizabeth does not want Ashley to think of her as dead? Does Jerry have a right to deny her existence to Ashley?
4. How does Dr. Torres believe Ashley will be best served going forward? Will her trust in her father be irreparably damaged if she discovers her mother is alive?
5. What moral views of parenthood does Dr. Torres bring to this scenario? Did Elizabeth forfeit respect for parental status by leaving Ashley? Generally speaking, does a mother have a right to know about her child? Or does Jerry have a right to continue raising his child on his terms (and with his stories)?

Ethical Course of Action

Directive per APA Code

Standard 6.01 (5) directs Dr. Torres to document his work in such a way as to be in compliance with the law. In a situation as described in this vignette, Dr. Torres needed to have documented that he had legal authorization to engage in treatment with Ashley. Now that a supposedly deceased mother has reappeared, Dr. Torres should ensure he acquires whatever documentation is needed to give him authorization to engage in treatment and to document that Elizabeth has a legal right to treatment information about Ashley.

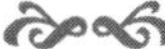

Dictates of One's Own Conscience

If you were Dr. Torres, after getting over the surprise of meeting a supposedly deceased person, what would you do?

1. Feel betrayed by Ashley's father, and withdraw from the case.
2. Request that both Jerry and Elizabeth furnish you with legal documentation to untangle the question of parental rights before making any changes.
3. Invite Elizabeth to schedule a session with Jerry for the purpose of determining your role in this family drama.
4. Invite Elizabeth to schedule a session without Jerry to get further information about Ashley, making it clear that you will not be releasing any information.
5. Tell both Jerry and Elizabeth that your role is to protect Ashley's interests and, as such, you will not reveal treatment information to either parent until legal status is determined through the courts.
6. Tell both parents that your clinical opinion is that children most often fare best if there is open access to both mother and father after a family dissolution. Therefore, you will facilitate Elizabeth's reintegration

back into Ashley's life regardless of the legal status of Elizabeth at this point.

7. Tell Elizabeth that until she can produce legal proof of parental rights you will have no contact with her about Ashley.
8. Start exploring the topic of her mother with Ashley in session to determine the impact of discovering that her mother is alive.
9. Do a combination of the previously listed actions.
10. Do something that is not previously listed.

If you were Dr. Torres practicing in the Netherlands, after getting over the surprise of meeting a supposedly deceased person, what would you do?

1. Request legal documentation from Elizabeth of her parental status and request legal documentation from Jerry of Elizabeth's death.
2. If evidence is provided of Elizabeth's status as Ashley's parent, then inform both Jerry and Ashley that you will undertake examination to determine a course of action that best protect Ashley's welfare.

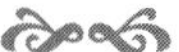

STANDARD 6.02: MAINTENANCE, DISSEMINATION, AND DISPOSAL OF CONFIDENTIAL RECORDS OF PROFESSIONAL AND SCIENTIFIC WORK

> (a) Psychologists maintain confidentiality in creating, storing, accessing, transferring, and disposing of records under their control, whether these are written, automated, or in any other medium.

A CASE FOR STANDARD 6.02 (A): "I Want the Money, But . . ."

Judith is a 32-year-old white female who was hospitalized and diagnosed with depression with psychotic features. Judith was transferred to day treatment 3 months ago. Her treating psychologist at the day treatment facility is Dr. Peterson. Judith does not work. She gets by on funds from welfare and lives in a subsidized low-income housing apartment. Judith confesses to Dr. Peterson that, though she could work, she feels overqualified for minimum wage jobs so will not take work that is beneath her abilities. In violation of her low-income housing rules, Judith lives with her boyfriend, Gerald. In treatment sessions, Judith complains of and is concerned about Gerald, who experiences many life obstacles. When these obstacles get the better of Gerald, he turns to alcohol for solace. When he drinks he often becomes violent. Judith's focus in therapy is "Tell me what to do for Gerald."

Judith brings a "release for confidential information" from the office of Social Security Disability Insurance (SSDI) to her session with Dr. Peterson. Judith says she has applied for SSDI, and they have to have Dr. Peterson's records. But she asks Dr. Peterson not to say anything about Gerald living with her or that she could work but does not want to work. Judith reports that if the government finds out about these issues she would lose her current welfare support and would also lose the low-income apartment if the truth is revealed about Gerald.

Issues of Concern

Standard 6.02 charges that Dr. Peterson would need to create confidential records of his work with Judith. If Gerald has been the content focus of Judith's sessions, Dr. Peterson would most likely have entered information about Judith's living arrangements or her capacity to work. Standard 6.02 also gives Dr. Peterson authority and responsibility to regulate access to confidential patient records. However, the request from Judith is essentially for Dr. Peterson to either redact parts of the record or to re-create a completely different record.

APA Ethics Code

Companion General Principle

Principle E: Respect for People's Rights and Dignity

> Psychologists respect . . . the rights of individuals to privacy [and] confidentiality. . . Psychologists are aware of and respect cultural, individual, and role differences, including those based on . . . socioeconomic status and consider these factors when working with members of such groups.

Principle E encourages Dr. Peterson to respect Judith's right to privacy and confidentiality, which means Judith has a right to determine what Dr. Peterson can or cannot say about her to outside entities like the Social Security Administration. In acknowledging differences, Principle E establishes that Dr. Peterson takes into account the values and mores regarding how the system views those belonging to the United State's subculture of poverty.

Principle A: Beneficence and Nonmaleficence

> Psychologists strive to benefit those with whom they work and take care to do no harm. In their professional actions, psychologists seek to safeguard the welfare and rights of those with whom they interact professionally and other affected persons...

Judith is clearly telling Dr. Peterson that if the full record were released then she believes she would be harmed. Would Dr. Peterson need to act on Judith's belief of harm in order to uphold the value of nonmaleficence?

Principle C: Integrity

> Psychologists seek to promote accuracy, honesty, and truthfulness in the ... practice of psychology. In these activities psychologists do not ... engage in fraud ... or intentional misrepresentation of fact.

Principle C advocates for Dr. Peterson to be accurate and truthful in all aspects of his professional activities. If Dr. Peterson agrees to alter the record for the purpose of deception, then he may have violated the value of integrity by engaging in fraud against the U.S. government. However, if Dr. Peterson redacts the record, would he be participating in fraud or subterfuge, or would he be respecting Judith's right to privacy and confidentiality?

Companion Ethical Standard(s)

Standard 4.01: Maintaining Confidentiality

> Psychologists have a primary obligation ... to protect confidential information ..., recognizing that the extent and limits of confidentiality may be regulated by law or established by institutional rules or professional ... relationship.

Standard 4.01 charges Dr. Peterson to protect information obtained from Judith through the course of treatment with Dr. Peterson. Given that Dr. Peterson works for and is providing treatment to Judith through the day treatment facility, the institution may have policies and procedures that regulate Dr. Peterson's response to Judith's request.

Standard 4.05: Disclosures

> (a) Psychologists may disclose confidential information with the appropriate consent of ... the individual client...

Standard 4.05 allows for Dr. Peterson to break confidentiality under the condition that Judith gives consent for such action. By having Judith sign a release of information she has given Dr. Peterson such consent. What should Dr. Peterson do when Judith gives him partial consent for release of information? Does it matter that Judith's intent for not releasing parts of the record is for deception?

Standard 3.04: Avoiding Harm

> Psychologists take reasonable steps to avoid harming their clients/patients ... and to minimize harm where it is foreseeable and unavoidable.

Standard 3.04 is the enforceable companion to Principle A: Nonmaleficence. Standard 3.04 directs Dr. Peterson to "take reasonable steps" not to inflict harm on to Judith. Do such reasonable steps involve either altering or redacting the record?

Standard 4.04: Minimizing Intrusions on Privacy

> (a) Psychologists include in ... reports and consultations, only information germane to the purpose for which the communication is made.

If Dr. Peterson were to follow the directive of Standard 4.04 (a), he would then write a summary that speaks to Judith's mental status. Is it possible to give an accurate account of Judith's ability to function without reference to the nature of her relationship with Gerald?

Legal Issues 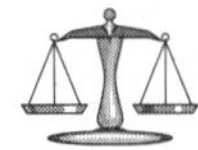

California

> *Cal. Community Mental Health Services § 5328 (West 2003). Confidentiality of records; authorized disclosures.*
>
> All information and records obtained in the course of providing services ... shall be confidential...

Information and records shall be disclosed only in any of the following cases:

. . . (c) To the extent necessary for a recipient to make a claim, or . . . for aid, insurance, or medical assistance to which he or she may be entitled.

Virginia

18 Va. Admin. Code § 125-20-150 (2010). Standards of practice.

. . . B. Persons licensed by the board shall:

. . . 5. Avoid harming patients or clients . . . and minimize harm when it is foreseeable and unavoidable.

. . . 9. Keep confidential their professional relationships with patients . . . and disclose client records to others only with written consent. . .

California allows release of Judith's confidential records under the category of Dr. Peterson submitting a claim for aid on behalf of a client. California is silent on the content of the records thus released. Virginia also allows for Dr. Peterson to release confidential records with Judith's written request but also is silent on the content of thus released records. In either state, Dr. Peterson would hold to the principle of not harming Judith to guide his decision about what content to include in a summary of the treatment to date. Sending a summary may not be viewed as sufficient for obtaining SSDI. Dr. Peterson should prepare Judith for the possibility that a treatment summary may be insufficient and help her develop another course of action to obtain a disability evaluation from another clinician who is not in a treatment relationship with her.

Cultural Considerations

Global Discussion

Code of Ethics: Netherlands

III.1.2 Honesty.

III.1.2.1 Avoidance of deception.

The psychologist refrains from any form of deception in his professional conduct.

III.2.5 Record.

III.2.5.1 Restriction of the record to relevant information.

When compiling records, the psychologist only collects and retains information which is germane to and serves the purposes of the professional relationship.

III.2.5.2 Information in the record about other persons than the client.

If it is necessary to include in the record information pertaining to other persons than the client, then this shall be done in such a way that, for reasons of confidentiality of this information, it may be temporarily removed should the client request an examination of the record.

There is a seeming conflict between two key principles of the Netherlands code: (1) honesty and (2) record. Psychologists are charged with "refraining" from any form of deception in their professional conduct, presumably including record keeping and submission of treatment notes to third parties. However, as stated in III.2.5.2, if there is information in Judith's record about Gerald and Judith requests it, Gerald's information may be "temporarily removed." When Dr. Peterson began treating Judith, and when she first mentioned Gerald, he felt that it was clinically relevant enough to include that information in the treatment records. Even if Dr. Peterson was vigilant about including only enough detail to accurately represent the content of the sessions, in keeping with Article III. 2. 5. 1, he would have would have included information about Gerald. Now that Judith has returned with a request to redact certain information, Dr. Peterson must weigh the client's rights under Article III 2.5.2 to have that information "temporarily" removed against the clear directive of Article III. 1.2.1, the avoidance of deception. Redacting a clinical record for purposes of deception is against the letter and intent of both of these portions of the Netherlands code.

American Moral Values

1. How does Dr. Peterson weigh the priorities Judith's situation presents? Is her relationship to Gerald worth concealing facts in order to obtain SSDI? Is Judith's relationship to Gerald worth working to save, for both Judith and Dr. Peterson? Does Judith need to take a job, no matter how qualified she believes herself to be?
2. How does Dr. Peterson assess Gerald's role in Judith's life? Does he judge him to be a destructive presence, as an alcoholic who at times gets violent with Judith? Would Dr. Peterson refuse to conceal Gerald's living with Judith as an incentive for her to leave him? At what point does Dr. Peterson believe a therapist must support a client's relationship choice? How would he ultimately help them both live productive, sustainable lives?

3. What does Dr. Peterson think of Judith for refusing jobs out of a feeling of superiority? Is this a harmful feeling of entitlement? Does she need a better "work ethic" in order to lead a successful life? What if Judith's refusal is an indirect expression of self-respect and a quest for respect? Will criticizing Judith help her rebound better?
4. What are Dr. Peterson's ideas about SSDI? Is it a program that more deserve to get, or is it an abused safety net? Does he believe the intake information is fair to ask of applicants? Could concealing info about Gerald be justifiable by the view that the testing is absurd anyway?
5. What is the risk to Dr. Peterson for giving false information on this application? What is the risk to Judith for doing so? Should Dr. Peterson review with Judith what those consequences could be? Might Dr. Peterson hesitate to argue with her about this application because of her present condition?

Ethical Course of Action

Directive per APA Code

Standard 6.02 places the responsibility of creating, accessing, and transferring of confidential records for Judith onto Dr. Peterson. Standard 4.05 allows Dr. Peterson to transfer Judith's confidential records with consent from Judith. Standard 4.04 directs Dr. Peterson to only release that part of the confidential information germane to the work of SSDI. It is possible Dr. Peterson would not need to mention Gerald in his summary of information regarding Judith's ability to work. Depending on Dr. Peterson's assessment of Judith's claim to being able to work but choosing not to work, this piece of information may be of benefit to Judith for SSDI. In conclusion, Principle C would lead Dr. Peterson to be accurate and truthful in what he puts into Judith's record while selecting only information that is relevant for the summary letter to SSDI.

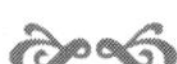

Dictates of One's Own Conscience

If you were Dr. Peterson, besides trying to determine what the Social Security Administration wants, what would you do?

1. Ask Judith what exactly the Social Security Administration wants.
2. Call the Social Security Administration, and ask what exact information they need from you for their work.
3. Tell Judith to get the records from the hospital if she wants nothing mentioned about her claim that she could work but chooses not to work.
4. Tell Judith that you will redact the records and that the Social Security Administration may ask you why you redacted the records.
5. Tell Judith that you will redact the records and that the Social Security Administration may ask Judith why she wanted the records redacted.
6. Tell Judith that you cannot lie and not tell the Social Security Administration about her refusal to work or her relationship with Gerald.
7. Tell Judith that she could find another psychologist who would not tell the Social Security Administration about her problems with Gerald.
8. Tell Judith to go to another psychologist and not talk about Gerald, thus no such information would be in the records.
9. Tell Judith that if she ends her relationship with Gerald that you would enter that information in the records.
10. Do a combination of the previously listed actions.
11. Do something that is not previously listed.

If you were Dr. Peterson working in the Netherlands, besides trying to determine what the Social Security Administration wants, would you tell Judith that you cannot alter a clinical record for purposes of deception?

STANDARD 6.02: MAINTENANCE, DISSEMINATION, AND DISPOSAL OF CONFIDENTIAL RECORDS OF PROFESSIONAL AND SCIENTIFIC WORK

. . . (b) If confidential information concerning recipients of psychological services is entered into databases or systems of records available to persons whose access has not been consented to by the recipient, psychologists use coding or other techniques to avoid the inclusion of personal identifiers.

A CASE FOR STANDARD 6.02 (B): Everyone Is Considered the Same

Much time and money has been spent on getting new practice software installed in the university's counseling clinic. The impetus for new database software is to enable students to access clinic functions through the internet, thus eliminating the congestion of waiting for a computer at the clinic to schedule treatment rooms and to enter chart notes. With much relief Keith, a 2nd-year graduate psychology student, accessed the clinic database from home. Expecting to see the list of his patients, Keith was surprised that the new software allowed him to access *all* clinic client files. The next day Keith asked the clinic administrator if his password might be set improperly because he was able to access all of the clinic's client records. The clinic administrator replied, "There is no problem with your password. Everyone accessing all client records is normal. Since we all work for the same clinic and access to the database is password protected, we are fine. Clinic records are not confidential between clinic personnel, including between student therapists."

At his next supervision session, Keith asked Dr. Gray, "Should I tell Judy, my client, that Samuel can see her chart records now?" Samuel is another student therapist who is a personal friend of Judy's boyfriend.

Issues of Concern

There are five players in this vignette— (1) the university clinic, (2) Keith, (3) Judy, (4) Dr. Gray, and (5) Samuel. The university clinic's database system makes Judy's chart notes "available to persons—namely Samuel, friend known to Judy—whose access has not been consented to by the recipient" and has not used "coding or other techniques to avoid the inclusion of personal identifiers." Thus the university's clinic has violated the directives of Standard 6.02 (b). Keith, to be in compliance with Standard 6.02, is correct in inquiring of his supervisor about how best to comply with Standard 6.02 (b).

Dr. Gray is responsible for Keith's work. Part of that responsibility is to make sure that Keith complies with all the directives of the American Psychological Association (APA) Ethics Code.

APA Ethics Code

Companion General Principle

Principle E: Respect for People's Rights and Dignity

> Psychologists respect . . . the rights of individuals to privacy . . .

Principle E encourages Keith to respect Judy's right to privacy by allowing Judy to decide who is to have access to her confidential information. To meet the highest ideal of Principle E, Keith would need to inform Judy of the clinic's records policy of allowing all student therapists access to all client files and allow her to make choices in response to those policies.

Principle C: Integrity

> . . . Psychologists strive to keep their promises and to avoid unwise or unclear commitments . . .

We presume Keith explained confidentiality and limits of confidentiality to Judy at the beginning of treatment. Judy would most likely receive the information on confidentiality as a promise from Keith that only people she has agreed to would have access to her treatment information.

Companion Ethical Standard(s)

Standard 2.05: Delegation of Work to Others

> Psychologists who delegate work to . . . supervisees . . . take reasonable steps to . . . (2) authorize only those responsibilities that such persons can be expected to perform competently . . . with the level of supervision being provided; and . . . (3) see that such persons perform these services competently.

Standard 2.05 (3) designates Dr. Gray as the person who is responsible for Keith's work. As such, Dr. Gray is the licensee who has delegated the work of keeping Judy's records confidential to Keith.

Standard 4.01: Maintaining Confidentiality

> Psychologists have a primary obligation and take reasonable precautions to protect confidential information obtained through or stored in any medium, recognizing that the extent and limits of confidentiality may be regulated by . . . institutional rules . . .

Standard 4.01 places the responsibility of keeping Judy's information confidential onto Keith. Since Keith is under supervision from Dr. Gray, it is ultimately Dr. Gray's responsibility to assure confidentiality of Judy's information. The caveat inserted in Standard 4.01 is that Dr. Gray and Keith are only responsible up to the limits set by the university clinic. Since it is the university clinic's policy that all records are accessible to all personnel working at the clinic, Dr. Gray and Keith have complied with the dictates of Standard 4.01.

Standard 1.03: Conflicts Between Ethics and Organizational Demands

> If the demands of an organization . . . for whom they are working conflict with this Ethics Code, psychologists clarify the nature of the conflict, make known their commitment to the Ethics Code, and to the extent feasible, resolve the conflict in a way that permits adherence to the Ethics Code.

Standard 1.03 directs both Dr. Gray and Keith to point out the clinic's violation of Standard 6.02 (b). In addition, Standard 1.03 directs Dr. Gray and Keith to make a statement to the clinic administer that they are committed to uphold the directives of Standard 6.02. Further, Standard 6.02 then charges Dr. Gray and Keith to negotiate with the clinic to make changes to clinic policy or protocol regarding staff access to client records.

Legal Issues 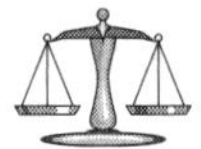

Georgia

> *Ga. Comp. R. & Regs. 510-5-.04 (2010). Maintenance and retention of records.*
>
> . . . (3) The psychologist shall store . . . records of patients and clients in such a manner as to ensure their confidentiality.

Hawaii

> *Haw. Code R. § 16-98-34 (2010). Unethical practice of psychology.*
>
> . . . (d) Safeguarding information about an individual that has been obtained by the psycholoisgt in the course of . . . practice . . . is the primary obligation of the psychologist. Such information shall not be communicated to others unless certain important conditions are met:
>
> . . . (2) Information obtained in clinical . . . relationships may be discussed only for professional purposes and only with persons clearly concerned with the case[;] . . . every effort shall be made to avoid undue invasion of privacy. . .

Both Georgia and Hawaii places the primary responsibility of keeping client information confidential on the psychologist. In this case, the psychologist is Dr. Gray who has delegated it to Keith, the graduate student. Neither state allows Dr. Gray to deviate from this obligation. If the clinic were located in either Georgia or Hawaii, Dr. Gray would be in violation of the law.

Cultural Considerations

Global Discussion

Code of Ethics: Netherlands

> III.2.5.5 Access to the record.
>
> The psychologist ensures that records are stored in such a way that no one can gain unauthorised access to them, thus safeguarding the confidentiality of the enclosed information.

The Netherlands code holds the psychologist responsible for storing records and to ensure that "unauthorized" persons may not have access to those records. It also discusses records concerning multiple persons, meaning software programs that keep records of more than one client. The Netherlands code states that these records must be available to appropriate persons named in the records but must be stored in such a way that only the named individual can access his or her records. This means only Keith should see the records of his clients and that the data must be stored in such a way that such crossover information among different people named is simply not available. In the Netherlands, this clinic would be in violation of both the letter and intent of the respective code.

American Moral Values

1. How does Dr. Gray evaluate the clinic's access policy? How important is it for therapists to have access to other therapists' files? Does it place too much of a burden on the computer system to have different levels of access? Should student therapists have a different level of access than the other psychologists?
2. If access is not to be limited by password, should Dr. Gray advise Keith to use coding for all his files? Does Keith need training about how to code effectively?
3. Will recommending coding be a response solely to Keith's problem, or should Dr. Gray advocate for coding by everyone practicing in the clinic? Is it his responsibility as Keith's advisor to set an example by

fighting for this principle? How will that fight, or a change in policy, affect Dr. Gray's relations with colleagues in the clinic?

4. What is Judy owed in terms of consent and confidentiality? Should she be told about the access policy, if only that her file was fully accessible before Keith coded his files? How should Dr. Gray interpret Keith's question about Samuel? Is it sufficient to inform Judy about the general policy, instead of giving a specific warning about her boyfriend's friend? Could Keith possibly be motivated by jealousy toward Judy's boyfriend? If mentioning Samuel leads her to quit therapy, would announcing that risk have been worth it?
5. To what degree would coding resolve the possible conflict between Judy and Samuel? Will Samuel, if he knows Judy is in therapy, try to access her file? Even if Keith codes his files, would Samuel be able to infer which was hers?

Ethical Course of Action

Directive per APA Code

The university clinic policy allowing all clinic personnel to have access to all client files is a violation of Standard 6.02 (b) unless clients have consented to such access. Given Keith's surprise at having access to all client files, it is safe to presume the university clinic has not followed the directives of Standard 6.02 (b). Thus in order to be in compliance with the directive of Standard 6.02 (b), Dr. Gray needs tell Keith to get written consent from Judy for all clinic personnel to access her files.

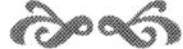

Dictates of One's Own Conscience

If you were Dr. Gray, knowing that asking Judy's consent to enact clinic's records policy would jeopardize treatment by violating Principle C and Principle E, what would you do?

1. Tell Keith to do the following:
   a. Develop a client consent form for you to review.
   b. Have Judy sign a consent form for all staff to potentially access her records.
   c. Avoid talking to Judy about this problem until further notice from you.
   d. Since it is clinic policy, decide he does not have to do anything about the situation with Judy.
   e. Make a hard copy of all information in Judy's records and then delete all of Judy's information from the clinic database.
2. Talk to the clinic administrator to request the following:
   a. Immediately suspend the use of new software until the problem of universal access is resolved.
   b. Create a memo that is sent to all staff and student therapists for an honor system of not looking at any client files besides the clients they are treating.
   c. Change the software so students cannot see other students' client files.
   d. Create a different password for each therapist so that only the student and supervisor can access the student therapist's files.
   e. File a formal complaint that the clinic is in violation of Standard 6.02 of the APA Ethics Code.
3. Tell the clinic administrator the following:
   a. You are authorizing your students to stop entering chart notes till software problem with confidentiality is fixed.
   b. You are requesting that students delete all of their client files from the clinic software files.
4. Do a combination of the previously listed actions.
5. Do something that is not previously listed.

If you were Dr. Gray working in a school that was located in the Netherlands, what would you do?

1. Tell Keith to stop entering chart notes until the software problem with confidentiality is fixed.
2. Tell Keith to copy all files onto their own computer, that is to be password protected, and delete all of their client files from the clinic software files.
3. Let the clinic administrator know that you have given Keith such a directive until the software is changed/fixed or the clinic changes its policy regarding records access.

STANDARD 6.02: MAINTENANCE, DISSEMINATION, AND DISPOSAL OF CONFIDENTIAL RECORDS OF PROFESSIONAL AND SCIENTIFIC WORK

. . . (c) Psychologists make plans in advance to facilitate the appropriate transfer and to protect the confidentiality of records and data in the event of psychologists' withdrawal from positions or practice.

A CASE FOR STANDARD 6.02 (C): Should Have Paid the Bill

Dr. Fisher, after many years of a lucrative forensic psychology practice, has decided to take a yearlong sabbatical. He and his wife, an art historian, will live in England where he will study at the Tavistock Clinic while she examines gravestones around England and Europe. Before leaving, Dr. Fisher arranged for the transfer of all confidential records to a secure storage unit and gave the keys to his office partner, Dr. Ramirez. Months into the sabbatical year, a letter arrived for Dr. Fisher, care of Dr. Ramirez. The correspondence with appropriate signed release of information requested records for an ex-patient. Dr. Ramirez, with storage locker key in hand, went to retrieve the record. Upon arriving to the storage unit, Dr. Ramirez found that her key did not work. The storage center manager said that the contents of the storage unit were auctioned off last month. State law allows storage facilities to auction off the contents of any storage unit for which payment has not been received for 45 days. Apparently the electronic payment didn't go through because the credit card had expired and no new renewal date was provided to the storage facility. In addition, the purchaser's identity and contact information are, by law and by policy of the storage center, confidential and unavailable.

Issues of Concern

In the event a psychologist stops his/her practice for any reason, Standard 6.02 (c) directs psychologists to do two things (1) to plan for the appropriate transfer of records and (2) to protect the confidentiality of records. Dr. Fisher, in accordance with the directive of Standard 6.02 (c), made plans for the transfer of records from himself to Dr. Ramirez when he withdrew from his practice to go to England. Also in accordance with Standard 6.02 (c), Dr. Fisher protected the confidentiality of the client's records by placing his records in a secure storage unit under lock and key. Dr. Fisher made arrangements for automatic withdrawal of fees from his credit card; he had no need to take further action on this matter.

Time passes, life events evolve, and credit card expiration dates arrive. Now not only has confidentially been breached but there is no apparent way to retrieve the records.

APA Ethics Code

Companion General Principle

Principle E: Respect for People's Rights and Dignity

> Psychologists respect the . . . rights of individuals to privacy . . .

In order for Drs. Fisher and Ramirez to uphold the value of respecting the right of Dr. Fisher's clients to privacy as outlined in Principle E, they must address the breach of privacy with the loss of the records.

Principle B: Fidelity and Responsibility

> . . . Psychologists . . . accept appropriate responsibility for their behavior, and seek to manage conflicts of interest that could lead to exploitation or harm.

Principle E establishes that in matters that are clearly the responsibility of a psychologist, he/she accepts such responsibility for the consequences of their behavior. Protecting the privacy of client records is an expected standard for psychologists to uphold. Thus Principle E encourages Dr. Fisher and Dr. Ramirez to take responsibility for their behavior by continuing to address this emerging problem.

Companion Ethical Standard(s)

Standard 4.01: Maintaining Confidentiality

> Psychologists have a primary obligation and take reasonable precautions to protect confidential information obtained through or stored in any medium . . .

Standard 4.01 unquestionably places the burden of keeping client records secure on Dr. Fisher. Depending on the agreement between Dr. Fisher and Dr. Ramirez, the responsibility may be extended to Dr. Ramirez.

Standard 2.05: Delegation of Work to Others

> Psychologists who delegate work to employees . . . take reasonable steps to . . . (2) authorize only those

> responsibilities that such persons can be expected to perform competently . . . and . . . (3) see that such persons perform these services competently.

Standard 2.05 (2) directs Dr. Fisher to make sure the storage unit could perform the task of keeping the contents of the storage unit secure. Section (3) of Standard 2.05 dictates that Dr. Fisher needs to monitor the situation to ensure that the service of the storage unit is done competently, which means the storage unit continues to keep the records secure. Dr. Fisher complied with section (2) of Standard 2.05 but violated the directive for section (3) of Standard 2.05.

Legal Issues 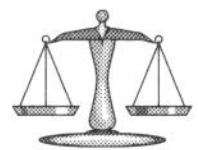

Indiana

> *Ind. Code Ann. § 16-39-7-1 (LexisNexis Supp. 2010). Maintenance of health records by providers . . .*
>
> . . . (b) A provider shall maintain the original health records . . . for at least seven (7) years.
>
> (c) A provider who violates subsection (b) commits an offense for which a board may impose disciplinary sanctions. . .
>
> (d) A provider is immune from civil liability for destroying . . . a health record in violation of this section if the destruction . . . [of] the health record occurred in connection with a disaster . . . unless the destruction . . . was due to negligence by the provider.

Kansas

> *Kan. Admin. Regs. § 102-1-10a (2010). Unprofessional conduct.*
>
> . . . (m) failing to maintain and retain records . . .
>
> *Kan. Admin. Regs. § 102-1-20 (2010). Unprofessional conduct regarding recordkeeping.*
>
> (a) Failure of a psychologist to comply with the recordkeeping . . . shall constitute unprofessional conduct.
>
> . . . (c) Retention of records. If a licensee is the owner or custodian of client . . . records, the licensee shall retain a complete record for the following time periods, unless otherwise provided by law. . .

In both Indiana and Kansas, the responsibility of keeping records confidential falls on Dr. Fisher. It was due to his negligence in keeping up with the payment for the storage unit that the client's confidentiality was breached. Dr. Fisher has engaged in unprofessional conduct in both jurisdictions.

Cultural Considerations

Global Discussion

Canadian Code of Ethics for Psychologists

> Privacy I.41. Collect, store, handle, and transfer all private information . . . in a way that attends to the needs for privacy and security. This would include having adequate plans for records in circumstances of one's own . . . termination of employment . . .

Canada's code states that there must be "adequate" plans in place for keeping records private and secure in case of a psychologist's termination, which again Dr. Fisher correctly did. Therefore, regardless of the outcome of the records in the storage facility, Dr. Fisher was in compliance with the letter of the Canadian code. Canada is silent on the extent, duration, or depth of the responsibility of the transferring psychologist, or of the one receiving the records or client care.

American Moral Values

1. What recourse is there for Dr. Fisher to retrieve his property? Does he have a legal argument for why his storage unit should not have been auctioned off or at least why the purchaser's information should not be confidential? What could be in the files that would be important enough for a court to step in and track down the unit's purchaser?
2. What if the files are gone? What does Dr. Fisher do for his clients' compromised confidentiality?
3. What was Dr. Ramirez's responsibility in this situation? Was she assumed to be responsible for making sure the storage facility was keeping Dr. Fisher's things?
4. How will Dr. Fisher's sabbatical play into the resolution of this problem? Is it seen by parties involved to be a type of vacation or more of a career move? Would those two different views result in different judgments about the lapsed storage fee? Was this an "on the job" mistake or an abandoned responsibility for the sake of traveling and living overseas?

Ethical Course of Action

Directive per APA Code

Dr. Fisher followed and met the directives of Standard 6.02 (c). He did make plans for the transfer of records from himself to Dr. Ramirez when he withdrew from his practice to go to England. Dr. Fisher also protected the confidentiality of the client's records by placing them in a secure storage unit under lock and key. However, he did not continue to monitor the situation and thus violated the directives of Standard 2.05 (3).

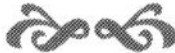

Dictates of One's Own Conscience

If you were either Dr. Fisher or Dr. Ramirez, enacting the highest ideals of responsibility, what would you do?

1. As Dr. Ramirez, you would do as follows:
   a. Contact Dr. Fisher to inform him of the breach of confidentiality.
   b. Contact the manager of the storage unit to see if there is any way to retrieve the contents of the unit.
2. As Dr. Fisher, you would do as follows:
   a. Contact the credit card company to confirm that fees have been paid to the storage unit as previously arranged.
   b. Request that Dr. Ramirez do you the favor of continued investigation into possible solutions.
3. Contact the state to see how long records need to be kept to determine whether you need to do anything about retrieving the records.
4. Contact all of your clients to inform them of the breach of confidentiality.
5. Ask the storage center manager to contact the people who purchased the contents of the storage unit to see if they are willing to have you contact them.
6. Offer to pay the winner of the auction for the content of the storage unit.
7. Ask the storage unit to inform the purchaser what the unit contained.
8. Contact an attorney to explore possible avenues:
   a. Retrieve the records by obtaining a court order to identify who took the contents of the locker and what occurred to those contents.
   b. Send a demand letter to ensure that all confidential information is destroyed.
9. Do a combination of the previously listed actions.
10. Do something that is not previously listed.

If you were either Dr. Fisher or Dr. Ramirez, with a practice in Canada, you would contact the clients to let them know of the unfortunate incident.

STANDARD 6.03: WITHHOLDING RECORDS FOR NONPAYMENT

Psychologists may not withhold records under their control that are requested and needed for a client's/patient's emergency treatment solely because payment has not been received.

A CASE FOR STANDARD 6.03: A Difficult Client

Kelly has been in outpatient psychotherapy with Dr. Watson for the past 2 years. Kelly is a 35-year-old white female living with her parents. She has reported a long history of bipolar episodes since age 21. Kelly's relationship with Dr. Watson has been tempestuous with many terminated and restarted therapy sessions, missed and rescheduled appointments, frequent complaints about Dr. Watson's rates and her bill, and repeated demands to see records of treatment. Kelly's treatment bill has been unpaid for the past 6 months. Each time Dr. Watson discusses the unpaid bill with her, Kelly cancels her next appointment. Kelly then repeatedly phoned the office billing staff to complain. Dr. Watson finally instructed the office staff to refer Kelly to her and not to respond to anything pertaining to Kelly's case. The correspondence in regards to Kelly's case then was sent only to Dr Watson and was no longer handled by front office staff.

Upon returning from a 2-week long vacation, Dr. Watson found a voice mail and a letter with a signed release for Kelly's records from the local hospital. Kelly had made a serious suicide attempt and had been hospitalized.

Issues of Concern

Standard 6.03 requires psychologists to release patient records, regardless of the financial status, if it is needed for emergency treatment. For a variety of reasons, which included nonpayment for services rendered, Dr. Watson's office had stopped responding to anything pertaining to Kelly. The office arrangement of having Dr. Watson alone in charge of responding to Kelly works when Dr. Watson is present. However, the system failed when Dr. Watson was absent. Since Dr. Watson's office did not respond to a request for records in the emergency hospitalization, Dr. Watson was technically in violation of Standard 6.03. Is Dr. Watson still as culpable if she did not intentionally violate Standard 6.03 by disregarding a request for records during an emergency? Or is she just as culpable because she established a system of response to Kelly based on Kelly's nonpayment of fees which resulted in withholding of records in an emergency?

APA Ethics Code

Companion General Principle

Principle B: Fidelity and Responsibility

> Psychologists uphold professional standards of conduct, clarify their professional roles and obligations, accept appropriate responsibility for their behavior, and seek to manage conflicts of interest that could lead to . . . harm. . .

Principle B is meant to prompt Dr. Watson to make clear what role she will play in Kelly's life and how she will respond to Kelly's contacts with her and her office. Principle B urges Dr. Watson to keep the ideal of doing no harm in mind as she executes her role as a psychologist.

Principle D: Justice

> Psychologists recognize that fairness and justice entitle all persons to access to and benefit from the contribution of psychology and to equal quality in the process, procedures and services being conducted by the psychologist. . . Psychologists exercise reasonable judgment and take precautions to ensure that . . . the boundaries of their competence . . . do not lead to . . . unjust practices. . .

Principle D speaks to Kelly's being entitled to treatment under the idea of fairness. It is possible that Dr. Watson is not competent to handle the difficulties that Kelly faces. In Dr. Watson's incompetent handling of a difficult case, Kelly may be unfairly denied psychological services.

Companion Ethical Standard(s)

Standard 6.04: Fees and Financial Arrangements

> . . . (d) If limitations to services can be anticipated because of limitations in financing, this is discussed with the recipient of services as early as is feasible. . .

Standard 6.04 (d) instructs Dr. Watson to discuss with Kelly the consequences of nonpayment, such as discontinuation of therapy with Dr. Watson.

Standard 2.01: Boundaries of Competence

> (a) Psychologists provide services . . . with populations and in areas only within the boundaries of their competence, based on their education, training, supervised experience, consultation, study, or professional experience.

It is possible that Dr. Watson has reached the limits of her competency in treating Kelly and that is why Kelly's behavior is not being contained. If so, Standard 2.01 (a) indicates it is unethical for Dr. Watson to continue treating Kelly.

Standard 10.10: Terminating Therapy

> (a) Psychologists terminate therapy when it becomes reasonably clear that the client . . . is not likely to benefit . . . by continued service. . .
>
> . . . (b) Psychologists may terminate therapy when threatened or otherwise endangered by the client/patient or another person with whom the client/patient has a relationship. . .
>
> . . . (c) Except where precluded by the actions of clients/patients or third-party payors, prior to termination of services, suggestions for alternative care should be provided. . .

Standard 10.10 (a) allows Dr. Watson to end treatment with Kelly if Dr. Watson thinks further treatment will not benefit Kelly. It is unclear as to whether treatment with Dr. Watson is no longer helpful to Kelly. It is apparent that Kelly's behavior is disruptive to Dr. Watson's schedule and to the office staff. It is not clear whether Kelly's behavior allows Dr. Watson to terminate therapy under specifications of Standard 10.10 (b). Regardless of whether Kelly thinks she is still in treatment with Dr. Watson or not, it may be helpful for

Dr. Watson to raise the possibility that conditions for Standard 10.10 (a) have been met. If Dr. Watson is thinking of ending her professional relationship with Kelly, Standard 10.10 (c) tells Dr. Watson to provide Kelly with treatment alternatives.

Standard 6.04: Fees and Financial Arrangements

> . . . (e) If the recipient of services does not pay for services as agreed, and if psychologists intend to use collection agencies or legal measures to collect the fees, psychologists first inform the person that such measures will be taken and provide that person an opportunity to make prompt payment.

Should Dr. Watson become tired of not having her bills paid and decide to have a collection agency handle Kelly's outstanding bill with the office, Standard 6.04 (e) says Dr. Watson should let Kelly know of this before actually sending the account to collections.

Legal Issues 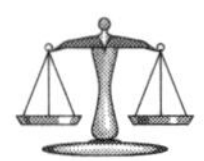

Kentucky

> *201 Ky. Admin. Regs. 26:145 (2010). Code of conduct.*
>
> Section 3. Competence.
>
> . . . (4) Referral. The credential holder shall make or recommend referral to other professional, . . . if a referral is clearly in the best interests of the client.
>
> . . . (7) Continuity of care. The credential holder shall make arrangements for another appropriate professional . . . to provide for an emergency need of a client . . . during a period of his or her foreseeable absence from professional availability.
>
> Section 5. Client Welfare.
>
> (1) Providing explanation of procedures. The credential holder shall give a truthful, understandable, and appropriate account of the client's condition to the client. . . The credential holder shall keep the client fully informed as to the treatment, or other procedure, and of the client's right to freedom of choice regarding services provided.
>
> . . . (2) Termination of services.
>
> (a) If professional services are terminated, the credential holder shall offer to assist the client in obtaining services from another professional.
>
> (b) The credential holder shall:
>
> 1. Terminate a professional relationship if the client is not benefiting from the services; and
>
> 2. Prepare the client appropriately for the termination.

Maryland

> *Md. Code Regs. 10.36.05.07 (2010). Client welfare.*
>
> A. A psychologist shall:
>
> . . . (2) Make arrangements for another appropriate professional to deal with emergency needs of the psychologist's clients as appropriate, during periods of anticipated absences from professional availability.
>
> . . . F. Termination of Services. A psychologist shall:
>
> (1) Make or recommend referral to other professional, . . . if the referral is clearly in the best interest of the client; and
>
> (2) Unless precluded by the actions of the client, terminate the professional relationship in an appropriate manner, notify the client in writing of this termination, and assist the client in obtaining services from another professional, if:
>
> (a) It is reasonably clear the client is not benefiting from the relationship. . .

Kentucky requires that Dr. Watson keep Kelly informed about her treatment and the need to end treatment. She also must facilitate a transfer of care for Kelly when it is determined that Kelly's course of treatment with Dr. Watson is finished. Kentucky is silent about whether Kelly's current status with Dr. Watson's office meets the conditions for transfer of care. Kelly appears to not be treatment compliant with Dr. Watson's treatment regime, and she needs to be terminated and transferred. If this is the case, Dr. Watson is in violation of the Kentucky laws regarding timely transfer of the client and failing to inform Kelly about the need for termination and transfer.

In Maryland, Dr. Watson failed to make an appropriate arrangement for Kelly's care if she needed care during the period Dr. Watson was absent from the practice. In addition, Kelly is no longer benefiting from Dr. Watson's care. Dr. Watson failed to notify Kelly in writing of her change of status from an active to closed treatment case. In the same letter, Dr. Watson also should include the names of other psychologists who might better serve her. He also would further discharge his obligation to assist Kelly by offering in the letter to assist Kelly in obtaining services from another professional if she would like further assistance.

Cultural Considerations

Global Discussion

The Professional Board for Psychology Health Professions Council of South Africa:
Ethical Code of Professional Conduct (April 2002)

> 4.6. Withholding information/reports/record for non-payment.
>
> Psychologists shall not withhold . . . records under their control that are requested and imminently needed for a client's treatment or court case because they have not received payment.

Of all the codes currently available in English, the United States and South Africa are the only two codes which state specifically that client records may not be withheld because of a lack of payment. The U.S. code allows records to be withheld for nonpayment except in emergencies, and South Africa's code specifies that treatment records needed for court or further treatment may not be withheld for nonpayment. One is left to wonder at ethical differences between a stance that says, "If you need your records, unless it's a dire emergency, you must pay first to access them" versus "If you need treatment records or records that could assist you in a court case, I will release them." If Dr. Watson was practicing in South Africa, she certainly would be in violation of this portion of the code—presumably, if Kelly has been checked into a hospital, she is in need of further treatment and has a right to access her records, regardless of the status of her bill.

American Moral Values

1. Does Kelly's suicide attempt, as an emergency, force Dr. Watson to release Kelly's records? Would it be morally possible to judge Kelly's action as manipulative? Or does a suicide attempt suspend normal judgments about behavior? Is there any way Dr. Watson can raise the issue of payment in the aftermath of this incident, or will that seem petty to the parties involved?
2. Is Dr. Watson confident in her treatment and her method of addressing Kelly's failure to pay? To some degree, does she deem Kelly obtaining her records a "victory" in an ongoing power struggle? Will the suicide attempt continue Kelly's pattern of behavior? Without necessarily denying records outright, can Dr. Watson do anything to address that pattern? Or will the hospital pick that up from the records?
3. What is Dr. Watson's relationship with the hospital? Does she feel that Kelly will get adequate treatment there? Does she believe Kelly will continue the same pattern with hospital billing? Would it be her responsibility to let the hospital know about that pattern, or is it fully described in the records?
4. At what point is it acceptable for Dr. Watson to bring up the issue of payment with Kelly? Is getting the payment simply a matter of squaring the books, or will Dr. Watson be pursuing this with therapeutic aims in mind, to help Kelly learn she is responsible and must face consequences? Should Dr. Watson work through some third party, since she could be considered an opposing party to Kelly?

Ethical Course of Action

Directive per APA Code

Standard 6.03 requires psychologists to release patient records, regardless of the financial status, if it is needed for emergency treatment. As Dr. Watson's office did not respond to a request for records in an emergency hospitalization, Dr. Watson is in violation of Standard 6.03. Standard 10.10 allows for Dr. Watson to have brought the professional relationship to a close, thus preventing the conditions under which Standard 6.03 was violated.

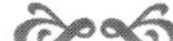

Dictates of One's Own Conscience

If you were Dr. Watson, what would you do upon returning from vacation and discovering that you had been contacted by the hospital about Kelly?

1. Contact the hospital immediately.
2. Coordinate with hospital for care of Kelly after discharge.
3. Contact Kelly's parents to explore the best course of action to ensure appropriate treatment for Kelly.
4. Send the hospital a copy of Kelly's records without further contact with Kelly or the hospital.

5. Contact Kelly to do the following:
   a. Find out what happened.
   b. Tell her that it is best for her to stay in the hospital because you think that she is not benefiting from treatment with you.
   c. Terminate treatment since she now has another treatment provider.
   d. Make a referral for other psychologists to provide treatment.
   e. Tell Kelly that in addition to ending treatment with her, you will be sending her account to collections.
   f. Invite Kelly for one more session after discharge from the hospital to discuss the concern that she was not benefiting from the work that was being provided, and provide information for alternative treatment providers.
   g. Negotiate and establish a payment plan if treatment is to continue with you.
6. Change office policy about responding to anything concerning Kelly.
7. Do a combination of the previously listed actions.
8. Do something that is not previously listed.

If you were Dr. Watson practicing in South Africa, what would you do upon returning from vacation and discovering that you had been contacted by the hospital about Kelly?

1. Immediately contact the hospital to provide Kelly's record.
2. Set up a better system for monitoring phone messages during times away from the office.

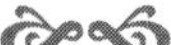

STANDARD 6.04: FEES AND FINANCIAL ARRANGEMENTS

(a) As early as is feasible in a professional or scientific relationship, psychologists and recipients of psychological services reach an agreement specifying compensation and billing arrangements.

A CASE FOR STANDARD 6.04 (A): But How Are We Supposed to Get Paid?

Dr. Ellis opens an envelope from Ralph, an ex-patient whose account is overdue. Expecting a payment, Dr. Ellis was unprepared for a complaint letter with a demand for a cease and desist order for further attempts to collect unpaid fees. At the time of treatment with Dr. Ellis, Ralph worked in the position of a group home attendant for a mental health residential facility. Part of the job payment was room and board for Ralph to live in the group home with the patients. Ralph claimed that Dr. Ellis has breached confidentiality by sending his fee statement to Ralph's previous place of employment, where the person who took over his position opened the mail. The fee statement contained Dr. Ellis's office name, Ralph's *Diagnostic and Statistical Manual of Mental Disorders* (*DSM–IV*) diagnostic code, the dates of service, and fees owed. Ralph threatened to report Dr. Ellis to the psychology disciplinary board if Dr. Ellis attempted any subsequent contact. On review of records, Ralph had signed a fee agreement for Dr. Ellis to provide Ralph with monthly financial statements instead of payment receipts at the end of each session. Further, the only address Dr. Ellis's office had for Ralph was at the group home. Ralph had not informed Dr. Ellis that he had changed jobs since ending treatment with Dr. Ellis.

Issues of Concern

Standard 6.04 requires that Dr. Ellis make arrangements with Ralph for payment of services. It appears that Dr. Ellis's standard office procedure is to send out monthly statements. Ralph agreed to this at the time of intake, according to the signed fee agreement Dr. Ellis has on file from Ralph. Up to this point, all is in accordance with the directives of Standard 6.04. Accidental breaches like this one with Ralph may be especially alarming to all concerned, especially because they take the psychologist by surprise.

APA Ethics Code

Companion General Principle

Principle E: Respect for People's Rights and Dignity

> Psychologists respect the . . . rights of individuals to privacy [and] confidentiality.

Principle E affirms the value of privacy and confidentiality. It is the expectation that psychologists endeavor to assure client confidentiality in order to support Principle A: Nonmaleficence.

Companion Ethical Standard(s)

Standard 4.01: Maintaining Confidentiality

> Psychologists have a primary obligation and take reasonable precautions to protect confidential information obtained through or stored in any medium. . .

Transitioning from an aspirational value of protecting people's rights to an enforceable one such as confidentiality, Standard 4.01 makes such protection mandatory. Does Dr. Ellis's mailing of the bill to Ralph, in accordance with their mutually established fee agreement, still transgress against Standard 4.01? Was there any way for Dr. Ellis to have foreseen this breach of confidentiality?

Standard 6.02: Maintenance, Dissemination and Disposal of Confidential Professional and Scientific Work

> (a) Psychologists maintain confidentiality in . . . accessing . . . records under their control. . .

Standard 6.02 (a) makes explicit that Standard 4.01 extends to records. Per Standard 6.02 (a), it was Dr. Ellis's responsibility to maintain the confidentiality of Ralph's records, and certainly fee statements are part of the records.

Standard 4.05: Disclosures

> (a) Psychologists may disclose confidential information with the appropriate consent of . . . the individual client . . . unless prohibited by law.
>
> . . . (b) Psychologists disclose confidential information without the consent of the individual only . . . where permitted by law for a valid purpose such as to . . . (4) obtain payment for services from a client/patient, in which instance disclosure is limited to the minimum that is necessary to achieve the purpose.

Exceptions to Standards 4.01 and 6.02 (a) occur when clients consent to such release of confidential information. When Ralph signed the fee agreement at the beginning of treatment that explicitly gave Dr. Ellis permission to send monthly fee statements to his residential address, Dr. Ellis is released from the directives of Standard 4.01 and 6.02.

Even if Dr. Ellis's fees agreement did not explicitly contain a statement about sending out monthly fee statements, Standard 4.05 (b) allows Dr. Ellis to breach confidentiality without Ralph's consent for the purpose of collecting payment for services rendered.

Legal Issues 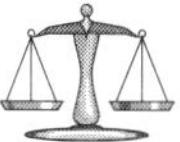

Michigan

> *Mich. Admin. Code r. 338.2515 (2010). Prohibited conduct.*
>
> Rule 15. Prohibited conduct includes, but is not limited to, the following acts or omissions by any individual covered by these rules:
>
> . . . (h) Willful or negligent failure to arrange for the continuity of necessary therapeutic service.

Minnesota

> *Minn. R. 7200.4700 (2010). Protecting the privacy of clients.*
>
> . . . Subp. 6. Statements for Services.
>
> A psychologist shall instruct the staff to inquire of clients and to comply with the wishes of clients regarding to whom and where statements for services are to be sent.
>
> *Minn. R. 7200.5200 (2010). Fees and statements.*
>
> . . . Subp. 2. Itemized Fee Statement.
>
> A psychologist shall itemize fees for all services for which the client . . . is billed and make the itemized statement available to the client. The statement shall identify at least the date on which the service was provided, the nature of the service, the name of the individual providing the service, and the name of the individual who is professionally responsible for the service.

In both jurisdictions, Dr. Ellis has not violated the law by the inadvertent disclosure of information due to Ralph not changing his address. Dr. Ellis did not willfully or negligently fail to arrange continuity of care. Neither jurisdiction has laws related to collection after treatment termination.

Cultural Considerations

Global Discussion

Czech-Moravian Psychological Society Code of Ethics

> 2.2. All professional activities . . . must be expressed in precise form (an agreement, a contract; including mutual agreement on eventual remuneration) from which it must be evident that the recipient of professional services has approved them.

Dr. Ellis has not violated this portion of the Czech-Moravian code, as he did express a contract in "precise form" with Ralph, and has documented Ralph's agreement to the amount of fees and the mailing of statements to Ralph's address with Ralph's signature.

American Moral Values

1. Does Dr. Ellis have a defense against Ralph's complaint? Was the problem sending the bill to the address given by Ralph, or was the problem the information disclosed on the bill? Does Dr. Ellis hold himself responsible for the information being seen by Ralph's coworker? Is Ralph owed anything?
2. What responsibility does Dr. Ellis attach to Ralph? Was it Ralph's responsibility to have mail forwarded to a new address or alert Dr. Ellis to his new address? Was it Ralph's responsibility to alert Dr. Ellis before that he did not want the bill to include the information it did?
3. What is the best way to settle accounts with Ralph? What counts as seeking subsequent "contact"? Does Dr. Ellis fear Ralph's threat more than dropping the issue? Is there a third party who could reach him by phone or in another fashion in order to arrange some plan of being paid? Are there legal means Dr. Ellis would consider employing? Does Dr. Ellis apologize to Ralph? Is that something that could have legal ramifications?
4. How does Dr. Ellis proceed with his own billing policy in the future? What information should be included on bills? Should he ask clients which address they prefer and warn them to consider the privacy of mail at that address? Should he have them agree to update their contact information at agreed upon intervals?
5. How does Ralph's position as caseworker at the mental health clinic affect Dr. Ellis's decision? Does Ralph earn more respect from him for working in an allied field, leading Dr. Ellis to think of him as more of a colleague? Does he sympathize with Ralph more for having that career? Does he expect more of Ralph in terms of knowing how billing would work? Is he more afraid of Ralph's threats because Ralph would know the procedures and codes on which a report to the disciplinary board would be based?

Ethical Course of Action

Directive per APA Code

Breaches of confidentiality are disturbing to clients and psychologists alike. It is unfortunate that Ralph's confidential information was exposed inadvertently. However, it appears that in Dr. Ellis's faithful adherence to the directives of Standard 6.04, he did not willfully violate Ralph's confidentiality. It also appears that Dr. Ellis did not violate any of the other standards by the handling of Ralph's fee statement.

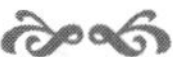

Dictates of One's Own Conscience

If you were Dr. Ellis, knowing that Ralph is upset but you have not violated any ethics standards, what would you do?

1. Presuming that the most recent letter contained Ralph's new address, contact Ralph to discuss the matter.
2. Send a copy of Ralph's signed consent to monthly fee statements in return mail, and ask Ralph what arrangements will be made to pay the remaining fees on his account.
3. Figure the outstanding bill is not worth the trouble with Ralph, and stop sending monthly fee statements to Ralph.
4. Change your office policy and procedure about how to do the following:
   a. Include a statement regarding handling of outstanding fees after termination of services.
   b. Remit monthly statements so as to not include information about Dr. Ellis's credential nor the *DSM–IV* diagnostic code.
   c. Provide sufficient information in the informed consent documents to stress the importance of current addresses of clients/address changes being made in writing to ensure prompt and confidential communication.
5. Do a combination of the previously listed actions.
6. Do something that is not previously listed.

If you were Dr. Ellis practicing in Czech-Moravia, the previously listed options would still apply since the guideline for fee statement and collection is not substantially different from those listed by the APA Ethics Code.

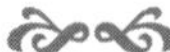

STANDARD 6.04: FEES AND FINANCIAL ARRANGEMENTS

(b) Psychologists' fee practices are consistent with law.

A CASE FOR STANDARD 6.04 (B): Who Pays for My Service?

Dr. Harrison charges a standard fee of $150 per 50-minute session for outpatient psychotherapy. The office policy is for patients to pay the insurance co-pay on the day of service, and the office will bill the patient's insurance for the remainder of the charge. Dr. Harrison has chosen not to join HMO panels but does participate in insurance panels without being a preferred provider.

Kathy, a new patient, says she prefers to pay out of pocket for now because she is applying for life insurance. Kathy reasons and thus proposed to Dr. Harrison that since Dr. Harrison's office will not be using staff time to collect from insurance that Kathy should benefit from the arrangement by paying the standard HMO fee of $97 per session.

Issues of Concern

Standard 6.04 (b) specifies that a psychologist's fee policy should be consistent with the law. How would Dr. Harrison find out if what Kathy suggested is actually consistent with the law? If it is lawful for psychologists to charge $150 per session and receive payment of $97 from HMO panels, why would it not be lawful for Dr. Harrison to receive $97 from Kathy? Why should patients who do not use their insurance be penalized by paying more?

APA Ethics Code

Companion General Principle

Principle D: Justice

> Psychologists recognize that fairness and justice entitle all persons to access to and benefit from the contributions of psychology . . .

Principle D suggests that Dr. Harrison treat all her clients fairly and justly. Is it fair for clients who do not use insurance to pay a higher rate? Is it justice for Dr. Harrison to receive different rates of payment depending on whether clients use insurance?

Principle C: Integrity

> Psychologists seek to promote accuracy, honesty, and truthfulness in the science, teaching, and practice of psychology. In these activities psychologists do not steal, cheat, or engage in fraud, subterfuge, or intentional misrepresentation of fact.

Principle C encourages psychologists not to "steal, cheat, or engage in fraud." Is it cheating Kathy to have to pay $150 for not using her insurance, or is it fraudulent to charge insurance $150 per 50-minute session while charging Kathy $97 per session?

Companion Ethical Standard(s)

Standard 6.01: Documentation of Professional and Scientific Work and Maintenance of Records

> Psychologists create . . . records . . . relating to their professional . . . work in order to . . .
>
> (4) ensure accuracy of billing and payments. . .

Standard 6.01 (4) dictates that Dr. Harrison keep records of services provided, fees charged, and payments made. In the creation and maintenance of such records, Dr. Harrison does engage office staff. The same amount of office staff time is used to create documents for insurance or for private pay situations. Although it may take a bit less time if no follow-up is necessary for insurance payment, it is probably not substantially enough time to support Kathy's argument for being charged a reduced fee.

Legal Issues 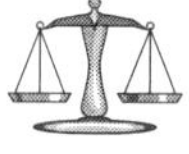

Missouri

> *Mo. Code Regs. Ann. tit. 20, § 2235-5.030 (2010). Ethical rules of conduct.*
>
> . . . (11) Remuneration.
>
> (A) Financial Arrangements.
>
> 1. All financial arrangements shall be made clear to each client in advance of billing.

> 2. The psychologist shall not mislead or withhold from any client, prospective client or third-party payor information about the cost of his/her professional services.
>
> 3. The psychologist shall not exploit a client or responsible payor by charging a fee that is excessive for the services performed. . .

Nebraska

> *172 Neb. Admin. Code §§ 156-009 (2010). 009 Fees for services.*
>
> A psychologist shall solicit or obtain fees for professional service in an appropriate manner consistent with the laws of the State of Nebraska. Unprofessional conduct includes but is not limited to:
>
> . . . 009.03 Division of fees, or agreeing to split or divide the fees received for professional services with any person for bringing or referring a patient.

Neither jurisdiction's law precludes the arrangement suggested by Kathy. Nor is it exploitative to the insurance companies as the contractual arrangement that exists between the provider and the companies do not apply to those clients not covered by the policies.

Cultural Considerations

Global Discussion

Code of Ethics for the Psychologist: Spain

> ***Article 55.*** Psychologists must refrain from accepting financial retribution that may devalue the profession or be in unfair competition.
>
> ***Article 58.*** The Official College of Psychologists may elaborate guidelines of minimum fees for each professional service according to the nature, length and other features of each service within the practice of Psychology.

If Dr. Harrison is practicing in Spain, she might be in violation of Article 55 in that it may be seen to be in "unfair competition" with insurance companies if Dr. Harrison simply does not bill them for services rendered. Fees in Spain are to contain a minimum that is based on the nature and length of the service, not necessarily whether or not the patient in question has insurance. Therefore, if Dr. Harrison's fees have minimums based on length and type of service, she would not be in violation of Article 58. Provided that Dr. Harrison is adhering to minimum fees established by the College of Psychologists in Spain and not undercutting or underbidding her professional colleagues by accepting discounts or other devalued fees, Dr. Harrison seems to be fully in compliance with Spain's code.

American Moral Values

1. What are the principles at work in a negotiation with Kathy over price? Is Kathy just trying to pay a fair price, considering it is out of pocket? Or is there an issue with Kathy's ability to pay? If Kathy's issue is the ability to pay, then shouldn't a payment plan be worked out? If the issue is not the ability to pay, then should Dr. Harrison negotiate over a fair price?
2. Does Dr. Harrison have other patients who pay out of pocket? If so, will negotiating with Kathy mean that those other patients deserve discounts, too? Is negotiating itself a different exercise than a payment plan? Does Dr. Harrison want negotiating to be a broader office policy if a patient requests it? Will it make the office seem too much like a business?
3. Assuming Dr. Harrison does negotiate with Kathy, is her request fair? How should services be computed to account for less office work with insurance? Is this fair to the office? On the other hand, how much does Dr. Harrison feel she deserves to be paid?
4. How does Dr. Harrison factor in Kathy's life insurance application? Would refusing Kathy's request mean Kathy would abandon her application? Does Dr. Harrison believe that life insurance policies unfairly judge applicants with mental health problems? Would that belief lead her to accept Kathy's plan until her policy is in place?
5. How does this decision bear on Dr. Harrison's decision not to join HMO panels or be a preferred provider?

Ethical Course of Action

Directive per APA Code

Standard 6.04 (b) directs Dr. Harrison to the law of her state to determine what to do with Kathy's proposal, regardless of what Dr. Harrison thinks of the health insurance industry. If Dr. Harrison was practicing in Nebraska or Missouri, she would enter into the arrangement proposed by Kathy since it is legal.

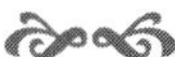

Dictates of One's Own Conscience

If you were Dr. Harrison, faced with a client like Kathy, what would you do? Here are examples of possible actions:

1. Say that you do not participate in any HMO or preferred provider networks so what Kathy is suggesting does not apply.
2. Say that if Kathy is willing to produce all necessary paperwork for documentation, then you are willing to accept a lower payment.
3. Investigate your contracts with various insurance panels to ascertain whether you would be breaching your contract with them, and then contact Kathy back with your answer.
4. Do a combination of the previously listed actions.
5. Do something that is not previously listed.

If you were Dr. Harrison practicing in Spain, faced with a client like Kathy, what would you need to consider?

1. Do not bargain for fees since it would devalue the service provided by psychologists.
2. Refer Kathy to the College of Psychologists to collectively puzzle out how best to consider HMO reimbursement rates.

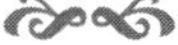

STANDARD 6.04: FEES AND FINANCIAL ARRANGEMENTS

(c) Psychologists do not misrepresent their fees.

A CASE FOR STANDARD 6.04 (C): Cheaper to Buy in Bulk

At the recommendation of other members of the local chamber of commerce and in keeping with practices of other service organizations in town, Dr. Gibson offered an introductory six-session treatment package. This package entails six 50-minute outpatient psychotherapy sessions for $600 paid at the beginning of the first session *or* a traditional fee for service paid at $150 per session.

Issues of Concern

What if a client pays the $600 for six sessions and then does not want to continue after the first session? Does Dr. Gibson keep the whole $600 since the advertisement was clear that the discounted fee is a package, not per session? If Dr. Gibson does keep the whole $600, has she just charged someone $600 per session? Has Dr. Gibson misrepresented her per session fee, thus violating Standard 6.04 (c) through the offering of a six-session package deal?

APA Ethics Code

Companion General Principle

Principle D: Justice

> Psychologists recognize that fairness and justice entitle all persons to . . . equal quality in the processes [and] procedures . . . being conducted by psychologists.

Is it a violation of the spirit of Principle D, specifically fairness and justice, that clients unable to afford $600 up front would pay substantially more per session than those with sufficient disposable income to purchase the discounted package?

Principle C: Integrity

> Psychologists seek to promote accuracy, honesty, and truthfulness in the science, teaching, and practice of psychology. In these activities psychologists do not engage in . . . intentional misrepresentation of fact.

Principle C encourages psychologists not to "intentionally misrepresent" any element of her work. Is it a misrepresentation of her per session fees to offer a cash discounted six-session package deal?

Companion Ethical Standard(s)

Standard 6.04: Fees and Financial Arrangements

> . . . (b) Psychologists' fee practices are consistent with law. . .

Dr. Gibson has not violated Standard 6.04 (b) per se, unless the state she practices in specifically prohibits such practice. If Dr. Gibson established her package price in coordination with other psychologists in town who are members of the chamber of commerce and did coordinate the package price, then it would be considered price fixing and thus a violation of antitrust laws that may be in existence for the state.

Standard 6.06: Accuracy in Reports to Payors and Funding Sources

> In their reports to payors for services . . . , psychologists take reasonable steps to ensure the accurate reporting of the . . . fees, charges, or payments . . .

If the purchaser of the six-session package were to use their health insurance to reimburse themselves for the therapy sessions, to be in compliance with the directives of Standard 6.06, which fee should she report to the insurance company? To be consistent with 6.04 (b), if Dr. Gibson were practicing in Missouri or Nebraska, as discussed in the previous vignette, she would need to report her per session fee of $150 to the insurance company and charge the purchaser of her chamber of commerce package $100 per session. If Dr. Gibson did so, would she be in violation of Standard 6.04 (c)?

Legal Issues 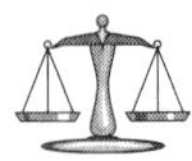

Nevada

> *Nev. Admin. Code § 641.210 (2010) . . . Professional fees . . .*
>
> A psychologist:
>
> . . . 3. Shall not mislead or withhold from a patient, . . . who will be responsible for payment of the psychologist's services, information concerning the fee for the professional services of the psychologist.

New Jersey

> *N.J. Admin. Code § 13:42-10.10 (2010). Financial arrangements with clients and others.*
>
> (a) A licensee shall inform clients of the financial arrangements for psychological services. Such financial arrangement(s) should be in writing. . . The information provided to the client shall include, but not be limited to:
>
> 1. The fee for services or the basis for determining the fee to be charged . . .
>
> 2. Whether the licensee will accept installment payments or assignment of benefits from a third party payor.

In both jurisdictions, as long as the client knew and consented to one of the two financial arrangements before service began, Dr. Gibson could proceed. Adequate written disclosure about the options should be made available in advance of the services beginning. In New Jersey, Dr. Gibson should specify with the purchaser of the chamber of commerce introductory offer package whether it is possible to use their insurance reimbursement in conjunction with the special rate.

Cultural Considerations

Global Discussion

Code of Ethics for the Psychologist: Spain

> ***Article 28.*** Psychologists must not take advantage of the situation of power that may arise from their status to claim special working conditions or payments exceeding those obtainable in normal circumstances.

If Dr. Gibson was practicing in Spain, she would be in violation of Article 28 because by demanding an upfront cash payment of $600, prior to informed consent to treatment or prior to a client's certainty that they wish to complete a full six sessions with her, Dr. Gibson has likely taken "advantage of the situation of power," which arose from her status. If the client cancels treatment before the six sessions have elapsed, Dr. Gibson would certainly be receiving money "exceeding those obtainable in normal circumstances."

American Moral Values

1. How does Dr. Gibson view being paid as a therapist? How much does she consider her practice to be a business that needs to survive through whatever honest marketing and product packaging will yield enough sales? What does changing the value of each session imply about her treatment? Will it, for example, cast a shadow over her treatment itself, perhaps suggesting she would cater her treatment to get a better purchase from the client?
2. Does the package imply a commitment to making therapy fit into a number of sessions divisible by six? Does that harm the idea of therapy (would a physical therapist offer to rehab a knee with a six session package)? What if six sessions are not needed? What if the prospective client does not know enough about therapy to begin with to make an informed decision?
3. Does this package as advertised present psychologists in a bad light? How does this work with insurance?

How does it relate to patients' ability to pay? Does it exclude someone who would not be able to muster that much money at once?

Ethical Course of Action

Directive per APA Code

Standard 6.04 dictates that Dr. Gibson should not misrepresent her fees. As long as the specifics of refund for unused sessions are in the fees agreement, Dr. Gibson has not violated the directives of Standard 6.04.

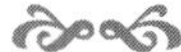

Dictates of One's Own Conscience

If you had joined your local chamber of commerce and were in receipt of business advice to offer cash discount bulk sessions, what would you do?

1. Figure out your refund policy on the cash discount package, and then offer it on a limited pilot basis.
2. Check in with insurance companies to see if this violates any terms of your agreement with them. If not, offer the cash discount package.
3. Do not act on the suggestion for bulk discount sessions. Explain to the chamber of commerce members that psychotherapy is medical treatment and cannot be prequantified into predetermined sessions.
4. Do a combination of the previously listed actions.
5. Do something that is not previously listed.

If you were Dr. Gibson practicing in Spain and had joined your local chamber of commerce and were in receipt of business advice to offer cash discounted bulk sessions, your course of action would be very clear. Your fees must be consistent with other established fees specified by psychologists and in keeping with "normal circumstances." Therefore, you would decline to act on such advice and to decline such an invitation from the chamber of commerce.

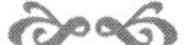

STANDARD 6.04: FEES AND FINANCIAL ARRANGEMENTS

. . . (d) If limitations to services can be anticipated because of limitations in financing, this is discussed with the recipient of services as early as is feasible.

A CASE FOR STANDARD 6.04 (D): Cost Containment

Dr. McDonald signed a contract with a local managed care company. This managed care company oversees Beverly's insurance benefit. The company authorized an initial 12 sessions for the treatment with necessity for a summary report at the end of the 10th session in order to authorize additional sessions. Beverly is a 20-year-old white female who was hospitalized after a suicide attempt. She was discharged from an inpatient hospital 2 days prior to her first appointment with Dr. McDonald. As the sessions progressed, Dr. McDonald realized that Beverly's father owns a large local construction company. At Dr. McDonald's suggestion, Beverly inquired into the contractual relationship between the managed care company and the construction company. Beverly reported her insurance's outpatient benefits package for mental health treatment covers 50 sessions per year with very good reimbursement rates. However, the contract specifies that should reimbursement go beyond 20 sessions per year the managed care company will discuss the case with the construction company's human resources (HR) department. Beverly does not have the financial resources to pay Dr. McDonald's fees without insurance coverage.

Issues of Concern

Standard 6.04 directs Dr. McDonald to discuss the limitations of treatment imposed by financial arrangements as early as possible. Following the directive of Standard 6.04, Dr. McDonald does explore the fees and the insurance arrangements with Beverly. Due to the contractual arrangement between the managed care company and the company paying for the insurance, confidential information would be shared. Should Beverly not wish to expose herself to the risk of having her father knowing of her treatment progress, then Dr. McDonald would need to discuss the limitations of treatment with Beverly.

APA Ethics Code

Companion General Principle

Principle D: Justice

Psychologists recognize that fairness and justice entitle all persons to access to and benefit from the contributions of

> psychology and to equal quality in the . . . services being conducted by psychologists.

Principle D stands on the idea that services from psychologists are not limited to only those with good and confidential insurance coverage or those who can pay out of pocket.

Principle E: Respect for People's Rights and Dignity

> Psychologists respect the . . . rights of individuals to privacy, confidentiality, and self-determination.

Principle E would have Dr. McDonald protect Beverly's right to privacy and confidentiality. Sensitive to practices which compromise a client's right to privacy, Dr. McDonald was right to have Beverly check into the contract between the HMO and the construction company.

Companion Ethical Standard(s)

Standard 10.01: Informed Consent to Therapy

> (a) When obtaining informed consent to therapy[,] . . . psychologists inform clients/patients as early as is feasible in the therapeutic relationship about the . . . fees, involvement of third parties, and limits of confidentiality and provide sufficient opportunity for the client/patient to ask questions and receive answers.

Standard 10.01 requires that Dr. McDonald discuss the fee arrangement with Beverly. Since Beverly is choosing to use her insurance, then Standard 10.01 directs Dr. McDonald to discuss with Beverly the limits of confidentiality in using her insurance.

Standard 4.02: Discussing the Limits of Confidentiality

> (a) Psychologists discuss with persons . . . (1) the relevant limits of confidentiality and (2) the foreseeable uses of the information generated through their psychological activities.

As directed by Standard 4.02, the discussion should include specifics of the avenues through which Beverly's information might be accessible by her father or employees of her father's company without her consent. It is feasible that if the company was large enough and the HR department quite professional, then the HR review of special cases might not compromise confidentiality. However, given that Beverly's father is the head of the company and presumably would have unfettered access to HR reports, it is possible he might wish to know something about how Beverly is doing and request reports from HR regarding exceptions made for extending treatment sessions, thus breaching Beverly's confidentiality.

Standard 4.05: Disclosures

> . . . (b) Psychologists disclose confidential information without the consent of the individual . . . , or where permitted by law for a valid purpose such as to . . . (4) obtain payment for services from a client/patient, in which instance disclosure is limited to the minimum that is necessary to achieve the purpose.

Standard 4.05 allows Dr. McDonald to submit confidential information to the insurance company without consent for specific information for the purpose of obtaining payment. Should the insurance company or the HMO company require very detailed accounts of the sessions then Dr. McDonald would be obligated to provide such information without permission from Beverly.

Standard 6.06: Accuracy in Reports to Payors and Funding Sources

> In their reports to payors for services . . . psychologists take reasonable steps to ensure the accurate reporting of the nature of the service provided . . . , the fees, charges, or payments, and where applicable, the identity of the provider, the findings, and the diagnosis.

Should Beverly continue use of her insurance, Dr. McDonald—as dictated by Standard 6.06—would need to report, at a minimum, dates and type of services provided, findings of treatment, and diagnosis.

Standard 3.12: Interruption of Psychological Services

> Unless otherwise covered by contract, psychologists make reasonable efforts to plan for facilitating services in the event that psychological services are interrupted by factors such as . . . the client's . . . financial limitations.

If Beverly chooses not to use her insurance because of the limits of confidentiality, then Standard 3.12 asks Dr. McDonald to plan for "facilitating services," which in this case would most probably mean a referral to a clinic with a sliding fee scale.

Standard 10.10: Terminating Therapy

> (a) Psychologists terminate therapy when it becomes reasonably clear that the client/patient . . . is being harmed by continued service. . .

> . . . (c) Except where precluded by the actions of . . . third-party payors, prior to termination psychologists provide pre-termination counseling and suggest alternative service providers as appropriate. . .

Standard 10.10 (a) directs Dr. McDonald to have a conversation with Beverly to determine how much harm may come with continued use of her insurance, given the limits of confidentiality accompanying its use. It is likely Dr. McDonald and Beverly may jointly decide that the risk of harm through the breach of confidentiality is too great for continued treatment. Then, echoing the directive of Standard 3.12, Standard 10.10 (c) calls for an orderly and planned transition from Dr. McDonald's service to another provider.

Legal Issues 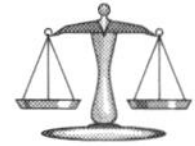

New Mexico

> *N.M. Code R. § 16.22.2.14 (2010). Fees and statements.*
>
> . . . D. Fees and financial arrangements. As early as is feasible in a professional . . . relationship, the psychologist and the patient . . . should reach an agreement specifying the compensation and the billing arrangements.
>
> . . . (2) If limitations to services can be anticipated because of the client's finances, the psychologist should discuss such anticipated limitations with the . . . client.

New Jersey

> *N.J. Admin. Code § 13:42-10.10 (2010). Financial arrangments with clients . . .*
>
> A licensee shall inform clients of the financial arrangements for psychological services. Such financial arrangements should be in writing . . .
>
> 1. . . . (c) Where payment of the usual fee would be a hardship, a licensee may adjust the fee, or shall assist clients to find other sources or make appropriate referrals for provision of the needed services.
>
> *N.J. Admin. Code § 13:42-10.11.1 (2010). Purpose and scope.*
>
> (a) This subchapter . . . limits the scope of and establishes procedures by which clients may authorize licensees to disclose confidential information upon the request of an insurer or other third-party payor . . .
>
> *N.J. Admin. Code § 13:42-10.11.4 (2010). Stage I: Information to be provided to the third party payor.*
>
> (a) A Stage I inquiry. . . The licensee shall provide the information set forth below directly to the third party payor.
>
> (b) Within 10 days of receipt of the authorization required . . . , the treating psychologist shall provide the third party payor with basic client information limited to the following. The information provided shall be marked "Confidential" and forwarded to the attention of the specific individual designated in the authorization, if any.
>
> 1. Administrative information, defined as the client's name, age, sex, address, educational status, identifying number within the insurance program, date of onset of difficulty, date of initial consultation, dates and character of sessions (individual or group) and fees;
>
> 2. Diagnostic information, defined as . . . the type found in . . . the current version of the DSM . . . ;
>
> 3. Status of the client (voluntary or involuntary; inpatient or outpatient);
>
> 4. The reason for continuing psychological services, limited to an assessment of the client's current level of functional impairmant and level of distress. Each aspect shall be described as "none," or by the term mild, moderate, severe or extreme; and
>
> 5. Prognosis, limited to an estimate of the minimal time during which treatment might continue.

If Dr. McDonald was practicing in New Mexico, he would be in compliance with the dictates of New Mexico administrative code. Dr. McDonald would revise the compensation and billing arrangements within his disclosure agreement to address the fact that the managed health care company would have access to the confidences that arose during the services at the end of 20th session.

If Dr. McDonald were practicing in New Jersey, it appears he has to inform the licensing board of the insurance company's request for any information that exceeds what is described in Stage I. It also appears that Dr. McDonald has another entity that reviews the legitimacy of insurance company requesting confidential material. In this case, Dr. McDonald would inform Beverly and the HMO that before any additional information is sent to the HMO, the board will need to be involved.

Cultural Considerations

Global Discussion

Singapore Psychological Society:
Code of Professional Ethics

> Principle 12. Renumeration.
>
> Financial arrangements in professional practice are in accord with professional standards that safeguard the best interest of the client and the profession.

1. In establishing rates for professional services, the psychologist is to consider carefully both the ability of the client to meet the financial burden and the charges made by other professional persons engaged in comparable work.

2. The psychologist in clinical or counselling practice must not take improper financial or other advantage of clients.

3. A psychologist does not accept a private fee or any other form of remuneration for professional work with a person who is entitled to those services through an institution or agency. The policies of a particular agency may make explicit provision for private work with its clients by members of its staff, and in such instances the client must be fully apprised of such policies.

If Dr. McDonald was practicing in Singapore, he has satisfied the mandate of Principle 12:1, wherein he is obligated to set fees which are comparable to other persons in his profession and give careful consideration to the financial impact of treatment on his client, Beverly. It also seems that Dr. McDonald is working very diligently to meet the mandates of Principle 12:2, by not seeking to take financial advantage of clients. However, Dr. McDonald is at risk of violating Principle 12:3, which demands that if a client can have treatment through an agency, then he cannot accept a private fee or other payment for those services. Singapore's code seems to state that if an institution or agency, such as an insurance company, entitles a client to services, than Dr. McDonald is obligated to allow his client to use those services and not take other forms of payment. Moreover, if Beverly is entitled to use her insurance benefit for therapy, then referring her to a low-cost sliding scale clinic may also violate this part of Singapore's code.

American Moral Values

1. How does Dr. McDonald view what he has found out about Beverly's health insurance? Will the contract between her father's company and the managed care company jeopardize her ability to pay if the treatment goes beyond 20 sessions? Will her father owning the company make it likely that his company will pay what they must to get her treatment? What should Dr. McDonald tell Beverly about what to expect from her coverage?
2. How does Dr. McDonald avoid taking advantage of the information he has? Is Beverly reporting her financial resources with her father's resources in mind? Does Dr. McDonald have unfair leverage in some way over the companies?
3. What role does Beverly's suicide attempt play in the decision about fighting for her to get adequate sessions? Given that a family member owns the company through which Beverly is insured, will there be an unreasonable amount of fear that not covering Beverly risks her becoming suicidal again?
4. Are there local implications for Dr. McDonald's treatment and the decision to cover it, given that both companies are local? Are there close-knit connections between people in both companies and Dr. McDonald's practice that could be conduits for information about Beverly's case? How can Dr. McDonald act as fairly and objectively as he would have without knowing the information he now has? Or is it a more important community value to show he recognizes special circumstances and particular people's situation?

Ethical Course of Action

Directive per APA Code

Standard 6.04 (d) requires that Dr. McDonald talk to Beverly about what happens at the end of the first 20 sessions. In this discussion, Standards 10.01 and 4.02 directs Dr. McDonald to address the possibility of Beverly's father having access to the reports Dr. McDonald sends into the insurance company for payment.

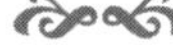

Dictates of One's Own Conscience

If you were Dr. McDonald, what next steps might you take once you found out the reporting arrangement between the HMO and purchasing company?

1. Recommend Beverly end treatment with you and transfer her case to another private psychologist.
2. Recommend Beverly end treatment with you, and refer Beverly to a publicly subsidized clinic with a sliding fee scale.
3. Figure out exactly what information the HMO requires for Beverly to use her insurance to pay for services and submit the sufficient amount of information.
4. Offer Beverly a lower rate to avoid breaching confidentiality by accessing insurance.

5. Enact whatever Beverly wants to do about the potential breach of confidentiality.
6. Contact the HMO to negotiate a special arrangement to access all 50 sessions per year without repeated request for reauthorization.
7. Contact the HR department, and request that no review of this case be conducted due to the identity of the insurer.
8. Do a combination of the previously listed actions.
9. Do something that is not previously listed.

If Dr. McDonald were practicing in Singapore and you found out the reporting arrangement between the HMO and purchasing company, what would you do?

1. Tell Beverly that you have to use her insurance for payment of services.
2. Talk to Beverly about the implications of needing to get reauthorization.
3. Suggest that Beverly talk to her father about the situation and possibly revise the company policy in regards to herself.

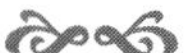

STANDARD 6.04: FEES AND FINANCIAL ARRANGEMENTS

> ... (e) If the recipient of services does not pay for services as agreed, and if psychologists intend to use collection agencies or legal measures to collect the fees, psychologists first inform the person that such measures will be taken and provide that person an opportunity to make prompt payment.

A CASE FOR STANDARD 6.04 (E): Who Is Paying the Bills?

Dr. Cruz was retained to conduct a child custody evaluation. It is his office policy that no reports for custody evaluations are released until all fees are paid in full. Mr. Lawrence and Mrs. Natasha are aware of the payment policy and signed in agreement of the fee arrangement. Dr. Cruz conducted separate psychological evaluations of Mr. Lawrence, the father, and Mrs. Natasha, the child's mother. Mrs. Natasha, a Russian immigrant, needed additional evaluative time. Neither the husband nor the wife objected to incurring the additional cost of Dr. Cruz's time. When the evaluation was completed and the final charges were sent separately to Mr. Lawrence and Mrs. Natasha, Mr. Lawrence paid his portion. Mrs. Natasha reported that Mr. Lawrence would pay for the whole evaluation because she had no source of income. Mr. Lawrence contested, saying he had made no such offer. He thought Mrs. Natasha was playing one more of her tricks to make him look bad, and he refused to be manipulated by her anymore. After 6 months of negotiations that resulted in no additional payment, Dr. Cruz notified Mr. Lawrence and Mrs. Natasha that he intended to turn the account over to a collection agency. In response, Mr. Lawrence countered with an intention to report Dr. Cruz for substandard work because they still had not received a report nearly 7 months after they first started the evaluation.

Issues of Concern

Standard 6.04 (e) addresses one possible course of action should clients not pay their fees. After 6 months of negotiating within the context of a contentious divorce, it is not unreasonable that Dr. Cruz wishes this matter to be brought to a close by handing over the whole thing to a collection agency. Following the specifics of Standard 6.04 (e), Dr. Cruz notifies Mr. Lawrence and Mrs. Natasha that their account will be turned over to a collection agency. Does Mr. Lawrence have any grounds for charges of malpractice?

APA Ethics Code

Companion General Principle

Principle A: Beneficence and Nonmaleficence

> ... Because psychologists' ... professional judgments and actions may affect the lives of others, they are alert to and guard against ... financial ... factors that might lead to misuse of their influence.

Principle A calls Dr. Cruz's attention to consider the effects of his decision to withhold the report. At a minimum, Dr. Cruz has some leverage to get payment for services rendered. In the worst case, withholding the report may delay his former clients' divorce. It is unpredictable how such a delay will affect the well-being of the children.

Principle D: Justice

> Psychologists recognize that fairness and justice entitle all persons to access to and benefit from the contributions of psychology and to equal quality in the processes, procedures, and services being conducted by psychologists.

Has Dr. Cruz upheld the value of justice espoused in Principle D by providing equitable time in the evaluation? By spending equitable time to ensure equal quality, Dr. Cruz may have unfairly penalized Mrs. Natasha by charging her more than Mr. Lawrence. Might it have been fair to charge both husband and wife equal amounts regardless of how much time was spent with whom during the evaluation? Does Dr. Cruz need to consider the possibility that Natasha is in fact unable to pay for services? Might he also consider whether his refusal to provide the custody evaluation disempowers or unwittingly colludes with Mr. Lawrence?

Companion Ethical Standard(s)

Standard 9.03: Informed Consent in Assessments

> (a) Psychologists obtain informed consent for assessments. . . Informed consent includes an explanation of . . . fees . . . and sufficient opportunity for the client/patient to ask questions and receive answers.

Dr. Cruz has complied with the dictates of Standard 9.03 by discussing his fee policy and obtaining a signed agreement for the fee arrangement from both parents.

Standard 6.03: Withholding Records for Nonpayment

> Psychologists may not withhold records under their control that are requested and needed for a client's/patient's emergency treatment solely because payment has not been received.

Given that the current situation with the divorcing couple does not involve emergency treatment for either Mr. Lawrence or Mrs. Natasha and the custody report is probably not crucial even if one of them were in need of emergency treatment, Standard 6.03 holds no sway in this case.

Legal Issues 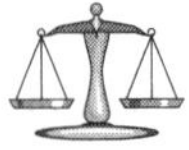

Tennessee

> *Tenn. Code § 63-2-101 (2010). Release of . . . records.*
>
> (a) (1) Notwithstanding any other provision of law to the contrary, a health care provider shall furnish to a patient . . . a copy or summary of such patient's medical records, at the option of the health care provider, within ten (10) working days upon request in writing by the patient or such representative.
>
> (2) If a provider fails to comply with the provisions of subdivision (a)(1), proper notice shall be given to the provider's licensing board or boards, and the provider may be subject to disciplinary actions that include sanctions and a monetary fine.

Texas

> *22 Tex. Admin. Code § 465.15 (2010). Fees and financial arrangements.*
>
> (a) General Requirements.
>
> . . . (3) Licensees shall not withhold records solely because payment has not been received unless specifically permitted by law.
>
> *22 Tex. Admin. Code § 465.18 (2010). Forensic services.*
>
> . . . (c) Describing the Nature of Services. A licensee must document in writing that subject(s) of forensic evaluations . . . have been informed of the following:
>
> . . . (6) The people . . . to whom psychological records will be distributed;
>
> (7) The approximate length of time required to produce any reports or written results. . .
>
> *22 Tex. Admin. Code § 465.22 (2010). Psychological records, test data and test protocols.*
>
> . . . (c) Access to Records and Test Data.
>
> . . . (7) Access to records may not be withheld due to an outstanding balance owed by a client for psychological services provided prior to the patient's request for records. However, licensees may impose a reasonable fee for review and/or reproduction of records and are not required to permit examination until such fee is paid. . .

In Tennessee, it appears that Dr. Cruz would be found in violation of the law if he withheld the records. The defense lawyer for Dr. Cruz may persuade the licensing board that the report is not a health care record but rather a report created for legal purposes. As a result, the defense lawyer would contend the licensing board should not apply the law related to the release of health care records to records created for a legal case. It remains unclear about how the Tennessee licensing board will rule. However, Dr. Cruz could have avoided any ambiguity by only proceeding with the evaluation after an advance fee for the evaluation was provided.

If in Texas, withholding the report is permitted by law. It appears that Dr. Cruz has met the requirements for prior notice to clients requesting forensic services. If Dr. Cruz were practicing in Texas, he might reconsider his plan to refer the case to collection. Such a practice will likely trigger Mr. Lawrence's urge to up the confrontation by reporting Dr. Cruz to the psychology licensing board.

Cultural Considerations

Global Discussion

Singapore Psychological Society:
Code of Professional Ethics

> Principle 12. Renumeration.
>
> Financial arrangements in professional practice are in accord with professional standards that safeguard the best interest of the client and the profession.

The Singapore code is silent on whether or not psychologists are able to release confidential information to an outside agency expressly for the purpose of collecting overdue fees. Provided that Dr. Cruz is safeguarding the "best interest of the client and the profession" by turning this past due account over to an outside agency, he would not be in violation of Singapore's code.

American Moral Values

1. How does Dr. Cruz view his roles in Mr. Lawrence and Mrs. Natasha's situation? Is his main job to procure the money from them, given the nature of their relationship and the opportunity to divert attention from their own troubles with each other? Does Dr. Cruz have any guilt over allowing the divorcing couple to promise the payment in the way they did? Was it not predictable such an arrangement could turn problematic? Does Dr. Cruz feel the need to make up for that? Does he himself feel exploited by Mr. Lawrence and Mrs. Natasha, possibly as a diversion from their own difficulties?
2. Would releasing the report be surrendering to Mr. Lawrence's pressure? What difference would it make if he released the report and sent the matter to the collection agency? Would it change the premise of Mr. Lawrence's complaint?
3. Does Dr. Cruz consider how the couple's children are affected by an ongoing dispute? Should he help to figure out who between Mr. Lawrence and Mrs. Natasha is responsible for the remaining amount? Would that be another session, or should he try to help them in a private conversation? Does that exceed his professional boundaries; if so, how will that affect his career?

Ethical Course of Action

Directive per APA Code

Dr. Cruz has met all requirements of Standard 6.04 (e) in his attempt to obtain payment for services already rendered. After 6 months of negotiating within the context of a contentious divorce, Dr. Cruz may wish to bring the matter to a close by turning the whole thing over to a collection agency. Following the specifics of Standard 6.04 (e), Dr. Cruz notifies Mr. Lawrence and Mrs. Natasha that their account will be turned over to a collection agency. Having followed the directives of Standard 9.03 (a) with a signed fee agreement, the ethics complaint about the evaluation taking too long may not be upheld by the licensing board in light of the fee dispute and the facts surrounding the fee dispute.

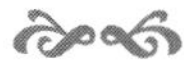

Dictates of One's Own Conscience

If you were Dr. Cruz, given the threat from Mr. Lawrence, regardless of whether Mr. Lawrence has grounds to win a malpractice complaint, what would you do?

1. Knowing that even though Mr. Lawrence has no grounds for winning a case and realizing it may cost you more money to defend against such a charge than the amount owing on the case, decide to call it a loss and turn over the custody report to the divorcing couple.
2. Knowing that you have done nothing wrong, send the file on to the collection agency after noting that such an action will likely result in aggravating the parties and result in an ethics complaint.
3. Decide that the continued holding of the report is delaying the divorce and adversely affecting the children. Release the report and turn the account over to a collection agency after noting that such an action will likely result in aggravating the parties and result in an ethics complaint.
4. Call Mr. Lawrence to discuss payment options that may assist the parents (especially Mrs. Natasha, if she is truly unable to pay) in meeting their obligations.
5. Revise the section of the evaluation based on this new piece of information regarding Mr. Lawrence making a threat.

6. Do a combination of the previously listed actions.
7. Do something that is not previously listed.

If you were Dr. Cruz practicing in Singapore, given the threat from Mr. Lawrence, regardless of whether Mr. Lawrence has grounds to win a malpractice complaint, what would you do?

1. In the best interest of the profession, decide not to send the case to collection to avoid a complaint from being filed in retribution.
2. Do not allow Mr. Lawrence to bully either yourself or his wife, so revise the report with the additional information about Mr. Lawrence's conduct subsequent to the formal forensic evaluation.
3. After the revision, release the report.

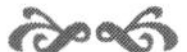

STANDARD 6.05: BARTER WITH CLIENTS/PATIENTS

> Barter is the acceptance of goods, services, or other nonmonetary remuneration from clients/patients in return for psychological services. Psychologists may barter only if (1) **it is not clinically contraindicated**, and (2) the resulting arrangement is not exploitative.

A CASE FOR STANDARD 6.05 (1): A Leaky Toilet

Dr. Ortiz practices in a small town situated in a rural part of the state. For the past year, he has been treating Nicholas, who, among other difficulties, displays a pervasive sense of entitlement that negatively affects his relationships with coworkers and family. Nicholas is $1,000 behind on his bill.

One day after work, Dr. Ortiz arrived home to discover that his upstairs toilet had sprung a leak and flooded the main floor of his house. The insurance adjuster informed him the only approved contractor for flood damage in the area is Nicholas & Co., and the insurance company will cover all expenses after the $500 deductible is paid directly to the contractor. Should Dr. Ortiz elect to engage a nonapproved contractor, whose total fee may be upwards of $5,000, depending on the extent of the damage?

When Dr. Ortiz contacts Nicholas & Co., he discovers the owner is his client, Nicholas. Nicholas assures him of immediate high-quality work, a speedy cleanup of his home, and suggests a barter arrangement in which Dr. Ortiz considers Nicholas's therapy bill paid in full for the insurance deductible.

Issues of Concern

The payment arrangement proposed by Nicholas is one of barter. Standard 6.05 specifies two conditions under which Dr. Ortiz should not enter into a bartering relationship with Nicholas. In this case, bartering may be clinically contraindicated because forgiving $500 of Nicholas's debt to Dr. Ortiz may theoretically play into Nicholas's sense of entitlement. However, what does a psychologist do when living in a rural town with regard to meeting the needs of clients and taking care of his personal life? If Dr. Ortiz does not engage Nicholas & Co., he would end up spending upwards of $5,000 in addition to possibly not collecting on the $1,000 owed by Nicholas. Is it considered a violation of Standard 6.05 if the arrangement exploits the psychologist, not the client? Nicholas essentially wants his $1,000 debt wiped away for what would be a $500 deductible by Dr. Ortiz. This means Dr. Ortiz is out $500, and Nicholas gets a $500 free ride.

APA Ethics Code

Companion General Principle

Principle A: Beneficence and Nonmaleficence

> . . . When conflicts occur among psychologists' . . . concerns, they attempt to resolve these conflicts in a responsible fashion that avoids or minimizes harm.

Would or could the proposed bartering scenario cause a conflict between Dr. Ortiz and Nicholas? Does such a conflict cause the kind of harm that impinges upon the principle of nonmaleficence?

Principle C: Integrity

> . . . Psychologists strive to . . . avoid unwise or unclear commitments.

Implied in the arrangement proposed by Nicholas is a promise from Dr. Ortiz not to seek reimbursement for the remaining $500 that Nicholas owes. Principle C cautions Dr. Ortiz against making unwise or unclear commitments. How might the barter proposed by Nicolas be unwise and/or unclear?

Companion Ethical Standard(s)

Standard 3.05: Multiple Relationships

> (a) A multiple relationship occurs when a psychologist is in a professional role with a person and . . . (3) promises to enter into another relationship in the future with the person. . . A psychologist refrains from entering into a multiple relationship if the multiple relationship could reasonably be expected to impair the psychologist's objectivity, . . . in performing his . . . functions as a psychologist. . . Multiple relationships that would not reasonably be expected to cause impairment . . . are not unethical.

Nicholas and Dr. Ortiz have one existing relationship, that of treating psychologist and patient/client. Nicholas is proposing Dr. Ortiz go into a second relationship with him, that of a homeowner and construction contractor. The current circumstance meets the definition of multiple relationships as defined in Standard 3.05 (a) (3). Per Standard 3.05, such an arrangement is not categorically prohibited. However, Dr. Ortiz is cautioned to refrain from such multiple relationships. It is permissible if Dr. Ortiz believes the arrangement would not impair his objectivity, competence, or effectiveness in his treatment of Nicholas. What are the probabilities the arrangement would not negatively affect Dr. Ortiz's assessment of Nicholas?

Standard 6.04: Fees and Financial Arrangements

> . . . (d) If limitations to services can be anticipated because of limitations in financing, this is discussed with the recipient of services as early as is feasible. . . (e) If the recipient of services does not pay for services as agreed, and if psychologists intend to use collection agencies or legal measures to collect the fees, psychologists first inform the person that such measures will be taken and provide that person an opportunity to make prompt payment.

A debt of $1,000 is sizable. Per the directives of Standard 6.04 (d), most psychologists would be discussing options that may include temporary reduction of session frequency. Since Nicholas has accumulated such a large outstanding debt to Dr. Ortiz, condition for Standard 6.04 (e) now exists. Nicholas is now proposing an arrangement for payment that could forestall Dr. Ortiz from terminating treatment and sending the case to collection.

Legal Issues 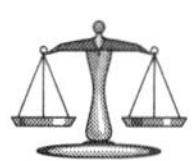

Vermont

> *26 Vt. Stat. § 3016 (2010). Unprofessional conduct.*
>
> . . . (9) Conduct which violates the "Ethical Principles of Psychologists and Code of Conduct" of the American Psychological Association, effective December 1, 1992, or its successor principles and code.

Virginia

> *18 Va. Admin. Code § 125-20-150 (2010). Standards of practice.*
>
> . . . B. Persons licensed by the board shall:
>
> . . . 11. Inform clients of . . . fees [and] billing arrangements . . . before rendering services. Inform the consumer prior to the use of collection agencies or legal measures to collect fees and provide opportunity for prompt payment. Avoid bartering goods and services. Participate in bartering only if it is not clinically contraindicated and is not exploitative . . .

As Vermont adopts the APA Ethics Code in its entirety, the arrangement would be contraindicated in light of Standard 6.05. Virginia's also uses similar language as APA Ethics Code for barter, and the clinical circumstances of the case would indicate that any bartering arrangement would be counter indicated and unethical.

Cultural Considerations

Global Discussion

The Professional Board for Psychology Health Professions Council of South Africa:
Ethical Code of Professional Conduct (April 2002)

> 4.8. Barter with clients.
>
> Barter is the acceptance of . . . services . . . from clients in return for psychological services. Psychologists may barter only if (1) it is not professionally contraindicated, (2) the resulting arrangement is not exploitative, and (3) it is the client's only mode of remuneration for the service provided.

It would appear that because of Nicholas's sense of entitlement it may be clinically unwise to allow this trade to take place. If Nicholas has another way to pay his therapy bill, then Dr. Ortiz would be in violation of South Africa's code by accepting such an arrangement.

American Moral Values

1. Would a barter relationship between Nicholas and Dr. Ortiz harm their client–therapist relationship,

even with a one-time job? Would it in fact be a one-time job, or would Nicholas expect Dr. Ortiz to call on him for similar work in the future? As the only contractor recommended by the insurance company, what if Nicholas & Co. is the only good choice locally? Would this arrangement set a bad precedent, both in coercing Dr. Ortiz to hire Nicholas and possibly feeding Nicholas's sense of entitlement?

2. How would refusing Nicholas's work affect Dr. Ortiz's relationship in the small town? Could it be seen as an un-neighborly action, especially if Nicholas is in trouble financially? Should Dr. Ortiz reflect on the different demands of the professional, detached ethos of the city compared to that of the interconnected, more personally bound system of a small town? Does Dr. Ortiz have strong moral associations about the virtues and faults of each?

3. Does negotiating about any type of work, barter or no, fit with the therapeutic relationship? Is it needlessly competitive? How does it differ from working out a reasonable payment schedule?

4. Does Dr. Ortiz consider his house troubles his personal business? Would he find it appropriate to have a client work on his house? Would it lead to disclosures and vulnerabilities that a client would exploit? Or would it show trust that would help assuage a client with fears about therapists and therapy in general?

Ethical Course of Action

Directive per APA Code

Standard 6.05 directs Dr. Ortiz not to accept Nicholas's barter proposal if it is clinically contraindicated. Accepting Nicholas's proposal meets the condition for Standard 3.5 (a) (3) and thus would place Dr. Ortiz in multiple relationships with Nicholas—one of treating psychologist/patient and another of homeowner/general contractor. The specifics of the arrangement proposed by Nicholas bolster his sense of entitlement, thus would be clinically contraindicated, per Standard 6.05.

However, not accepting Nicolas's proposal could propel them into foreshortened treatment based on financial difficulties, per Standard 6.04 (d) and (e). Such a condition would also be clinically contraindicated. In addition, the financial impact of not engaging Nicholas & Co could potentially cost Dr. Ortiz upwards of $6,000. Arguably this would negatively impact Dr. Ortiz's objectivity in his dealings and treatment of Nicholas.

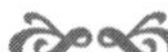

Dictates of One's Own Conscience

If you were Dr. Ortiz, faced with a soggy and quickly molding home and in an exploitative situation, what might you do?

1. Contact the insurance company to discuss further options without revealing the reasons for alternative arrangements.
2. Consider it a cost of doing business in a small town, and pay for repairs out of pocket with another contractor.
3. Consider Nicholas's proposal as "grist for the mill," and discuss evidence of Nicholas exploiting the situation for his own benefit.
4. Decline Nicholas's proposal to commingle two business dealings.
   a. Engage Nicholas & Co. to do the clean-up work, and pay him the $500 deductible.
   b. Engage Nicholas & Co. to do the clean-up work, and continue to seek reimbursement for $1,000.
   c. Engage Nicholas & Co. to do the clean-up work, and offer to deduct $500 from his bill with you.
5. Do a combination of the previously listed actions.
6. Do something that is not previously listed.

If Dr. Ortiz were practicing in South Africa, he would be in violation of 4.8 if he engaged in barter with Nicholas. Thus it is quite clear that Dr. Ortiz needs to decline accepting Nicholas's proposal for barter and engage another company for the repair work.

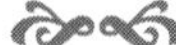

STANDARD 6.05: BARTER WITH CLIENTS/PATIENTS

> Barter is the acceptance of goods, services, or other nonmonetary remuneration from clients/patients in return for psychological services. Psychologists may barter only if (1) it is not clinically contraindicated, and **(2) the resulting arrangement is not exploitative**.

A CASE FOR STANDARD 6.05 (2): A Thank-You Gift

Mary is a psychology intern doing a rotation in a hospital emergency room. She is often called upon to do evaluations in an emergency room setting and then follow up with short-term treatment. The day following a crisis intervention and evaluation of a young girl who was assaulted, the receptionist called Mary to come to the front office. Upon arrival, a large Russian family presented Mary with a compact state-of-the-art TV/DVD for her office. They told Mary they chose the gift knowing the day before Mary had stayed in the emergency room for hours waiting with their daughter. They told Mary, "This is for all those hours you have to spend in the hospital to do your good deed." The interpreter then said to Mary, "The family is very poor so they took great pride in getting enough money to give you such an expensive gift. It is a measure of their appreciation and respect for you and it would be an insult to the family for you not to accept the gift."

Issues of Concern

There are three issues of concern in this situation. One is regarding therapy with clients who are culturally different. The second concerns receiving gifts. The third is regarding barter. In some cultures, goods may be considered an expression of gratitude, an expression of intimacy, a form of payment for services rendered, or a bribe. For some clients, it may be a way to equalize the power imbalance between themselves and the psychologist. The situation calls for Mary to determine how to interpret the gift and whether it is exploitative of the client.

APA Ethics Code

Companion General Principle

Principle E: Respect for People's Rights and Dignity

> Psychologists are aware of and respect cultural, individual, and role differences, including those based on . . . ethnicity, culture, national origin, . . . and socioeconomic status and consider these factors when working with members of such groups.

To abide by the principle of respect for people's rights and dignity, the psychologist in this situation needs to act in such a way so as to be aware that the gift has a different meaning and that the culturally specific meaning of the gift from the client group is of importance. A response that simply states the hospital or the psychologist is not able to accept the gift ignores the cultural aspect of the gift.

Companion Ethical Standard(s)

The APA 2002 Ethical Principles of Psychologists and Code of Conduct does not specifically address gifts, either receiving or giving. Though not part of the APA 2002 Ethical Principles of Psychologists and Code of Conduct, APA does provide for guidelines in providing therapy with clients from different cultural backgrounds.

The APA Guidelines for Providers of Psychological Services to Ethnic, Linguistic, and Culturally Diverse Populations (APA, 1990) Guideline

> **Section 2** (a): Psychologists acknowledge that ethnicity and culture impacts behavior and take those factors into account when working with various ethnic/racial groups.
>
> **Section 4:** Psychologists respect the roles of family members and community structures, hierarchies, values, and beliefs within the client's culture.
>
> **Section 4b:** Clarification of the role of the psychologist and the expectations of the client precede intervention. Psychologists seek to ensure that both the psychologist and client have a clear understanding of what services and roles are reasonable.

Though not part of the code, APA guidelines are of equal importance because guidelines give more specific parameters for treatment of specific populations. The combined directive of 2 (a) and 4 (b) would point to the psychologists need to clarify the cultural significance of the gift.

Legal Issues 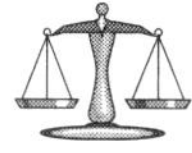

Ohio

> *Ohio Admin. Code 4732:17 (2010). Rules of professional conduct.*
>
> . . . (D) Remuneration
>
> (1) Financial arrangements

> . . . (c) A psychologist . . . shall not exploit a client . . . by entering into an exploitative bartering arrangement in lieu of a fee.
>
> . . . (2) Improper arrangements
>
> (a) A psychologist . . . shall neither derive nor solicit any form of monetary profit or personal gain as a result of his/her professional relationship with clients . . . beyond the payment of fees for psychological services rendered. However, unsolicited token gifts from a client are permissible.

Washington

> *Wash. Admin. Code § 246-924-364 (2009). Fees.*
>
> (1) A psychologist may participate in bartering only if . . .
>
> . . . (b) The bartering relationship is not exploitive.

Neither the Ohio nor the Washington laws specifically address services to culturally diverse clients. Neither does the Washington law address gifts. The one section of the Washington law that might be relevant to the situation in the vignette is related to barter. This section would apply only if the client is engaging in a bartering relationship and believes that the TV/DVD is payment for the services of the psychology intern.

However, Ohio does address gifts. If the psychologist was practicing in Ohio, the psychologist may accept an unsolicited gift. The issue would not be one of whether accepting gifts is permissible but whether a gift that was clearly beyond the means of the giver is consider a "token gift." One should consider that the family was from a society that paid for medical/healer services through gifts and evaluate whether the payment of a TV/DVD was exploitative in terms of whether the equivalent dollar value exceeded what the hospital would have charged the patient for the services rendered the night before in the emergency room.

Cultural Considerations

Global Discussion

Canadian Code of Ethics for Psychologists

> Principle IV. Responsibility to society.
>
> IV.15. Acquire an adequate knowledge of the culture, social structure, and customs of a community before beginning any major work there.
>
> IV.16. Convey respect for and abide by prevailing community mores, social customs, and cultural expectations in their . . . professional activities, provided that this does not contravene any of the ethical principles of this code.

Although it is silent on the issue of barter or of gift-giving, directives regarding cultural and social contexts are included as guiding principles within the main body of the Canadian code. Rather than being a companion standard or aspirational guideline (and thus not enforceable), the CPA seems to be more explicit in their expectations that psychologists consider how culture impacts ethical behaviors. Provided that it does not violate other principles of the code, if Mary was in Canada, she would be obligated to "abide by" the cultural expectations of her client's family and accept the gift.

American Moral Values

1. Does Mary consider gifts to be an expression of intimacy? Does the greater value of the gift indicate a greater degree of intimacy? Would accepting such an expensive gift suggest that Mary is willing to enter into a more intimate relationship with her client's family? Does Mary worry that the client and her family could then expect a greater degree of influence with her?
2. Does Mary consider gifts to be an expression of gratitude, as it is in many cultures? Does the value of the gift indicate the level of appreciation from the giver to the recipient? Could such an expensive gift indicate that the family recognizes the importance of Mary's work for the daughter? Does Mary consider the impact of her decision on how psychologists might be esteemed in a specific ethnic community?
3. Does Mary consider the gift to be a form of payment? Does she judge that the family comes from a barter culture in which goods are accepted as payment for services? What is her responsibility in explaining how gifts are usually not used in this manner in an American medical context?
4. What kind of relationship does Mary believe this gift sets up? Does accepting a gift indicate that one has taken a client's problems seriously—that Mary has taken to heart both the client and her problems? Does refusing a gift cause a loss of respect or trust? Will the family be shamed if the gift is refused? Who best determines whether or not the gift is exploitative or harmful, the family or the psychology intern?

Ethical Course of Action

Directive per APA Code

Standard 6.05 (2) pertains to barter. It is unclear whether the TV/DVD should be considered payment, thus barter, or a gift, would be not applicable for Standard 6.05 (2). If the TV/DVD were considered barter, than it is clearly exploitative of the client if in addition to the cost of the TV/DVD the client would also have to pay the hospital emergency room fee.

If the TV/DVD is considered a gift, then the question to ask oneself is whether the TV/DVD could be considered a token gift, regardless of whether the judgment of token is based on the means of the giver, or on the perception of the receiver.

It is possible that the TV/DVD is, for the Russian family, neither an offer of barter nor a gift. In such, case the APA Guidelines for Providers of Psychological Services to Ethnic, Linguistic, and Culturally Diverse Populations (APA, 1990) directs Mary and the hospital to clarify the cultural significance of the gift.

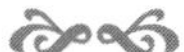

Dictates of One's Own Conscience

If you were Mary, faced with a room full of people, an interpreter, and other hospital staff immediately outside the room, what would you do?

1. Explain to the interpreter that you would get in trouble because it would be considered exploitative for you to accept the gift.
2. Explain that you do not represent the hospital, and ask to be excused so you could call a financial representative of the hospital to discuss the matter with the family.
3. Explain the American value of gifts as indication of intimacy and that it is inappropriate for you to hold an intimate relationship with the family.
4. Discuss and arrive at an agreement with the family regarding the meaning of the gift for the giver and the receiver.
5. Negotiate for a gift of lesser monetary value that may be much more culturally valuable for the hospital, such as a plaque from the community expressing appreciation for the services of the hospital.
6. Do a combination of the previously listed actions.
7. Do something that is not previously listed.

If you were Mary practicing in a hospital in Canada, you would have only one option—to "abide by" the cultural expectations of her clients' family and accept the gift.

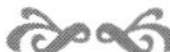

STANDARD 6.06: ACCURACY IN REPORTS TO PAYORS AND FUNDING SOURCES

> In their reports to payors for services or sources of research funding, psychologists take reasonable steps to ensure the accurate reporting of the nature of the service provided or research conducted, the fees, charges, or payments, and where applicable, the identity of the provider, the findings, and the diagnosis.

A CASE FOR STANDARD 6.06: A Dying Wish

Dr. Gomez is working in her first postgraduate job at a cancer care clinic. The first payment of her $150,000 school loan is due now. For the past 9 months, Dr. Gomez has continued to treat Mr. Sam, even though he became nonambulatory and then entered into hospice care. Payment for out-of-office therapy sessions was paid through Mr. Sam's insurance company. Through the work of therapy, Mr. Sam had resolved many of his difficult relationships with his adult children and other family members. He felt very grateful, and one of his wishes before dying was to express that gratitude by giving Dr. Gomez a gift of any amount of money she named. He asked that Dr. Gomez give him an amount of funds she would like. Dr. Gomez replied to Mr. Sam that his insurance and his copay cover reimbursements for her services. In other words, there were no other payments necessary. Mr. Sam replied, "This is my dying wish and you can consider it as a thank you for job well done."

Issues of Concern

Standard 6.06 directs Dr. Gomez to accurately report to Mr. Sam's insurance company the service provided, charges for the services, and any payments made against those charges. Dr. Gomez and Mr. Sam's relationship is purely professional. Would any amount from Mr. Sam to Dr. Gomez need to be reported to the insurance company? Would it be a violation of Standard 6.06 if Dr. Gomez does not report the money from Mr. Sam? Does payment from Mr. Sam fall outside of the situation described in Standard 6.06 since Mr. Sam has specified the money to be a gift and not a payment for services rendered?

APA Ethics Code

Companion General Principle

Principle C: Integrity

> Psychologists seek to promote accuracy, honesty, and truthfulness in the . . . practice of psychology. In these activities psychologists do not . . . engage in . . . subterfuge, or intentional misrepresentation of fact. Psychologists strive to keep their promises and to avoid unwise or unclear commitments . . .

Principle C: Integrity is the underlying value of Standard 6.06. To enact the value of integrity, Dr. Gomez would need to truthfully and accurately represent to all parties all financial interactions between herself, Mr. Sam, and Mr. Sam's insurance company. In addition, she is cautioned against making an unwise commitment to Mr. Sam by agreeing to accept his gift.

Principle E: Respect For People's Rights and Dignity

> Psychologists respect . . . the rights of individuals to . . . self-determination. Psychologists are aware that special safeguards may be necessary to protect the . . . welfare of persons . . . whose vulnerabilities impair autonomous decision making.

Principle E also calls for Dr. Gomez to respect Mr. Sam's right to self-determination in deciding what to do with his money. At the same time, this respect for autonomy needs to be tempered with awareness that vulnerable populations may need special protections. Mr. Sam's situation of being a vulnerable elderly person confronting the end of his life makes him especially susceptible to people who seek personal financial gain at his expense.

Companion Ethical Standard(s)

Standard 6.04: Fees and Financial Arrangements

> (a) As early as is feasible in a professional . . . relationship, psychologists and recipients of psychological services reach an agreement specifying compensation and billing arrangements. . . (b) Psychologists' fee practices are consistent with law. . . (c) Psychologists do not misrepresent their fees.

It appears that Dr. Gomez has already discharged this directive by the note in the vignette that payment for out-of-office therapy sessions was paid through Mr. Sam's insurance company. Presumably Dr. Gomez's charges for psychotherapy sessions are in line with the law of the state or else the insurance company would have objected to fees that were outside the standard and ordinary charges. Would it be a misrepresentation if all of a sudden Mr. Sam is reimbursing Dr. Gomez for services well done, services for which charges have already been made and reimbursement has already been provided to Dr. Gomez?

Standard 3.05: Multiple Relationships

> (a) A multiple relationship occurs when a psychologist is in a professional role with a person and . . . (3) promises to enter into another relationship in the future with the person. . . A psychologist refrains from entering into a multiple relationship if the multiple relationship could reasonably be expected to . . . risk exploitation . . . to the person with whom the professional relationship exists. Multiple relationships that would not reasonably be expected to . . . risk exploitation . . . are not unethical.

Dr. Gomez would be entering into a multiple relationship, as defined by Standard 3.05 (a) (3), if she accepted the offer of a gift from Mr. Sam. While Standard 3.05 does not prohibit entering into a multiple relationship, it does provide some parameters. Standard 3.05 directs Dr. Gomez not to enter into a different relationship with Mr. Sam if it might cause or risk exploitation. Mr. Sam's proposal is an additional role of benefactor to the existing role of patient. Even if Mr. Sam does not see the monetary gift as exploitative, Mr. Sam's children may likely have a different opinion.

Legal Issues 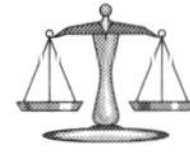

California

> *Cal. Bus. & Prof. Code § 475 (West 2010). Denial, suspension and revocation of licenses.*
>
> (a) Notwithstanding any other provisions of this code, the provisions of this division shall govern the denial of licenses on the grounds of:
>
> . . . (3) Commission of any act involving dishonesty, fraud or deceit with the intent to substantially benefit himself . . .

District of Columbia

> *17 District of Columbia Mun. Reg. § 6909. Code of professional conduct (2010).*

> 6909.1 A licensee . . . or graduate shall adhere to the standards set forth in the . . .
>
> "Ethical Principles of Psychologists and Code of Conduct" as published by the American Psychological Association.

California law is silent about whether a monetary gift from Mr. Sam would be considered payment for services rendered and reportable to the insurance company. If Dr. Gomez did not report Mr. Sam's extra payment, then it would be reasonable to consider the extra money as a gift from Mr. Sam to Dr. Gomez. If Dr. Gomez accepted Mr. Sam's gift, she would be engaging in an act that would substantially benefit herself and would be vulnerable to a licensing board infraction.

District of Columbia law adopts the APA Ethics Code in its entirety; the arrangement would be contraindicated in light of Standard 6.06.

Cultural Considerations

Global Discussion

Code of Ethics New Zealand: Psychological Society

> 4.4. Where information is gathered by a psychologist for use by a third party, the informed consent of those to whom the information refers is obtained and the recipient is informed by the psychologist of the need to protect confidentiality.

Dr. Gomez would be obligated under the New Zealand code to ensure that Mr. Sam has given his consent to having information released to the payor, and Dr. Gomez would need to inform the payor of the need for the safeguarding of Mr. Sam's confidential information. New Zealand's code is silent with regard to the accuracy or completeness of that information to third parties; it only mandates that the information released must be done with full consent and protection of confidentiality.

American Moral Values

1. What is Dr. Gomez's view of gifts from a client to a therapist? Are they acceptable if they are symbolic rather than monetarily valuable? Could Dr. Gomez ask for a very small gift as a mere token of his wish? Should she stay away from money and ask for a small memento or thank-you note that she could promise Mr. Sam she would keep? Would accepting such a gift be a kind act toward Mr. Sam?
2. How should Dr. Gomez think of her position relative to Mr. Sam's family? Could this gesture harm their relationship with their father, even before he dies? Does she have moral judgments about their respective relationships with Mr. Sam? Does she believe they have done enough to support him? Does she believe she was forced to play a role for the whole family, not just Mr. Sam? Could she collaborate with the family to resolve the situation (perhaps by assuring Mr. Sam she would accept something and then assuring the family that she will not accept money after he passes)?
3. Do Dr. Gomez's student loans factor into her moral deliberation? Does her performance merit something over and above her current pay? Does she believe therapists like her are not paid fairly for these kinds of situations? Does she believe the student loan system is unfair?
4. Does Mr. Sam's degree of wealth make a difference as to whether she would ask for a monetary gift? Would she be more or less willing to accept a gift from someone who could afford to give a lot of money? Would it be exploitative to believe that Mr. Sam could afford to give her a large sum and ask for it? Are there ways she could justify using a larger amount of money, such as naming something after Mr. Sam (e.g., a scholarship), when she herself has enough to give to charity?

Ethical Course of Action

Directive per APA Code

Following Principle C: Integrity, if Dr. Gomez considers any monetary payment from Mr. Sam as reimbursement for services rendered, then Dr. Gomez would need to report the payment to Mr. Sam's insurance company, per directive of Standard 6.06.

Following Principle E: Respect for People's Rights, Dr. Gomez would think that Mr. Sam has a right to do with his money as he sees fit. If Dr. Gomez accepts extra money from Mr. Sam and does not report the money as payment from Mr. Sam to the insurance company, then the monetary exchange is considered a gift. Gifts are not subject to the Standard 6.06 directive to report to the insurance company. However, accepting Mr. Sam's monetary gift would more than meet the conditions for multiple relationships as defined in Standard 3.05 (a) (3). If Dr. Gomez were practicing in California, she would be vulnerable to charges of exploitation and subject to denial of license.

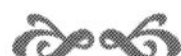

Dictates of One's Own Conscience

If you were Dr. Gomez, faced with large graduate school debt, perhaps a satisfying but not a very well-paying job, and the offer of a large monitory gift, what would you do?

1. Contact the insurance company and discuss how they would consider money from Mr. Sam to Dr. Gomez.
2. Ask Mr. Sam for a memorable but not expensive gift.
3. Contact Mr. Sam's children to discuss Mr. Sam's offer to see if they would consider it exploitative to accept perhaps a large amount of money from Mr. Sam.
4. Knowing the value of satisfying dying wishes, you would do the following:
   a. Tell Mr. Sam about the school loans, and ask that Mr. Sam decide how much to gift you.
   b. Tell Mr. Sam he should decide on the amount and you will accept the money graciously.
5. Do a combination of the previously listed actions.
6. Do something that is not previously listed.

If you were Dr. Gomez working in New Zealand, faced with large graduate school debt, perhaps a satisfying but not a very well-paying job, and the offer of a large monetary gift, what would you do?

1. Ask Mr. Sam for consent to report the offer of the gift to the insurance company.
2. If Mr. Sam does not give consent for release of such information, do not report additional monetary exchange to the insurance company.
3. Dr. Gomez should report the additional monetary payment from Mr. Sam to the insurance company.

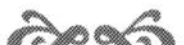

STANDARD 6.07: REFERRALS AND FEES

> When psychologists pay, receive payment from, or divide fees with another professional, other than in an employer–employee relationship, the payment to each is based on the services provided (clinical, consultative, administrative, or other) and is not based on the referral itself.

A CASE FOR STANDARD 6.07: Slicing the Pie?

Dr. Murray is a newly licensed psychologist who has moved to a new city to join a large group practice. The group practice partners keep 60% of fees collected by all members of the group for joint practice expenses. The joint expenses of the group practice consist of capital equipment, administrative staff who also does all of the client/insurance billing, a psychometrist who conducts intake sessions, and a marketing person who generates contracts and referrals.

As part of outreach to build his practice, Dr. Murray advertises to psychology students who are required to engage in personal therapy. He provides a discounted student rate of $50 per hour without insurance. Dr. Murray reasons that he generates the referrals for students, no insurance is billed, and neither group intake nor testing is done. Therefore the 60%/40% split for fees collected is unnecessary. Thus Dr. Murray has been keeping all of the fees generated from the discounted student sessions.

Issues of Concern

Standard 6.07 makes a distinction between fee splitting for services, such as use capital equipment or shared administrative staff versus fee splitting for referrals, which is considered in the same light as kickbacks. Fee splitting for services is ethical; kickback arrangements are not ethical. The arrangement described in the previous vignette is for services shared by the members of the group. Dr. Murray reasons that if he does not use these shared services, than he does not need to reimburse the group practice by splitting the fees collected from his client. Does this kind of reasoning fall under the purview of Standard 6.07? Would Dr. Murray's office partners think his reasoning was just?

APA Ethics Code

Companion General Principle

Principle A: Beneficence and Nonmaleficence

> When conflicts occur among psychologists' obligations . . . , they attempt to resolve these conflicts in a responsible fashion that avoids or minimizes harm. . .

Dr. Murray does not appear to have a conflict with his fee arrangements. However, his practice partners may perceive him to have fallen short of his obligation of paying for shared administrative services of the office. Could Dr. Murray's behavior in this situation be harmful to the other psychologists in the practice?

Principle B: Fidelity and Responsibility

> Psychologists establish relationships of trust with those with whom they work. They are aware of their professional . . . responsibilities . . . to the specific communities in which they work. Psychologists uphold professional standards of conduct, clarify their professional . . . obligations, accept appropriate responsibility for their behavior, and seek to manage conflicts of interest that could lead to exploitation or harm . . .

The community of concern in this vignette is the other psychologist with whom Dr. Murray works. It does not foster an atmosphere of trust when not everyone in the practice is contributing equally. Does Dr. Murray need to clarify his financial obligations to the practice group? Has Dr. Murray managed the conflict of interest between upholding his fiduciary responsibility to the group verses needing to increase his earnings?

Companion Ethical Standard(s)

Standard 1.04: Informal Resolution of Ethical Violations

> When psychologists believe that there may have been an ethical violation by another psychologist, they attempt to resolve the issue by bringing it to the attention of that individual . . .

Members of Dr. Murray's practice may consider his withholding payment for services to be in violation of his group obligation and in violation of the principle of fidelity and responsibility. If this is true, then the members of his group practice should bring this to his attention as directed by Standard 1.04.

Standard 3.06: Conflict of Interest

> Psychologists refrain from taking on a professional role when . . . financial . . . interests . . . could reasonably be expected to (1) impair their objectivity . . . in performing their functions as psychologists or (2) expose . . . [the] organization with whom the professional relationship exists to harm or exploitation.

It could certainly be argued that Dr. Murray's interest in increasing his own personal income is in conflict with his obligations as a professional member of the group practice and is exploitative of the other members of the group. If Dr. Murray was aware of the possibility that by recruiting and accepting doctoral students as clientele at a reduced fee would lead him to alter his fee-sharing arrangement, it would also impair his objectivity about his relationship with the other group members and exploit their office-sharing arrangement. Might it be argued that he should have refrained from seeking that market, per the directive of Standard 3.06?

Legal Issues 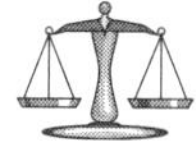

Hawaii

> *Haw. Code R. § 16-98-34 (2010). Unethical practice of psychology.*
>
> . . . (h) A psycholgist shall act with integrity in regard to colleagues in psychology. . .
>
> . . . (2) The welfare of . . . colleagues requires that psychologists in joint practice . . . make an orderly and explicit arrangement regarding the conditions of their association. . .
>
> (i) Financial arrangements in professional practice shall be in accord with professional standards that safeguard the best interest of the client and the profession:
>
> . . . (2) The psychologist in clinical or counseling practice shall not use relationships with clients to promote commercial enterprises of any kind for personal gain. . .

Indiana

> *868 Ind. Admin. Code 1.1-11-4 (2010). Professional practice; fees.*
>
> Sec. 4.
>
> . . . (e) A psychologist shall not divide a fee for professional services with any individual who is not a partner, employee, or shareholder in a corporation operating the psychology service unless:
>
> (1) the patient or client consents after full disclosure; and
>
> (2) the division of fees is made in proportion to the actual services performed and the responsibility assumed by each practitioner.

In Hawaii, Dr. Murray has not acted with integrity by failing to arrive at an arrangement with the group practice partners in regards to how he has treated his colleagues. If in Indiana, the group practice partners may have overreached by taking the vast percentage of the fee. The licensing board would likely entertain expert opinions about expenses in similar practices to determine whether the law was violated and the group practice partners overreached in their arrangement with Dr. Murray. No law exists in Indiana about whether Dr. Murray should have informed the group partners about his arrangement with the students.

Cultural Considerations

Global Discussion

Code of Ethics for the Psychologist: Spain

> ***Article 60.*** Psychologists must never receive any remuneration related to the passing of clients to other professionals.

Although Spain's code does not specifically address the "passing" of clients to one's self or keeping fees generated, it is likely that Dr. Murray would be in violation of the intent of the Spanish code in this instance. As he is generating his own referrals but works in a group setting where all fees are to be shared, Dr. Murray is "passing clients" to himself and receiving a fee for doing so; thus his actions place him in direct conflict with the intent and letter of this portion of the Spanish code.

American Moral Values

1. How does Dr. Murray separate his treatment of these graduates from normal services and fees for the practice? How do referrals, billing to insurance, and group testing make a difference for the fees he collects? Does Dr. Murray believe obtaining clients is the most important reason he benefits from joining the practice?
2. Does Dr. Murray's work with these graduate students involve office work from the practice's staff? Does someone handle the money he receives? Do they benefit from the 60%/40% split? Should they not get paid for those activities?
3. Would the partners approve of Dr. Murray using his office time to see patients whom he exempts from the agreed-upon percentage of fee distribution? What are the larger expectations between colleagues in the practice? Do other colleagues treat people with no insurance or special deals?
4. Does Dr. Murray's arrangement give him an incentive to continue treating these graduate students? Do they become moneymakers for him, or is his fee a courtesy deal he wants to extend as a help to students?

Ethical Course of Action

Directive per APA Code

Dr. Murray pays the other professionals in his group practice for shared expenses of administrative staff. This arrangement is deemed ethical as specified by Standard 6.07. Dr. Murray argues that if the clients he sees do not use the services of those shared administrative staff then he should not pay for those services. If he was practicing in Indiana, his line of reasoning would be supported by the law. If he were not practicing in either Hawaii or Indiana, he may be perceived as reneging on prior obligations and violating Standard 3.06 for not monitoring his actions so as to guard against eviscerating the agreement he practices under. Certainly Dr. Murray has violated the spirit of Principle B: Fidelity and Responsibility.

Dictates of One's Own Conscience

If you were a member of the group practice that invited Dr. Murray and you discovered his practice of withholding the agreed upon 60% of client fees for those graduate student clients, what would you do?

1. Per directive of Standard 1.04, approach Dr. Murray directly to attempt informal resolution.
2. Examine the validity of his reasoning. If indeed he does not use any group resources, then support a change in policy.
3. Reason that it is impossible to see clients without utilizing shared resources, at a minimum the office/heat/light, and consider Dr. Murray to be in violation of agreed-upon practice responsibilities.
4. Do a combination of the previously listed actions.
5. Do something that is not previously listed.

If you were practicing in Spain, you would have to resolve this matter without the guidance of the profession since Spain's code is silent on the matter of fee splitting.

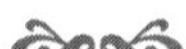

CHAPTER 7

Education and Training

Ethical Standard 7

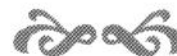

CHAPTER OUTLINE

- Standard 7.01: Design of Education and Training Programs
- Standard 7.02: Descriptions of Education and Training Programs
- Standard 7.03: Accuracy in Teaching
- Standard 7.04: Student Disclosure of Personal Information
- Standard 7.05: Mandatory Individual or Group Therapy
- Standard 7.06: Assessing Student and Supervisee Performance
- Standard 7.07: Sexual Relationships With Students and Supervisees

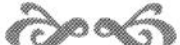

STANDARD 7.01: DESIGN OF EDUCATION AND TRAINING PROGRAMS

> Psychologists responsible for education and training programs take reasonable steps to ensure that the programs are designed to provide the appropriate knowledge and proper experiences and to meet the requirements for licensure, certification, or other goals for which claims are made by the program.

A CASE FOR STANDARD 7.01: What Do You Mean I'm Not Done Yet?

The Modern School of Professional Psychology has started a branch campus in another state. The school has replicated their standard curriculum. The school claims the program meets all requirements for American Psychological Association (APA) accredited clinical psychology programs, and students enrolled are eligible for state licensure upon graduation. The specific state licensure requirements are different from the home state of the Modern School of Professional Psychology. The home state requires a total number of supervised experience hours regardless of whether the hours are accrued at the pre- or postdoctoral level. The licensure in the new state specifically requires postdoctoral hours, regardless of the number of predoctoral experience hours. This semantic difference has generated some confusion and frustration among the students and the school. The students claim they have been misled to think they were eligible for licensure upon graduation. Conversely, the school claims they have not misled the students, and the statement that students upon graduation are eligible for licensure is accurate.

Issues of Concern

Standard 7.01 informs psychologists who are responsible for design of training programs to make sure students receive the knowledge and experience necessary for licensure. In this vignette, the credential in question is that of eligibility for state licensure. To meet the criterion set by Standard 7.01, the Modern School of Professional Psychology should have as requirement for graduation everything necessary for the students to be "eligible for state licensure upon graduation." It appears that the stated requirements for experience hours are different for the home campus and the new campus. Should the Modern School of Professional Psychology change their program design to meet the licensure requirements for each different campus in each state? Does the equivocation of "eligible" for licensure meet the directive of Standard 7.01?

APA Ethics Code

Companion General Principle

Principle C: Integrity

> Psychologists seek to promote accuracy . . . in the . . . teaching . . . of psychology. In these activities psychologists do not . . . engage in . . . intentional misrepresentation of fact.

Principle C would suggest psychologists who design training programs are upright citizens of the profession. The Modern School of Professional Psychology in keeping to a program design that has received accreditation from its home campus state is offering something that has produced good results. With the best of intentions, this same program claims that it may be less than accurate—at the very least misleading.

Principle B: Fidelity and Responsibility

> . . . They are concerned about the ethical compliance of their colleagues' . . . professional conduct. . .

It is not unusual that psychologists who are responsible for the design of a program are not involved in the development of public statements for advertisement of the program. Principle B suggests that psychologists working at the Modern School of Professional Psychology take responsibility for the school's marketing material.

Companion Ethical Standard(s)

Standard 5.01: Avoidance of False or Deceptive Statements

> (a) Public statements include . . . brochures [and] printed matter. . . Psychologists do not knowing[ly] make public statements that [are] . . . deceptive . . . concerning their . . . work activities or . . . organizations with which they are affiliated.

Standard 5.01 (a) makes it clear that if psychologists who work in the Modern School of Professional Psychology are responsible for or have oversight of any aspect of the program development and/or advertisement that they need to be meticulously accurate so as to avoid seeming deceptive.

Standard 5.02: Statements by Others

> Psychologists who engage others to create . . . public statements that promote their professional . . . activities retain professional responsibility for such statements.

Even as psychologists are not responsible for the development of marketing material to prospective students, Standard 5.02 does not absolve psychologists working for the Modern School of Professional Psychology from their ethical responsibility.

Standard 1.04: Informal Resolution of Ethical Violations

> When psychologists believe that there may have been an ethical violation by another psychologist, they attempt

to resolve the issue by bringing it to the attention of that individual if an informal resolution appears appropriate and the intervention does not violate any confidentiality rights that may be involved.

Presuming the faculty of the psychology program does not have absolute authority over all aspects of the school, Standard 1.04 directs psychologists to voice their objections if they see any violations. It may be that the admissions or marketing personnel were simply using the same tried and true advertising language when the Modern School of Professional Psychology used the phrase "eligible for state licensure upon graduation." It is also quite possible that neither the staff nor the faculty fully understand the nuanced differences between the two state's licensure requirements. Regardless, Standard 1.04 requires that those psychologists who did understand the nuanced differences bring the problem to the attention of whoever does have authority over advertisement material.

Legal Issues 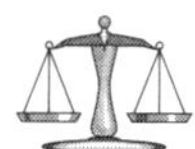

Illinois

Ill. Admin. Code tit. 68, § 1400.80 (2010). Unethical, unauthorized, or unprofessional conduct.

The Department may . . . take other disciplinary action, based upon its finding of "unethical, unauthorized, or unprofessional conduct" . . . to include, but is not limited to, the following acts or practices:

. . . h) The commission of any dishonest, corrupt, or fraudulent act which is substantially related to the functions or duties of a psychologist providing services or supervising psychological services . . .

Kansas

Kan. Admin. Regs. § 102-1-10a (2010). Unprofessional conduct.

. . . (h) misrepresenting the services offered or provided, which shall include the following acts:

. . . (4) knowingly engaging in fraudulent or misleading advertising . . .

In both jurisdictions, the licensing boards would find that the lack of clarity of the marketing statement " . . . upon graduation students are eligible for licensure) is accurate was misleading because of the knowledge about what the licensing laws required in the way of hours and how the program failed to meet that threshold. By not changing the marketing materials to correct the impression left by such a statement, the faculty members are likely to be viewed as acting unethically.

Cultural Considerations

Global Discussion

The Professional Board for Psychology Health Professions Council of South Africa: Ethical Code of Professional Conduct (April 2002)

9.1 Design of education and training programmes.

Psychologists responsible for education and training programmes shall seek to ensure that the programmes . . . provide the proper experiences, and meet the requirements for competency for which claims are made by the programme.

If a psychology program is being designed in South Africa, those responsible for doing so must "ensure" that the program is designed to provide sufficient experience to meet the competency and requirements that it claims to do. Therefore, if such a program claims that it is designed to allow graduates to be eligible for licensure upon its completion, it must be "competently" designed enough to do so.

American Moral Values

1. How does the school interpret its statement about eligibility for licensure? How does their published materials and recruitment speakers interpret "eligible" and "upon graduation"?
2. Is the school assuming that postdoctoral hours are students' responsibility? Do other schools make that assumption? Was it reasonable to expect students to make the same assumption in interpreting the requirements?
3. Is the school getting away with a deceptive description? Should it add a qualifying phrase about postdoctoral experience, at least for students in this state?
4. What should school representatives do about current students? What would be the best way to acknowledge and address their resentment? How should school officials anticipate this issue affecting student–administration relations on other issues?

5. What steps do students feel they are entitled to take to improve their situation? What kind of action preserves their professional standing? What action represents their interests more generally?

Ethical Course of Action

Directive per APA Code

Standard 7.01 addresses two areas of student's training: knowledge and experience. For the Modern School of Professional Psychology, Standard 7.01 establishes the criteria of student's training meet requirements for licensure in the state that the program is located. Standard 7.01 directs psychologists to "take reasonable steps" for ensuring that the design of the program meets requirements for licensure. To comply with the dictates of Standard 7.01 and Standard 1.04, those psychologists working in the Modern School of Professional Psychology should, at a minimum, have alerted the school to the needed program changes. Aspiring to the principle of integrity, psychologists would ensure that the new branch campus had a different curriculum, one that required a greater number of experienced hours before graduation. If the new branch campus was located in Illinois or Kansas, psychologists working there are at risk for violating administrative code and should disengage association with the program unless the public statement regarding licensure is changed.

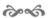

Dictates of One's Own Conscience

If you were working at the Modern School of Professional Psychology and were faced with the disgruntlement of the students, what would you do?

1. As faculty teaching in the psychology program, you would do as follows:
   a. Sympathize with the students.
   b. Direct the students to the dean.
   c. Tell the students that you have nothing to do with university marketing.
   d. Advise the students to take on a greater number of experience hours, regardless of the graduation requirements.
   e. Raise the problem with the marketing department.
   f. Suggest that the program be redesigned to fulfill the necessary experience hours in the state for licensure.
2. As a student in the psychology program, you would do as follows:
   a. Complain to fellow students.
   b. Raise the concern with your faculty advisor.
   c. Raise the concern with the dean.
   d. File a formal grievance, and demand compensation for the fact that you have done everything required for graduation and are still not eligible for licensure.
3. As a psychologist responsible for program design, you would do as follows:
   a. Alert the marketing department to the problem.
   b. Request that new recruitment material be developed that does not use possibly misleading language.
   c. Convene a work group to redesign the degree program so students do meet all licensure requirements at graduation.
4. Do a combination of the previously listed actions.
5. Do something that is not previously listed.

If you had designed the program in South Africa, which would you do?

1. Revise the program's advertising materials so that they do not claim to render graduates "license eligible" upon graduation.
2. Change the program requirements to ensure they include all of the necessary supervised clinical hours required for licensure eligibility.

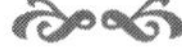

STANDARD 7.02: DESCRIPTIONS OF EDUCATION AND TRAINING PROGRAMS

Psychologists responsible for education and training programs take reasonable steps to ensure that there is a current and accurate description of the program content (including participation in required course- or program-related counseling, psychotherapy, experiential groups, consulting projects, or community service), training

> goals and objectives, stipends and benefits, and requirements that must be met for satisfactory completion of the program. This information must be made readily available to all interested parties.

A CASE FOR STANDARD 7.02: The Missing Professor

The Modern School of Professional Psychology is proud of their nationally renowned forensic psychology concentration that has been going for the past 2 years. This is a wildly popular focus track and has been generating strong interest from top-notch applicants. Recruitment and all other published material prominently mention the training sequence. A substantial number of students have chosen the program specifically to receive training from Dr. Dunn. He is the nationally known forensic psychologist. All is going well until the sudden death of Dr. Dunn in a diving accident during the summer holiday. Upon learning of Dr. Dunn's death, Dr. Perkins, the chair of the department, realized she must communicate with the faculty and the current student body regarding this tragedy. As she was outlining her public statement, the head of the admissions department came in with a mock-up design of the next year's marketing materials for the psychology program. Prominently featured in the materials are Dr. Dunn and several of his students, who are quoted as saying very positive things about the forensic concentration. The head of admissions reminded the chair that these materials must be approved for printing by the end of this week, and any changes to them at this point, other than small edits, could result in thousands of dollars of wasted time and materials and greatly delay the advertising material that the program sorely needs.

Issues of Concern

Standard 7.02 asks the Modern School of Professional Psychology to have "a current and accurate description of the program content." Presumably all published material includes a description of the forensic track. Also, presumably students are in the forensic track pipeline in order to meet graduation requirements. However, would allowing next year's marketing material to go to press with Dr. Dunn prominently featured violate Standard 7.02? Is it possible for Dr. Perkins to stop the publication of the marketing material?

In addition, through no fault of the Modern School of Professional Psychology, they are now unable to implement the program as described. Furthermore, the students are now unable to engage in the forensic training and graduate in a timely manner. Has the Modern School of Professional Psychology violated the directives of Standard 7.02?

APA Ethics Code

Companion General Principle

Principle C: Integrity

> Psychologists seek to promote accuracy . . . and truthfulness in the . . . teaching . . . of psychology. In these activities psychologists do not . . . engage in . . . intentional misrepresentation of fact.

Integrity guides psychologists to assure published materials are accurate. Through no fault of their own, the Modern School of Professional Psychology is now in a position where they cannot fulfill the obligation of offering the forensic courses uninterrupted. Does Principle C now guide psychologists to take further steps in their efforts to meet their responsibility to the students?

Companion Ethical Standard(s)

Standard 7.01: Design of Education and Training Programs

> Psychologists responsible for education and training programs take reasonable steps to ensure that the programs are designed to provide the appropriate knowledge and proper experiences, and to meet the requirements for licensure, certification, or other goals for which claims are made by the program.

Should the program have built in a redundancy design to ensure that students receive the knowledge and experience necessary to graduate? Does Standard 7.01 pertain to program design and not to timely offering of courses and experience placements that ensure unencumbered progress through the degree plan?

Legal Issues 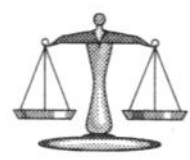

Kentucky

> *201 Ky. Admin. Regs. 26:145 (2010). Code of conduct.*
>
> . . . Section 8. Representation of Services.

> ... (4) False or misleading information. The credential holder shall not include false or misleading information in a public statement concerning professional services offered.

Maryland

> *Md. Code Regs. 10.36.05.05 (2010). Representation of services and fees.*
>
> (2) A psychologist may not:
>
> ... (c) Make public statements that contain:
>
> (i) False, fraudulent, misleading, or deceptive statements;
>
> (ii) Partial disclosures of relevant facts that misrepresent, mislead, or deceive; or
>
> (iii) Statements that create false or unjustified expectations of favorable results ...

Unfortunate events happen—events that are beyond anyone's control. And when such a tragic event as the death of a faculty member occurs, it is understandable that published statements released prior to the accident would not accurately reflect the current circumstances. The school would not be deemed at fault for its inability to provide current students with the type of training claimed in the printed material at the time of their admissions. However, if the school were in Kentucky or in Maryland, the inclusion of Dr. Dunn in the publication of next year's marketing material would likely be deemed misleading at best.

Cultural Considerations

Global Discussion

Hong Kong Psychological Society:
Professional Code of Practice

> Chapter 5: Teaching and training in psychology.
>
> 5.5. Members must make every effort to ensure that published information concerning any educational programme in which they have a teaching or organizing role is accurate and not misleading, especially with respect to expectations of and possible benefits to participants.

If this situation had occurred in Hong Kong, through no foreseeable fault of its own, the program's administration would find itself in violation of this portion of code. At the time the information regarding the forensic program was published, it was accurate and contained relevant information regarding the "possible benefits" to the students, namely, studying with a renowned expert in the field of forensic psychology. However, with the death of Dr. Dunn and the future of the forensic program now uncertain, the administration is called upon to correct the published information regarding the program or risk being out of compliance with this portion of code. Hong Kong's code does not specify how or to what extent "every effort" must be made but only that program administrators do so.

American Moral Values

1. Where does the Modern School of Professional Psychology draw the line between promoting the school and its programs and promoting an individual instructor? Does Dr. Dunn's death make their promotional material false in terms of ranking, popularity, etc.? Assuming they publish new material for applicants, what can they promote about their program that is still true? Are there values, principles, and interests that the program will continue to pursue?
2. What do new applicants deserve in terms of disclosure of this news? Would announcing it on the school's website be sufficient, or should the school e-mail those who have applied already?
3. Where does student responsibility lie in this case? Is it fair to expect that students stay informed about the programming at the schools to which they apply—especially when they make final decisions about where to attend? Is it reasonable for them to be expected to check in with the school before they accept in order to make sure nothing has happened to the faculty that had attracted them to the school?
4. Had the school hired a superstar professor in another program, would they have edited material in order to announce that fact? If not, could the school fairly say that "things happen" sometimes for the better or sometimes for the worse?
5. Have websites and other electronic media changed the standards for the question of publicity and promotion? Could applicants get a newsfeed in order to be assured they are receiving up to the minute news from the school? How quickly would the school be expected to announce this news?

Ethical Course of Action

Directive per APA Code

Standard 7.02 asks the Modern School of Professional Psychology to have "a current and accurate description of the program content," which it does.

Standard 7.02 does not address the manner or the timeliness in which the Modern School of Professional Psychology implement the program as described in their materials. Even if the reason for why the students are not able to engage in the forensic training were under the school's control (such as the untimely death of Dr. Dunn), the Modern School of Professional Psychology has not violated the directives of Standard 7.02.

If the institution allows next year's published marketing material to include Dr. Dunn in the program, then Dr. Perkins would be in violation of Standard 7.02.

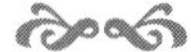

Dictates of One's Own Conscience

If you were Dr. Perkins, faced with the untimely accidental death of Dr. Dunn, what would you do about previous printed material and next year's marketing material?

1. Send notification to all current students through established channels for announcements to the students and to other members of the university of Dr. Dunn's accident.
2. Correct previously printed material regarding course offerings by notifying students enrolled in Dr. Dunn's course for the next quarter regarding cancellation of the course and the reasons for such cancellation
3. Request that all web-based material related to Dr. Dunn's participation in the training program be revised to accurately reflect the fact that Dr. Dunn is no longer with the university.
4. Reason that the marketing material for next year is essentially in press and that regardless of whether Dr. Dunn is teaching or not, the program will continue to have forensic psychology classes, therefore approve next year's marketing material as is.
5. Reason that next year's marketing material will be published after Dr. Dunn's accidental death is known, thus request that the marketing material for next year be modified to accurately reflect current faculty.
6. Do a combination of the previously listed actions.
7. Do something that is not previously listed.

Dr. Perkins, working in Hong Kong, to comply with Chapter 5.5 of the ethics code, would need to notify her superior, most probably the dean, to correct current and future published information regarding the program.

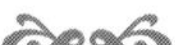

STANDARD 7.03: ACCURACY IN TEACHING

(a) Psychologists take reasonable steps to ensure that course syllabi are accurate regarding the subject matter to be covered, bases for evaluating progress, and the nature of course experiences. This standard does not preclude an instructor from modifying course content or requirements when the instructor considers it pedagogically necessary or desirable, so long as students are made aware of these modifications in a manner that enables them to fulfill course requirements.

A CASE FOR STANDARD 7.03 (A): Understandable Modifications

Dr. Hudson is an assistant professor in a clinical psychology program. She teaches a practicum seminar with a maximum enrollment size of five students. At the end of the first day of classes, three students each individually requested to drop the class and requested that the program add another section of the practicum seminar for them. Upon inquiry, the students separately said that they felt uncomfortable being in such an intense class with Emily, an African American student in the class who was always bringing up race and discrimination. The school informed the students that adding another section after the start of a semester is not possible. Dr. Hudson informed the students that not only is the course required for graduation but she is changing the syllabus for the three students who had requested to transfer to another section. For those three students, there would be two additional assignments that would involve (1) writing a paper examining the manifestations of institutional racism in psychology programs and (2) keeping and then submitting a weekly ongoing journal of their daily personal experience about their acts of racial micro-aggressions in general and specifically against the one African American student in their program.

Issues of Concern

Standard 7.03 (a) requires that course syllabi include the content that will be covered and how students will be evaluated. Standard 7.03 (a) allows for changes in syllabi as long as those changes are designed and communicated to students in such a manner that students are able to successfully fulfill the requirements of the course. Dr. Hudson engaged in two changes. She changed the requirements of the class, but then she intended to apply the changes selectively to three of the five enrolled students. Is the addition of the paper for only three students ethical? Does Standard 7.01 (a) allow Dr. Hudson to require different assignments based on the differences in student's levels of competency? Is the addition of a paper for only three students punitive? Or is it pedagogically necessary?

APA Ethics Code

Companion General Principle

Principle E: Respect for People's Rights and Dignity

> . . . Psychologists are aware of and respect cultural . . . and role differences, including those based on . . . race, ethnicity, culture . . . and consider these factors when working with members of such groups. Psychologists try to eliminate the effect on their work of biases based on those factors, and they do not knowingly participate in or condone activities of others based upon such prejudices.

Dr. Hudson is called upon to respect the role differences between professor and student. At the same time, Dr. Hudson is to respect individuals, who are those enrolled in her class, regardless of race, ethnicity, and culture. In this vignette, Dr. Hudson is called upon to work with two different ethical conundrums: (1) engaging the culture of racism exhibited in the request of the three students and (2) finding ways of redirecting the student's activities that are based on racial prejudice so the rights and dignity of all can be furthered.

Companion Ethical Standard(s)

Standard 3.04: Avoiding Harm

> Psychologists take reasonable steps to avoid harming their . . . students . . . and to minimize harm where it is foreseeable and unavoidable.

More likely than not, the program and faculty espouse the idea that it is good for the European American students to have minority students in the classroom so the white students are exposed to diversity. It is unclear as to whether it is of benefit for non–European American students to be in a classroom with European American students who discriminate based on race. Will being in the seminar with the three students who do not want to be in the same class with her because of race harm Emily? Would it be less harm to Emily if she were given a choice to choose a different seminar section so she would not have to endure the foreseeable difficulties?

Standard 3.01: Unfair Discrimination

> In their work-related activities, psychologists do not engage in unfair discrimination based on . . . race, ethnicity, culture, . . . or any basis proscribed by law.

Standard 3.01 reflects Principle E: Respect. Standard 3.01 directs Dr. Hudson not to engage in unfair discrimination based on culture. Is it permissible for Dr. Hudson to engage in discrimination that is based on the U.S. culture of racism but only if the discrimination is fair and justified? The justification for differential assignments may be to uphold Standard 3.01, Standard 3.04, and Principle E. Arguably, the fairness of assigning different assignments is based on sound pedagogy.

Standard 2.01: Boundaries of Competence

> . . . (b) Where scientific or professional knowledge in the discipline of psychology establishes that an understanding of factors associated with . . . race, ethnicity [and] culture . . . is essential for effective implementation of their services . . . , psychologists have or obtain the training, experience, consultation, or supervision necessary to ensure the competence of their services. . .

If the term *service* as used in Standard 2.01 (b) includes teaching, then Dr. Hudson is required to be competent in teaching the subject content of the practicum seminar, and the students, inclusive of African Americans at the graduate level. All programs are cognizant of needing to have faculty who are competent to teach the content area, thus it is safe to assume that Dr. Hudson is properly credentialed with commensurate experience to teach the practicum seminar. Most graduate programs do not think teaching non–European American students requires special training. If Dr. Hudson has not had special training to teach non–European American students or has not sought consultation or supervision to develop her competency, then Dr. Hudson would be in violation of Standard 2.01 (b).

Legal Issues 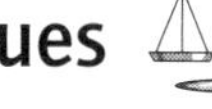

Michigan

Mich. Admin. Code r. 338.2515 (2010). Prohibited conduct.

Rule 15. Prohibited conduct includes, but is not limited to, the following acts or omissions by any individual covered by these rules:

(a) Engaging in harassment or unfair discrimination based on . . . race, ethnicity, culture, . . . or any basis proscribed by law.

Minnesota

Minn. R. 7200.5400 (2010). Welfare of students, supervisees, and research subjects.

A psychologist shall protect the welfare of psychology students . . . and shall accord the students . . . the client rights listed in parts 7200.4700 and 7200.4900.

Minn. R. 7200.4900 (2010). Client welfare.

. . . Subp. 3. Stereotyping. A psychologist shall consider the client as an individual and shall not impose on the client any stereotypes of behavior, values, or roles related [to] . . . race, . . . which would interfere with the objective provision of psychological services to the client.

It is doubtful that the licensing board of either jurisdiction would view Dr. Hudson's "differential assignments" for the three students who have returned to the class as breaking the law. The laws of both jurisdictions focus on whether Dr. Hudson has engaged in harassment or discriminatory behavior due to stereotyping or prejudice. The facts of the vignette support the change in pedagogy due to the evidence that emerged about the three students' multicultural naïveté.

Cultural Considerations

Global Discussion

The Professional Board for Psychology
Health Professions Council of South Africa:
Ethical Code of Professional Conduct (April 2002)

9.3. Accuracy and objectivity in teaching.

9.3.2. When engaged in teaching . . . , psychologists shall recognise the power they hold over students, . . . and therefore shall make reasonable efforts to avoid engaging in conduct that is personally demeaning to such persons and shall ensure that their constitutional rights are upheld.

This portion of South Africa's code is clear with regard to teaching responsibilities of psychologists. However, each student in this scenario might have a different standard of what is "personally demeaning" to them, and it may differ from the standards the professor is using. At issue here is the professor's treatment of the students, not the students' behavior toward one another. Would Dr. Hudson possibly be in violation of the code by assigning different and extra work to the three students who spoke out and not the other two? Is it a misuse of her professorial power to single out some students for an assignment and not others? Is Dr. Hudson herself white or is she a person of color, and what, if any, impact does this have on the decisions she may make in this scenario? If her three students find the extra assignments and the implicit implication that they are being assigned such work because they have a deficiency with regard to race sensitivity, would that be "personally demeaning" to them? Would it be "personally demeaning" to the African American student if no action is taken by Dr. Hudson? Should Dr. Hudson provide extra assignments to everyone in the class, with the understanding that all are members of a racist culture and the other two students who remained silent may or may not also practice or hold beliefs which could be termed *microaggression*? If Dr. Hudson cannot remain objective in this situation, could it be argued from this portion of code that she must either consult with a colleague or in some way bring her own conduct into compliance with what it directs her to do?

American Moral Values

1. What is the purpose of the practicum seminar? Will this purpose differ for each student, or are there common skills students must acquire? If so, how does the extra assignment tie into the skills being taught to everyone else in the seminar? Will this extra work be incorporated into the regular class, or will Dr. Hudson conduct extra sessions with these three students alone?
2. What is Dr. Hudson's goal for the three students in relation to the rest of the class? Is the extra assignment being meted out as a punishment? Does it represent a requirement for them to earn back a place in the class? Is it meant to redress what appears to be unfair judgments about an African American student? Does

Dr. Hudson believe the weekly journal will help them understand issues of race and racial intimidation better?

3. Is it permissible to assign extra work to only some students in a class? What does Dr. Hudson believe are fair ground rules for a class? Is she within her rights to change requirements as she sees fit? On what principle would she object to a professor singling out an African American student with two assignments on paranoia and conspiracy theories after that student complained about racism?

4. What is Dr. Hudson's vision for discussions in the seminar? Does she want to encourage constructive discussions without intimidation between students? Does she believe her reaction to these three students will work toward that?

5. How will Dr. Hudson's action affect the other students in the class? Will Dr. Hudson's perspective be attributed to the African American student? Will it be said that the student pressured Dr. Hudson and the school to take that action? Will that student's experience be improved by having the three students return to the class, especially on these terms?

6. How will the practicum address issues of race? Will Dr. Hudson introduce the topic, or will students have to raise it? Will she provide instruction about institutional racism, or will the three students be expected to research and integrate the topic on their own? What if they argue there is no institutional racism in the program or express resentment in their journals? By what measure will these assignments be evaluated?

7. Are there other measures Dr. Hudson could take to address these students' reactions to discussions about race and discrimination? Could some of these be outside the class?

Ethical Course of Action

Directive per APA Code

The topic of concern for this vignette is Dr. Hudson's modifications of the requirements for the course and applying these modifications differentially. Standard 7.03 (a) allows for modifications if such changes are pedagogically necessary or desirable and if the students are informed of the modifications in such a way that allows the students to fulfill the new course requirements. Since Dr. Hudson had sound pedagogical reasons for modifying the course requirements, the dictates of Standard 7.03 (a) have been met. Standard 7.03 (a) is silent about whether course requirements may be differentially applied to students in the class. Requiring more work from the three students who filed complaints gives the appearance of retribution. Yet, no sound pedagogical evidence for imposing the additional work on the two other students emerged from the circumstances of the interactions.

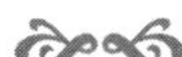

Dictates of One's Own Conscience

If you were Dr. Hudson, faced with half of your class wanting out because of interpersonal conflict, what would you do?

1. Follow the directive of Standard 2.01(c) and do some self-education on the topic.
2. Consult with colleague(s) about how to handle the situation.
3. Suggest that Emily transfer to another seminar for her protection.
4. Talk to Emily about the student's complaints regarding her in-class behavior, make it clear that the complaints appear to be acts of micro-aggression, and ask her how she can feel supported in general during the class.
5. Ask the three students to talk to Emily individually, and discuss with Emily their curiosity about her experience of being the lone African American among European Americans.
6. Hold an in-class discussion on the topic of race.
7. Hold an in-class discussion about some of the students requesting transfers out of the class.
8. Do a combination of the previously listed actions.
9. Do something that is not previously listed.

If you were Dr. Hudson, teaching in South Africa and faced with half of your class wanting out because of interpersonal conflict based on race, might you recognize the high probability that demeaning interactions involving everyone would repeatedly arise if these three students stayed in the seminar and grant their request to transfer out of the class?

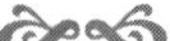

STANDARD 7.03: ACCURACY IN TEACHING

... (b) When engaged in teaching or training, psychologists present psychological information accurately.

A CASE FOR STANDARD 7.03 (B): Mandatory Reporting

Philip is in a human sexuality class with Professor Gardner. The class is discussing treatment of clients with HIV and other sexually transmitted diseases. Philip has just taken the orientation workshop at a clinic that is unrelated to the class but is a place he will work. At the clinic, he was told psychologists are mandatory reporters of sexually transmitted diseases. He raised the question about how best to handle the clinical implications of reporting clients with sexually transmitted diseases. Professor Gardner said, "It is a rumor that always floats around the hallways of the school that you have to contact people when a client has HIV or other sexually transmitted diseases. Please don't spread rumors about needing to report or contact client's sexual partners when you find out they have HIV."

Issues of Concern

Standard 7.03 directs psychologists to be accurate about the information they teach. If Philip was wrong and was indeed spreading an unfounded rumor about a situation where psychologists are mandated to report, then Dr. Gardner was right to correct him. Philip would naturally be confused as to what he should do when he encounters a client who is diagnosed with a communicable sexually transmitted disease. Regardless of whether Dr. Gardner is correct in her information, the manner in which she responded to Philip may preclude further exploration to determine the accuracy of the information.

APA Ethics Code

Companion General Principle

Principle C: Integrity

Psychologists seek to promote accuracy . . . in . . . teaching . . . psychology. In these activities psychologists do not . . . engage in . . . intentional misrepresentation of fact.

Principle C guides psychologists to be accurate in the teaching of psychology. To implement the value of integrity, Dr. Gardner would either need to be absolutely sure about her facts, or keep open to the possibility that Philip may be correct or seek to uncover the facts to resolve the question about mandated reporting for sexually transmitted diseases.

Companion Ethical Standard(s)

Standard 2.01: Boundaries of Competence

(a) Psychologists . . . teach . . . in areas only within the boundaries of their competence, based on their education, training, supervised experience, consultation, study, or professional experience.

Presumably Dr. Gardner is competent to teach the subject matter of human sexuality. It is necessary for Dr. Gardner to be knowledgeable about state mandatory reporting laws to teach the course. If the Modern School of Professional Psychology is a clinical program, competency in teaching human sexuality may require accurate knowledge about state mandatory reporting laws.

Standard 3.03: Other Harassment

Psychologists do not knowingly engage in behavior that is harassing or demeaning to persons with whom they interact in their work based on factors such as those persons' age, gender, gender identity, race, ethnicity, culture, national origin, religion, sexual orientation, disability, language, or socioeconomic status.

Philip's demographic characteristics are not known. Hopefully Dr. Gardner's demeaning manner in response to Philip's statement is not based on any of the possible statuses listed in Standard 3.03. Additionally, Standard 3.03 was not written in a manner as to imply harassing or demeaning behavior may be acceptable as long as those acts are not based on status factors.

Legal Issues 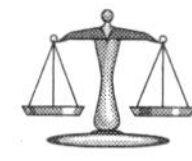

Missouri

Mo. Code Regs. Ann. tit. 20, § 2235-5.030 (2010). Ethical rules of conduct.

... (3) Competence.

(A) Limits on Practice. The psychologist shall limit practice and supervision to the areas in which competence has been gained through professional education, training derived through an organized training program and supervised professional experience. . .

(B) Maintaining Competency. The psychologist shall maintain current competency in the areas in which s/he practices, . . . in conformance with current standards of scientific and professional knowledge.

. . . (8) Welfare of Supervisees, Clients, Research Subjects and Students.

(A) Welfare of Supervisees and Students. The psychologist shall not harass . . . a . . . student in any way. . . The psychologist as a teacher shall recognize that the primary obligation is to help others acquire knowledge and skill. The psychologist shall maintain high standards of scholarship by presenting psychological information . . . accurately. The teaching duties of the psychologist shall be performed on the basis of careful preparation so that the instruction is accurate, current and scholarly.

Montana

Mont. Admin. R. 24.189.2305 (2009). Practice of psychology.

(1) In regard to conduct in the integrity of the profession, a licensee:

. . . (b) shall not provide any services in the practice of psychology except those services within the scope of the licensee's education, training, supervised experience or appropriate professional experience;

(c) shall not participate in activities in which it appears likely that the psychologist's skills or data will be misused by others, unless corrective mechanisms are available.

. . . (5) In regard to education, a licensee:

(a) shall present psychological information accurately and with a reasonable degree of objectivity, when engaged in teaching or training . . .

In both jurisdictions, Dr. Gardner's dismissive, perhaps harassing remark violated the laws that require her to conduct her teaching in a competent manner and maintain that competency. Assuming that a mandatory reporting duty existed within these jurisdictions, her failure to cite the law accurately could lead to her students acting wrongfully.

Cultural Considerations

Global Discussion

The Professional Board for Psychology Health Professions Council of South Africa: Ethical Code of Professional Conduct (April 2002)

9.3 Accuracy and objectivity in teaching.

9.3.1. When engaged in teaching . . . , psychologists shall present psychological information accurately and with a reasonable degree of objectivity.

Professor Gardner seems to be out of compliance with this portion of South Africa's code, as she has not presented psychological–legal information regarding the duties of mandated reporting accurately and may in fact be seen to have impaired objectivity, depending upon the reasons for her inaccurate information that she has presented. If the main reason behind Professor Gardner's stance contains some sort of bias, either in agreement with or against the duties of psychologists as mandated reporters, she has allowed her objectivity in this matter to be impaired. If the main reason for the inaccurate teaching were her own ignorance or lack of understanding of the topic, in that case, while troubling, she would not be necessarily seen to have impaired objectivity; however, she is still presenting information inaccurately. South Africa's code does not specify how to correct such an error, but it could be argued that she is nonetheless responsible for disseminating accurate information to her students, which she has clearly failed to do.

American Moral Values

1. What is Professor Gardner's relationship with the clinic? Should she be informed about what instructions are being given at orientation? Is there a problem in the relationship that has led to this discrepancy in information?
2. How does the issue of HIV enter into Professor Gardner's perspective? Are her concerns about rumors due to the many false rumors that circulated from the time HIV/AIDS became a well-known health problem? What response would best serve those concerns?
3. Professor Gardner dismisses Philip's question as akin to spreading a rumor, which would be considered unprofessional behavior. Does she owe Philip an

apology for that insinuation? Should she have asked on what basis he was assuming sexually transmitted diseases had to be reported?

4. What will be the effect of Professor Gardner's remarks be on the whole class? Will it undermine her credibility? Did she seem needlessly curt and dismissive? Does she need to rebuild trust and rapport with her class after her remarks?

Ethical Course of Action

Directive Per APA code

Standard 7.03 directs psychologists to be accurate in the information they teach. Standard 7.03 requires that Dr. Gardner accurately know and represent what the mandatory reporting requirements are for the state in which she is teaching.

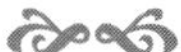

Dictates of One's Own Conscience

If you were Dr. Gardner, faced with a student who reported something that was contrary to your understanding, what would you do?

1. Suggest that Philip cite the exact law or administrative code to support his claim.
2. Cite the exact state law or administrative code to support your claim that psychologists are not mandatory reporters of communicable sexually transmitted diseases.
3. Assign the homework for everyone in the class to look at all situations in which psychologists are mandatory reporters, then hold a discussion on Standard 7.03 and how the class as a whole might handle a situation in which there is a difference of opinion of a topic.
4. Do a combination of the previously listed actions.
5. Do something that is not previously listed.

If you were Dr. Gardner, faced with a student who reported something that was contrary to your understanding, the previously listed options would still apply since the accuracy in teaching is not substantially different from those listed by the APA Ethics Code.

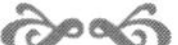

STANDARD 7.04: STUDENT DISCLOSURE OF PERSONAL INFORMATION

> Psychologists do not require students or supervisees to disclose personal information in course- or program-related activities, either orally or in writing, regarding sexual history, history of abuse and neglect, psychological treatment, and relationships with parents, peers, and spouses or significant others except if (1) the program or training facility has clearly identified this requirement in its admissions and program materials or (2) the information is necessary to evaluate or obtain assistance for students whose personal problems could reasonably be judged to be preventing them from performing their training or professionally related activities in a competent manner or posing a threat to the students or others.

A CASE FOR STANDARD 7.04: Psychologist, Know Thyself

Paula is a 2nd-year graduate student in the clinical program at the Modern School of Professional Psychology. She is in a human sexuality class with Professor Berry. Professor Berry has given the assignment of writing a personal sexual history paper. This is to include a follow-up in class discussion about how the student's past sexual history impacts their work as a treating psychologist. Paula is very uncomfortable with the assignment. She grew up in a family where her stepfather sexually molested her older sister and had been sexually provocative with Paula. During her adolescent years, Paula abused alcohol and was sexually promiscuous for a brief period of time. She is fearful that if any of this information was revealed to her professor or her classmates in the course of the class, it would adversely affect her graduate school career. Paula has let the professor know of her discomfort and requested a different assignment. Professor Berry told Paula that she should withdraw from the class and take it another quarter when he was not teaching the human sexuality class.

Issues of Concern

In general, Standard 7.04 prohibits the type of assignments required by Professor Berry. In its specificity, Standard 7.04 allows for such an assignment under two conditions: (1) if the program clearly states the requirement for self-examination and/or (2) if the student is exhibiting some personal problems. In the absence of Paula giving any indications that any of her personal problems are interfering with her graduate studies, the assignment of writing a personal sexual history paper is in violation of Standard 7.04. However, if the Modern School of Professional Psychology indicates in their published material that revealing personal information is necessary to successfully navigate the degree program, then such assignments are permissible under Standard 7.04. Should Professor Berry require Paula to participate in therapeutic exercises within the context of the course requirements? Does the alternative offered by Professor Berry seem reasonable?

APA Ethics Code

Companion General Principle

Principle E: Respect for People's Rights and Dignity

> Psychologists respect the dignity and worth of all people, and the rights of individuals to privacy, confidentiality, and self-determination. Psychologists are aware that special safeguards may be necessary to protect the rights and welfare of persons or communities whose vulnerabilities impair autonomous decision making.

Due to the power differential among professors and students, students are a category of people who are vulnerable to exploitation in a variety of ways. Principle E hopes Professor Berry would respect Paula's right to privacy and self-determination in what she chooses to reveal of her private life and her sexual history. Professor Berry appears to be invoking Paula's right to self-determination by suggesting that she can withdraw from the course. Professor Berry's suggestion does not appear to take into account the possible effects of withdrawing from the course, such as a delayed graduation or negative impact to Paula's reputation.

Principle A: Beneficence and Nonmaleficence

> . . . In their professional actions, psychologists seek to safeguard the welfare and rights of those with whom they interact professionally and other affected persons. . . Because psychologists' . . . actions may affect the lives of others, they are alert to and guard against personal . . . factors that might lead to misuse of their influence. . .

Principle A gives professors who are also psychologists a primary goal of being a benefit to students and "other affected persons" who would be future clients. If Professor Berry were being guided by the principle of beneficence, the aim of the assignment would be to benefit the student and their future clients. Professor Berry might argue that for the benefit of future clients, future psychologists need to be aware of and guard against their own sexual biases and urges. Even if Professor Berry's reason holds substance, in ignoring Paula's situation, Professor Berry appears to overlook the second value of nonmaleficence. Additionally, there is the appearance of Professor Berry possibly misusing his influence and giving a specific assignment that has hues of voyeurism.

Companion Ethical Standard(s)

Standard 7.05: Mandatory Individual or Group Therapy

> (a) When individual or group therapy is . . . [a] course requirement, psychologists responsible for that program allow students in . . . graduate programs the option of selecting such therapy from practitioners unaffiliated with the program. . . (b) Faculty who are . . . responsible for evaluating students' academic performance do not themselves provide that therapy.

Though Professor Berry's assignment is not for Paula to participate in in-class group or individual therapy, for Paula it may be akin to giving a testimonial or participating in self-help group therapy. For Paula, and maybe other students, the assignment may feel like course-mandated therapy, which is prohibited per Standard 7.05 (a). It is possible that Paula and other students may think Professor Berry will evaluate more positively those papers and presentations that are more intimate or revealing. Adhering to Standard 7.05 (b) protects students from such pressures, regardless of how Professor Berry may actually evaluate each student's work.

Standard 3.04: Avoiding Harm

> Psychologists take reasonable steps to avoid harming their . . . students . . . and to minimize harm where it is foreseeable and unavoidable.

Standard 3.04 is the companion to the nonmaleficence portion of Principle A. Regardless of Professor Berry's intentions, Standard 3.04 requires Professor Berry to examine the possibility that the assignment may be harmful and without sufficient redeeming benefit to warrant such an exercise. Standard 3.04 also requires Professor Berry to explore other pedagogical methods to achieve the same results with the possibility of producing less harm.

Standard 1.03: Conflicts Between Ethics and Organizational Demands

> If the demands of an organization with which psychologists . . . are working conflict with this Ethics Code, psychologists clarify the nature of the conflict, make known their commitment to the Ethics Code, and to the extent feasible, resolve the conflict in a way that permits adherence to the Ethics Code.

Paula has a conflict between meeting the organizational demands in the form of completing Professor Berry's assignment required to pass the course and her rights as outlined in Standard 7.04 and implied in Standard 7.05. Standard 1.03 directs Paula to object to the assignment.

Standard 1.04: Informal Resolution of Ethical Violations

> When psychologists believe that there may have been an ethical violation by another psychologist, they attempt to resolve the issue by bringing it to the attention of that individual, if an informal resolution appears appropriate . . .

Paula's situation appears to meet the specifications as explained in Standard 1.04. To follow the dictates of Standard 1.04, Paula is to bring her problem to the attention of Professor Berry, which she has done. Up to this point Paula has followed the directives of Standard 1.04.

Standard 1.05: Reporting Ethical Violations

> If an apparent ethical violation . . . is likely to substantially harm a person . . . and is not . . . resolved properly [per standard 1.04], psychologists take further action appropriate to the situation. Such action might include referral to . . . the appropriate institutional authorities. . .

Paula has made the proper first steps as specified in Standard 1.04 to resolve this conflict between her personal well-being and the course requirements by speaking to Professor Berry directly. Unfortunately, Professor Berry's response does not provide the proper resolution of Paula's concerns. Thus, per Standard 1.05, Paula is to take further action appropriate to the situation. Actions that may be appropriate to the situation might include contacting her academic advisor, the chair of the program, or the school's ombudsperson.

Legal Issues 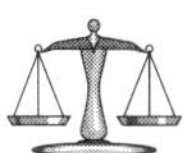

Nebraska

> *172 Neb. Admin. Code § 156-006 (2010). Regulations defining unprofessional conduct by a psychologist.*
>
> 001 ADOPTION. The Board hereby adopts the Ethical Standards of Psychologists of the American Psychological Association as the Code of Professional Conduct for the practice of Psychology in Nebraska . . .

New Jersey

> *N.J. Admin. Code § 13:42-10.13 (2010). Conflicts of interest; dual relationships.*
>
> . . . (d) A licensee shall not enter into any dual relationship. Examples of such dual relationships include, but are not limited to [,] . . . students. . .
>
> (e) A licensee who recognizes the existence of a conflict of interest or dual relationship shall take action to terminate the conflict or the dual relationship.

In both jurisdictions, it is unlikely that a licensing board would find that Professor Berry broke the law if the program clearly specified that self-examination and/or public discussion "regarding sexual history, history of abuse and neglect, psychological treatment, and relationships with parents, peers, and spouses or significant others" would occur during coursework within the program. Without the specificity, it is possible that a licensing board may interpret the assignment to involve a dual relationship in which Professor Berry's assignment is self-serving rather than pedagogical.

Cultural Considerations

Global Discussion

Code of Ethics: Netherlands

> Psychologist and the working environment.
>
> III.4.6.3 Assistance and support to colleagues, students and supervisee.
>
> The psychologist applies his expertise and experience to assist and support . . . students . . . in any way he can, enabling them to engage in professional activity in a

competent and ethical manner. He refrains from activities which could be detrimental to these persons in this regard.

If Paula and Professor Berry were in the Netherlands, this scenario could be interpreted according to this code in several ways. If the purpose of Professor Berry's assignment is to be better able to "engage . . . in a competent and ethical manner," especially as he is screening students who will begin to work in the school's clinic, it could be argued that he is upholding this portion of the code. However, if Paula feels that this assignment is not helpful for her professional development and is in fact "detrimental" then she would likely assess Professor Berry as being in violation of this portion of code. Arguably, although the Netherlands code is silent regarding motivation of psychologists who teach, the issues at hand here have to do with the intention of Professor Berry and what he hopes his students will gain from such an assignment. If it would be detrimental to Paula to reveal her personal history in a group setting, and if any potential harm or retribution may occur related to her revelations, then that potential outcome may be seen as too harmful to justify under the obligation of "assisting and supporting" students. If, however, such an assignment is seen as assisting students in their ethical and professional development by allowing them an experience of revealing painful history in front of peers and professors and thus know better what therapeutic work entails, then it may be argued that such activities are justifiable and not in violation of the code.

American Moral Values

1. What are Professor Berry's principles for requiring the disclosure and discussion of each student's personal sexual history? Is making this history public part of the process, or is the goal just to make students aware of how sexual history could affect the therapy they provide? If it is the latter, is there a different way to meet that goal than the one Professor Berry has proposed?
2. Has Professor Berry fully considered the effect on students of narrating their respective histories for the class? Is this therapeutically advisable? Is this class serving as a form of therapy, and if so, to what degree? Has Professor Berry assumed a therapist's role in addition to an instructor's?
3. What is Professor Berry assuming about sexual history and the proper format for discussing it in a class? Would post-traumatic stress disorder (PTSD) sufferers recovering from war be required to share a personal history with violence? Is Professor Berry attempting to open up a taboo subject because he believes its repression causes more suffering than its disclosure? Would reflection and communication about loaded topics such as sexuality be better worked within psychotherapy rather than as part of the pedagogy of a doctoral psychology program?
4. What kind of class atmosphere is Professor Berry trying to create? Will it be possible to have the trust needed for students to be honest about their histories? What if two of the students have had sex with each other? What if one of the students considered it nonconsensual? What if the threat of disclosure, even to a lone professor, leads to the minimization and dissimulation about the experiences?
5. Is Professor Berry's recommendation to Paula a form of coercion? Could this coercion be seen as sexually harassment, for her or other students who need to take this class? Does Professor Berry gain personal pleasure out of students exposing their histories to him rather than serving any legitimate pedagogical purpose?

Ethical Course of Action

Directive per APA Code

If the published material about the program clearly specifies such self-examination and/or public discussion "regarding sexual history, history of abuse and neglect, psychological treatment, and relationships with parents, peers, and spouses or significant others," then Professor Berry is able to assign the writing and presentation of a student's personal sexual history. If the published material speaks in generalities about the possibility students may be required to discuss material of a personal nature in the program, then Professor Berry's assignment violates the intended protection of Standard 7.04. To uphold the value of respect in Principle E, the Standard 3.04 of avoiding harm, and to prevent Paula from taking the next step directed by Standard 1.05, Professor Berry could consider designing an alternative assignment or allowing students those options explicated in Standard 7.05.

Dictates of One's Own Conscience

If you were either Professor Berry or Paula or another student in the same class having witnessed the exchange between Paula and Professor Berry, what might you do?

1. As the professor teaching the class, I would do the following:
   a. Encourage Paula to face her personal demons and do the assignment.
   b. Encourage Paula to face her personal demons by writing the paper as assigned, but give her the option of presenting on something else or presenting the paper to her personal psychotherapist.
   c. Design another assignment for Paula, and require that she go into personal therapy to confront her personal demons before being allowed to treat clients.
   d. Require that Paula present you with some alternative equivalent assignment.
   e. Tell Paula to take her complaint to the chair of the program if she does not want to take the class as designed.
2. As Paula, a student who is uncomfortable with the assignment, I would do the following:
   a. Talk to your psychotherapist about your feelings and thoughts.
   b. Talk to your academic advisor to help resolve this accordingly.
   c. Talk to your fellow students for a reality check on your own emotional response to the assignment.
   d. Check the schedule of classes to see if it is possible to take the course from another professor without unduly upsetting your own graduation timeline.
3. As a fellow student, I would do the following:
   a. Talk to Paula, and encourage her to stay in the class but not do the assignment as in-depth so as to avoid the feared harm to both herself and her graduate career.
   b. Support Paula, and encourage her to voice the concerns that most other students also have regarding the inappropriateness of the assignment.
   c. Think that Professor Berry is preparing students to meet the rigors of doing therapy, thus Paula is oversensitive and should drop the class.
   d. Think that Paula does not belong in a clinical psychology program if she is not able to face her own demons.
4. As the advisor and/or chair of the program, I would do the following:
   a. Talk directly with Professor Berry, reminding him of the relevant ethical codes, and propose an option to the assignment such as to turn in the paper to her psychotherapist.
   b. Support Professor Berry's right to craft his class in any manner he chooses as long as he does not violate any of the ethics standards.
5. Do a combination of the previously listed actions.
6. Do something that is not previously listed.

If this course were occurring in the Netherlands, Paula and Professor Berry might engage in a conversation to ascertain the benefit to Paula in completing Professor Berry's assignment. Based on the specifics of the conversation, if it was determined that completion of the assignment would be detrimental to Paula, than Professor Berry, to comply with section III.4.6.3 of the Netherlands code of ethics, would arrange for alternative assignment.

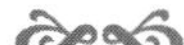

STANDARD 7.05: MANDATORY INDIVIDUAL OR GROUP THERAPY

(a) When individual or group therapy is a program or course requirement, psychologists responsible for that program allow students in undergraduate and graduate programs the option of selecting such therapy from practitioners unaffiliated with the program.

(b) Faculty who are or are likely to be responsible for evaluating students' academic performance do not themselves provide that therapy.

A CASE FOR STANDARD 7.05 (a) & (b): The Hollywood Blonde Syndrome

After a year of coursework in her doctoral degree program, Phyllis found herself sitting in group class. Her group class is designed as a participatory learning experience where the students hold weekly group therapy sessions for 1.5 hours with Professor Matthews in the role of group leader. No disclosures about Standard 7.05: Mandatory Individual or Group Therapy have occurred, and no option for alternative assignments were offered. Halfway into the quarter, Phyllis witnessed two students in a heated discussion during class. Professor Matthews made an interpretation: "Lupe, do you think you might be upset at Norma because you are jealous since she is slim and pretty with long blonde hair? Might this be your internalized oppression showing through?" (Lupe is a first-generation immigrant with parents who are from Mexico.)

Issues of Concern

For this vignette, there are several issues of concern. One is the question of supervisory responsibility of the course instructor Professor Matthews. Second is Phyllis's responsibility when witnessing a professional conflict and a failure of meeting the standard of competency. The third issue of concern is the profession's collective responsibility of nonoppressive and nondiscriminatory practice in all settings in which psychologists work. Standard 7.05 requires that students be given options to opt out of participation in course-based group therapy. Given that Professor Matthews has ignored the dictates of Standard 7.05, what then are the rights of the students in revealing personal information when a seemingly inappropriate question has been asked by an authority figure?

APA Ethics Code

Companion General Principle

Principle E: Respect for People's Rights and Dignity

> Psychologists respect the dignity and worth of all people. . . . Psychologists are aware that special safeguards may be necessary to protect the rights and welfare of persons . . . whose vulnerabilities impair autonomous decision making.

Phyllis, Norma, Lupe, and the others in the class, in their position as students with little power, are vulnerable. Because of this vulnerability, Professor Matthews is specially charged to protect their dignity by assuring students they have the right to not participate in course-based group therapy.

Principle B: Fidelity and Responsibility

> Psychologists . . . are concerned about the ethical compliance of their colleagues' scientific and professional conduct.

Phyllis, being a psychologist-in-training and thus subject to the authority of the APA Ethics Code, should be concerned with the ethical violations of professors and fellow students. Principle B hopes that Phyllis becomes involved in the interchange between Professor Matthews, Lupe, and Norma.

Principle D: Justice

> Psychologists exercise reasonable judgment and take precautions to ensure that their potential biases, the boundaries of their competence, and the limitations of their expertise do not lead to or condone unjust practices.

To abide by Principle D: Justice, might Phyllis find herself being concerned about the well-being of her fellow students if she viewed the professor's comments as racially discriminatory toward Lupe? To help ascertain whether or not she is unfairly ascribing discriminatory overtones to Professor Matthews's question, might Phyllis ask this companion question: "Why did Professor Matthews not ask Norma, the blonde-haired student, if it is her racism being manifested?"

Companion Ethical Standard(s)

Standard 3.01: Unfair Discrimination

> In their work-related activities, psychologists do not engage in unfair discrimination based on . . . ethnicity . . .

By asking the question and directing it to Lupe without asking a companion question of Norma, it is quite possible Professor Matthews is engaging in unfair discrimination based on Lupe's ethnicity. If so, Standard 3.01 has been violated. Such a violation establishes a possible group norm/pressure for students to divulge personal information without consent, which has a high probability of students feeling victimized.

> Guidelines on Multicultural Education, Training, Research, Practice, and Organizational Change for Psychologists (APA, 2003)
>
> ***Guideline 2.*** To recognize the importance of multicultural sensitivity/responsiveness, knowledge, and understanding about ethnically and racially different individuals. (APA, 1990, p. 25)

Did Professor Matthews's comment fail to meet the second multicultural guideline, which encourages psychologists to understand the nuances of handling racial issues? If Professor Matthews was white, might this be an example of his racial/ethnicity bias? If Professor Matthews was not white, might this be an example of internalized racial/ethnic oppression? Understanding that it is not Phyllis who engaged in discriminatory behavior, Phyllis could be considered a collaborator in unfair discrimination if she remained silent following Professor Matthews's comment? How might Phyllis respond in the moment to uphold the spirit of the previously referenced principles?

Standard 2.01: Boundaries of Competence

> (a) Psychologists . . . teach . . . in areas only within the boundaries of their competence, based on their education, training, supervised experience, consultation, study, or professional experience.

If Professor Matthews did not give students the option of choosing alternative therapy because he was unaware of the directives of Standard 7.05, then he would be demonstrating incompetence regarding the topic of teaching a group therapy class at the psychology graduate level.

Standard 1.04: Informal
Resolution of Ethical Violations

> When psychologists believe that there may have been an ethical violation by another psychologist, they attempt to resolve the issue by bringing it to the attention of that individual, if an informal resolution appears appropriate . . .

Witnessing violations of Standard 7.05: Mandatory Individual or Group Therapy and noncompliance with Principles B and D, and possible racially discriminatory behavior, Phyllis might find herself considering how best to address her concerns within the context of her own status as a student. Section 1.04 of the code would direct Phyllis to speak directly to Professor Matthews. As a student, what safeguards might Phyllis wish for in order to protect herself from any possible negative repercussions?

Legal Issues 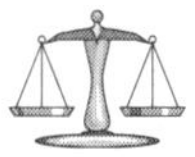

Idaho

> *Idaho Rules of State Board of Psychologists Examiners § 24.12.601(1993).*
>
> . . . (b) The licensed supervising psychologist exercising PROFESSIONAL control shall:
>
> . . . (ii) Establish and maintain a level of supervisory contact sufficient to be readily accountable in the event that professional, ethical, or legal issues are raised . . .

Arkansas

> *074-00-1 Ark. Code R. § 6.3 (2009).*
>
> A. Supervision of Students. Students who are enrolled in a program of study . . . shall be supervised in any and all practice of the profession of psychology, in keeping with the regulations for training students in the practice of psychology, and shall be the responsibility of the Psychologist supervisor, both site and academic.

Both of the licensing boards in Idaho and Arkansas would recognize Dr. Matthews as the supervisor in light of his teaching the group class. If Phyllis was attending a training program located in either Idaho or Arkansas, she could suggest to the supervising psychologist that the law was not sufficiently met in the ways discussed in the above sections regarding the code.

Cultural Considerations

Global Discussion

The Professional Board for Psychology Health Professions Council of South Africa:
Ethical Code of Professional Conduct (April 2002)

> Chapter 9: Teaching, training and supervision.
>
> 9.52 Mandatory individual or group therapy or experiential activities.
>
> Psychologists shall not impose . . . group therapy as a mandatory programme requirement. Where it is recommended in a programme, psychologists associated with that programme allow students . . . the options of (1) recusing themselves from such a therapeutic experience, or (2) selecting such therapy outside the programme . . . faculty who are or are likely to be responsible for evaluating students . . . performance do not themselves provide the therapy.

If this class were being taught in South Africa, it would be in violation of this portion of code, which clearly says that group therapy may not be "imposed" and even in situations where it is "recommended" that students be given a clear option for removing themselves from such an experience. Further, because the instructor who made the interpretation during group therapy was the same instructor who would then be in charge of evaluating student performances, the intent and letter of this portion of code has been violated substantially. Even if all the students had agreed to such an experience and rejected possible other equivalent learning experiences, the group leader and the instructor/evaluator should not have been the same person. South Africa's code is clear: You may not demand that students take part in individual or group therapy as part of a requirement to complete a psychology program. Clearly, the instructor involved in this scenario would be in violation of South Africa's code.

American Moral Values

1. Are the professor's comments to Lupe an unfair attack cloaked in the terms of therapy? Is the suggestion that Lupe shows racially based jealousy a discriminatory attack on a nonwhite person? Or does the professor believe it is worth making a provocative hypothesis if it leads Lupe to understand the sources of her reaction?
2. Does this remark's possible offensiveness outweigh the benefits of therapeutic dialogue (which attempts to draw out unstated or subconscious motives)? How does Professor Matthews weigh the moral benefits of therapy against the pain of discrimination by race (sex, class, sexual orientation, etc.)?
3. Does the race of the professor change the moral equation of these remarks? What if the professor were Latino and had published work on internalized oppression and beauty standards? Would the remarks toward Lupe still function as discriminatory or stigmatizing behavior? How can therapy aim at deep-seated racist attitudes while not indulging in gratuitous, painful remarks? How can a group therapy class address race while maintaining respect for each person's identity and experience?
4. Do the professor's remarks interpret Lupe in a sexist fashion? Would a Latino male have been accused of being jealous of a white male's appearance? How can this issue be addressed in tandem with the issue of race?
5. What are the implications of the professor's remarks for the whole class? What action will best serve all students' ongoing training in group therapy? Will allowing the remark to pass by without comment reinforce a racist atmosphere?
6. What administrative intervention does the professor deserve for this remark? Is there a punishment that would be appropriate?
7. What are the implications of the professor serving as both academic evaluator and therapist? Is this role threatening for students who might be inclined to disagree with the instructor's interpretations?

Ethical Course of Action

Directive per APA Code

Standard 7.05 is very clear in that Phyllis, Norma, and Lupe should not find themselves in the position described in the vignette. Professor Matthews is in violation of Standard 7.05 (a) by not having informed students they had the option of choosing to fulfill the participatory part of the group therapy class through attendance in group therapy sessions not associated with the training program. Professor Matthews is also in violation of Standard 7.05 (b) by both conducting the group therapy sessions and giving the course grade.

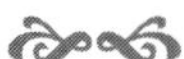

Dictates of One's Own Conscience

If you were Professor Matthews, Phyllis, Norma, Lupe, or a student in the same class having witnessed the exchange between Dr. Matthews and Lupe, what might you do?

1. As the training program, I would do the following:
   a. Seriously consider recommending that students take the ethics class early in their training.
   b. Expect that with knowledge of standards for training that students would be able to help monitor ethical delivery of the curricula.
2. As a student in this class, I would do the following:
   a. Knowing the standard regarding group or individual therapy, the students might have objected to the design of the class and thus prevented such a situation as the one previously described.
   b. Once in the situation, students like Phyllis, in the spirit of engaging in informal resolution of ethical violations, might consider functioning as a coleader by helping each person in the class discuss the meaning of the professor's comment.
   c. Intervene to protect Lupe from answering Professor Matthews's question.
   d. Notify Professor Matthews that he is in violation of Standards 7.04, 7.05a, and 7.05b.
   e. Write to the APA Div 42 ethical dilemma advice column for further advice.
   f. Report Professor Matthews's actions to the department chair or other administrator with supervisory responsibility over Professor Matthews.

3. As Professor Matthews, I would take possible cues from students and pause before proceeding.
4. Do a combination of the previously listed actions.
5. Do something that is not previously listed.

If you were Professor Matthews, Phyllis, Norma, Lupe, or a student in a program located in a South Africa class having witnessed the exchange between Dr. Matthews and Lupe, the previously listed options would still apply since the guideline for course-based group therapy is not substantially different from those listed by the APA Ethics Code.

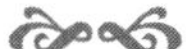

STANDARD 7.06: ASSESSING STUDENT AND SUPERVISEE PERFORMANCE

(a) In academic and supervisory relationships, psychologists establish a timely and specific process for providing feedback to students and supervisees. Information regarding the process is provided to the student at the beginning of supervision.

A CASE FOR STANDARD 7.06 (A): The Application Lie

Tina, a 2nd-year student in a doctoral clinical psychology program, is assigned her first case through the university training clinic. Tina's client, Clarence, is pursuing a master's degree in a counseling program. In the course of treatment, it came to light that Clarence had omitted the fact that he has had a conviction for domestic violence (DV) in his application to enter the program. Tina thinks that Clarence should not be in the counseling field since he did not reveal his DV conviction during the application process of the program. He has been physically abusive in the past. Tina took her concerns to Dr. Wagner, her clinical supervisor. Together with her supervisor, it was decided that Clarence's information was collected in the course of psychotherapy and thus is confidential and should not be released to the master's degree program.

The information regarding his past DV conviction surfaced in one of Clarence's classes. Clarence claims the university had not asked for information on the application regarding past legal offenses; in addition, the university knows the information because he disclosed the information while receiving treatment at the university's student counseling center from Tina to address the DV problem. The chair of the master's degree program, Dr. Willis, a psychologist, suggested to Tina's supervisor that she be given an unfavorable assessment for not reporting Clarence's lying on his application and his perpetrator status to the proper university authorities.

Issues of Concern

The dilemma is whether Tina and Dr. Wagner made an ethically sound decision in deciding not to reveal Clarence's history. Another dilemma is whether the university can use this information against either Clarence or Tina. Standard 7.06 (a) specifies that supervisors let students know how and when the student will be evaluated. Following the directive of Standard 7.06 (a), Dr. Wagner and Tina should have had a conversation about how Tina will be evaluated for her clinical work. Presumably that conversation did not include that part of Tina's evaluation would be based on complaints from faculty. The question relevant to Standard 7.06 (a) raised by Dr. Willis's request is whether criteria for performance evaluation should be changed after an incident has occurred that suggests the criteria were insufficient. Two secondary questions are raised by Dr. Willis's charge of Tina's misdeed: one is whether supervisees should be negatively affected for following their supervisor's recommendation and secondly, whether information collected at the school clinic belongs to the school and should have been shared with Clarence's master's degree program. Is such information privileged to the client and inaccessible by the school's academic department?

APA Ethics Code

Companion General Principle

Principle C: Integrity

. . . Psychologists strive to keep their promises and to avoid unwise or unclear commitments. . .

The establishment of a supervisory relationship is premised on how the student will be evaluated. Dr. Wagner essentially promised he would evaluate Tina's performance based on preestablished criteria. Secondarily, Tina upheld Principle C by keeping information from Clarence confidential, as required. She also consulted as required.

Principle D: Justice

> Psychologists recognize that fairness and justice entitle all persons to access to and benefit from the contributions of psychology and to equal quality in the processes, procedures, and services being conducted by psychologists. Psychologists exercise reasonable judgment and take precautions to ensure that their potential biases, the boundaries of their competence, and the limitations of their expertise do not lead to or condone unjust practices.

Equal quality, the value espoused in Principle D, would lead Dr. Wagner to reason that regardless of the setting of services, psychologists protect client's rights. Unless Clarence was notified in advance that confidentiality did not exist between the school clinic and the school's academic programs, equal quality of service would lead Dr. Wagner and Tina to protect Clarence's confidentiality. Might Tina's opinion about perpetrators of DV or Dr. Willis's bias influence their actions toward Clarence?

Principle E: Respect for People's Rights and Dignity

> Psychologists respect the dignity and worth of all people, and the rights of individuals to privacy, confidentiality, and self-determination.

Psychologists' respect of people's right to privacy and confidentiality require that Tina protect Clarence's information. Dr. Wagner's action appeared to have been based on Principle E.

Companion Ethical Standard(s)

Standard 4.01: Maintaining Confidentiality

> Psychologists have a primary obligation and take reasonable precautions to protect confidential information obtained through . . . any medium, recognizing that the extent and limits of confidentiality may be regulated by law or established by institutional rules or professional . . . relationship.

Standard 4.01 directs Tina and Dr. Wagner to keep Clarence's information confidential, which means not to divulge Clarence's past DV conviction to his academic program. Standard 4.01 allows for permeability of information from Tina to the academic program if "established by institutional rules." Such a condition of Standard 4.01 allows Tina to tell Dr. Willis about Clarence's DV conviction if the university had an established policy that academically relevant information gathered through psychotherapy be communicated to the student's academic degree program.

Standard 4.02: Discussing the Limits of Confidentiality

> (a) Psychologists discuss with persons . . . with whom they establish a . . . professional relationship . . . (1) the relevant limits of confidentiality and . . . (2) the foreseeable uses of the information generated through their psychological activities. . . (b) Unless it is not feasible or is contraindicated, the discussion of confidentiality occurs at the outset of the relationship and thereafter as new circumstances may warrant.

Standard 4.02 (a) and (b) requires that Tina let Clarence know the limits of confidentiality. If the school had an established policy that academically relevant information gathered through psychotherapy be communicated to the student's academic degree program, then Tina should have let Clarence know at the very beginning of treatment. Based on the information contained in the vignette, it appears that the clinic had no such policy in place.

Standard 5.01: Avoidance of False or Deceptive Statements

> . . . (b) Psychologists do not make false, deceptive, or fraudulent statements concerning (1) their . . . experience. . .

The intent of the word *experience* in Standard 5.01 (b) (1) probably does not refer to past legal problems unless the application's questions are drafted in such a manner that would require disclosure about crimes, such as those related to dangerous behavior directed at others. The expectation is that psychologists do not make false or deceptive statements. Absence of a statement, as in Clarence not revealing his past convictions because the application did not request such information, may be deceptive. In as far as Clarence is not in a psychology program, none of the APA Ethics Code applies to him or to his academic degree program.

Legal Issues 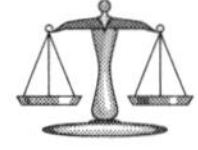

New Mexico

> *N.M. Code R. § 16.22.2.10 (2010). Patient welfare.*
>
> . . . **J. Avoiding harm.** Psychologists take reasonable steps to avoid harming . . . others with whom they work, and minimize harm where it is foreseeable and unavoidable.

New York

> *N.Y. Comp. Codes R. & Regs. tit. 8, § 29.1 (2010). General provisions.*
>
> a. Unprofessional conduct shall be the conduct prohibited by this section. . .
>
> . . . 5. failing to exercise appropriate supervision over persons who are authorized to practice only under the supervision of the licensed professional.

In both jurisdictions, the ethics board would be unlikely to hold that Tina or Dr. Wagner broke the laws. Tina followed the supervision suggestions of Dr. Wagner. The context did not call for any mandatory reporting to occur under the law. Dr. Wagner rightly supervised Tina to protect the confidences of her client.

Cultural Considerations

Global Discussion

The Professional Board for Psychology
Health Professions Council of South Africa:
Ethical Code of Professional Conduct (April 2002)

> 9.6 Assessing performance.
>
> 9.6.1. In academic and supervisory relationships, psychologists shall establish an appropriate process for providing feedback to students, supervisees and trainees.
>
> 9.3. Accuracy and objectivity in teaching.
>
> 9.3.2. When engaged in teaching or training, psychologists shall recognise the power they hold over students, supervisees and trainees and therefore shall make reasonable efforts to avoid engaging in conduct that is personally demeaning to such persons and shall ensure that their constitutional rights are upheld.

The key difference between the codes of the United States and South Africa is demarcated by ". . timely and specific" (United States) versus ". . appropriate" (South Africa). South Africa's code is silent with regard to the speed or specificity of information that could reasonably be considered appropriate. It can be argued that psychologists themselves are responsible for establishing the process of supervisory and academic feedback. Although this allows for greater variance of supervisory styles between psychologists and those they supervise and teach, psychologists are still clearly obligated to follow both the law, the code of ethics, and to uphold the Constitutional rights of those over whom they have power.

Some important things for Dr. Wagner to consider, keeping in mind the standards of 9.3.2. and 9.6.1 would be as follows: Which course or courses of action meets both the need for an appropriate feedback process for his student Tina, while also protecting both Tina and her client from any action or conduct which could be considered to be demeaning?

American Moral Values

1. Was a conviction for DV something that Clarence misrepresented on his application, or did he simply not include it? Was it a piece of information he was required to put on his application? Did this play a part in Tina and her supervisor's decision, or were they solely concerned with confidentiality? Does confidentiality outweigh the possible harm of Clarence becoming a therapist without this coming to light?
2. What authority does the head of the psychology program have in Tina's evaluation? Does the fact that Tina made her decision with her supervisor absolve her of responsibility? Does the head have the right to establish that Tina should have reported Clarence's DV past?
3. What is the importance of Clarence's application in relation to his ability to become a therapist? If an answer to a question on his application involved deception, is the problem more that he lied to get into the program, or that having committed DV renders him unfit for the program? Is there a way to address the serious implications of Clarence's situation and still keep him in the program? Are misrepresentations on an application cause for immediate dismissal? Are therapists required to tell the school if a client reveals that their application was inaccurate?
4. Does Clarence represent a threat to the university community? Does his DV record make him unfit for university involvement, much less the pursuit of a master's degree in clinical psychology?
5. What kind of information would Tina and her supervisor have thought serious enough to reveal to the university? Would a rape conviction have been sufficient? A murder conviction? What kind of possible danger would a client pose in order to cross that threshold of confidentiality and invoke the need to make a report to the university?

Ethical Course of Action

Directive per APA Code

Following the directive of Standard 7.06 (a), Dr. Wagner and Tina should have had a conversation about how Tina will be evaluated for her clinical work. Dr. Willis is at liberty to request Dr. Wagner consider the situation with Clarence in his final evaluation of Tina. On the principle of integrity to keep his promise of how Tina would be evaluated and following the dictates of Standard 7.06 (a), Dr. Wagner should not change the criteria by which Tina is evaluated.

Unless the school clinic had a policy that required Tina to report Clarence to his academic degree program, Dr. Wagner's advice for Tina to protect Clarence's confidences is in keeping with Standard 4.

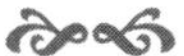

Dictates of One's Own Conscience

If you were either Tina or Dr. Wagner, what would you do?

1. As Dr. Wagner, you would do as follows:
   a. Double-check on clinic policy regarding limits of confidentiality between the academic programs and clinic cases.
   b. Evaluate Tina negatively if she did not follow my directive and kept Clarence's information confidential.
   c. Evaluate Tina negatively since Dr. Willis had a complaint against Tina.
   d. Complain about Dr. Willis's interference with my work as a supervisor.
2. As Tina, you would do as follows:
   a. Know that I acted in accordance with best practice by upholding confidentiality and consulted with my supervisor.
   b. Feel unjustly treated if Dr. Wagner acted on Dr. Willis's request and gave me a negative evaluation, and file a formal grievance within the university and with the licensing board of the jurisdiction regulating Dr. Wagner and Dr. Willis.
3. Do a combination of the previously listed actions.
4. Do something that is not previously listed.

If you were Dr. Wagner or Tina in a university clinic somewhere in South Africa, the previously listed options would still apply since the guideline for student evaluation asks for "appropriate" feedback, which is less specific than "timely and specific" as required by the APA Ethics Code.

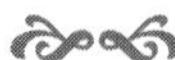

STANDARD 7.06: ASSESSING STUDENT AND SUPERVISEE PERFORMANCE

> . . . (b) Psychologists evaluate students and supervisees on the basis of their actual performance on relevant and established program requirements.

A CASE FOR STANDARD 7.06 (B): The Annual Review

Ruby, a graduate student in a clinical psychology program, was late in submitting two major assignments for Dr. Watkins's class. Ruby met with Dr. Watkins to explain that she is experiencing anxiety and depression due to childhood abuse that was triggered by some of the class material. Ruby reported having difficulty becoming stabilized on her psychotropic medications and asked whether it would be possible to obtain an extension on the assignments. Dr. Watkins granted Ruby the extension, and Ruby eventually completed all assignments satisfactorily. At the end of the year, Ruby's annual review letter said, "Ruby was late in submission of her assigned work due to acute reemergence of her depression and anxiety disorders." Ruby objected to the language of this annual review letter.

Issues of Concern

Standard 7.06 (b) directs the program to evaluate Ruby on her performance, not on her reasons for a delayed performance or the intent behind the action. Standard 7.06 (b) would have allowed Dr. Watkins to make comment about the timeliness of the assignments. Does Standard 7.06 (b) allow Dr. Watkins to make statements regarding the reason behind the tardy assignment?

Should Ruby's professor have included on her evaluation the fact that she has had some anxiety and depression? Isn't the evaluation about the actual performance of the student? Should the assessment be based on actual performance or turning in the work on time?

APA Ethics Code

Companion General Principle

Principle E: Respect for People's Rights and Dignity

> Psychologists are aware of and respect . . . role differences . . . and consider these factors when working with members of such groups. Psychologists try to eliminate the effect on their work of biases based on those factors, and they do not knowingly participate in or condone activities of others based upon such prejudices.

Per Principle E: Respect, Dr. Watkins and the faculty in their annual review deliberations, are to be sensitive to "role differences" between faculty and students. Principle E suggests that the faculty safeguard sensitive information regarding a student. Although the standards do not provide the same safeguards for student confidentially as they do for clients, sharing sensitive student information about a clinical condition may blur the boundary of remaining a professor rather than a clinician. Professors do not conduct multiple measure evaluative practices to arrive at a clinical finding as a clinician would.

Principle B: Fidelity and Responsibility

> Psychologists . . . are aware of their professional . . . responsibilities to . . . the specific communities in which they work. Psychologists uphold professional standards of conduct, clarify their professional roles and obligations, accept appropriate responsibility for their behavior, and seek to manage conflicts of interest that could lead to exploitation or harm. . . They are concerned about the ethical compliance of their colleagues' scientific and professional conduct.

Principle B suggests that Ruby, as a psychologist-in-training, takes on the value of honoring her responsibilities. As a student, it is Ruby's responsibility to turn in all course assignments on time. Part of Ruby's responsibility is to manage her own emotional problems in such a manner that she is able to meet her professional obligations. If Ruby was not able to meet her professional obligations, then she should be prepared to accept appropriate responsibility, which may include some type of academic reprimand if she had not acted responsibly. By seeking an extension, didn't Ruby act responsibly?

Companion Ethical Standard(s)

Standard 7.06: Assessing Student and Supervisee Performance

> (a) In academic . . . relationships, psychologists establish a timely and specific process for providing feedback to students. . . Information regarding the process is provided to the student at the beginning of supervision.

Standard 7.06 (a) allows Dr. Watkins and the faculty to comment on Ruby's work at preestablished times, such as the end of the quarter and at annual review. The timing and process of the feedback is in congruence with Standard 7.06 (a).

Standard 3.04: Avoiding Harm

> Psychologists take reasonable steps to avoid harming their . . . students . . . and to minimize harm where it is foreseeable and unavoidable.

Depending on the use of annual review letters, a certain amount of harm may be done to Ruby. Aside from the probability that Ruby may feel hurt or betrayed by Dr. Watkins for violating a confidence, real future harm may be done if the annual review resides permanently in the student's academic file because it is difficult to know all the situations for which Ruby may need to use the academic file. Stigma still exists for mental health issues. Would the file be viewed differently by future readers if Ruby's postponement of her assignment had been due to an excused delay to complete the assignment due to her recovery from a bad case of the flu?

Standard 7.04: Student Disclosure of Personal Information

> Psychologists do not require students . . . to disclose personal information in course . . . related activities, either orally or in writing, . . . except if . . . (2) the information is necessary to evaluate or obtain assistance for students whose personal problems could reasonably be judged to be preventing them from performing their training or professionally related activities in a competent manner. . .

Standard 7.04 allows Dr. Watkins access to personal information in order to evaluate Ruby's work. It is reasonable for Dr. Watkins to expect to know why Ruby needed an extension in order to decide whether to grant the extension for the assignment. Thus Ruby's information regarding her mental and emotional status falls well within the parameters of Standard 7.04.

Legal Issues 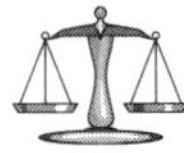

Ohio

Ohio Admin. Code 4732:17-01 (2010). General rules of professional conduct pursuant to section 4732.17 of the revised code.

... (B) Negligence:

(1) A psychologist ... shall be considered negligent if his/her behaviors toward his/her ... students, in the judgment of the board, fall below the standards for acceptable practice of psychology ...

... (G) Confidentiality:

... (2) Protecting confidentiality ...

... (d) A psychologist ... shall safeguard the confidential information obtained in the course of practice, teaching, research, or other professional duties...

Oklahoma

Okla. Admin. Rules, Title 575:10-1-10. (2010). A code of ethics for psychologists.

(a) Adoption of "Ethical Principles of Psychologists and Code of Conduct." The "Ethical Principles of Psychologists and Code of Conduct," 2002 revision, of the American Psychological Association (APA) is adopted by the Board in its entirety as part of its Code of Ethics.

In both jurisdictions, Dr. Watkins would likely be found to have broken the laws. The personal information that Ruby revealed to Dr. Watkins should not be considered in evaluating Ruby's performance within the class or the program. The expectation would be that Dr. Watkins protects the confidential information disclosed by Ruby.

Cultural Considerations

Global Discussion

The Professional Board for Psychology
Health Professions Council of South Africa:
Ethical Code of Professional Conduct (April 2002)

9.6 Assessing performance.

9.6.1. Psychologists shall evaluate students, supervisees and trainees on the basis of their actual performance on relevant and established programme requirements that are objectively determined.

If Dr. Watkins was evaluating Ruby's performance in South Africa, she would need to evaluate Ruby's work using "established" program requirements and be assured those requirements were created "objectively." In other words, are they designed with the commonly understood professional obligations and competencies of a psychologist in mind, and are they fairly and uniformly applied, or are the standards used arbitrarily depending upon the situation? It is unclear from the vignette whether a program requirement includes the necessity of a student to be relatively untroubled by past family abuse or psychological distress,or whether or not a student can be in good standing in the program while being treated for psychological conditions with therapy and psychotropics. It is likely that timeliness and quality of work are program requirements that can and should be expected, but it is not clear to what degree an evaluation of a student can be based upon personal characteristics, life stressors, or biopsychological factors such as imbalances in one's medications.

At issue here is the understanding that all such "personal" factors, including physical, emotional, and mental health have an impact on a student's performance and possible work with clients, and as such, could arguably be the purview of the professor to include in the evaluation. What is curious about psychological "illness" versus a purely medical illness is the stigma attached—if Ruby had been late with her assignments because she ran out of insulin and went into shock for a few days, would that have been included in her evaluation? Are psychological factors seen to be the responsibility or failing on the part of the student, even when that student is in a psychology program? Is it fair for programs to include information in evaluations that is personal and potentially stigmatizing, under the rubric of it being a relevant program requirement? Did the program clearly state that one of the requirements was for students not to have medication imbalances or life events that could potentially affect the timeliness of their work?

Just as the South Africa code specifies that its mandates only apply to one's professional role as a psychologist, do students receive the same sort of distinction—problems in one's personal life only become a concern when they impact one's professional decisions or actions? In this case, while it is true that Ruby's work is late and that this seems a reasonable piece of information to include in her evaluation, speculation or inclusion of possible causative reasons that carry with them their own stigma and potential harm to Ruby's career seem unwarranted in this situation and potentially harmful. Only if all students are held to a similar standard as Ruby would it seem that this would be an objective program requirement.

American Moral Values

1. What does Dr. Watkins think the purpose of an annual review letter is? Does it need to inform colleagues of the reasons for Ruby's extension, especially when these pertain to mental health issues? Why is such mental health information appropriate and useful to share in this document?
2. Do faculty members need to explain the reason for extensions? Would Dr. Watkins have shared Ruby's problems if they had just come up in a private conversation, with no reference to an assignment?
3. Did Ruby trust Dr. Watkins not to share private information with others? Did Dr. Watkins understand that expectation, or does she believe Ruby cannot make that demand?
4. Provided that Dr. Watkins did feel the need to mention Ruby's mental health struggles, was "depression and anxiety disorders" the best way to describe them in the letter? Does that summary give enough context to what set off her struggles? Do colleagues need to know about adjustments in medication? Will it have an adverse impact on the way other faculty relate to and evaluate Ruby's work?
5. Does Dr. Watkins regret giving Ruby her extension? Is this a type of warning to Ruby that her problems cannot continue to be an excuse for late work? Is it a way to show that late work requires some kind of excuse in order to be accepted?

Ethical Course of Action

Directive per APA Code

Standard 7.06 (b) directs the program to evaluate Ruby on her performance, not on her reasons for a delayed performance or the intent behind the action. Standard 7.06 (b) would have allowed Dr. Watkins to comment about the timeliness of the assignments. Standard 7.06 (b) does not allow Dr. Watkins or the faculty to make statements regarding the reason behind the tardy assignment. The reference to Ruby's "depression and anxiety disorder" in the annual review letter, if solely based on the tardy assignment, violates Standard 7.06 (b).

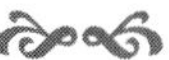

Dictates of One's Own Conscience

If you were Dr. Watkins and the faculty was faced with a student who is not managing her emotional problems, what would you do with the annual review?

1. To be fair and honor the other students who did manage their lives in such a way as to turn in their assignments on time, do not grant Ruby the extension. Explain to Ruby that to function as a psychologist she needs to be able to manage her health (physical or mental) in a professional and prompt manner that does not interfere with her work.
2. To be fair and honor the other students who did manage their lives in such a way as to turn in their assignments on time and given that you did give Ruby an extension, then let Ruby know that the reason for the extension will be noted in the assessment somewhere.
3. Act on the policy of the student handbook that delineates the nature of annual review. With the student handbook in hand, meet with Ruby before the annual letter is sent.
4. Argue with your colleagues that Standard 7.06 (b) does not allow any comments regarding Ruby's emotional health.
5. Argue with colleagues that something should be placed in the annual review letter that noted Ruby was proactive in discussion with Dr. Watkins and in her requests for additional time to complete class assignments.
6. Let Ruby know that though the letter confined the statement to late assignments, the faculty considered her overall ability to function in the program as directed by Standard 7.04 and decided to restrict the scope of their comment to the assignment. However, Ruby should know that the faculty is concerned about her overall ability to manage her depression.
7. Do a combination of the previously listed actions.
8. Do something that is not previously listed.

If you were Dr. Watkins and the faculty working in South Africa, faced with a student who is not managing her emotional problems, you could determine her performance was inadequate based on the standard that professionals are timely in their products. Comments beyond the timeliness of assignment would be a violation of the South African code.

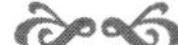

STANDARD 7.07: SEXUAL RELATIONSHIPS WITH STUDENTS AND SUPERVISEES

> Psychologists do not engage in sexual relationships with students or supervisees who are in their department, agency, or training center or over whom psychologists have or are likely to have evaluative authority.

A CASE FOR STANDARD 7.07: The Home Office

Dr. Olsen is a well-respected clinical psychology professor with many student admirers. He is also the current subject of an ethics investigation. The investigation was started when faculty in his department became alarmed by the stories of troubled students visiting his home office for evening appointments. Dr. Olsen's contract has come up for renewal, and as the school does not offer tenure to faculty, it is permissible for professors to be replaced, sometimes with little notice. Dr. Olsen enjoys good evaluations from many of his students, and his colleagues report that he is easy to work with, although unorganized. Dr. Olsen has also been a key and outspoken advocate of a shared governance system of university administration, something the president and academic dean have opposed. On the day of his annual review, Dr. Olsen found himself in a meeting with not just the chair of the department but also the dean and a human resources (HR) staff member. He was told that his services are no longer needed as faculty and that he has 1 day to pack his office and leave the premises.

Issues of Concern

Does inviting students to visit his home office in the evening constitute a multiple relationship, sexual or not? If students interpret such invitations as opening the door for possible romantic relationships, then has Dr. Olsen violated Standard 7.07? Even if he has not engaged in any romantic or sexual activities, has Dr. Olsen engaged in multiple relationships by offering therapy? If he has indeed engaged in romantic relationships but not sexual in nature, has Dr. Olsen violated Standard 7.07? And regardless of whether Dr. Olsen has engaged in multiple relationships with students, does the hint of such possibility give the university an easy excuse for terminating employment of a troublesome faculty member?

APA Ethics Code

Companion General Principle

Principle B: Fidelity and Responsibility

> Psychologists . . . are aware of their professional . . . responsibilities . . . to the specific communities in which they work. Psychologists uphold professional standards of conduct, clarify their professional roles and obligations, accept appropriate responsibility for their behavior, and seek to manage conflicts of interest that could lead to exploitation or harm.

Principle B directs Dr. Olsen to be aware of his professional responsibility to the students and to his colleagues. If Dr. Olsen is not romantically involved with troubled students but offering psychotherapeutic services or friend relationships to these problematic students, might he be violating professional standards by engaging in multiple relationships?

Companion Ethical Standard(s)

Standard 1.08: Unfair Discrimination Against Complainants and Respondents

> Psychologists do not deny persons employment . . . based solely upon . . . their being the subject of an ethics complaint. This does not preclude taking action based upon the outcome of such proceedings or considering other appropriate information.

If the termination of the contract with Dr. Olsen was based solely on the internal ethics investigation, then the university acted prematurely and violated Standard 1.08.

Standard 3.08: Exploitative Relationships

> Psychologists do not exploit persons over whom they have supervisory, evaluative, or other authority such as . . . students. . .

If Dr. Olsen was engaged in providing psychotherapeutic sessions or extending personal friendship to students, might he be exploiting his faculty position to get more business for his practice or personal attention from impressionable people? If Dr. Olsen was engaged in sexual relationships with students in his home office, then he would clearly be in violation of Standard 7.07.

Standard 7.05: Mandatory Individual or Group Therapy

> . . . (b) Faculty who are responsible for evaluating students' academic performance do not themselves provide therapy.

If Dr. Olsen was engaged in providing psychotherapeutic sessions to students, and these were students over whom he had evaluative authority, Dr. Olsen would be in violation of Standard 7.05.

Standard 3.05: Multiple Relationships

> (a) A multiple relationship occurs when a psychologist is in a professional role with a person and (1) at the same time is in another role with the same person...
>
> ...A psychologist refrains from entering into a multiple relationship if the multiple relationship could reasonably be expected to impair the psychologist's objectivity, competence, or effectiveness in performing his or her functions as a psychologist, or otherwise risks exploitation or harm to the person with whom the professional relationship exists...
>
> ...Multiple relationships that would not reasonably be expected to cause impairment or risk exploitation or harm are not unethical...

Regardless of what Dr. Olsen was doing with the students in his home office, unless it was to teach an independent studies course, he has engaged in multiple relationships. Though it is not necessarily a violation to engage in such multiple relationships, Standard 3.05 (a) (1) does advise caution.

Legal Issues 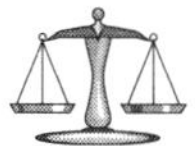

Pennsylvania

> *49 Pa. Code § 41.61 (2010). Code of ethics.*
>
> Principle 7. Professional relationships.
>
> (e) Psychologists do not exploit their professional relationships with ... students ... sexually or otherwise...

Rhode Island

> *R.I. Rules and Regulations For Licensing Psychologists (R-5-44-PSY) (2010).*
>
> Section 10.0 Denial, Suspension or Revocation of License - Violations
>
> ... 10.2 The Board shall have the power to ... discipline a psychologist upon proof that the person:
>
> ... (7) has willfully or repeatedly violated any of the ethical principles governing psychologists and the practice of psychology, ... provided however that those ethical principles shall be of a nationally recognized standard.

In both jurisdictions, Dr. Olsen's behavior would be viewed as having established multiple relationships with his students. Such relationships would be found exploitive and a violation of the laws.

Cultural Considerations

Global Discussion

Canadian Code of Ethics for Psychologists

> Principle II: Responsible caring.
>
> II.28. Not encourage or engage in sexual intimacy with students ... with whom the psychologist has an evaluative or other relationship of direct authority...
>
> Principle III: Integrity in relationships.
>
> III.31. Not exploit any relationship established as a psychologist to further personal ... interests at the expense of the best interests of their ... students... This includes, but is not limited to ... taking advantage of trust ... to encourage or engage in sexual intimacies.

In as much as Dr. Olsen's invitation for "troubled" students to come to his house after hours for appointments could be seen as an encouragement to engage in intimacy, sexual or otherwise, he could be in violation of Canada's code. It might also be argued that by inviting so-called troubled, likely more vulnerable students to his private home instead of his campus office he might be "taking advantage of trust or dependency" to develop a relationship with his students. Regardless of whether Dr. Olsen is genuinely interested in the welfare of his troubled students and wishes to provide them with personal support at his home, or whether he is grooming vulnerable students with the intention of encouraging sexual intimacy, at question here is what is in the best interest of the students, not the psychologist.

Even if incorrect or overly Victorian, there is a clear cultural understanding of the message of intimacy conveyed by an invitation to someone's personal space, such as their home, versus requesting a meeting at a neutral space or workspace on campus. The psychologist making such a request must be aware of the implications and the appearance of that request and relationship to others in the department, and weigh whether or not it is in the best interests of the student to do so. As much as the students are responsible for their actions and decisions as well, the balance of power and possible exploitation is in the hands of the psychologist. Sadly, troubled students who may be perceived as more vulnerable can be (and often are) targets for exploitative relationships of all kinds and are more likely to welcome attention that others would be offended or alarmed by. Unless Dr. Olsen has a long-standing policy of meeting all students in his home at night, regardless of their degree of vulnerability, he risks opening himself to the perception that his actions are unusual, possibly exploitative, and encouraging of a relationship that is outside the established norms of a professor–student relationship.

American Moral Values

1. How does Dr. Olsen interpret the decision not to renew his contract? Does he believe it stems from his political advocacy for shared governance, the accusations of sexual relationships with his students, or both? Given evaluations and feedback he has received up until now, what was his estimation of his chances to be renewed?
2. How does Dr. Olsen view his relationship to students? Does a strong relationship with students entail evening visits to his office, or do those visits invite speculation of inappropriate conduct? Is the purpose of these visits therapeutic, academic, or physical? To what degree is each of them, or some combination thereof, acceptable? What types of problems does Dr. Olsen want to address for these students?
3. What were the stories that faculty had heard about "troubled students"? Were students complaining about these visits? Did faculty discuss this issue with Dr. Olsen? Did Dr. Olsen need to explain these visits to colleagues? Did these stories harm the department and/or the school if they spread beyond them?
4. How does Dr. Olsen's position on governance affect his standing at the school? Given that no faculty members have tenure, how does faculty opposition to administration usually play out? How many faculty members who fought the administration have not been renewed when their contract ran out?
5. The demand to leave in 1 day seems more severe than a refusal to renew. Is Dr. Olsen facing charges of inappropriate conduct? How will this charge affect his career? Does he need legal representation?

Ethical Course of Action

Directive per APA Code

If Dr. Olsen was providing psychotherapy in these evening appointments with the students, then he would be in violation of Standard 7.05. If he was engaging in romantic and/or sexual relationships with students in these evening appointments, he would be in violation of Standard 7.05. Regardless of how students interpret an invitation for his home office appointments, Dr. Olsen has entered into multiple relationships as defined in Standard 3.05 (a) (1). Regardless of the nature of the evening appointments, multiple relationships are not prohibited in of themselves. Finally, regardless of the outcome of the ethics investigation, the university has violated Standard 1.08 if the ethics investigation is the sole grounds on which the employment contract was terminated.

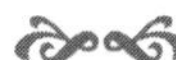

Dictates of One's Own Conscience

If you were the chair of the program, faced with a faculty being investigated for possible ethics violation and at the same time generating some animosity in advocating for shared governance, how might you approach a reappointment situation?

1. Verbally reprimand Dr. Olsen for having students go to his home office, and advise that he stop such practices.
2. Write a letter to Dr. Olsen requesting that he stop meeting students in his home office, and confine all of his meetings with students to his university office.
3. Tell Dr. Olsen that the situation at this university has become tenuous, and advise Dr. Olsen to seek employment elsewhere.
4. Argue with the dean and HR to give Dr. Olsen the option to resign from his post as faculty.
5. Do a combination of the previously listed actions.
6. Do something that is not previously listed.

If you were the chair of a program in Canada, faced with the previously described situation, you might choose to write a letter to Dr. Olsen requesting that he stop meeting students in his home office and confine all of his meetings with students to his university office as a first step to a discipline proceeding.

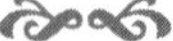

CHAPTER 8

Research and Publication

Ethical Standard 8

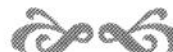

CHAPTER OUTLINE

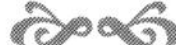

STANDARD 8.01: INSTITUTIONAL APPROVAL

When institutional approval is required, psychologists provide accurate information about their research proposals and obtain approval prior to conducting the research. They conduct the research in accordance with the approved research protocol.

A CASE FOR STANDARD 8.01: Two Masters

Clara is a graduate student on an internship with an interest in suicide. She considers herself extremely fortunate to have gotten a rotation with the county coroner's office. Under the tutelage of the coroner, Dr. Anderson, Clara has had the opportunity to accompany her to crime scene investigations and attend psychological autopsies, as well as complete training sessions in how to conduct psychological autopsies.

For her dissertation, Clara proposes to examine the effect of a psychological autopsy on family members. Her study calls for follow-up interviews of family members in cases where psychological autopsies were performed and in cases where they were not performed. Clara submits her dissertation proposal to the university's institutional review board (IRB). She receives notice that permission to interview family members has been declined. The IRB cited insufficient safeguards to protect the family members from re-traumatization. Clara then resubmits her proposal including additional safeguards for the interviewees and awaits the IRB's review.

While Clara is awaiting the IRB's response, Dr. Anderson informs Clara that the office is especially busy and assigns her the case of a recent teen death. Dr. Anderson notes that it is unclear as to whether cause of death is a result of suicide or accidental death and tells Clara to conduct a psychological autopsy and to interview the surviving family members. She also tells Clara to audio record these interviews for supervision review. Clara is unable to get an expedited response from the IRB to give her permission to interview these family members.

Issues of Concern

Standard 8.01 names psychologists, regardless of training status, as responsible for obtaining approval prior to conducting research. Clara is required by Standard 8.01 to obtain approval from the IRB to interview family members of suicide victims. At the same time, psychology interns are under supervision, and as supervisees, they are required to carry out the directives of their supervisor. In this case, if Clara were to follow the directives of Standard 8.01, then she would not conduct the family interviews. However, if Clara were to follow the directives of her supervisor, then she would conduct and record the family interviews.

Timing of the IRB review process is not under the control of researchers. What if Clara conducts the interviews as directed by her supervisor, and in the middle of the interview process, she receives approval from the IRB to proceed with her research? In such an event, would Clara be ethically correct in using this current case for her research?

APA Ethics Code

Companion General Principle

Principle B: Fidelity and Responsibility

> Psychologists uphold professional standards of conduct, clarify their professional roles and obligations, accept appropriate responsibility for their behavior, and seek to manage conflicts of interest that could lead to exploitation or harm.

Principle B guides Clara to uphold the professional standard of only conducting research activities that have been approved by the IRB. Principle B, in the same sentence, also guides Clara to clarify her professional roles and obligations. In order for Clara to adhere to this aspirational goal, she would need to be clear about the possible divergent responsibilities in her role as an intern versus her role as a researcher.

Companion Ethical Standard(s)

Standard 3.05: Multiple Relationships.

> (a) A multiple relationship occurs when a psychologist is in a professional role with a person and . . .
>
> (1) at the same time is in another role with the same person. . . A psychologist refrains from entering into a multiple relationship if the multiple relationship could reasonably be expected to impair the psychologist's . . . effectiveness in performing his or her functions as a psychologist, or otherwise risks exploitation or harm to the person with whom the professional relationship exists. Multiple relationships that would not reasonably be expected to cause impairment or risk exploitation or harm are not unethical.

When Clara interviews family members for her research, she is in the role of a researcher and at the same time in the role of a coroner who is an agent of the legal system. This dual role meets the definition of multiple relationships as specified in Standard 3.05 (a) (1). Standard 3.05 does not categorically prohibit such multiple relationships. It asks that Clara make a judgment call to determine whether entering into such a dual role would create foreseeable negative situations. Would she conduct the interview and be tempted to later use the family for her research without having implemented the additional safeguards for re-traumatization that are likely to be ordered by the IRB?

Standard 2.05: Delegation of Work to Others

> Psychologists who delegate work to . . . supervisees, or research . . . assistants[,] . . . take reasonable steps to . . . (2) authorize only those responsibilities that such persons can be expected to perform competently on the basis of their education, training, or experience, either independently or with the level of supervision being provided.

Though Dr. Anderson is not a psychologist, she is directing the work of a psychology intern. Most states allow for a portion of psychology interns' work to be done under someone who is equivalently credentialed, such as a medical doctor. As Clara's supervisor, it is Dr. Anderson's responsibility to determine Clara's competency in deciding the level of independence to give her. In this case, Dr. Anderson has given Clara the autonomy to conduct independent interviews, with the ability to allow for detailed scrutiny through the audio recordings.

10.01: Informed Consent to Therapy

> . . . (c) When the therapist is a trainee and the legal responsibility for the treatment provided resides with the supervisor, the client/patient, as part of the informed consent procedure, is informed that the therapist is in training and is being supervised and is given the name of the supervisor.

A psychological autopsy does not fall under the purview of therapy, thus Standard 10 does not apply. As an intern, all of Clara's work in the coroner's office is under the legal responsibility of Dr. Anderson. From the perspective of borrowed competency, Standard 10.01 does inform this situation. In the position of supervisee, Clara is to perform work of the coroner's office as directed by Dr. Anderson. In this case, following Dr. Anderson's directive, Clara is to conduct and audio record the interviews.

Standard 1.03: Conflicts Between Ethics and Organizational Demands

> If the demands of an organization . . . for whom they [psychologists] are working are in conflict with this Ethics Code, psychologists clarify the nature of the conflict, make known their commitment to the Ethics Code, and take reasonable steps to resolve the conflict consistent with the General Principles and Ethical Standards of the Ethics Code.

In multiple relationship situations, it is common to have conflicting demands. Standard 8.01 directs Clara not to audio record nor conduct the interviews until approval from the IRB is received; the demand from Standard 10.01 is for Clara to follow her supervisor's directive of conducting and audio recording the psychological autopsy. When psychologists are caught in such a conflict, Standard 1.03 directs Clara to voice her dilemma to both the university's IRB and to Dr. Anderson, and to make clear to all that her primary obligation is to follow the directives of the APA Ethics Code.

Standard 9.03: Informed Consent in Assessments

> (a) Psychologists obtain informed consent for . . . evaluations . . . services, as described in Standard 3.10, Informed Consent, except when (1) testing is mandated by law or governmental regulations.

When Clara engages in psychological autopsy, she is conducting an evaluation as mandated by the authority of the coroner's office to investigate any cause of death. Therefore, Clara does not need informed consent from the family of the deceased for interviews. Per Standard 9.03, not only does Clara not need the assent of the university IRB, but she does not even need the consent of the family members to proceed with the interviews.

Legal Issues 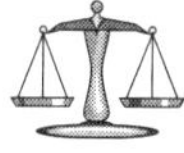

California

> *Cal. Code Regs. tit. 16, § 1387.1 (West 2010). Qualifications and Responsibilities of the Primary Supervisors.*
>
> (d) Primary supervisors shall be responsible for ensuring compliance at all times by the trainee with the provisions of the Psychology Licensing Law and the regulations adopted pursuant to these laws.
>
> (e) Primary supervisors shall be responsible for ensuring . . . compliance with the Ethical Principles and Code of Conduct of the American Psychological Association.
>
> (f) Primary supervisors shall be responsible for monitoring the welfare of the trainee's clients. . .

(h) Primary supervisors shall be responsible for monitoring the performance and professional development of the trainee.

Colorado

Colo. Rev. Stat. Ann. § 12-43-202(West 2010). Practice Outside of or Beyond Professional Training, Experience, or Competence.

Notwithstanding any other provision of this article, no . . . unlicensed psychotherapist is authorized to practice outside of or beyond his or her area of training, experience, or competence.

Colo. Rev. Stat. Ann. § 12-43-222 (West 2010). Prohibited Activities—Related Provisions.

(g) Has acted or failed to act in a manner that does not meet the generally accepted standards of the professional discipline under which such person practices. . .

California and Colorado are both silent on the matter of institutional approval for conducting research with human subjects. On the matter of competence and responsibility, both California and Colorado designate the responsibility to the supervisor—in this case, Dr. Anderson. This means Clara should follow the directives of Dr. Anderson in conducting and taping the interviews.

Cultural Considerations

Global Discussion

Hong Kong Psychological Society: Professional Code of Practice

Chapter 6: Research in Psychology.

6.1. In planning a psychological . . . investigation, Members shall undertake a careful evaluation of the ethical issues involved. . . The responsibility for ensuring ethical practice in research remains with the principal investigators and cannot be shared. They are also responsible for the ethical treatment of research participants by collaborators . . . [and] students[,] . . . all of whom incur similar obligations.

6.10. Members who supervise students in research shall ensure that their supervisees conduct research in accordance with professional and ethical requirements.

Chapter 4: Employment in Organizations.

4.2. Materials prepared by Members as a part of their regular work under the specific direction of the . . . organization normally become the property of the employing . . . organization. Such materials are released for use or publication by Members in accordance with the policies of authorization, assignment of credit and related matters which have been established by the . . . organization.

4.5. When Members employed by an . . . organization cannot ensure that information recorded by them will not be communicated to others, they shall exercise considerable discretion in regard to the form and content of the record, and consider whether they should advise the clients of this matter.

If Clara's interviews are to end up as part of her dissertation work, standard 6.1 guides Clara, as the principal investigator, to "ensure ethical practices" and "ethical treatment" of all participants by herself and Dr. Anderson. If Dr. Anderson was a psychologist instead of a medical doctor, then, as directed by 6.10, Dr. Anderson would assign Clara to those procedures for which she has been adequately trained. As Dr. Anderson is not bound by the ethics code for psychologists, this standard offers guidance; it does not impose obligation.

Hong Kong's code is silent regarding a specific body such as an IRB, unless the standards in Employment in Organizations are used as equivalent. If so, then any interviews done at the behest of an institution (4.2) remains the property of that institution. Next (4.5), it instructs Clara to be cautious in recording information provided by "clients" if she cannot guarantee their privacy, presuming "clients" and "research participants" are synonymous in Hong Kong's code. Finally (6.1), Clara is responsible for ensuring compliance to the code. If Clara decides that the most ethical course for the participants is to not have their psychological autopsies recorded before IRB approval, then she must take responsibility for explaining this to Dr. Anderson. If she decides that as an intern, she is obligated to relinquish control of the information and research to that institution, Clara could perform the psychological autopsy as requested and go forward, as she has received the proper training.

American Moral Values

1. Would Clara conduct her interview differently depending on whether it was for her research or not? Can she in good conscience conduct an interview as a researcher while working under the auspices of Dr. Anderson and the coroner's office? Is she aiming to provide the same service that Dr. Anderson does?

2. How does Clara interpret the IRB's objection to psychological autopsies? Is there a larger moral objection to them in general? Will survivors of such deaths be re-traumatized regardless of the research purposes and methodology? Should Clara reconsider the practice as a whole and talk about it with Dr. Anderson? Should she ask for a justification from Dr. Anderson? Does she owe the IRB a notification that she is conducting an interview under her supervisor's orders?

3. How does Clara, as a student of psychology, regard Dr. Anderson's work as a coroner? How are coroners seen by Clara's other advisors and colleagues? Is the IRB's judgment shaped by the fact that her proposal involves work through a coroner's office? Is there an assumption that psychologists should be more sensitive to trauma than the coroner's office and the rest of the legal system?

Ethical Course of Action

Directive per APA Code

Clara is in an inherently conflictual situation, as referenced by Standard 3.05 (a) (1). In relation to the family and friends of the person who appears to have committed suicide, she could be viewed as both someone who represents the office of the coroner and who is a graduate psychology student conducting research for her dissertation. Standard 1.03 directs Clara to make known to both the university's IRB and to her supervisor, Dr. Anderson, the nature of this multiple relationship and the divergent demands inherent in the situation. Beyond attempts to expedite the work of the IRB, Standard 8.01 clearly prohibits Clara from starting the research without IRB approval. If she resided in either of the two states, neither California nor Colorado State law addresses research consent. Without approval, Clara cannot use this case in her research. Clara is able to conduct the psychological autopsy as directed by Dr. Anderson if Clara does not use this case for her dissertation.

Dictates of One's Own Conscience

If you were Clara, would you:

1. Plead with the IRB to expedite a review, telling the IRB that appropriate cases do not emerge often, and if you are not able to use this current case for your dissertation, your graduation may be unduly delayed?
   a. Stall the interview until you hear from the IRB?
   b. Start the interview as appropriately demanded by the coroner?
   c. Ask the IRB to allow for admission of this current case should the IRB decide that your revised plan is acceptable?
2. Consider conducting a psychological autopsy of this case as a practice run for your dissertation, and proceed to conduct the interviews with full knowledge that no part of this case can be used for your dissertation?
3. Think that if IRB approval is received at any time when this case is open, there's reason that approval was received and would you use all audio recordings of this case for your dissertation after notifying the IRB of such a plan of action?
4. Ask Dr. Anderson if you can delay starting the investigation of this case pending notification from the IRB about the use of this case in your dissertation?
5. Proceed with your revised research protocol with this case, reasoning that no one would know or care that you started early once you receive IRB approval?
6. Combinations of the above-listed possible courses of action?
7. Or one that is not listed above?

If you were Clara and held an internship in Hong Kong, what would you do?

1. Function only as a psychology intern when conducting work under the direction of Dr. Anderson and let the family members know that you are doing the investigation as part of the coroner's office?
2. Discuss the situation with Dr. Anderson that all recording of the investigation belongs to the coroner's office, not to the principal investigator of any research?

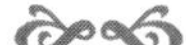

STANDARD 8.02: INFORMED CONSENT TO RESEARCH

(a) When obtaining informed consent as required in Standard 3.10, Informed Consent, psychologists inform participants about (1) the purpose of the research, expected duration, and procedures; (2) their right to decline to participate and to withdraw from the research once participation has begun; (3) the foreseeable consequences of declining or withdrawing; (4) reasonably

> foreseeable factors that may be expected to influence their willingness to participate such as potential risks, discomfort, or adverse effects; (5) any prospective research benefits; (6) limits of confidentiality; (7) incentives for participation; and (8) whom to contact for questions about the research and research participants' rights. They provide opportunity for the prospective participants to ask questions and receive answers.

A CASE FOR STANDARD 8.02 (A): How Are We Doing?

The Modern School of Psychology in the New Center University conducts a survey of student satisfaction once every 2 years. The first part of the survey is an anonymous questionnaire. The second part of the survey is an in-depth, in-person interview to clarify responses from the questionnaire. The participants for the interview are students who are randomly selected from a list of students enrolled in the doctoral psychology program. The interviewees are assured that their participation is voluntary, that individual responses will be kept confidential, and that only consolidated information will be released.

Gail was selected for an interview. She says that simple deletion of her name does not assure confidentiality because of the specificity of the information she is being asked to talk about and the smallness of the community in which the program exists. In addition, she is also concerned that her identity will not be kept confidential since the signed consent form is the property of the program and any faculty can look up which students were interviewed. Gail is not assured that confidentiality is protected nor is she assured that she will escape retribution if she says anything negative about the program. In addition, having just completed her research methods course, she also questions the validity of the interview. Gail thinks the subject's responses will not be accurate because students will self-monitor and could delete all negative feedback.

Issues of Concern

Standard 8.02 (a) directs psychologists to obtain consent from subjects for research. The questions relevant for this situation are (1) whether the program needs IRB approval, (2) whether the project needs subject consent, and (3) whether the project needs signed subject consent. Standard 8.02 directs the researcher to give Gail fair warning and asks Gail to make an informed choice. If, once given fair warning, Gail decides to participate, the assumption is that she has knowingly agreed to incur possible negative consequences. In this case, though there is an offer of anonymity by deletion of names, given the smallness of the community, the implication is that should Gail decide to proceed with the interview, she should assume the faculty will know it is Gail who is making negative statements.

The assumption behind the need for protection of anonymity is the power differential between professors and students. In the normal course of degree progress, students make decisions as to how much and when to complain about their professors or degree program. In the case of a student interview initiated by the program, Gail does not have the freedom to decide how much to complain based on the specifics of any given situation and set of circumstances.

APA Ethics Code

Companion General Principle

Principle A: Beneficence and Nonmaleficence

> In their professional actions, psychologists seek to safeguard the welfare and rights of those with whom they interact professionally.

In the spirit of Principle A: Beneficence and Nonmaleficence, the psychology program would protect Gail from possible harm. The task of this research project is to discover and understand the specific problematic concerns students experience. Striving to meet the aspirational goal of nonmaleficence, the program would address Gail's concern by a careful examination of the research design and not dismiss Gail's fear of possible retribution.

Companion Ethical Standard(s)

Standard 3.10: Informed Consent

> (a) When psychologists conduct research[,] . . . they obtain the informed consent of the . . . individuals . . . except when conducting such activities without consent . . . as otherwise provided in this Ethics Code.

If the program's survey of student satisfaction is considered research, then Standard 3.10 directs the program to obtain informed consent. This project may not meet the definition of research that needs consent under Standard 8.05 (1) (a).

Standard 8.05: Dispensing With Informed Consent for Research

> Psychologists may dispense with informed consent only (1) where research would not reasonably be assumed to create distress or harm and involves (a) the study of normal educational practices . . . conducted in educational settings.

Given that this project is concerned with normal educational practices, it could be reasoned that Standard 8.05 (1) (a) applies and the student interviews could proceed without obtaining subject consent for participation. When a student signs up for a degree program, the student has consented to engage with the activities of the degree program, including providing feedback to the degree program regarding the student's level of satisfaction with his or her educational experience. Alternatively, it could be argued that since voluntary participation in in-depth individual interviews specifically regarding problem areas of the degree program could create distress and harm, then conditions for Standard 8.05 (1) (a) do not apply. Thus, the project would require subject consent.

Standard 7.02: Descriptions of Education and Training Programs

> Psychologists . . . take reasonable steps to ensure that there is a current and accurate description of the program content . . . and requirements that must be met for satisfactory completion of the program. This information must be made readily available to all interested parties.

If the program includes a description of the biannual survey in the recruitment materials that were available for prospective students, would such a practice eliminate the need to comply with Standard 8.05 (1) (a)? Does such a description make the activity of individual in-depth student interviews a normal educational practice? If forewarning students in the recruitment material makes interviews a normal educational practice, could the program mandate students to participate in such random interviews?

Standard 2.04: Bases for Scientific and Professional Judgments

> Psychologists' work is based upon established scientific and professional knowledge of the discipline.

The knowledge available regarding the bias needs to dictate the design of studies. Gail's criticism appears to be a legitimate concern (Heppner, Wampold, & Kivlighan, 2008). To grant protection from adverse consequences of participation, might the program not ask students to sign a subject consent form? Instead of having subjects give written consent, could the program ask the interviewers to sign a document attesting to the fact that informed consent was discussed and the subjects, without giving any names, provided the interviewer with verbal consent for the interview? Neither Standard 8.02 (a) nor Standard 3.10 specifies whether that consent needs to be a written document signed by the subject.

Legal Issues 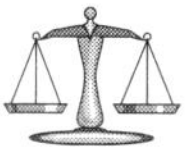

Florida

> *Fla. Admin. Code Ann. r. 64B19-19.006 (2010). Confidentiality.*
>
> (1) One of the primary obligations of psychologists is to respect the confidentiality of information entrusted to them by service users. Psychologists may disclose that information only with the written consent of the service user. . . If there are limits to the maintenance of confidentiality, however, the licensed psychologist shall inform the service user of those limitations. . . Similar limitations on confidentiality may present themselves in educational . . . situations, and in each of the circumstances . . . the licensed psychologist must obtain a written statement from the service user which acknowledges the psychologist's advice in those regards.

> *Florida Statute 490.009 (2010). Discipline.*
>
> (1) The following acts constitute grounds for denial of a license or disciplinary action, as specified in s. 456.072(2):
>
> (l) Making misleading, deceptive, untrue, or fraudulent representations in the practice of any profession licensed under this chapter.
>
> (r) Failing to meet the minimum standards of performance in professional activities when measured against generally prevailing peer performance, including the undertaking of activities for which the licensee is not qualified by training or experience.

Hawaii

> *Haw. Code R. § 16-98-34 (2010). Unethical Practice of Psychology.*
>
> (d) Safeguarding information about an individual that has been obtained by the psychologist in the course of

teaching, practice, or investigation is a primary obligation of the psychologist. Such information shall not be communicated to others unless certain important conditions are met.

(1) Information received in confidence may be revealed only after careful deliberation and where there is a clear and imminent danger to an individual . . . and then only to appropriate professional workers or public authorities. . .

(e) The psychologist shall respect the integrity and protect the welfare of the person or group with whom the psychologist is working.

(1) The psychologist in . . . education . . . in which conflicts of interest may arise among various parties . . . shall define the nature and direction of the psychologist's loyalties and responsibilities and keep all parties concerned informed of these commitments;

(2) When there is a conflict among professional workers, the psychologist shall be concerned primarily with the welfare of any client involved and only secondarily with the interest of the psychologist's own professional group. . .

(m) The psychologist shall assume obligations for the welfare of the psychologist's research subjects, both animal and human.

(1) Only when a problem is of scientific significance and it is not practicable to investigate it in any other way is the psychologist justified in exposing research subjects . . . to physical or emotional stress as part of the investigation;

(2) When a reasonable possibility of injurious after-effects exists, research may be conducted only when the subjects or their responsible agents are fully informed of this possibility and agree to participate nevertheless;

(3) The psychologist shall seriously consider the possibility of harmful after-effects and avoid them, or remove them as soon as permitted by the design of the experiment.

Both Florida and Hawaii emphasize the importance of keeping confidential the information psychologists obtain through the course of their work. Neither Florida nor Hawaii differentiates between information obtained through treatment and that obtained through research. Hawaii places an additional burden on psychologists to protect the welfare of the research subjects, in addition to keeping information confidential. If the psychology program were located in Florida or Hawaii, the program would be obligated to address Gail's concerns and alter the project to assure absolute anonymity of the students being interviewed.

Cultural Considerations

Global Discussion

Singapore Psychological Society:
Code of Professional Ethics

Principle 16: Research Precautions

The psychologists assume obligations for the welfare of their research subjects, both animal and human.

1. Only when a problem is of scientific significance and it is not practicable to investigate it in any other way is the psychologist justified in exposing research subjects, whether children or adults, to physical or emotional stress as part of an investigation.

2. When a reasonable possibility of injurious after-effects exists, research is conducted only when the subjects . . . are fully informed of this possibility and agree to participate nevertheless.

3. The psychologist seriously considers the possibility of harmful after-effects and avoids them, or removes them as soon as permitted by the design of the experiment.

If the school is conducting the satisfaction survey in Singapore, the school is not under any obligation to require a written record of informed consent, but they must ensure that participants are "fully informed" (2) of any possible negative after-effects of the research, and they cannot proceed with the interviews until the participants have been informed and agree, nonetheless, to proceed with the interview. No written record of such consent seems to be required by Singapore's code. Finally, psychologists conducting research attempt to foresee and remove possible harmful effects of their research (3), or move to do so as quickly as possible after the interview is conducted. Therefore, the school could eliminate the written record of consent, provided that the participants were told the possible risks and agreed to move forward anyway.

American Moral Values

1. Is there a way of securing informed consent without a signature? Can there be a verbal attestation of consent so that no identification would be on the form?
2. If Gail is worried about identifying information, does a signature matter? Isn't the real issue what she chooses to reveal about the program? Is a thorough and detailed evaluation even possible for a close-knit

community or institution, where particular members' stories are widely known?

3. Are there particular conflicts with faculty that Gail owes it to the school to address for future students? How does Gail assess the risk of being identified? What is the risk of retribution in light of how faculty have responded to earlier student complaints? Is there a way that Gail can preempt retribution by talking about it with fellow students? Is there another forum for complaint or criticism?

4. Should the program continue in-depth interviews? Can subjects trust who the interviewer is and what the relationships are among the interviewer, the dean, the faculty, and so forth? How do they address Gail's concern with self-monitoring? Is there a depth and quality of feedback that only one-on-one questioning can elicit from subjects?

5. What decisions are seen to depend on this survey? Does Gail owe it to the school and its future students to point out the program's flaws and virtues?

Ethical Course of Action

Directive per APA Code

Standard 3.10 specifies that informed consent is to be obtained. Standard 8.02 specifies the types of information psychologists are to include when obtaining informed consent from subjects. The part that may be of the most relevance to this situation is one that is actually missing from the standards. Neither Standard 3.10 nor Standard 8.02 specifies that a subject's informed consent necessarily needs to be proven through a signed document. To meet the requirements of Standards 3.10 and 8.02, the program may require the interviewer to attest to the fact that informed consent was obtained verbally from the subject, with no specification of an individual's name.

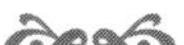

Dictates of One's Own Conscience

If you were the program administrator overseeing this project, would you

1. Argue that the study is part of the normal educational process and thus does not need consent? Proceed with interviewing Gail, letting her know that what she says or does not say is left to her discretion?

2. Argue that the study is beyond the normal educational process since only randomly selected students are asked to participate in the interview, and ask Gail to consent with full knowledge that faculty could discover the identities of the students interviewed?

3. Move on to another subject, looking for a student who would not object to participation under the conditions specified?

4. Require that the interviewer attest to the fact that the subject received information for informed consent, but not have the subject be self-identified through signing an informed consent form?

If you were Gail, the student requested for an interview, which of these would you do?

1. Go ahead with the interview,
   a. self-monitoring to say only positive comments about the graduate program and your professors.
   b. reason that your professors are all psychologists functioning under the ethics code and thus would not engage in retaliatory actions, and say whatever is on your mind, be it positive or negative.
   c. sign the informed consent under a different name.
   d. only if the interviewer agrees to use a fake name for you.
2. Decline, claiming you are
   a. overwhelmed with class work and think nothing more of the matter.
   b. writing a letter to the university's IRB requesting IRB review of the study.
3. Combinations of the above-listed actions.
4. Or one that is not listed above.

If you were the school administrator working in a school located in Singapore, you would require that the interviewer attest to the fact that the subject received information for informed consent, but not have the subject be self-identified through signing an informed consent form.

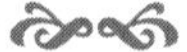

STANDARD 8.02 (B): INFORMED CONSENT TO RESEARCH

> . . . (b) Psychologists conducting intervention research involving the use of experimental treatments clarify to participants at the outset of the research (1) the experimental nature of the treatment; (2) the services that will or will not be available to the control group(s) if appropriate; (3) the means by which assignment to treatment and control groups will be made; (4) available treatment alternatives if an individual does not wish to participate in the research or wishes to withdraw once a study has begun; and (5) compensation for or monetary costs of participating including, if appropriate, whether reimbursement from the participant or a third-party payor will be sought.

A CASE FOR STANDARD 8.02 (B): We Will Be Famous

Miguel, a 7-year-old European American male, is reported to be disruptive in school. His teachers complain that he is inappropriately loud in the classroom, disorganized, in constant motion, and is rough during recess with other kids. Joanne, Miguel's mother, was referred by their pediatrician to First Start, an early education and intervention program for children with disabilities, for further testing in order to rule out a possible diagnosis of attention deficit hyperactivity disorder (ADHD). Dr. Jackson, the psychologist at First Start, is a 37-year-old single European American male who specializes in ADHD diagnosis and treatment in children.

After the first testing session with Dr. Jackson, Miguel asks his mother, Joanne, if Grandpa ever touched her private parts. Later, Miguel asks his mother if she has sex with Grandpa or with his uncle. Somewhat alarmed, Miguel's mother asks him why he is asking her these kinds of questions. Miguel replies that Dr. Jackson had asked him about these things during their session. Joanne is concerned and contacts Dr. Harris, director of First Start.

Dr. Harris calls a meeting with Dr. Jackson to discuss Joanne's concerns. Dr. Jackson responds by saying that many of the children he has evaluated for ADHD seemed to exhibit symptoms reflective of a repressed maternal intrapsychic conflict around sexuality. He further notes that based on his clinical practice, and his hypothesis that ADHD in children is directly linked to repressed maternal sexual conflict, he has developed a structured interview protocol for diagnosing childhood ADHD. Dr. Jackson acknowledges that this protocol is experimental, but refutes that he needed to discuss this protocol with Dr. Harris or obtain approval from the agency's institutional review board before its use. Dr. Jackson reasons that he was providing clinical treatment, not conducting research. He further indicates that his work is being written up for publication in a single case design study demonstrating the effectiveness of the clinical intervention. He suggests that not only did he not need to follow research procedures, but his work will also bring prestige to the agency.

Issues of Concern

What constitutes intervention research? Is it an accurate or reasonable claim that when activities are restricted to clients who are requesting treatment, then those activities are not subject to the rules and regulations of research? It seems that Dr. Jackson's claim is disingenuous if he is seeking to publish his work. If indeed Dr. Jackson's work were usual and customary for the assessment and treatment of ADHD, then there would be neither need nor audience for publication. However, if Dr. Jackson sincerely did not believe his work was innovative, and was not intending to publish his work, would his claim to not need institutional review be reasonable and accurate?

APA Ethics Code

Companion General Principle

Principle B: Fidelity and Responsibility

> Psychologists . . . are concerned about the ethical compliance of their colleagues' scientific and professional conduct.

Dr. Harris, being director of an agency, presumably has supervisory responsibility over Dr. Jackson. When Dr. Harris requests a meeting with Dr. Jackson, she is, at a minimum, basing her actions on Principle B. In the best of all possible worlds, someone in the agency would have known of Dr. Jackson's activities well before clients are affected.

Companion Ethical Standard(s)

Standard 9.03: Informed Consent in Assessments

> (a) Psychologists obtain informed consent for assessments, evaluations, or diagnostic services... Informed consent includes an explanation of the nature and purpose of the assessment . . . and sufficient opportunity for the client/patient to ask questions and receive answers...
>
> (b) Psychologists inform persons with questionable capacity to consent . . . about the nature and purpose of the proposed assessment services, using language that is reasonably understandable to the person being assessed.

Congruent with Dr. Jackson's claim that he was providing treatment, not conducting research, he should have followed the directives of Standard 9.03 (a) by obtaining informed consent for assessment from Joanne; and he should have informed Miguel of the nature and purpose of the assessment per Standard 9.03 (b).

Standard 9.01: Bases for Assessments

> (a) Psychologists base the opinions contained in their . . . evaluative statements . . . on information and techniques sufficient to substantiate their findings.

The basis of any concluding statement from Dr. Jackson needs to rest on techniques deemed adequate to support the findings. Using an instrument that is not normed or generally used, and thus does not meet the professional standards, is not considered sufficient evidence to support any finding. Dr. Jackson's unconventional use of his own instrument that has not been tested is in violation of Standard 9.01 (a).

Standard 2.04 Bases for Scientific and Professional Judgments

> Psychologists' work is based upon established scientific and professional knowledge of the discipline.

To the casual lay observer, psychologists make inquiries on topics that do not seem to be linked. Someone could ask why a psychologist is asking him or her to look at blots of ink when he or she is seeking treatment for depression. Similarly, one could reasonably ask whether Dr. Jackson should make a connection between disruptive classroom behaviors from a 7-year-old and a family history of incest. If there were evidence of such a causal link in the published literature, then Dr. Jackson's line of questioning to Miguel would comply with Standard 2.04. However, to date, no known publication points to a direct causal link between the phenomenon of disruptive classroom behavior and incest. In the absence of such knowledge, Dr. Jackson's line of questioning is in violation of Standard 2.04.

Legal Issues 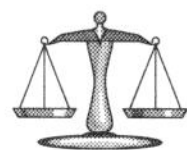

Indiana

> *868 Ind. Admin. Code 1.1-11-4.1 (2010). Relationships within professional practice.*
>
> (l) A psychologist shall exercise reasonable care and diligence in the conduct of research and shall utilize generally accepted scientific principles and current professional theory and practice. New or experimental procedures, techniques, and theories shall be utilized only with proper research safeguards, informed consent, and peer review of the procedures or techniques.

Kansas

> *Kan. Admin. Regs. § 102-1-1(2010). Definitions.*
>
> (b) "Client" or "patient" means a person who meets either of the following criteria:
>
> (1) Is a recipient of direct psychological services within a relationship that is initiated either by mutual consent of the person and a psychologist or according to law . . .
>
> *Kan. Admin. Regs. § 102-1-10a (2010). Unprofessional conduct.*
>
> (e) failing to obtain informed consent, which shall include the following acts:
>
> (1) Failing to obtain and document, in a timely manner, informed consent from the client or legally authorized representative for clinical psychological services before the provision of any of these services... This informed consent shall include a description of the possible effects of treatment or procedures when there are known risks to the client or patient;
>
> (2) Failing to provide clients or patients with a description of what the client or patient may expect in the way of tests . . . and
>
> (3) Failing to inform clients or patients when a proposed treatment or procedure is experimental...

(n) improperly engaging in research with human subjects, which shall include the following acts:

(1) Failing to consider carefully the possible consequences for human beings participating in the research;

(2) Failing to protect each participant from unwarranted . . . harm;

(3) Failing to ascertain that the consent of the participant is voluntary and informed.

In Kansas, Dr. Jackson would clearly have violated laws regarding treatment of research participants. It is less clear for Indiana. However, neither state addresses the issue of what constitutes research. Dr. Jackson's argument is that he is engaged in treatment and does not have to follow research protocol.

Cultural Considerations

Global Discussion

Code of Ethics for Psychologists: Netherlands

III.2 Respect.

III.2.1.2 Respect for the mental and bodily integrity of those involved.

The psychologist respects the mental and bodily integrity of those involved and does not prejudice their dignity. He only infringes on the privacy of those involved to the extent that this is strictly germane to the purposes of the professional relationship.

III.3 Competence.

III.3.3.5 Justification of professional acting.

The psychologist has to be able to justify his professional acting in the light of the state of science at the time of the professional acting in question, as it is shown from professional literature.

III.4 Responsibility.

III.4.1 The quality of professional conduct.

III.4.1.3 Adequate professional and ethical standards.

The psychologist imposes high professional standards and ethical norms on his professional practice. He acts in accordance with acknowledged scientific views. To the best of his ability, he strives for the advancement of such norms and standards in his professional field.

Dr. Jackson has "infringed on . . . privacy" beyond what is germane for assessment of Miguel for ADHD, a violation of III.2.1.2. The causal link between familial incest and ADHD is unproven, undocumented, speculative, and potentially harmful to families upon whom such a theory is imposed; therefore, Dr. Jackson's decisions and actions are not supported by scientific standards or current practice, a violation of III.3.3.5 and III.4.1.3. To be in compliance, Dr. Jackson would need to immediately stop asking clients, particularly children, about parts of their family history not germane to the clinical problem at hand, and not attempt to apply his interview protocol.

American Moral Values

1. What does Dr. Harris believe Dr. Jackson owed to Miguel and his mother in terms of information about his approach? Is the problem with Dr. Jackson's treatment that it is experimental and not yet supported by current research? Should he alert ADHD referrals about the experimental character of his approach? Does Dr. Harris believe Dr. Jackson is hiding the character of his approach in order to keep his clients?
2. Is the sexual character of Dr. Jackson's hypothesis part of what makes his approach objectionable? Are children like Miguel prepared to discuss the questions Dr. Jackson is asking, whether with a therapist or a parent? Does this approach interfere with different families' ways of teaching their children about sex? Are the psychological effects of these questions worth the treatment of ADHD?
3. What are Dr. Harris's views about appropriate sexual education? If Dr. Jackson were pursuing an experimental approach based on physical activity and relaxation exercises, would Dr. Harris take the same tack with Joanne's misgivings?
4. At what point does Dr. Harris believe a family should explore alternative treatments for ADHD? Does she believe Miguel's family is in a position to decide the best treatment for Miguel? Could their desperation lead to a rash decision?
5. How does Dr. Harris evaluate Dr. Jackson's defense that the IRB need not be informed about his approach? Can an experimental approach require institutional approval even if a particular case will not be used in any publication? What are the criteria for when such oversight can be invoked?

Ethical Course of Action

Directive per APA Code

Standard 9.03 (a) directs Dr. Jackson to inform Joanne about the assessment services. Standard 9.03 (b)

son to have talked to Miguel about
ess. In obtaining informed consent,
have discussed his use of his own
ct the assessment.
ing an instrument that is not usual
hological assessments. Therefore,
lies. At the beginning of the assess-
son should have informed Joanne
quired for disclosure by Standard
nne's complaints, it appears that
ation of Standard 8.02 (b).
ormed of the deviations from
ractice in assessment, Dr. Harris
vene based on Principle B and
(a).

Dictates of One's Own Conscience

If you were Dr. Harris, faced with a staff psychologist admitting to using his own unvalidated assessment interview protocol, which of these would you do?

1. Order Dr. Jackson to stop using his ADHD interview protocol.
2. Have Dr. Jackson reassess Miguel using the usual and customary assessment instruments.
3. Facilitate further education for Dr. Jackson on ethics and on test construction.
4. Start disciplinary proceeding for Dr. Jackson.

If you were Joanne, faced with questionable behavior from the assessing psychologist, which of these would you do?

1. Request another psychologist to take over the assessment.
2. Make a formal complaint against Dr. Jackson.

If you were Dr. Jackson, faced with inquiry from Dr. Harris and Joanne, which action would you choose?

1. Defend the validity of the ADHD structured interview protocol.
2. Defend the procedure based on the fact that informed consent was obtained from Joanne.
3. Offer to submit the interview protocol for institutional review.
4. Develop a research study for use of your ADHD structured interview protocol.
5. Offer to apologize to Joanne, explain things to Miguel, and proceed with finishing the assessment using established instruments.
6. Combinations of the above-listed possible courses of action.
7. Or one that is not listed above.

If First Start were in the Netherlands, and you were Dr. Harris, faced with a complaint from Joanne about Dr. Jackson, which of these would you do?

1. Request that Dr. Jackson submit his justification for his actions with Miguel.
2. Regardless of the justification for his assessment of Miguel, request that Dr. Jackson demonstrate his understanding of how he behaved with respect to Joanne's "mental integrity."
3. Until such time that Dr. Jackson is able to provide justification to your satisfaction, reassign Miguel to another psychologist in the clinic.
4. Request that Dr. Jackson cease using his own ADHD interview protocol until such time that you are able to adequately review his justifications.

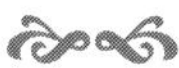

STANDARD 8.03: INFORMED CONSENT FOR RECORDING VOICES AND IMAGES IN RESEARCH

Psychologists obtain informed consent from research participants prior to recording their voices or images for data collection.

A CASE FOR STANDARD 8.03: Out of Money

Marcus is a psychology graduate student working with Dr. White. Dr. White has written a textbook on counseling skills and uses it to teach his class. In preparation for writing the second edition of his textbook, Dr. White wants to know what students actually learn from his textbook in contrast to the class lectures. In order to obtain this information, he asks Marcus to interview the students in his counseling skills class and audio record these sessions.

Dr. White had the students sign a subject consent form stipulating that in order to protect the students' anonymity, Dr. White would not have access to the voice recordings and the interviews would be transcribed by an outside transcription service. The consent form also specified that the transcripts would be reviewed by Marcus to redact any identifying information before Dr. White has access to them.

However, due to budgetary constraints, Dr. White is now unable to pay for an outside transcription service. He has decided to have the transcriptions of the taped interviews done by a departmental work-study student, and asks Marcus to deliver the recordings to this student.

Issues of Concern

Following the directive of Standard 8.03, Marcus and Dr. White obtained consent from interview subjects before recording. In addition, Marcus and Dr. White, following the directive of 8.02 (a) (6), specified the limits of confidentiality by stating that the interviews would be transcribed by an outside transcription service. The assumption was that transcribers employed at a service independent of the university would not know the individuals involved in the study. In addition, the follow-up step of redacting identifying information would assure anonymity of the interviewee. However, having students who work in the department transcribe the interviews instead suggests that the interviewee's identity may not be kept confidential because work-study students may very well know the interviewee. Also, having the interviews openly accessible within the department runs the risk of other students, staff, and faculty having access, albeit accidentally. The relevant question in this situation is, what happens when the researcher does not follow the plan as specified in the informed consent? In such a situation, does Dr. White changing the conditions for the transcription mean that the previously signed consent becomes nullified? Does the research project need to go back to the subjects for re-consent? How far can subsequent research procedures and protocol deviate from those specified in subject consent before subjects need to be re-consented?

APA Ethics Code

Companion General Principle

Principle C: Integrity

> Psychologists strive to keep their promises and to avoid unwise or unclear commitments.

A signed consent is a form of promise from the researcher. When psychologists deviate from the activities specified in the consent signed by the interviewees, they essentially break their promise. Principle C: Integrity suggests that psychologists aspire to keep their promises to the people with whom they work, be they research subjects, students, or patients. Is Dr. White's change of plan regarding who transcribes the interviews egregious enough to constitute a breach of promise?

Principle B: Fidelity and Responsibility

> Psychologists establish relationships of trust with those with whom they work... They are aware of their professional and scientific responsibilities to society and to the specific communities in which they work... They are concerned about the ethical compliance of their colleagues' scientific and professional conduct.

Keeping promises is an element of trust. When a psychologist does not keep the trust of the subjects by violating aspects of the informed consent, then the willingness of other future subjects and the integrity of other psychologists conducting research are compromised. Dr. White's lack of upholding the terms of the informed consent has wide-ranging effects on the community of researchers.

Marcus is part of the research community. He was the person who, by implication of being the interviewer, made the promise of confidentiality. Principle B suggests that Marcus should be concerned with Dr. White's proposed course of action.

Companion Ethical Standard(s)

Standard 8.01: Institutional Approval

> [P]sychologists . . . obtain approval prior to conducting the research. They conduct the research in accordance with the approved research protocol.

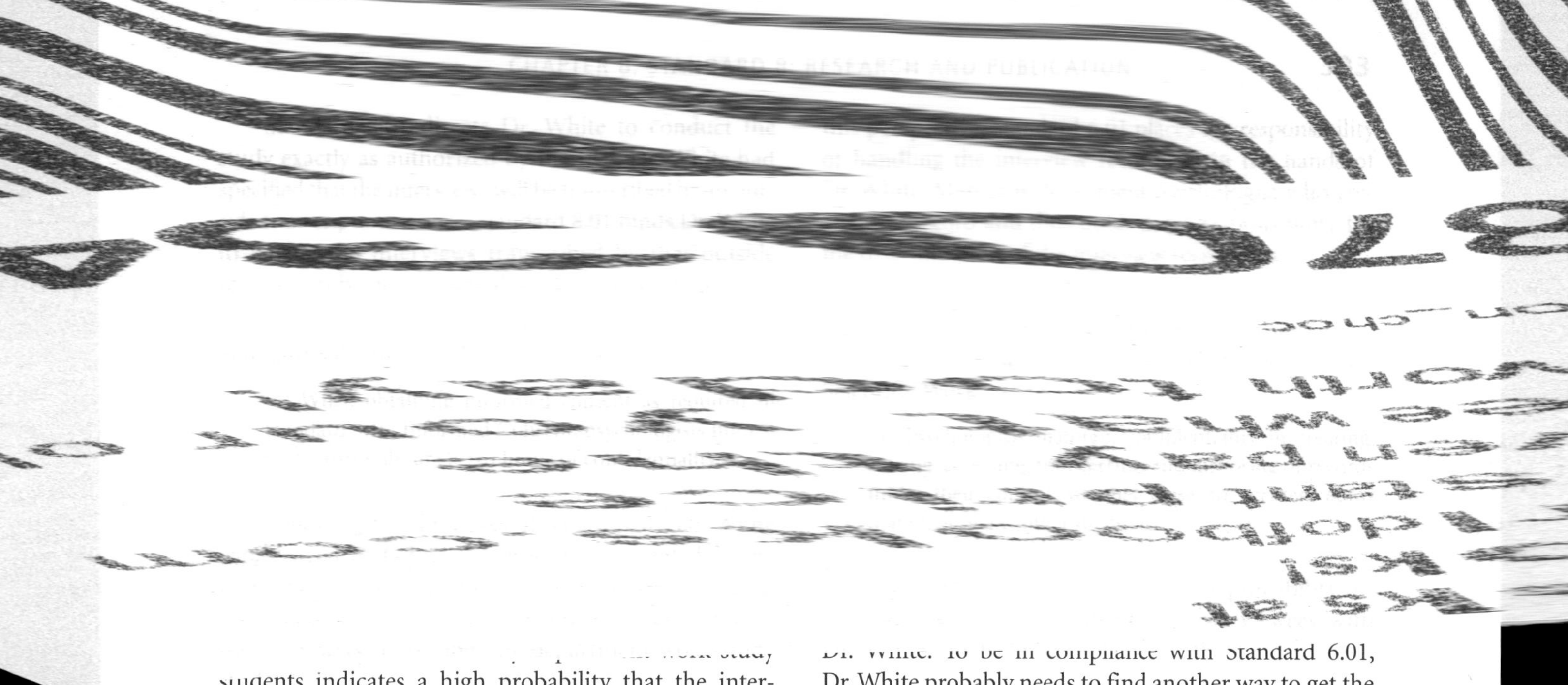

students indicates a high probability that the interviewee's identity will not be kept confidential.

Standard 2.05: Delegation of Work to Others

> Psychologists who delegate work to . . . research . . . assistants . . . take reasonable steps to . . . (2) authorize only those responsibilities that such persons can be expected to perform competently on the basis of their education, training, or experience, either independently or with the level of supervision being provided; and (3) see that such persons perform these services competently.

Marcus, being the graduate student, performs the work for this study under the direction and supervision of Dr. White. Standard 2.05 specifies that Dr. White assure Marcus's work is competently performed. Standard 2.05, by implication, does not consider Marcus to be responsible for his work performed in Dr. White's research study under Dr. White's supervision.

Standard 6.01: Documentation of Professional and Scientific Work and Maintenance of Records

> Psychologists create, and to the extent the records are under their control, maintain, disseminate, store, retain, and dispose of records and data relating to their professional and scientific work in order to . . . (2) allow for replication of research design and analyses, (3) meet institutional requirements . . . and (5) ensure compliance with law.

Since Dr. White is the principal investigator, all parts of the research project data are under his care. From

Dr. White. To be in compliance with Standard 6.01, Dr. White probably needs to find another way to get the interviews transcribed.

Standard 1.03: Conflicts Between Ethics and Organizational Demands

> If the demands of an organization . . . for whom they are working are in conflict with this Ethics Code, psychologists clarify the nature of the conflict, make known their commitment to the Ethics Code, and take reasonable steps to resolve the conflict consistent with the General Principles and Ethical Standards of the Ethics Code.

Marcus, aspiring to Principle B and C, is placed in a position to either comply with the organization's demand for him to hand over the interviews to a work-study student, or uphold the promise he made to the interviewees to guard their identity from Dr. White. Following Standard 8.02 and Principle B and C, Marcus would defy Dr. White's request to transfer possession of the recordings of the interview to the work-study student for transcription. Finding himself in such a dilemma, Standard 1.03 directs Marcus to voice his concerns and reiterate his commitment to the code. In the final analysis, whatever resolution is negotiated between Marcus and Dr. White, Marcus is directed to uphold all of the sections of the APA Ethics Code. In this case, it means Marcus has responsibility to keep his promise that neither Dr. White nor anyone else associated with the organization has access to non-redacted interview material.

Standard 1.04: Informal Resolution of Ethical Violations

> When psychologists believe that there may have been an ethical violation by another psychologist, they attempt to resolve the issue by bringing it to the attention of that individual, if an informal resolution appears appropriate and the intervention does not violate any confidentiality rights that may be involved.

Standard 1.04 directs Marcus to take an additional step of saying to Dr. White that he is violating principles and standards specified in the APA Ethics Code.

Legal Issues 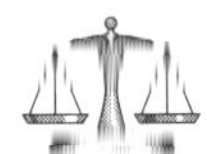

Kentucky

201 Ky. Admin. Regs. 26:145 (2010). Code of Conduct.

Section 1. Definitions.

(2) "Confidential information" means information . . . obtained by a credential holder in a professional relationship. . .

(6) "Professional service" means all actions of the credential holder in the context of a professional relationship with a client.

Section 6. Welfare of Supervisees and Research Subjects.

(1) Welfare of supervisees. The credential holder shall not exploit a supervisee.

(2) Welfare of research subjects. The credential holder shall . . . comply with all relevant statutes and administrative regulations concerning treatment of research subjects.

Section 8. Representation of Services.

(4) False or misleading information. The credential holder shall not include false or misleading information in a public statement concerning professional services offered.

Maryland

Md. Code Regs. 10.36.05.02 (2010). Definitions.

A. In this chapter, the following terms have the meanings indicated.

B. Terms Defined.

(2) "Client" means the individual . . . that the psychologist provides, or has provided, with professional services.

Md. Code Regs. 10.36.05.05 (2010). Representation of Services and Fees

(1) A psychologist may not:

(2) Make public statements that contain:

(i) False, fraudulent, misleading, or deceptive statements;

(ii) Partial disclosures of relevant facts that misrepresent, mislead, or deceive. . .

B. Informed Consent. When conducting research . . . a psychologist shall . . .

(2) In research, make clear to the client . . .

(c) All aspects of research including any risks and consequences of the research that will reasonably be expected to influence willingness to participate;

(d) The right to withdraw from treatment or research at any time.

Md. Code Regs. 10.36.05.07 (2010). Client Welfare.

A. A psychologist shall:

(1) Take appropriate steps to disclose to all involved parties' conflicts of interest that arise, with respect to a psychologist's clients, in a manner that is consistent with applicable confidentiality requirements. . .

B. Exploitation. A psychologist may not:

(1) Exploit or harm . . . research participants . . . [or]

(3) Exploit the trust and dependency of . . . students . . . and subordinates.

Md. Code Regs. 10.36.05.08 (2010). Confidentiality and Client Records.

A. A psychologist shall:

(1) Maintain confidentiality regarding information obtained from a client in the course of the psychologist's work . . .

(3) Safeguard information . . . research . . .

(4) Release . . . confidential information only as permitted or required by law. . .

B. Legal and Ethical Limits. A psychologist shall inform:

(3) Research participants of any limits to confidentiality as part of the informed consent.

A research subject consent form is a public document. Once distributed, Dr. White is bound to the content of the consent form. To act in any other manner would constitute false or misleading information for Kentucky and be viewed as exploitative in Maryland. In addition, both Kentucky and Maryland treat information obtained from research subjects with the same regard for confidentiality as information obtained from a treatment client. As a result, if Marcus or Dr. White assigned transcription of the voice-recorded interviews to anyone in the department, such an action would be a violation of both confidentiality and their public statements contained in the consent form.

Cultural Considerations

Global Discussion

Hong Kong Psychological Society:
Professional Code of Practice

> 2. Relationships with clients.
>
> *Consent: 2.1.0.* All monitoring and all video or photographic recordings of professional procedures involving other persons should be made with the explicit agreement of the participants or legal guardian, both with regard to the making of the recording and to the subsequent conditions of access to and use of it.

For Dr. White and Marcus to alter the conditions under which original consent was given is a violation of Hong Kong's code.

American Moral Values

1. Would Dr. White's subject consent form be violated by having a student in the department transcribe the interviews? Is such a student more likely to know the interviewees than an outside transcriber? Does it even matter if the student knows the interviewees, given that the original terms of consent are not being upheld? If Dr. White came up with a way for the student not to be able to identify the interviewees, would another consent form still be necessary?
2. What is Marcus's duty to the interview subjects? Is it to make sure they have an exact understanding of how confidentiality was maintained, or is it to make sure they receive the same degree of confidentiality to which they agreed? Can a consent form be considered intact if the same level of confidentiality is maintained, or must subjects agree to the exact conditions spelled out in the contract?
3. Dr. White has already entrusted one graduate student, Marcus, with redacting the interview material to mask interviewees' identity. How much risk does a second student's involvement pose for the interviewees being identified? Is there a way that Marcus can redact the recordings, or play them in the transcriber's presence, so that the identity of the interviewee does not make its way into the transcription that Dr. White receives? Or is it enough of a problem that another student will hear the interviews?
4. Is Marcus responsible for the use of these recordings, knowing what he does about the original consent form? Should he view Dr. White as the primary investigator and let him deal with the problem of consent? Unless Marcus says something, will anyone else know there was a change to the terms of consent? What does Marcus owe to the research community in the field? Should he refuse to give over the recordings until Dr. White takes measures for proper consent?
5. What is Marcus's professional relationship to Dr. White? Can he voice his concerns directly to Dr. White, or does he need to go to higher authorities? How will those authorities and Dr. White likely react to his objections?
6. How important does Marcus consider Dr. White's textbook and class to be? How does he weigh the loss of important feedback and improvement to Dr. White's work if these interviews go unused?

Ethical Course of Action

Directive per APA Code

Standard 8.03 specifies that Dr. White is to obtain informed consent before recording the interview. Standard 8.02 specifies that the subjects are to be told how the interview information is to be handled. Standard 8.01 specifies that Dr. White is not to deviate from previously approved procedures.

Standards 1.03 and 1.04 direct Marcus to point out to Dr. White the problems with his giving the recorded interviews to the departmental work-study student.

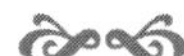

Dictates of One's Own Conscience

If you were Marcus, beyond voicing your concern, which of these would you do?

1. Give Dr. White the interviews under the knowledge that all research data belongs to the principal investigator and that it is the responsibility of the principal investigator to assure confidentiality, not you.

2. Reason that since you are the one who conducted the interviews, the data belong to you; thus, you
   a. refuse to compromise the confidentiality of your data by giving it to the departmental work-study student.
   b. refuse to recognize that Dr. White has any authority in the matter, and assert that he does not have a right to the data.
3. Assert that Dr. White does not have the right to access the interviews per the agreement approved by the IRB, and therefore you
   a. refuse to give up possession of the recorded interviews.
   b. suggest reapplication to the IRB accommodating budgetary access.
   c. suggest re-consent from the students.
4. Combinations of the above-listed possible courses of action.
5. Or one that is not listed above.

If the school was in Hong Kong and you were Marcus working for Dr. White, would you comply with the directives of the ethics code and refuse to consent to Dr. White's request for the voice recordings of the student interviews?

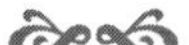

STANDARD 8.03: INFORMED CONSENT FOR RECORDING VOICES AND IMAGES IN RESEARCH

> Psychologists obtain informed consent from research participants prior to recording their voices or images for data collection unless (1) the research consists solely of naturalistic observations in public places, and it is not anticipated that the recording will be used in a manner that could cause personal identification or harm.

A CASE FOR STANDARD 8.03 (1): The BBQ—Part I

The Modern School of Psychology in the New Center University has a very small café in the building. The café contracts with a local organic vegetarian catering service. The students take pride in this and tout that this is evidence of the school's support for socially sustainable living.

Professor Garcia teaches social psychology. For the class, he assigns the students to undertake some type of naturalistic observation. Later, he assists students in preparing a manuscript about their research to publish in social psychology journals, while serving as one of the coauthors. Three of Professor Garcia's social psychology students, Lucille, Clifford, and Jamie, recognized that, although they are vegetarian when in school, none of them had actively decided to eat a vegetarian-only diet outside of school. They perceived that the school's support of vegetarianism by offering only vegetarian meals in the café felt somewhat oppressive. For their social psychology course project, Jamie, Clifford, and Lucille decided to find out whether people would choose to rebel against "political correctness" when given a chance. One way to find this out is to give people a chance to choose whether to be politically correct (i.e., vegetarian) or not by giving them a choice of a meat-based or vegetarian meal. To test this out, they decided to observe people's reaction to the availability of meat. They chose to host a BBQ in front of the school café on the next sunny day. In order to capture the reactions of faculty and students when meat is an available option at the café, the students set up a video recorder on the patio.

It did not take much time or effort to discover that Lucille, Clifford, and Jamie were hosting the BBQ to fulfill their social psychology course requirement. That afternoon, the chair of the psychology department received several complaints about the social psychology experiment and proceeded to ask Professor Garcia whether the students and he had obtained permission from the institutional review board to conduct this experiment.

Professor Garcia tells the department chair that indeed he had sent all of the students information about how to obtain exemptions from IRB approval because the research designs were all taking place in public space for naturalistic observation. The IRB had reviewed the design and found that exemption would be possible.

Issues of Concern

Standard 8.03 (1) specifies that all research subjects need to consent to having their images or voices recorded, except when the study consists of naturalistic observation in a public place. It is assumed that people would not expect privacy in public areas. Researchers are not invading or probing into confidential areas when the data is obtained in such a way that participants do not expect privacy. Is video recording people's eating behavior in a large shopping mall different from video recording people's behavior in a relatively small community? To some extent, people expect to meet others whom they know in the setting of the school café. Would people expect higher levels of privacy in a small café in their workplace versus in a café at a large shopping mall? Is it really public behavior to video record people eating and interacting in a small community? The question is whether bringing in meat violates the condition of a naturalistic setting, and whether a café inside a private establishment is considered a public place.

APA Ethics Code

Companion General Principle

Principle A: Beneficence and Nonmaleficence

> In their professional actions, psychologists seek to safeguard the welfare and rights of those with whom they interact professionally.

The conditions and assumptions where psychologists are allowed to conduct research without subject consent are ones where no harm would be expected from the research activity. Indeed, there is no expectation that observing anonymous individuals' public behavior, where people do not expect any privacy, would violate anyone's privacy, and thus it would not be expected to produce harm.

Companion Ethical Standard(s)

Standard 3.04: Avoiding Harm

> Psychologists take reasonable steps to avoid harming their . . . research participants . . . and to minimize harm where it is foreseeable and unavoidable.

Standard 3.04 is the operationalization of Principle A: Beneficence and Nonmaleficence. Following the line of reasoning in which people would expect all of their behavior to be observed in public places, would Professor Garcia or any of the members of the IRB have reason to believe the researchers would be harming anyone when recording people in a naturalistic setting? Or is the introduction of meat into the setting an alteration of that naturalistic setting, thus qualifying as an experimental condition?

Standard 3.10: Informed Consent

> (a) When psychologists conduct research . . . they obtain the informed consent of the individual or individuals using language that is reasonably understandable to that person or persons.

If the introduction of meat into the school café constitutes a research experiment and the private café inside the school building cannot be considered a naturalistic setting, then Lucille, Clifford, and Jamie would have violated Standard 3.10 by not obtaining subject consent.

Legal Issues 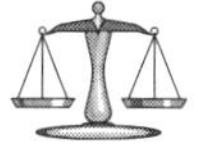

Michigan

> *Mich. Admin. Code r. 338.2515 (2010). Prohibited Conduct.*
>
> Rule 15. Prohibited conduct includes, but is not limited to, the following acts or omissions by any individual covered by these rules[:] . . .
>
> (c) Taking on a professional role when . . . professional . . . relationships could impair the exercise of professional discretion or make the interests of a . . . student secondary to those of the licensee.

Minnesota

> *Minn. R. 7200.5400 (2010). Welfare of Students, Supervisees, and Research Subjects.*
>
> A psychologist shall protect the welfare of . . . research subjects and shall accord the . . . human research subjects the client rights listed in parts 7200.4700 and 7200.4900.
>
> *Minn. R. 7200.4700 (2010). Protecting the Privacy of Clients.*
>
> Subpart 1. In general.
>
> A psychologist shall safeguard the private information obtained in the course of . . . research. . . [P]rivate information is disclosed to others only with the informed written consent of the client.
>
> Subp. 2. Disclosure without written consent.

> Private information may be disclosed without the informed written consent of the client when disclosure is necessary to protect against a clear and substantial risk of imminent serious harm being inflicted by the client on the client or another individual. In such case the private information is to be disclosed only to appropriate professional workers, public authorities, the potential victim, or the family of the client.
>
> *Minn. R. 7200.4900 (2010). Client Welfare.*
>
> Subpart 1. Providing explanation of procedures.
>
> A client has the right to have and a psychologist has the responsibility to provide, on request, a nontechnical explanation of the nature and purpose of the psychological procedures to be used... The psychologist shall establish procedures to be followed if the explanation is to be provided by another individual under the direction of the psychologist.
>
> Subp. 2. Statement of competence; clients' rights.
>
> A psychologist shall . . . make available as a handout . . . a statement that consumers of psychological services offered by psychologists licensed by the state of Minnesota have the right:
>
> A. to expect that a psychologist has met the minimal qualifications of training and experience required by state law . . .
>
> F. to privacy as defined by rule and law . . .
>
> I. to be free from exploitation for the benefit or advantage of the psychologist.

In Michigan, Professor Garcia's interests in the pedagogy of his social psychology class would be viewed as secondary to those interests of the research subjects who are unaware that their privacy interests would be violated. In Minnesota, the laws regulating the welfare of research subjects are no different from the laws regulating clients of psychologists. The research protocol systematically violated several laws related to providing informed consent and adequate disclosures about the welfare interests of the research subjects.

Cultural Considerations

Global Discussion

Canadian Code of Ethics for Psychologists

> Principle I: Respect for the dignity of persons.
>
> I.8. Respect the right of research participants . . . to safeguard their own dignity.
>
> I.25. Provide new information in a timely manner, whenever such information . . . is significant enough that it reasonably could be seen as relevant to the original or ongoing informed consent.

The Canadian code does not specify naturalistic versus controlled settings for experimentation, only that respect for the rights and dignity of all in that research process be protected and safeguarded. The participants, willing or not, must be allowed to safeguard their own rights and dignity. Therefore, informing the café diners that they are part of an experimental condition and allowing them to have choice and control over their own participation seem warranted. The addition of meat into an experiment involving a vegetarian community is significant and could reasonably be expected to be relevant to those participants. Fully informed consent by those participants becomes both necessary and prudent in order to comply with Canada's code.

American Moral Values

1. What defines public space? Is the premise of public space that basically anyone can be there, and therefore that one's behavior can be observed by anyone who is there? If so, is the café used by the whole school, or is it a more restricted, "safe" space almost exclusively used by the department? Is there a reasonable expectation by department members that they will be observed by people they know? Does observation in a smaller, communal space mean easier identification or more intimate exposure than a true public space? What if public space means anyplace where one's action could be observable, regardless of who or how many people are there? How is the café different from an empty waiting room, or an elevator with a security camera?
2. What defines naturalistic observation? Is the recording of people choosing what to eat an invasive observation, like zooming in on a credit card number or a pill bottle label? Or is it more like viewing a crowd, where particular people are not the focus? Will this video show people easily identified by other department members? Given today's technology, is there any public space where particular people can be recorded without being recognized?
3. What cultural and political significance do food choice and eating carry in this experiment? How much of oneself does food choice communicate? Level of education about what is healthy, self-control,

political awareness, class (in terms of what food is affordable), and refinement of taste? Given the premise of the research—that vegetarianism is more like a political ideology than a dietary preference—what is the implied political motive of these observations? Is it to determine how many hypocrites the department has, to show the gap between stated values and actual preferences? Is it to undermine vegetarianism as a viable choice?

4. How can this experiment gain the consent of all involved? Will it be possible to gain the consent of members after they have been recorded? Will they demand to see what the video shows? How will this affect the results? Should a member of a psychology department be self-aware enough to know that experiments are possible anywhere, or should the person expect that colleagues maintain a strict standard of consent with each other?
5. What are the complaints being registered in the department? What process should be used to address these complaints? What complaints can be anticipated, and how will the department handle them in terms of the experiment going forward?
6. How does this experiment fit in with other "naturalistic observation" experiments carried out in different places by other faculty? Is the psychology department just getting a taste of its own medicine, so to speak?

Ethical Course of Action

Directive per APA Code

The fact that those anonymous individuals were able to identify Lucille, Clifford, and Jamie within a matter of hours speaks to the fact that the school café is not a public space. The fact that complaints arose, presumably about the presence of meat because the students had not had a chance to even let anyone know the lunch scenes were to be recorded, would suggest that this situation was not naturalistic. Despite the seeming public nature of the setting, the BBQ was in violation of Standard 3.10 because subject consent was not obtained and in violation of Standard 8.03 (1) for failing to meet the conditions for the exceptions to subject consent.

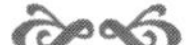

Dictates of One's Own Conscience

If you were Professor Garcia on the receiving end of the inquiry, which of these would you do?

1. Contact Lucille, Clifford, and Jamie to find out what exactly occurred at the café.
2. Defend the integrity of the classroom assignment.
3. Justify the project by citing the approval from the university's IRB.

If you were the chair of IRB, which of these actions would you take?

1. Immediately reread the application to see what was authorized.
2. Contact the members of the review committee to determine if anyone had any thought that the project would generate any harm.
3. Ask to see the exact nature of the complaints.

If you were the students, which action would you choose?

1. Cite Standard 8.03 (1) to justify your project.
2. Tell everyone that there was no intent to harm and that you do not see that anyone was harmed by being observed in a public place.
3. Ask Professor Garcia why the project was authorized if it was not completely okay.
4. Combinations of the above-listed actions.
5. Or one that is not listed above.

If you were Professor Garcia teaching social psychology in a psychology program located in Canada, you would not be in such a situation because Canada does not give exceptions for subject consent in naturalistic settings.

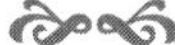

STANDARD 8.03: INFORMED CONSENT FOR RECORDING VOICES AND IMAGES IN RESEARCH

> Psychologists obtain informed consent from research participants prior to recording their voices or images for data collection unless . . . (2) the research design includes deception, and consent for the use of the recording is obtained during debriefing.

A CASE FOR STANDARD 8.03 (2): Disappointment

Dr. Martin works for the Establishment for a Responsible Society, a social research organization. The great recession of 2008–2010 generated a growing interest in finding out what people's perception is of their economic stability. It is hypothesized that people will save more money if they do not feel economically stable, but how economically unstable do people feel?

In order to determine people's perception of economic insecurity, Dr. Martin's team of researchers decides to contact people by randomly dialing telephone numbers within a large, metropolitan, midwestern city. The subjects are told that they have been randomly selected and have won a $1,000 reward for shopping at and supporting a local chain of grocery stores. To claim the prize, all the subjects needed to do was to give their consent for the reward team to come to the front door of their home and video record the subject receiving the prize money.

Dr. Martin, a cameraperson, and an attractive well-groomed assistant go to the front door of the subject's home. The subjects are videotaped as the assistant holds the envelope while Dr. Martin asks, "What are you going to do with the money?" A debriefing session occurs immediately after the video-recorded interview. In this debriefing session, the subjects are told that they have just participated in a research study and that there is no $1,000 reward, but they would receive $100 for their participation if they give consent for use of the video recording.

Issues of Concern

Standard 8.03 (2) gives exception to the need for subject consent prior to video or audio recordings. For research that involves deception, it is necessary to the condition that subjects cannot know the nature of the research, and thus they cannot give informed consent before being recorded. Dr. Martin's research design seems to be following the requirements for Standard 8.03 (2) in terms of obtaining consent for using the video recordings during debriefing. However, the receipt of the $100 seems to be dependent on subjects giving consent for recording. Is it coercive to make a reward contingent on permission to use the recordings?

APA Ethics Code

Companion General Principle

Principle C: Integrity

> In situations in which deception may be ethically justifiable to maximize benefits and minimize harm, psychologists have a serious obligation to consider the need for, the possible consequences of, and their responsibility to correct any resulting mistrust or other harmful effects that arise from the use of such techniques.

As with any research that involves deception, the primary consideration is calculating the benefit to society against the risk of harm to the subjects. Principle C: Integrity urges psychologists to make amends to subjects when such deception is used. Has Dr. Martin's research design met the spirit of Principle C during the debriefing phase of the data collection?

Companion Ethical Standard(s)

Standard 8.07: Deception in Research

> (a) Psychologists do not conduct a study involving deception unless they have determined that the use of deceptive techniques is justified by the study's significant prospective scientific, educational, or applied value and that effective nondeceptive alternative procedures are not feasible.

Standard 8.07 (a) requires Dr. Martin to ask the question of whether the same information could be obtained without the use of deception. The rationale behind the design of the study is that if people perceived personal economic stability, then unexpected extra money may be spent on luxury items instead of basic items like paying utility bills. If one believed that one cannot really know how one will spend unanticipated income unless and until one is confronted with the situation, this assumption thus justifies the need for deception as required by Standard 8.07 (a).

Standard 8.07: Deception in Research

> . . . (b) Psychologists do not deceive prospective participants about research that is reasonably expected to cause . . . severe emotional distress.

A significant number of people were either unemployed or underemployed during the years following

2007. For those individuals and families, $1,000 may have been a significant amount of money that could make the difference in crucial household items such as paying for utilities or catching up on a mortgage that is in arrears. The anticipation of receiving $1,000 may prompt individuals to spend money between receiving the phone call and Dr. Martin's visit. Significant financial and emotional harm could have been inflicted on the subjects. Does the possibility of such an occurrence meet the requirement that prohibits deception as specified in Standard 8.07 (b)?

Standard 8.06: Offering Inducements for Research Participation

> (a) Psychologists make reasonable efforts to avoid offering excessive or inappropriate financial or other inducements for research participation when such inducements are likely to coerce participation.

If any of Dr. Martin's subjects were in dire financial difficulty, $100 would most likely be experienced as coercive to giving consent for use of video recordings. Would it seem less coercive if subjects were offered the some amount of financial reward regardless of whether consent for use of video recordings was given?

Legal Issues

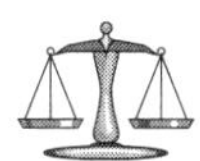

Missouri

> *Mo. Code Regs. Ann. tit. 20, § 2235-5.030 (2010). Ethical Rules of Conduct.*
>
> (8) Welfare of Supervisees, Clients, Research Subjects, and Students. . .
>
> (B) Welfare of Clients and Research Subjects. . .
>
> 18. Deception and debriefing. The psychologist shall not deceive human participants about the experience of participating in a study, especially those aspects that subjects might find negative, such as . . . unpleasant emotional experiences. Any deceptive aspects of a study shall be explained at the conclusion or earlier. Before conducting such a study, psychologists have a special responsibility to determine whether—
>
> A. The use of deceptive techniques is justified by the study's prospective scientific, educational, or applied value; and
>
> B. Alternative procedures are available that do not use concealment or deception.

Montana

> *Mont. Admin. R. 24.189.2309 (2009). Professional Responsibility.*
>
> (2) In regard to respect for others, a licensee:
>
> (a) shall not exploit persons over whom they have . . . authority such as . . . research participants.

In both jurisdictions, the potential harm to the credibility of psychology may have occurred because the participants could feel unduly deceived and were particularly vulnerable because of financial difficulty, which made the deception particularly alluring. Missouri's section on deception is essentially the same as the APA Ethics Code and thus requires the determination of whether the study's prospective scientific value justifies the deception. In Montana, the focus of the law revolves around preventing exploitation of the research participants. Montana's licensing board would have to determine whether Dr. Martin's research design was exploitative of the research subjects.

Cultural Considerations

Global Discussion

Code of Ethics for the Psychologist: Spain

> IV: On Research and training.
>
> ***Article 36.*** When research requires the psychologist to resort to deception or tricks, he or she must ensure that this will not cause long-term harm to any of the subjects and must always inform them of the nature and experimental need for the deception at the end of the session or research.

It is difficult to know exactly what, if any, potential long-term harm could come to study participants who have been promised significant amounts of money and are then informed that this has been deceptive. There is a risk of material harm if subjects have anticipatorily "spent" sums of money of which they will then be deprived. Potentially, those participants willing to have psychologists come to their personal home under the auspices of awarding money are those most likely to be in need of that money; therefore, they are less likely to be able to resist giving consent in order to obtain some amount of money, even a much lower sum.

The experimenters seem to have upheld the part of Article 36 which states that they must "inform" participants about the need for and nature of the deception they have undergone. Regardless of the nature of the debriefing, and the nature of possible coercion in consenting to have their recordings used, the potential for long-term harm to these participants is significant enough to place these researchers in violation of Spain's Code, regardless of the thoroughness of the final debriefing. These experimenters have violated the first part of Article 36, which is to only resort to deception if they can reasonably predict that such deception will not cause long-term harm.

American Moral Values

1. Which people should give consent for this experiment? Should it be all those who are initially called, or just those who accept the prize, or only the ones who accept the $100? What level of participation, with what amount of time and inconvenience, requires recognition that this is an experiment? Should any participant who agrees to the prize, regardless of whether he or she gives video consent, be given $100?
2. What kind of deception is needed in order to obtain the information regarding feelings about economic security and saving? How important is that information compared to the negative effects the deception may have on research subjects? Is there a difference between deceiving a subject who has consented to be in an experiment about its purpose, and deceiving a subject about whether he or she is participating in an experiment at all? In other words, does this experiment bypass the requirement for informed consent to participate in a research experiment at the beginning?
3. Is it right to offer $100 only to those who consent to their video footage being used? What is owed to those who do not give their consent, but who were put through the inconvenience and embarrassment of having the offer turn out to be false? Should any participant who agrees to the prize, regardless of whether he or she gives video consent, be given $100? Or is the deception more akin to a radio prank, where the victim is not legally required to get money? Is $100 generous compensation for a video interview and the disappointment of not winning $1000?
4. In deciding whether this experiment justifies its deception, should Dr. Martin believe this approach will eliminate self-monitoring in responses? With a video camera and attractive assistant handing them an envelope, would subjects try to muster up a lottery-winner response? Would their stated plans for the money be the same as if they received a notice in the mail? Might people distort their true intentions under the assumption they will receive local publicity, or perhaps out of embarrassment of being exposed as a bad spender?
5. What is the Establishment of a Responsible Society? What policy positions do they intend to advance? Is Dr. Martin's team looking for a specific conclusion from their interviews? How does one measure a state of economic security in this moment of surprise?
6. How does the condition of consent screen the selection of subjects? Will someone's willingness to accept $1000 and the attention of a camera crew depend on the percentage of one's income it represents, just as it would for accepting $100 in exchange for video footage? How much can one gauge "economic security" if $1000 changes that state of mind for the winner? Does this risk making a spectacle out of those willing to take the money?
7. Does winning a contest distort the planning of the subjects? Is winning something like a lottery culturally tied to celebration with friends and family, instead of pure economic calculation? What harmful policy conclusions about savings, poverty, and incentives could arise through these and other distorted results?
8. Does this type of experiment trivialize the field of psychology, especially if the organization touts Dr. Martin's credentials in its publications and lobbying efforts? On the other hand, does Dr. Martin's work show the reach of psychological methods into important policy discussions, encouraging other psychologists to pursue other socially engaged experiments?

Ethical Course of Action

Directive per APA Code

Standard 8.03 (2) directs Dr. Martin to get subjects' consent for use of the recordings during debriefing. Standard 8.03 (2) is silent on the condition of a subject's obtaining financial incentives for participation contingent on consent for Dr. Martin to use the video recordings. The design of the experiment does not violate the directive as specified in Standard 8.03

(2), but does violate the spirit of Principle C: Integrity and Standards 8.06 and 8.07.

Dictates of One's Own Conscience

If you were a member of the institutional review board of the Establishment for a Responsible Society and you were responsible for review of the experiment, which of these would be your response to Dr. Martin?

1. Agree with Dr. Martin's reasons for use of deception, and authorize the experiment without changes.
2. Disagree with Dr. Martin's reasons for use of deception; think that the same information could be obtained without the use of deception, so move to deny authorization for the experiment.
3. Agree with Dr. Martin's reasons for use of deception, but request alteration of the condition of receiving $100 because you think it is coercive.
4. Though you agree with Dr. Martin's reasons for use of deception, you think the emotional pain and the risk of severe financial impact on certain subjects is too great to justify the experiment, and thus move to deny its authorization.
5. Combinations of the above-listed actions.
6. Or one that is not listed above.

If you were Dr. Martin working in Spain, you would not design such an experiment because the long-term harm would be too great to either justify it or pass the IRB review.

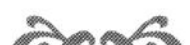

STANDARD 8.04: CLIENT/ PATIENT, STUDENT, AND SUBORDINATE RESEARCH PARTICIPANTS

> (a) When psychologists conduct research with clients/ patients, students, or subordinates as participants, psychologists take steps to protect the prospective participants from adverse consequences of declining or withdrawing from participation.

A CASE FOR STANDARD 8.04 (A): The Repeating Relationship

Dr. Thompson teaches basic counseling skills for a clinical psychology program. As part of the course requirements, students are asked to engage in practice interviews, take process notes on these sessions, and note any self-observations. In conjunction with teaching this class, Dr. Thompson plans to publish a textbook on pedagogical methods for teaching counseling skills. Dr. Thompson wishes to use the students' class assignments as part of her research for the textbook and asks students to sign a consent form giving her permission to use their assignments. The consent forms are distributed at the end of the class with the request that students mail in their consent forms *after* their final grades have been posted. This is to assure students that their agreement or refusal to participate will not adversely affect their grades. After final grades have been posted and the semester break begins, Dr. Thompson receives the signed subject consent forms from her students. Alicia is the only student in the class who did not sign the consent form.

The next semester, Dr. Thompson sees that Alicia is enrolled in the group therapy class she is scheduled to teach.

Issues of Concern

It appears that Dr. Thompson uses the classes' assignments as part of her research data. For the purpose of data analyses, she probably does not need to know who is linked with which paper. Whether a student participates in the study is not known until the course is completed and the grades are submitted. Therefore, regardless of whether students decline participation, their grades are not affected. Dr. Thompson apparently has attempted to meet the requirements of Standard 8.04 (a) to protect the students from adverse consequences of declining to participate in the professor's research project. However, despite the precautions taken in the counseling skills class, Alicia may experience some adverse consequence for declining participation in Dr. Thompson's research project. Neither Alicia nor Dr. Thompson foresaw the possibility that only one student would decline participation and that student then taking subsequent courses from Dr. Thompson. Is it possible for Dr. Thompson not to be affected by Alicia being the only student who refused participation?

Now that Dr. Thompson has evaluative authority over a student who declined to participate in her research, is it reasonable to expect that Alicia would not wonder whether Dr. Thompson has a negative opinion of her? Is it reasonable that Alicia's declining would have no effect upon Dr. Thompson's subsequent evaluation of Alicia?

APA Ethics Code

Companion General Principle

Principle A: Beneficence and Nonmaleficence.

> In their professional actions, psychologists seek to safeguard the welfare and rights of those with whom they interact. . . Because psychologists' scientific and professional judgments and actions may affect the lives of others, they are alert to and guard against personal . . . factors that might lead to misuse of their influence.

Principle A: Beneficence and Nonmaleficence is the value behind enacting safeguards to protect research participants as directed in Standard 8.04 (a).

Companion Ethical Standard(s)

Standard 7.06: Assessing Student and Supervisee Performance

> . . . (b) Psychologists evaluate students and supervisees on the basis of their actual performance on relevant and established program requirements.

It is possible that Alicia may feel retaliation if Dr. Thompson gives her anything but a glowing evaluation for the group class. Is it possible for Alicia to feel fairly assessed if Dr. Thompson adheres to the directives of Standard 7.06 (b) and gives Alicia an accurate but less-than-positive evaluation in the group class?

Standard 7.05: Mandatory Individual or Group Therapy

> (a) When . . . group therapy is a . . . course requirement, psychologists . . . allow students . . . the option of selecting such therapy from practitioners unaffiliated with the program.

It is not clear whether Dr. Thompson will include either a group therapy requirement or in vivo group process sessions in her group class. If she does in-class group process sessions, might it be possible that Alicia would feel inhibited, fearing that Dr. Thompson does not like her based on the counseling skills class? If so, might Alicia's inhibiting her own participation actually generate a negative evaluation from Dr. Thompson?

Standard 8.08: Debriefing

> . . . (c) When psychologists become aware that research procedures have harmed a participant, they take reasonable steps to minimize the harm.

If Dr. Thompson conducts a debriefing session with her students when classes resume, she could find out how Alicia feels about declining to participate in her research project and about now being evaluated by Dr. Thompson in group class. She could also investigate ways of minimizing harm.

Legal Issues 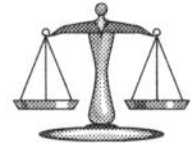

Nebraska

> *172 Neb. Admin. Code §§ 156-011 (2010). 011 Research With Human Participants.*
>
> A psychologist shall respect the dignity and welfare of human research participants, and shall comply with these regulations governing such psychological research.
>
> Unprofessional conduct includes but is not limited to:
>
> 011.01 Except in minimal risk research . . . failure to establish an agreement with research participants, prior to their participation, that clarifies the obligations and responsibilities of the psychologist and of the participant . . . failure to inform participants of all aspects of the research that might reasonably be expected to influence willingness to participate. . .
>
> 011.03 Failure to grant a participant the right to decline to participate in or to withdraw from the research at any time.
>
> 011.06 Failure to make reasonable efforts to detect and remove or correct undesirable consequences for the individual participants, including long-term effects.

Nevada

> *Nev. Admin. Code § 641.215 (2010). . . Care of . . . Research Subjects. (NRS 641.100).*
>
> A psychologist . . .
>
> 13. Shall, in the conduct of psychological research:
>
> (a) Respect the dignity and protect the welfare of his research subjects;

> (b) Comply with all relevant laws and regulations concerning the treatment of research subjects;
>
> (c) Fully inform each person who is a prospective subject of research . . . of any danger of serious after-effects before the person is used as a subject; and
>
> (d) Use reasonable efforts to remove any possible harmful after-effects of emotional stress as soon as the design of the research permits.

Nebraska law indicates that Dr. Thompson has engaged in unprofessional conduct by failing to remove or correct undesirable consequences for Alicia. A consideration is whether it was reasonable to anticipate the negative consequences for Alicia. Another consideration is whether Dr. Thompson could retrospectively correct the harm to Alicia due to her refusal to give consent for the use of her homework assignments in Dr. Thompson's research. It appears that Dr. Thompson has complied with all of the requirements for the Nevada law.

Cultural Considerations

Global Discussion

Hong Kong Psychological Society:
Professional Code of Practice

> 1: Introduction.
>
> d. Taking account of their obligations under the law, Members shall hold the interest and welfare of those in receipt of their services to be paramount at all times and shall ensure that the interests of participants in research . . . are safeguarded to the best of their ability.
>
> 6: Research.
>
> 6.4: A Member engaged in research in which there is a possibility of harmful effects to subjects must take steps to protect the subjects. . .
>
> 6.7: A Member must not use a position of authority to exert undue pressure on potential subjects for the purpose of securing their participation in a particular research project.

Dr. Thompson attempted to safeguard her human subjects by protecting their confidentiality, by ensuring an informed consent process was adhered to and carried out, and by making clear that students' participation was voluntary. Dr. Thompson could not be found in violation of either the intent or the letter of standards of items d and 6.4. She may, however, even unwittingly, be found in violation of 6.7 because her position of authority now has undue influence upon Alicia after she declined to participate in the research study. The difficulty now is that Dr. Thompson cannot ascertain the degree of her own influence over Alicia and Alicia's perception that her declination of participation will have some negative impact on their future student–instructor relationship.

American Moral Values

1. How does Dr. Thompson regard Alicia as both a student in her group therapy class and the only student not to participate in her research? Will the latter status affect how Dr. Thompson treats Alicia? Can Dr. Thompson determine that for herself? Is there any kind of safeguard or external check that Dr. Thompson could exercise to make sure Alicia was evaluated fairly? Would taking that trouble already adversely affect how Alicia's performance is assessed?
2. Does Dr. Thompson's judgment of Alicia depend on Alicia's assignment in the prior class? Was it a particularly good example to use for her book? Does Dr. Thompson believe there was a specific reason Alicia did not participate? Is there a need to clear the air with Alicia before the group therapy class proceeds?
3. Would questioning Alicia about her declination to participate cause more problems than it solves in terms of Dr. Thompson's relationship with her as a student? Should Dr. Thompson wait to see Alicia's manner and performance in the class before deciding to address the issue explicitly with her?

Ethical Course of Action

Directive per APA Code

Following the requirements of 8.04 (a) Dr. Thompson guarded against adverse consequences to students' grades by waiting until after grades are submitted before asking for students to participate in her study. However, despite the precautions taken in the counseling skills class to protect Alicia from any possible retribution for refusal to participate, Alicia finds herself in a situation where her refusal may influence Dr. Thompson's assessment of her course work again.

Following the directive of Standard 8.08, Dr. Thompson could hold a debriefing session with Alicia. If Dr. Thompson finds out that Alicia feels uneasy, she could implement Standard 8.08 (c) and take steps to minimize any real or feared harm. The problem in following the directive of Standard 8.08 (c) is that the very act of holding a meeting with Alicia to discuss the consequences of her not giving consent in the counseling skills class violates the nature of subjects being free to withdraw from a research project at any time. In addition, holding such a conversation conflicts with Principle A of Beneficence and Nonmaleficence in that the power differential between Dr. Thompson and Alicia is too great for Alicia to have a fair and honest discussion with her teacher.

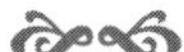

Dictates of One's Own Conscience

If you were Dr. Thompson, seeing Alicia on the roster for your group class immediately after learning she has declined to participate in your research study, which of these would you do?

1. Do nothing because it is of no consequence that Alicia declined participation.
2. Wonder why Alicia declined and what it suggests about her personality.
3. Notice Alicia's behavior in class in light of the knowledge that she declined participation in your research study.
4. Contact Alicia to invite her to have a conversation about your relationship in light of her declining to participate in the research study.
5. Meet with Alicia and state that in light of your concern that she may feel as if her not participating in the research would affect your evaluation of her in the group's class, her work will be evaluated independently by a colleague.
6. Combinations of the above-listed actions.
7. Or one that is not listed above.

If you were Dr.Thompson teaching in Hong Kong, you would attempt to ascertain the possible impact of your relationship with Alicia as your ongoing student in your current class so as not to use your position to exert undue influence.

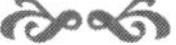

STANDARD 8.04: CLIENT/PATIENT, STUDENT, AND SUBORDINATE RESEARCH PARTICIPANTS

. . . (b) When research participation is a course requirement or an opportunity for extra credit, the prospective participant is given the choice of equitable alternative activities.

A CASE FOR STANDARD 8.04 (B): Grades Are Important

Professor Martinez is researching the differences in male versus female symptomology of anxiety disorders. Every semester, she offers her students the opportunity to earn 100 extra-credit points. Students who choose to earn the extra-credit points may either write additional papers or participate in the study she is conducting for her research. Each paper is worth 20 points, and students have the option of writing up to five papers in order to receive a total of 100 extra-credit points. The paper must be a review of the literature on a topic chosen by Professor Martinez and contain at least five references. For those who choose the option of completing the full research study, they are required to fill out a questionnaire that takes approximately 45 minutes to complete, participate in a 2-hour group interview, and engage in a 15-minute follow-up phone interview.

Suzanne is one of Professor Martinez's students. She failed the midterm exam and decides she would like to earn extra-credit points, so she signs up for the research study. The one available group interview time is on the Saturday of Suzanne's brother's bar mitzvah. She decides to talk to Professor Martinez about the time conflict. Professor Martinez says, "You can withdraw from the study with no penalty. However, without it you won't pass the class. How about the literature review papers?"

Issues of Concern

Having students participate in her study for extra credit makes Dr. Martinez's situation fall within the parameters of Standard 8.04 (b). This standard requires that Dr. Martinez give students opportunity for equitable alternative activities, which she does by providing the paper option. The question is whether five literature review papers are equivalent to the time and effort involved with the study participation. Participation in the study would have taken Suzanne 3 hours. It is very doubtful that anyone could find and read five articles and then write a summary of each topic within 3 hours. A secondary question is whether Dr. Martinez is obligated to open up an alternative time for Suzanne on the grounds of cultural accommodation.

APA Ethics Code

Companion General Principle

Principle E: Respect for People's Rights and Dignity

> Psychologists are aware that special safeguards may be necessary to protect . . . persons . . . whose vulnerabilities impair autonomous decision making. Psychologists are aware of and respect cultural . . . and role differences, including those based on . . . ethnicity, culture . . . [and] religion . . . and consider these factors when working with members of such groups. Psychologists try to eliminate the effect on their work of biases based on those factors.

By virtue of their subordinate and vulnerable states, students are not fully free to make autonomous decisions with dignity. Principle E would suggest that Dr. Martinez is fully aware of students' vulnerabilities and would not take advantage of their subordinate status for her own advantage. Suzanne is not fully free to choose attendance at her brother's bar mitzvah without untoward consequences. By not making special allowances for a very significant cultural event like a bar mitzvah, Dr. Martinez may be open to accusations of discrimination.

Principle D: Justice

> Psychologists recognize that fairness and justice entitle all persons to . . . equal quality in the . . . services being conducted by psychologists. Psychologists exercise reasonable judgment and take precautions to ensure that their potential biases . . . and the limitations of their expertise do not lead to or condone unjust practices.

Principle D suggests that Dr. Martinez should act in such a way that all of her students would be treated fairly. Equitable substitutions of assignments based on time or effort falls in the arena of fairness. It does not seem fair to give research participation that takes 3 hours the same point value as writing five papers, particularly as both the research study and the research paper topics are areas of Dr. Martinez's choosing and direct benefit.

Companion Ethical Standard(s)

Standard 3.01: Unfair Discrimination

> In their work-related activities, psychologists do not engage in unfair discrimination based on . . . ethnicity, culture . . . [and] religion.

Is it discriminatory of Dr. Martinez not to give special consideration for a bar mitzvah? Or might it be that in a teaching institution, regardless of what dates Dr. Martinez sets for the experiment, there would be someone with an equally legitimate reason for not being able to attend?

Standard 3.08: Exploitative Relationships

> Psychologists do not exploit persons over whom they have . . . evaluative . . . authority such as . . . students.

It seems highly probable that some students will need extra credit and will not be able to attend the study on the day assigned. Arguably, then, it is almost guaranteed that someone will be writing those extra-credit papers. Is it exploitative for Dr. Martinez to assign students to do the literature review for her own research?

Legal Issues 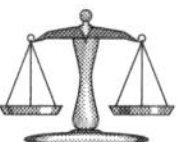

New Jersey

> *N.J. Admin. Code § 13:42-10.6 (2010). Research.*
>
> (a) A licensee shall observe research requirements consistent with accepted standards of practice including the following. . .
>
> 5. A licensee shall treat research participants ethically.

> *N.J. Admin. Code § 13:42-10.13 (2010). Conflicts of Interest; Dual Relationships.*
>
> (d) A licensee shall not enter into any dual relationship. . . [B]artering for any services provided by any current client shall also be prohibited.

New Mexico

> *N.M. Code R. § 16.22.2.10 (2010). Patient Welfare.*
>
> F. Exploitative relationships.

> (1) The psychologist shall not exploit persons over whom the psychologist has supervisory, evaluative, or other authority such as . . . research participants. . .
>
> **J. Avoiding harm.** Psychologists take reasonable steps to avoid harming their . . . research participants . . . and minimize harm where it is foreseeable and unavoidable.

N.M. Code R. § 16.22.2.11 (2010). Welfare of Supervisee and Research Subjects.

> **B. Welfare of research subjects.** The psychologist shall respect the dignity and protect the welfare of his research subjects, and shall comply with all relevant statutes and the board's regulations concerning treatment of research subjects.

New Jersey might consider that Dr. Martinez treated her student Suzanne unethically. The conflict of interest law would indicate that Dr. Martinez engaged in an exploitative relationship when she put her students into a bind. They could engage in 3 hours of being a research subject or not serve as a research subject and write five papers. Such an arrangement does not respect the students' time nor protect their welfare in terms of time and grades.

Cultural Considerations

Global Discussion

New Zealand Psychological Society Code of Ethics

> Principle I: Responsibility.
>
> 1.4. The welfare of research subjects . . . [and] students . . . takes precedence over the self-interest of psychologists.

Dr. Martinez's course assignments are inherently self-serving. The Code calls for psychologists' allegiance to lie with the welfare of their research subjects and students. Dr. Martinez is in violation of the intent and letter of this portion of the code, and she ought to revise her syllabus with assignments that are not blatantly self-interested, but rather meet the interests and educational needs of her students.

American Moral Values

1. How do Suzanne and Dr. Martinez view the two extra-credit options? Are they "equitable" in terms of time and effort? Is Suzanne being presented with a fair choice? Does she deserve a fair choice less than other students, having failed the midterm?
2. What is the value of these extra-credit assignments among the overall course goals? Given that the research study seems to require less time, is there an educational value that makes it worth the work of writing the papers? Should Dr. Martinez offer more extra-credit points for the paper assignment?
3. Is the study option a generous offer from Dr. Martinez, or is it just a way to use students to help her research? What topics is Dr. Martinez choosing for the literature review? Is this a way for students to read secondary literature in the course's material, or does it chiefly serve as a literature review for Dr. Martinez's own use?
4. Is Dr. Martinez being sufficiently accommodating for Suzanne's bar mitzvah conflict? Does Dr. Martinez appreciate the religious and cultural importance of this event? Should Dr. Martinez consider the fact that every Saturday could pose a conflict for Jewish students observing the Sabbath? If the paper assignment is not an equitable alternative, does Dr. Martinez owe Suzanne another way to participate in the research study? Should Dr. Martinez come up with a third alternative to meet Suzanne's situation?
5. What are Suzanne and Dr. Martinez's views about academic work and performance? Will Suzanne argue on principle for an extra-credit assignment that can help her pass, or does she believe that failing the midterm puts her at the mercy of Dr. Martinez? Does she blame herself for her failure in the midterm, or does she fault Dr. Martinez for being a bad teacher? Does Dr. Martinez believe students who protest the fairness of the extra-credit assignment are being insubordinate or ungrateful? Does Dr. Martinez believe that when she was a student, professors would have just failed students like Suzanne?
6. What example is Dr. Martinez setting for her students as a teacher? Do students think they are doing work in her field, or doing work for her? Will an exception for Suzanne upset students with equally compelling reasons not to make Saturday interview times?

Ethical Course of Action

Directive per APA Code

Participation in the study takes 3 hours. The time necessary to write a paper is variable and depends on students' individual abilities. However, it is highly improbable that anyone could write five papers in 3 hours. Assigning both activities 100 extra-credit points is not equitable. Dr. Martinez's extra-credit opportunities violate requirements for Standard 8.04 (b) as well as the spirit of Standard 3.08 and Principle D: Justice.

Whether Dr. Martinez acted in a prejudicial manner by not giving special consideration for a student to attend a bar mitzvah is more equivocal. If the alternative activity had truly been equitable, then Dr. Martinez's response may not have appeared so dismissive of a religious and cultural event.

Dictates of One's Own Conscience

If you were Suzanne, faced with Dr. Martinez's response to your difficulties, which of these would you do?

1. Point out to Dr. Martinez that it will take you much longer than 3 hours to write five papers.
2. Ask Dr. Martinez to reschedule the research experiment date.
3. Ask whether you could write one large paper with 25 references instead of five papers with 5 references each.
4. Offer to recruit more participants to Dr. Martinez's study if she would add another experiment date.
5. Cite Standard 8.04 (b).
6. Complain that Dr. Martinez should be more sympathetic to the importance of your brother's bar mitzvah.
7. Resolve to study for the final course exam, go to your brother's bar mitzvah, and not write the papers.
8. Combinations of the above-listed actions.
9. Or one that is not listed above.

If you were Suzanne attending a school in New Zealand and were faced with Dr. Martinez's response to your difficulties, which of these would you do?

1. Clearly know that Dr. Martinez is in violation of the New Zealand Psychological Society's Code of Ethics.
2. Have a conversation with Dr. Martinez about her violation of the ethics code.
3. Talk to the department chair about Dr. Martinez's violation of the ethics code.

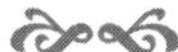

STANDARD 8.05: DISPENSING WITH INFORMED CONSENT FOR RESEARCH

> Psychologists may dispense with informed consent only (1) where research would not reasonably be assumed to create distress or harm and involves (a) the study of normal educational practices, curricula, or classroom management methods conducted in educational settings.

A CASE FOR STANDARD 8.05 (1) (A): What Is the Complaint?

The Modern School of Psychology in the New Center University has received a number of notes in their anonymous suggestion box complaining about their on-site training clinic. The dean has requested a report from the director of the clinic regarding the nature of student discontent.

Dr. Robinson, director of the clinic and a licensed psychologist, decided to conduct in-person interviews of all students who use the library on Friday afternoons. The interview questions revolved around students' perception of possible barriers they encounter in using the clinic. Soon after Dr. Robinson started interviewing students, student complaints began to appear in the anonymous suggestion box denoting the harassing nature of the interviews. The dean and the institutional review board inquire about (1) why Dr. Robinson did not submit a request for research and (2) the exact nature of the interviews. Dr. Robinson argues that he did not need permission to conduct the interviews, and thus did not need to submit an IRB application because the study is a normal educational practice that has no negative consequences for the students.

Issues of Concern

Dr. Robinson is aware of the conditions for exceptions to consent to research. It is true that the interviews are being conducted in an educational setting. It is also true that Dr. Robinson could argue that the interviews are being conducted at the request of the dean and that they serve pedagogical purposes rather than research interests.

Is it true that the interviews would not reasonably be assumed to create distress or harm? What if the cause of complaints is the clinic director? Might this create some distress?

Is it true that that being interviewed by the clinic director would not reasonably be assumed to create harm? What if the clinic director assigned cases or influenced access to the clinic work space or other parts of the operation that would affect the student clinicians? Might students feel harmed if after the interview they were no longer getting assigned desirable cases, the hours that they requested, and so forth?

Is it true that the interviews are part of the normal educational practice? Has the university routinely conducted student interviews regarding the clinic or any other aspect of its programming?

Is it true that a request from the dean is supported by an institutional regulation? It may feel like directives from the dean are regulatory and one has no option but to obey. Do such feelings justify not going through the IRB?

APA Ethics Code

Companion General Principle

Principle B: Fidelity and Responsibility

> Psychologists . . . are aware of their professional and scientific responsibilities to . . . the specific communities in which they work. Psychologists uphold professional standards of conduct, clarify their professional roles and obligations, accept appropriate responsibility for their behavior, and seek to manage conflicts of interest that could lead to exploitation or harm.

Dr. Robinson, being aware of his responsibility toward the dean, is probably being guided by the ideal of responsibility expressed in Principle E. This principle guides Dr. Robinson's attention to all members of the community in which he works, meaning he holds responsibility for the welfare of the students, his subordinates, and other staff and faculty. Principle E also suggests Dr. Robinson will clarify his role as faculty or administrator or researcher when he conducts his interviews with students.

Companion Ethical Standard(s)

Standard 3.04: Avoiding Harm

> Psychologists take reasonable steps to avoid harming . . . students . . . and to minimize harm where it is foreseeable and unavoidable.

Even if Dr. Robinson did not think any harm could be created by his following routine educational practices, students might perceive the possibility of harm. Dr. Robinson, in his multiple roles as faculty, administrator, and researcher, is required to avoid harming the students. Does lack of oversight by the IRB ignore the opportunity for others to help him figure out if possible harm was foreseeable?

Standard 7.06: Assessing Student and Supervisee Performance

> . . . (b) Psychologists evaluate students and supervisees on the basis of their actual performance on relevant and established program requirements.

If Dr. Robinson, in addition to his administrative responsibility as clinic director, also taught classes, he would be in a position of evaluating these same students. Conflating his faculty role with that of a researcher receiving confidential information from interviewees may compromise his ability to evaluate students based solely on actual performance.

Legal Issues 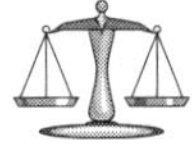

New York

> *N.Y. Comp. Codes R. & Regs. tit. 8, § 29.1 (2010). General Provisions.*
>
> b. Unprofessional conduct in the practice of any profession licensed . . . shall include:
>
> 1. willful or grossly negligent failure to comply with substantial provisions of Federal, State or local laws, rules or regulations governing the practice of the profession.

> *N.Y. Comp. Codes R. & Regs. tit. 8, § 29.12 (2010). Special Provisions for the Profession of Psychology.*
>
> a. Unprofessional conduct in the practice of psychology . . . shall also include the following:
>
> 1. . . . failing to inform prospective research subjects . . . fully of the danger of serious after-effects, if such danger exists, before they are utilized as research subjects.

Ohio

Ohio Admin. Code 4732:17-01 (2010). General Rules of Professional Conduct Pursuant to Section 4732.17 of the Revised Code.

(E) Multiple relationships. A multiple relationship exists when a psychologist . . . is in another relationship with the same person. . . Depending on the timing and nature of one's interactions before or after the establishment of a professional psychological role, multiple relationships can result in exploitation of others. . . Psychologists . . . actively identify and manage interpersonal boundaries to ensure that there is no exploitation of others. . .

(2) Prohibited multiple relationships. The board prescribes that certain multiple relationships are expressly prohibited due to inherent risks of exploitation.

Ohio Admin. Code 4732:17-02 (2010).

Ethics governing research . . . involves the professional practice of psychology . . . in which client welfare is directly affected.

(A) Ethical acceptability. In planning a study, the investigator has the personal responsibility to make a careful evaluation of its ethical acceptability, taking into account these principles for research with human beings. . .

(B) Treatment of participants. Responsibility for the establishment and maintenance of acceptable ethical practice in research always remains with the individual investigator. . .

(C) Full disclosure. Ethical practice requires the investigator to inform the participant of all features of the research that reasonably might be expected to influence willingness to participate, and to explain all other aspects of the research about which the participant inquires. Failure to make full disclosure gives added emphasis to the investigator's abiding responsibility to protect the welfare and dignity of the research participant. . .

(E) Freedom to decline. Ethical research practice requires the investigator to respect the individual's freedom to decline to participate in research or to discontinue participation at any time. The obligation to protect this freedom requires special vigilance when the investigator is in a position of power over the participant. . .

(G) Risk. The ethical investigator protects participants from . . . mental discomfort. . . If the risk of such consequences exists, the investigator is required to inform the participant of that fact, secure consent before proceeding, and take all possible measures to minimize distress.

New York created an expansive view as to what constitutes research. Given the rapidity with which students' complaints were filed, Dr. Robinson appears to have violated the New York statutes for research by failing to remove the harmful effects of the research before the study was launched. The likelihood that students would be feeling harmed appeared predictable from the multiple relationships. Unlike New York, Ohio has established very specific laws regarding the treatment of research subjects, none of which Dr. Robinson followed. Apparently, Dr. Robinson thought he had no reason to refer to or to comply with research law. In light of the specificity of the Ohio laws about research, Dr. Robinson was doing research and acted unethically.

Cultural Considerations

Global Discussion

The Professional Board for Psychology Health Professions Council of South Africa:
Ethical Code of Professional Conduct (April 2002)

> 10.5. Dispensing with informed consent.
>
> Before determining that planned research (such as research involving only anonymous questionnaires, naturalistic observations, or certain kinds of archival research) does not require the informed consent of research participants, psychologists shall consider applicable regulations and institutional review board requirements, and they shall consult with colleagues as appropriate.

Regardless of whether Dr. Robinson thought his interviews were exempt from informed consent, he has not consulted, nor has he considered, IRB regulations. Thus he is in violation of Standard 10.5. Presumably, if both the dean and the IRB are inquiring as to why no request for research was submitted in this case, it seems clear that Dr. Robinson has failed to consider the IRB requirements carefully enough, and failed to consult with colleagues.

American Moral Values

1. What is the exact purpose of Dr. Robinson's interviews? Does Dr. Robinson believe that his report should exonerate the clinic and cast doubt on student complaints, or does he suspect that the clinic needs to submit itself to necessary criticism through student input? Are his interviews meant to challenge student perceptions or help students elaborate about them?

2. What is the problem students are finding from the "harassing" interviews Dr. Robinson seems to be conducting? Is it that they fear their answers will not be confidential? Is his style of interviewing too aggressive? What is the possible "distress or harm" students could be experiencing here? Should Dr. Robinson stick to a preset list of questions, or does he need to press students to explain their misgivings and perceptions of the clinic? Should Dr. Robinson revise his list of questions?

3. Does the library constitute an appropriate "educational setting" for these interviews? Could interrupting studying in a more formal location (compared to, say, a cafeteria) create more anxiety than necessary? Do students feel pressured to answer questions even though they are preparing for exams, completing assignments, and so on?

4. What is the state of Dr. Robinson's relationship with the dean? What does Dr. Robinson believe he owes to his superior? Is the dean just trying to show students that something is being done about the clinic, or does Dr. Robinson feel the dean is criticizing how the clinic is being run? Should the dean supervise this effort and ask Dr. Robinson to submit a list of the questions he is asking? Does Dr. Robinson need a vote of confidence to proceed?

5. How does Dr. Robinson intend to undo the apparent damage his interviews have done to the clinic's relationship with some students? Is there another format for getting honest input about the clinic?

Ethical Course of Action

Directive per APA Code

Standards 8.05 (1) and (2) set the conditions under which psychologists conducting research with humans may forgo subject consent. Standard 8.05 (1) sets as a foundational requirement, above all other conditions, the specifiers that the research would not reasonably be assumed to create distress or harm; Standard 8.05 (2) stipulates when there is an expectation of harm that the experiment proceed only if it is allowable by law or regulations.

Dr. Robinson's activities seem to be missing some conditions that allow for dispensing with subject consent. Even without post-interview complaints from the students, it is reasonable to expect students' distress from any number of sources, such as the following: The source of the problem may be the clinic director, and thus students feel uncomfortable telling Dr. Robinson about how he is not performing his job. Or, Dr. Robinson probably has evaluative authority over the students, so students may feel fearful of retaliation. In the context of Standard 8.05 (1) (a), even allowing for Dr. Robinson's interviews being part of normal educational practices, the interviews did not meet the condition of "no reasonable expectation of harm." Conditions for Standard 8.05 (1) have not been met; Dr. Robinson was in violation of Standard 8.05 (1) and Standard 8.05 (1) (a).

Dr. Robinson probably caused some distress, based on the fact that there were follow-up complaints about the interviews, which means Dr. Robinson violated Standard 3.04 and may be poised to violate Standard 7.06.

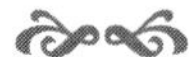

Dictates of One's Own Conscience

If you were the dean, faced with student complaints and Dr. Robinson's reasons for his actions, which of the following would you choose to do?

1. Ask the chair of the IRB to comment on Dr. Robinson's reasons for dispensing with application for IRB approval.
2. Ask Dr. Robinson to give evidence for his rationale for dispensing with IRB approval.
3. Consider the soundness of Dr. Robinson's rationale in the context of student complaints.
4. Excuse Dr. Robinson from the responsibility of investigating student complaints.
5. Assign investigation of student complaints to someone outside of the clinic or any departments that have direct interaction with the clinic.
6. Require Dr. Robinson to submit a study design and a request for approval to the IRB.
7. Require Dr. Robinson to obtain subject consent to interview without submission to the IRB.
8. Combinations of the above-listed actions.
9. Or one that is not listed above.

If you were directing a clinic in South Africa and you were Dr. Robinson, which of these would you do now?

1. Knowing the requirements of the ethics code, would you have consulted with the IRB and with colleagues before starting any approach that involved data collection?
2. Would you apologize to the dean and the IRB for having neglected this step and proceed to submit an application to the IRB for review and approval of the project?

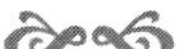

STANDARD 8.05: DISPENSING WITH INFORMED CONSENT FOR RESEARCH

> Psychologists may dispense with informed consent only (1) where research would not reasonably be assumed to create distress or harm and involves . . . (b) only anonymous questionnaires, naturalistic observations, or archival research for which disclosure of responses would not place participants at risk of criminal or civil liability or damage their financial standing, employability, or reputation, and confidentiality is protected.

A CASE FOR STANDARD 8.05 (1) (B): What Is Archival?

Dr. Rodriguez, faculty at the Modern School of Psychology in the New Center University, conducts a records review for his research. He is interested in whether the theoretical orientation of the supervisor necessarily dictates the theoretical orientation of the student therapist or the treatment technique utilized by the student. He has a list of supervising psychologists and their theoretical orientations from the vitae retained by university personnel records. A records review of cases consists of reading the treatment notes and watching archival treatment videos. Dr. Rodriguez did not think obtaining subject consent was necessary for this archival research. He submitted his research proposal to the New Center University's institutional review board, and the IRB agreed that no subject consent was necessary because the research activity only involved archival data.

Michelle and Calvin are graduate students who work for Dr. Rodriguez on the research project. Their task is to read the progress notes, watch the video recordings of treatment sessions, and rate the student therapist's activities in the sessions according to categories of theoretical orientation. Michelle read a treatment note from one student that appeared to indicate that his client was suicidal. This treatment note was not followed by any notation of supervisor instruction or treatment intervention in response to the client's suicidality. The client still is being treated by the student. Michelle and Calvin noticed that a pattern of nonresponsiveness to client suicidality by the same student therapist has occurred during the treatment of several different clients, although all of the other cases of this student's appeared to have terminated in the normal course of the clients making treatment gains. Michelle and Calvin report this to Dr. Rodriguez.

Issues of Concern

Per Standard 8.05 (1) (b), the condition Dr. Rodriguez uses for dispensing with subject consent is that the project involves only archival data. The members of the IRB agreed and the project was approved. Was Dr. Rodriguez or were the IRB members aware of the caveat in Standard 8.05 (1) (b) that places additional conditions on a review of archival information? To meet qualifications for archival research as stated in Standard 8.05 (1) (b), the review of the stored data should not violate the client's confidentiality or damage the student therapist or the supervisor by either putting them at risk of legal liability or hurting their professional standing.

The usual meaning of *archival* is that it refers to material stored for historical reference. Usually, a review of archival data is not expected to harm anyone since time has passed and events described in the records are no longer relevant. A literal meaning of *archive* is simply stored information, with no time reference. The records reviewed by Dr. Rodriguez's project may or may not concern people who are no longer practicing in the clinic, and thus the information gathered may or may not have real-time impact. Relevant questions regarding this situation include the following: Is the student therapist still actively treating clients in the clinic? Should Dr. Rodriguez identify the student to his or her supervisor or the student's graduate degree program? If Dr. Rodriguez was conducting the research in a state in which psychologists are mandatory reporters of intent to harm the self, would Dr. Rodriguez need to break confidentiality and report the situation to the police?

APA Ethics Code

Companion General Principle

Principle A: Beneficence and Nonmaleficence.

> When conflicts occur among psychologists' obligations or concerns, they attempt to resolve these conflicts in a responsible fashion that avoids or minimizes harm.

Principle A suggests psychologists should be of benefit to others, but at a minimum at least they are not to harm others. Depending on how Dr. Rodriguez decides to act to resolve the conflict of his duty to protect against harm to self versus keeping (archival) client confidentiality, the student may be harmed or this student's future clients may be harmed.

Principle B: Fidelity and Responsibility

> Psychologists . . . are aware of their professional and scientific responsibilities to society and to the specific communities in which they work. . . They are concerned about the ethical compliance of their colleagues' scientific and professional conduct.

Dr. Rodriguez as faculty has an obligation to monitor the clinical work of students. Being concerned about the behavior of this student's clinic work upholds the value of Principle B.

Companion Ethical Standard(s)

Standard 1.02: Conflicts Between Ethics and Law, Regulations, or Other Governing Legal Authority.

> If psychologists' ethical responsibilities conflict with law . . . psychologists clarify the nature of the conflict, make known their commitment to the Ethics Code and take reasonable steps to resolve the conflict consistent with the General Principles and Ethical Standards of the Ethics Code.

Here the conflict involves keeping to the integrity of the study, while having an awareness of the fact that students do not know their records are being viewed by the study investigators. Responsibility for the student's work and the duty to protect has arisen in this context. Standard 1.02 directs Dr. Rodriguez to take reasonable steps to resolve the conflicting demands in this situation in such a way that he acts consistently with the APA General Principles and Ethics Standards.

Standard 4.01: Maintaining Confidentiality

> Psychologists have a primary obligation . . . to protect confidential information obtained through . . . any medium, recognizing that the extent and limits of confidentiality may be regulated by law.

All members involved in this situation have an obligation to maintain client confidentiality. Imagine the client's surprise, alarm, and sense of betrayal if a stranger (as in Dr. Rodriguez) breaks confidentiality to enact the state's "duty to protect" law. Under what conditions might Dr. Rodriguez and the clinic adhere to both client confidentiality and duty to protect?

Standard 4.05: Disclosures

> . . . (b) Psychologists disclose confidential information without the consent of the individual only as mandated by law, or where permitted by law for a valid purpose such as . . . [to] (3) protect the client/patient, psychologist, or others from harm.

A psychologist license does not distinguish among practicing, teaching, or research. Laws refer to psychologists as one generic category. When state law mandates a duty to protect, that law pertains to any and all licensed psychologists as well as psychology students. And when laws cite psychologists as mandated reporters, it matters not whether that psychologist was engaged in researching archival data or actively providing treatment. In this circumstance, Michelle, Calvin, and Dr. Rodriguez are protected under Standard 4.05 (b) should they decide to break confidentiality and report the client if he or she is in active treatment.

Standard 1.04: Informal Resolution of Ethical Violations

> When psychologists believe that there may have been an ethical violation by another psychologist, they attempt to resolve the issue by bringing it to the attention of that individual.

In order to comply with Standard 1.04, Dr. Rodriguez, as the principal investigator, should bring the matter to the offending student's attention.

Legal Issues 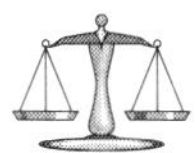

Pennsylvania

> *49 Pa. Code § 41.61 (2010). Code of Ethics.*
>
> Principle 9. Research with human participants. . .
>
> (d) Responsibility for the establishment and maintenance of acceptable ethical practice in research always remains with the individual investigator. The investigator is also responsible for the ethical treatment of research participants by . . . students[,] . . . all of whom, however, incur parallel obligations. . .
>
> (k) If research procedures result in undesirable consequences for the individual participant, the investigator has the responsibility to detect and remove or correct these consequences, including long-term effects.

Psychologists in Pennsylvania may disclose confidential information in filing a written application to the county administrator setting forth facts constituting reasonable grounds to believe a person is severely mentally disabled and in need of immediate involuntary treatment (42 Pa. Cons. Stat. Ann. § 7609 [West 2010]). In addition, on personal observation of the severely mentally disabled person, a physician or peace officer may take such a person to an approved facility for emergency examination (42 Pa. Cons. Stat. Ann. § 7302(a) [West 2010]); the facts of the case should suggest that the client is severely mentally disabled and in need of immediate treatment because the client lacks the capacity to exercise self-control, judgment, and discretion in the conduct of his or her affairs or in the client's social relations, or to care for personal needs, so that the client poses a clear and present danger of harm to others or to self. A clear and present danger to self is shown by establishing that within the past 30 days, the person has attempted suicide and there is a reasonable probability of suicide without adequate treatment, or the person has substantially mutilated or attempted to mutilate him- or herself and there is a reasonable probability of mutilation without adequate treatment (42 Pa. Cons. Stat. Ann. § 7301(b)(2) [West 2010]).

South Carolina

> *S.C. Code Ann. Regs.100-4 (2010). Code of Ethics.*
>
> F. Welfare of supervisees and research subjects. . .
>
> (2) Welfare of research subjects. The psychologist shall respect the dignity and protect the welfare of his/her research subjects and shall comply with all relevant statutes and administrative rules concerning treatment of research subjects.

The emergency admission procedures for South Carolina permit a psychologist who cannot gain access to a physician (to provide certification that a client requires involuntary treatment) to execute an affidavit for a probate court judge to issue an order of detention (S.C. Code Ann. § 44-17-430 [2002]). Also, a law enforcement officer can take the client into custody for an examination by a licensed physician to determine whether certification for involuntary commitment will occur, but the client must be mentally ill, which means "a person afflicted with a mental disease to such an extent that, for his own welfare or the welfare of others or of the community, he requires care, treatment or hospitalization" (S.C. Code Ann. § 44-22-10(1) [2002]). In addition, a likelihood of serious harm must exist and "because of mental illness there is (1) a substantial risk of physical harm to the person himself as manifested by evidence of threats of, or attempts at, suicide or serious bodily harm" (S.C. Code Ann. § 44-22-10(2) [2002]).

If Dr. Rodriguez was conducting the research project in Pennsylvania or South Carolina, he would have to conduct a careful assessment of whether the duty to protect existed in the case, and in light of the findings of the assessment, whether the research subject's client should be evaluated for involuntary treatment. Both jurisdictions have elected to create permissive duties about this issue. However, judicial activism has created uncertainty about how such a case would be viewed by the courts and perhaps the licensing boards. In Pennsylvania, under *Goryeb v. Commonwealth, Dep't of Pub. Welfare* (575 A.2d 545 [Pa. 1990]), psychologists are liable to third parties for negligent treatment of a person within their institutional realm who later does harm. It also is clear from *Bishop v. South Carolina Dep't of Mental Health* (502 S.E.2d 78, 82 [S.C. 1998]) that the South Carolina court also has engaged in judicial activism and did find a duty to warn existed in a case in which a patient was within the institutional control of the clinician. In light of the pattern of neglect across several other cases that went unidentified by the clinical supervisor, the licensing boards in both jurisdictions may find that both the clinical supervisor of the research subject and Dr. Rodriquez acted unethically if they did not engage in a contemporaneous evaluation of the person at risk who is within the control of the institution, once the person was identified by the research project as being at risk for suicide. Pennsylvania law makes it clear that the responsibility for addressing the dilemma at hand rests with Dr. Rodriquez and not with the students, Michelle and Calvin. Because the students identified the risk to their supervisor, South Carolina would likely hold Dr. Rodriquez responsible for the decisions that occurred subsequent to facts becoming known.

Cultural Considerations

Global Discussion

Canadian Code of Ethics for Psychologists

> Principle I: Respect for the dignity of persons.
>
> I.20. Obtain informed consent for all research activities that involve obtrusive measures, invasion of privacy, more than minimal risk of harm, or any attempt to change the behaviour of research participants.

Dr. Rodriguez and his students may be, albeit unwittingly, in violation of the letter and intent of Canada's code. Although the original intent of the archival study was to observe and record behavior of student therapists, not directly change it, Canada's code suggests that it was improper to dispense with informed consent. For a current student therapist, having one's chart notes read and filmed sessions observed without having given informed consent is an invasion of privacy. This invasion of privacy also extends to clients of the school, some of whom are likely community members, and in some cases may be fellow students. Dr. Rodriguez and his students must now weigh the consequences of not having obtained informed consent from students, and a potential "duty to warn" situation. Reporting a client's suicidality, or reporting a student therapist's failure to take action to the clinic or program dean, will have an immediate potential to "change the behavior of research participants."

American Moral Values

1. What is the purpose of the archival research that Dr. Rodriguez has assigned Michelle and Calvin? If it is to determine the theoretical orientation of a supervisor's students, why does Michelle need to examine how competently a student tracks suicidality? Has she crossed a line of archival research by delving into therapeutic faults rather than a theoretical stance? Or is one not able to track theoretical orientation accurately without some reference to how a student treats issues like suicidality?
2. Could Michelle's research, if shared with others, violate the standard of not damaging a subject's professional reputation? Could this subject even face civil or criminal liability if suicides were later committed by his clients? Should Dr. Rodriguez rethink his claim about subject consent given that these conditions apply?
3. How should Dr. Rodriguez, Michelle, and Calvin view the archival material for the student at issue? Is a lack of responsivity to suicidal tendencies an urgent enough issue to tell other faculty or the practice where this student now works? What if this flaw was addressed by the student's own supervisor long ago? What if Dr. Rodriguez, Michelle, and Calvin subsequently find out about suicides committed by this person's more recent clients? What position do they occupy to intervene?
4. If Dr. Rodriguez decided to investigate where this student works and inform various authorities (supervisor, police) of this archival material, what kind of precedent would this set? Does Dr. Rodriguez believe anyone's student treatment records should be investigated in order to ensure they are not presently putting clients in danger? Would Dr. Rodriguez want his own student treatment notes submitted to this standard?
5. How should Dr. Rodriguez instruct Michelle and Calvin going forward? Should he tell them that under no circumstance should they attend to possible treatment malpractice, but instead they should adhere strictly to theoretical orientation? Are there other scenarios where he would want his students to alert him to dangerous flaws in a person's performance?

Ethical Course of Action

Directive per APA Code

Standard 8.05 (1) (b) specifies conditions for dispensing with subject consent if the research involves archival data. The information uncovered in the archival research does not meet the specifics of the caveats given for Standard 8.05 (1) (b). The discovered information could place the offending student, the clinical supervisor, and Dr. Rodriquez at risk for civil liability and/or damage their reputations. Moreover, if there is a duty to protect, as in Pennsylvania and South Carolina, there is a risk of violating confidentiality (Standard 4.01) unless the standards for involuntary treatment are met. It appears that both Dr. Rodriguez and the IRB violated the conditions for Standard 8.05 (1) (b) in conducting this project.

Now that information is uncovered and subject consent has not been obtained, Dr. Rodriguez is obligated to uphold the state laws and Standard 4.01, which seem to place him in the circumstances described in Standard 1.02. Following the directive of Standard 1.04, at a minimum Dr. Rodriguez needs to alert the offending student to the situation, and the clinical supervisor, the student, and Dr. Rodriquez should review and document the contemporaneous facts of the case to determine whether the client in question remains at great risk for suicide. If Dr. Rodriguez were in Pennsylvania or South Carolina, it appears that Standard 4.05 (b) would allow for breach of confidentiality.

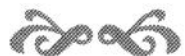

Dictates of One's Own Conscience

If you were Dr. Rodriguez, which of these would you do?

1. Consult with
   a. the chair of the IRB.
   b. the director of the clinic.
   c. the chair of the graduate program.
   d. the university's attorney.
   e. Dr. Rodriguez's malpractice carrier's attorney.
2. Read the chart entries for yourself to double-check the work of Michelle and Calvin.
3. Discuss the case with the supervisor to verify that an intervention was undertaken.
4. Review the archival videotape for the sessions in question to confirm accuracy of the chart notes.
5. Contact the offending student to discuss the situation.

If Michelle and Calvin's suspicions were verified after your personal assessment of the video recording, chart notes, conversations with the supervisor and with the offending student, and further discussions with the attorneys involved in the matter, would you

1. Request that the supervisor perform closer monitoring of the student in question?
2. Direct the student to contact his client and conduct a current mental status exam and suicidal risk assessment under close clinical supervision?
3. Recommend that the student be required to do remedial work on confidentiality, duty to protect, and assessment/interventions with suicidality?
4. Combinations of the above-listed actions?
5. Or one that is not listed above?

If you were Dr. Rodriguez and you were conducting this study in Canada, which of these would you do?

1. Stop the study immediately and seek informed consent from all current students who have active cases in the clinic.
2. Inform all students with active cases in the clinic that a research project with review of case records is being conducted.

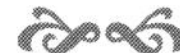

STANDARD 8.05: DISPENSING WITH INFORMED CONSENT FOR RESEARCH

> Psychologists may dispense with informed consent only (1) where research would not reasonably be assumed to create distress or harm and involves . . . (c) the study of factors related to job or organization effectiveness conducted in organizational settings for which there is no risk to participants' employability, and confidentiality is protected.

A CASE FOR STANDARD 8.05 (1) (C): The Informant

The new clinic supervisor at the Modern School of Psychology in the New Center University, Dr. Clark, was told to improve the clinic functioning for accreditation. Dr. Clark hears from his supervisees that they have many concerns about lax enforcement of ethics rules in the clinic.

Gail is in her final quarter as an intern in the clinic. Dr. Clark asks Gail to interview her fellow interns to ascertain the nature, extent, and specifics of the various rumored ethics violations. After Gail does so, she turns in a summary report to Dr. Clark that does not include the names of any interviewees.

The dean of the Modern School of Psychology and the upper administration of the New Center University learn of the existence of this report. Dr. Clark is told that the staff needs to understand the problematic nature of their practices and is urged to release the report written by Gail. Dr. Clark distributes Gail's summary report to the full clinic faculty and staff during a meeting. Dr. Clark then proceeds to discuss the specifics about the ethical violations contained in Gail's report.

Issues of Concern

The interviews were conducted to determine organizational effectiveness, they were conducted in an organizational setting, no interviewees were identified, and there is no direct threat to any specific person's employment. Have Dr. Clark and Gail met the conditions for dispensing with subject consent as enumerated in Standard 8.05 (1) (c)? Even if no interviewee's names were identified, is it possible that the interviewees revealed violations by others who were named in the interview? Is it possible that the identity of the clinic staff may be discernable from the report or from the specifics of the incidences? Finally, was it reasonable to expect a student being asked to report incidences of observed ethics violations would not be somewhat distressed?

APA Ethics Code

Companion General Principle

Principle E: Respect for People's Rights and Dignity

> Psychologists respect the . . . rights of individuals to privacy, confidentiality, and self-determination. Psychologists are aware that special safeguards may be necessary to protect the rights and welfare of persons or communities whose vulnerabilities impair autonomous decision making.

The value of respecting an individual's right to the privacy of their own thoughts and to self-determination in regards to what is said to whom, is expressed through obtaining subject consent. Gail's interviewees may have been led to believe that the information shared was for very limited distribution and may have revealed more specifics than they otherwise might have.

Companion Ethical Standard(s)

Standard 8.01: Institutional Approval

> When institutional approval is required, psychologists provide accurate information about their research proposals and obtain approval prior to conducting the research. They conduct the research in accordance with the approved research protocol.

When Dr. Clark asked Gail to gather information by interviewing clinic personnel, it is doubtful that either of them thought of this project as research. What constitutes research, and when does a project require institutional approval?

Standard 4.04: Minimizing Intrusions on Privacy

> (a) Psychologists include in written . . . reports . . . only information germane to the purpose for which the communication is made. . . (b) Psychologists discuss confidential information obtained in their work only for appropriate . . . professional purposes and only with persons clearly concerned with such matters.

Regardless of whether it is the privacy of a client or the privacy of research subjects at stake, psychologists do not reveal more information than necessary. Would Gail have included as much information if she had known how Dr. Clark was going to use the report?

Legal Issues 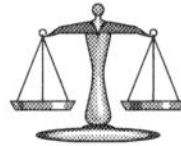

Texas

> *22 Tex. Admin. Code § 465.13 (2010). Personal Problems, Conflicts and Dual Relationships.*
>
> (a) In General. . .
>
> (3) Licensees do not exploit persons over whom they have supervisory evaluative authority such as students . . . [or] employees.

> *22 Tex. Admin. Code § 465.20 (2010). Research.*
>
> (a) Conducting Research.
>
> (1) Licensees who conduct research involving human research participants must obtain informed consent . . . including anticipated sharing . . . of personally identifiable research data and of the possibility of unanticipated future uses.

Virginia

18 Va. Admin. Code § 125-20-150 (2010). Standards of Practice.

B. Persons licensed by the board shall . . .

5. Avoid harming . . . students and others for whom they provide professional services and minimize harm when it is foreseeable and unavoidable. Not exploit or mislead people for whom they provide professional services. Be alert to and guard against misuse of influence. . .

14. Design, conduct and report research in accordance with recognized standards of scientific competence and research ethics.

It is quite probable that the licensing boards in both jurisdictions would find that Dr. Clark's request to Gail crossed the line from supervision to exploitation by having Gail act as an informant. Dr. Clark also would be in violation as a supervisor. The final use of the report indicates that the project should have been undertaken as research, with all of the safeguards established in Texas and Virginia for research that should have been followed by Dr. Clark.

Cultural Considerations

Global Discussion

Canadian Code of Ethics for Psychologists

Principle I: Respect for the dignity of persons.

I.20. Obtain informed consent for all research activities that involve . . . invasion of privacy, more than minimal risk of harm, or any attempt to change the behaviour of research participants.

I.36. Be particularly cautious in establishing the freedom of consent of any person who is in a dependent relationship to the psychologist (e.g., student, employee).

Dr. Clark and, indirectly, Gail are in violation of the letter and intent of I.20 and I.36 of the Canadian Code. Canada's Code is silent on dispensing with informed consent as part of organizational effectiveness. What 1.20 demands is that psychologists obtain informed consent for all activities designed to change behavior of research participants, which ultimately was the aim of Dr. Clark's request of Gail to interview student clinicians. Therefore, Dr. Clark is in violation of I.20 by not having informed consent secured by Gail or himself prior to the interviews of students. Next, Dr. Clark is in violation of Standard I. 36, which requires psychologists to attend carefully to power differentials. By asking Gail, an intern and student, to carry out the interviews, Dr. Clark did not attend to the dependent nature of Gail's relationship to him. Gail, by being a more experienced intern and potentially having perceived or actual evaluative authority over the other students, also neglected to attend to the dependent nature of the other interns.

American Moral Values

1. Have Dr. Clark and Gail taken enough precautions with their initial interviews to protect the confidentiality and employability of the interviewees? Has the purpose of this report changed now that the dean and others have demanded it be addressed to the staff? Did Dr. Clark foresee that his superiors could make this kind of request? Should he have taken precautions at a prior stage to account for the possibility?
2. How did these interviews serve Dr. Clark's purpose as the new clinic director? Did this piece of research cause distress to its subjects, given that ethics violations could cost them their jobs? Was there another way to find out how rules were enforced without using this type of interview format? Would subjects self-monitor with Gail, or did the fact that she was leaving soon help them air out their honest views?
3. What does it mean to Dr. Clark that the staff "has to understand" the ethics problems exposed by the report? Does Dr. Clark have the authority to conduct the review of the report alone with the clinic staff? Can he protect faculty and staff from having their jobs threatened by what the report itself revealed about the administrative and supervisory practices of the clinic? Can he ensure that the staff's individual comments will remain confidential among the faculty and staff members themselves, as well as with regard to the School of Psychology and university as a whole?
4. How will higher authorities in the school and university hold Dr. Clark accountable for changes based on the report? Should Dr. Clark demand independence in his handling of the report, including whatever meetings he holds to review it? Will the school's concerns over accreditation override Dr. Clark's demands? Has it hurt his position with the dean and others to have had Gail gather data and present the report?
5. What does Dr. Clark believe about the ethics violations reported by Gail's interviews? Are they structural problems stemming from how the clinic is set up? Are

they the result of a few unethical staff members? What kind of moral authority should he present as the new director, based on the problems he sees? Should he present himself as "cleaning house"? Should he be more of a cheerleader who wants to help everyone perform to a higher standard?

Ethical Course of Action

Directive per APA Code

When a project involves the gathering of information from humans, Standard 8.05 (1) (c) allows for not fully informing subjects of all those elements listed in Standard 8.02 if the topic is about organizational effectiveness. Dr. Clark's project appears to have met all of the conditions for Standard 8.05 (1) (c): The interviews were conducted to determine organizational effectiveness; they were conducted in an organizational setting; no interviewees were identified; and no direct threat to any specific person's employment was possible.

Yet there is a certain discomfort in how the information was used. The discomfort may come from subjects being unprepared for how Dr. Clark would use the information. There was potential for distress and possible harm to people's reputations if the clinic is relatively small and the information could reasonably identify individuals. This potential for distress and harm violates Standard 8.05 (1).

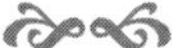

Dictates of One's Own Conscience

If you were Gail, sitting in the staff meeting, listening to how your report was being used, which of these would you do?

1. Think Dr. Clark is brave to confront the ethics violations publicly.
2. Want to distance yourself from the report because
   a. people's confidences were being betrayed.
   b. you told interviewees that the information was going to Dr. Clark only and not beyond.
   c. you assured interviewees that the information would not be shared publicly.
3. When it becomes apparent that your report is to be disseminated in the meeting, but before Dr. Clark has a chance to distribute your report, question Dr. Clark on the efficacy of sharing the report.
4. Feel uncomfortable during the meeting and talk to Dr. Clark in private afterward about the difficult position he put you in.
5. After the meeting, apologize privately and individually to your interviewees, telling them that you did not know Dr. Clark would publicly release the report.
6. Combinations of the above-listed possible courses of action.
7. Or one that is not listed above.

If you were Gail, interning in Canada, which of these would you do in the situation?

1. Question Dr. Clark's need to write a research proposal and obtain IRB approval at the first mention of data collection.
2. Decline Dr. Clark's suggestion to collect information from fellow interns on the grounds of the power differential.

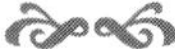

STANDARD 8.05: DISPENSING WITH INFORMED CONSENT FOR RESEARCH

Psychologists may dispense with informed consent only . . . (2) where otherwise permitted by law or federal or institutional regulations.

A CASE FOR STANDARD 8.05 (2): The Gift of Sleep

The Modern School of Psychology at the New Center University has received a study grant from the Foundation for Human Engineering. Dr. Lewis is the principal investigator. She has two graduate students working with her, Brittany and Clyde. The study is to determine the cognitive functioning of people whose jobs require unusually long shift work. Of particular interest are those who work in potentially physically dangerous situations. The Research Institute for Social Responsibility was able to gain access to a military installation where soldiers guard munitions stockpiles.

On a daily basis, Brittany and Clyde administer the Mini-Mental State Exam (MMSE) to soldiers at 6:00 a.m. and at 6:00 p.m. The Research Institute, in collaboration with the military installation, changes the length of the soldiers' shifts at random, affecting their sleep patterns.

Issues of Concern

Dr. Lewis's grant has been issued through the university for a study that requires the administration of the MMSE in a naturalistic work situation. Standard 8.05 (2) does not apply to her work. However, the subjects of her study are being assigned to different lengths of work shifts that interfere with sleeping patterns. The manipulation of their sleep and shifts is not within the scope of Dr. Lewis's study and is beyond her control. Yet it appears that the sleep deprivation and stress are very much a part of the study the granting agency wants conducted. Given the context of the study, does Standard 8.05 (2) apply? Standard 8.05 (2) allows Dr. Lewis to dispense with subject consent if there is a law or regulation that governs aspects of the study, which may be possible given the interface with the military. Could it be that for the administration of the MMSE, Dr. Lewis needs to obtain subject consent and that she needs to state a disclaimer regarding the manipulation of the soldiers' sleep and shift work?

APA Ethics Code

Companion General Principle

Principle C: Integrity

> In situations in which deception may be ethically justifiable to maximize benefits and minimize harm, psychologists have a serious obligation to consider the need for, the possible consequences of, and their responsibility to correct any resulting mistrust or other harmful effects that arise from the use of such techniques.

Principle C calls a psychologist's attention to the negative effects of deception. From Dr. Lewis, Brittany, and Clyde's point of view, they are simply conducting a straightforward study of cognition and stress with no manipulation or deception. From the subjects' perspective, it appears that Dr. Lewis is manipulating their shift length and rotations for the purpose of the study.

Companion Ethical Standard(s)

Standard 1.02: Conflicts Between Ethics and Law, Regulations, or Other Governing Legal Authority.

> If psychologists' ethical responsibilities conflict with . . . governing legal authority, psychologists clarify the nature of the conflict, make known their commitment to the Ethics Code and take reasonable steps to resolve the conflict consistent with the General Principles and Ethical Standards of the Ethics Code.

It is unclear how much Dr. Lewis was aware of the granting organization's ability to alter the research subjects' work schedule. Without the direct influence of the Research Institute for Social Responsibility on research subjects' work schedules, the study would not be research experimentation; it would be a survey of a naturalistic situation. Once Dr. Lewis, Brittany, or Clyde becomes aware of the direct influence that the Research Institute has on their subjects' work situation, Standard 1.02 requires them to make known the nature of their conflict and to take steps to resolve the conflict. The most drastic measure for resolution may necessitate full withdrawal from the grant.

Standard 3.04: Avoiding Harm

> Psychologists take reasonable steps to avoid harming their . . . research participants, and to minimize harm where it is foreseeable and unavoidable.

Once Dr. Lewis, Brittany, or Clyde becomes aware of the possibility that the entity associated with the study is manipulating the subjects' shifts and sleep schedules, it would be appropriate for the research team to consider whether their participation in the study is harming their subjects.

Legal Issues 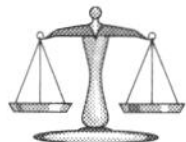

Washington

> *Wash. Admin. Code § 246-924-361 (2009). Exploiting Supervisees and Research Subjects.*
>
> (1) Psychologists shall not exploit persons over whom they have . . . evaluative . . . authority such as students . . . employees, research participants . . . [etc.].

> *Wash. Admin. Code § 246-924-366 (2009). Fraud, Misrepresentation, or Deception.*

> (1) The psychologist shall not use . . . misrepresentation, or deception . . . in conducting any other activity related to the practice of psychology.

California

> *Cal. Bus. & Prof. Code § 2960 (West 2010). Causes for Disciplinary Action.*
>
> Unprofessional conduct shall include, but not be limited to . . . (n) The commission of any dishonest, corrupt, or . . . fraudulent act.

Once the activity of Dr. Lewis's study is identified as deception, then the project is in violation of both Washington and California's laws, which prohibit any dishonest or deceptive behavior by psychologists. Neither jurisdiction defines what constitutes deception or dishonesty within the laws regulating psychologists. Such definition would be taken from laws related to civil and criminal fraud of the jurisdictions in order to determine whether deception and dishonesty applied to the research design.

Cultural Considerations

Global Discussion

Code of Ethics for the Psychologist: Spain

> ***Article 7.*** Psychologists must not, either on their own behalf or in collaboration with others, contribute to any practices that may violate individual liberty or physical or psychological integrity. Direct participation or cooperation in torture or maltreatment—apart from being a crime—is the gravest violation of the Psychologist's professional ethics. They must never participate in any way, nor as researchers, or advisors, or in concealment, or the practice of torture, or any other cruel, inhuman and degrading practices, whoever the victims may be, and regardless of their crimes or the accusations or suspicions against them, or the information that might be obtainable from them, nor situations of armed conflict, civil war, revolution, terrorism or whatever other motivations may be offered as justification for such practices.
>
> ***Article 15.*** When faced with a conflict between personal and institutional interests, psychologists must strive to act with the greatest impartiality.
>
> ***Article 37.*** Psychological research in normal situations, whether experimental or observational, must always be carried out with respect for the dignity of the individuals.

Dr. Lewis, Brittany, and Clyde have quite possibly become unwitting coconspirators in violations of several portions of Spain's Ethical Code, including Articles 7, 15, and 37. The original intent of the study was to research the impact of long shift work upon cognition, rather than directly alter sleep and work patterns, causing sleep deprivation. Sleep deprivation and the alteration of work and sleep schedules, especially without consent, is in violation of the soldiers' "liberty or physical or psychological integrity" (Article 7). Chronic sleep deprivation, without opportunity to consent or withdraw as a condition of one's work, has also been defined by the Geneva Convention and the Nuremberg Laws as an act of torture.

Dr. Lewis and her team are further obligated, under Article 15, to protect the interests of the individual soldiers from the interests of the institution, in this case, the military. Dr. Lewis is obligated, under the Spanish Code, to break their allegiance with the institution if violations of the rights of individuals occur. The use of deception, sleep deprivation, and alteration of work and sleep schedules on soldiers who cannot easily depart or seek remediation without retaliation qualifies as a conflict. Dr. Lewis and her team are mandated by Article 15 to protect the dignity of the soldiers more strongly than that of other populations, rather than seek to exploit them due to their availability and perceived organizational compliance to the regulations and culture of the military.

American Moral Values

1. What is the relationship between Dr. Lewis's study and the Research Institute? Is her administration of the Mini-Mental State Exam a morally distinct act from the institute's manipulation of sleep and shift length? Or does her study constitute an implicit endorsement of those methods?

2. What kind of consent does Dr. Lewis need from the soldiers? Do they simply need to consent to her Mini-Mental State tests? Does Dr. Lewis believe they would feel the same way about those tests if they knew how their sleep and shift times were being changed? Would they object if presented with the Research Institute's purposes? If so, is Dr. Lewis collaborating on a project that wrongly dispenses with consent?

3. What is the relationship between the Research Institute and the military? Why does Dr. Lewis believe the military is allowing her study? Could the military be looking into other aspects of sleep

deprivation other than soldier performance? Would Dr. Lewis be responsible for ulterior uses for this study? How much should Dr. Lewis investigate this issue? Will it undermine possibly constructive advances to be made with the help of the Research Institute?

4. How does this work reflect Dr. Lewis's views about psychologists working in collaboration with the government? Is this a good example to set for other psychologists? How will her colleagues judge her involvement with this project?

Ethical Course of Action

Directive per APA Code

The original scope of Dr. Lewis's study as funded by the Research Institute for Social Responsibility does not meet the conditions that allow for dispensing with research subject consent. Thus, per Standard 8.02 (a) and 3.10, Dr. Lewis would need her subjects' consent to be administered the MMSE.

The original scope of the study was not set up as an experimental condition. The full scope of the study actually involves manipulation of sleep patterns and length of time on duty, then sampling the solder's mental status at two set points in the day. The full scope of the study with military personnel may fall within the parameters of Standard 8.05 (2) and indeed allows the Research Institute for Social Responsibility to dispense with obtaining subject consent. Once Dr. Lewis, Brittany, or Clyde becomes aware of the full scope of the study, Principle C would suggest they would take measures to dispel misconceptions the soldiers may hold about Dr. Lewis's involvement in manipulating their shift assignments. Standard 1.02 would require that Dr. Lewis make known any problems she has with the full scope of the study, and take steps to minimize whatever harm that might come to the subjects in the study, per Standard 3.04.

Dictates of One's Own Conscience

If you were Brittany or Clyde, administering the MMSE to the soldiers, and it dawns on you that their sleep schedules are actually being manipulated, which of these would you do?

1. Tell Dr. Lewis of your suspicions.
2. Make further inquiries of the soldiers about what kind of alterations are being made to their duty shifts.
3. Ask Dr. Lewis for a copy of the grant to explore whether there is any possible connection between the soldiers' shift changes and your study.
4. Research the source of funds that support the Research Institute for Social Responsibility.
5. Make inquiries of the subjects' commander to further determine if the shift changes were coincidental or somehow linked to your study.

If, upon further inquiry, you discover that the Research Institute for Social Responsibility has intimate links to the military, would you

1. Think that you are paranoid and fabricating conspiracy theories where there are only coincidences?
2. Suggest to Dr. Lewis that there may be more to this study than what Dr. Lewis knows?
3. Do combinations of the above-listed actions?
4. Or one that is not listed above?

If you were Dr. Lewis and were conducting this project in Spain, and it dawns on you that the soldiers' sleep schedules are actually being manipulated, which of these would you do?

1. Immediately cease all data collection.
2. Seek to discuss the situation with the granting agency and the military to resolve the situation of exploiting the soldiers for the research.
3. End your affiliation with the military or granting agency if other solutions fail to resolve this particular situation.

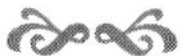

STANDARD 8.06: OFFERING INDUCEMENTS FOR RESEARCH PARTICIPATION

(a) Psychologists make reasonable efforts to avoid offering excessive or inappropriate financial or other inducements for research participation when such inducements are likely to coerce participation.

A CASE FOR STANDARD 8.06 (A): I'm Not Sleeping or Eating Regularly Anyways

Dr. Lee is under contract with a new biotechnology company. The research question is to find out the relationship between pain, and nutrition and sleep. Dr. Lee wants to determine people's subjective experience of pain in different states of nutrition and sleep deprivation. He decides to recruit individuals who would normally experience variability with regard to the amount of food and the amount of sleep they receive on a daily basis. Dr. Lee reasons that he has easy access to two groups of individuals who fit the research criteria—undergraduate students and homeless individuals. The research involves the completion of a questionnaire asking about the actual amount of food and sleep the individual has had in the previous 72 hours. The subject's perceived discomfort level is then measured by administering pressure through blood pressure cuffs. The participants are asked to rate the levels of pain and discomfort they are experiencing at different rates of pressure. To determine whether pain thresholds differ as nutrition and sleep vary, participants are invited to return on different days, up to 3 times within a week.

For their participation, the subjects are given $50 gift cards to the grocery store each time they come in. The gift card has no limitations regarding items purchased at the grocery store.

Issues of Concern

The ability to acquire $50 a day and up to $150 within a week offers a large sum to individuals who have no means of earning money. The ability to use the money with no restriction at a grocery store opens up a wide array of possibilities. For those who are homeless or poor, the financial incentive would most probably be enticing indeed, especially when participants only undergo a 30-second blood pressure cuff and the answering of some questions. Does Dr. Lee's research design violate Standard 8.06 (a)? Even if the financial incentive is of sufficient amount to be coercive, is there anything immoral about passing some wealth to individuals who naturally meet the unfortunate experimental criteria of not having regular sleep or food?

APA Ethics Code

Companion General Principle

Principle A: Beneficence and Nonmaleficence

> Psychologists strive to benefit those with whom they work and take care to do no harm.

Principle A states that psychologists try to be of benefit to others without doing harm. The possible harm from Dr. Lee's research experiment is the temporary experience of pain. Does this temporary pain outweigh the benefit society might derive from the knowledge gained through the experiment? Are there other sources of possible harm besides the pain?

Companion Ethical Standard(s)

Standard 3.04: Avoiding Harm

> Psychologists take reasonable steps to avoid harming their . . . research participants . . . and to minimize harm where it is foreseeable and unavoidable.

Standard 3.04 is the companion to Principle A: Beneficence and Nonmaleficence. There is no foreseeable harm from the pressure exerted through a blood pressure cuff, but there may be foreseeable harm through the unfettered use of $50–$150 at a grocery store. Grocery stores carry drugs and alcohol in addition to food items. Having access to these mind-altering items may be harmful to the participants.

Legal Issues 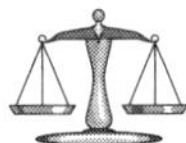

Colorado

> *Colo. Rev. Stat. Ann. § 12-43-222. (West 2010). Prohibited Activities—Related Provisions.*
>
> (j) Has exercised undue influence on the client . . . in such a manner as to exploit the client for the financial gain of the practitioner.

Florida

> *Florida Statute 490.009 (2010). Discipline.*
>
> (1) The following acts constitute grounds for denial of a license or disciplinary action, as specified in s. 456.072 (2)[:] . . .

> (m) Soliciting patients or clients personally, or through an agent, through the use of . . . undue influence.

Dr. Lee's research has targeted vulnerable subjects who are likely to engage in harmful behavior because of the incentive that is offered to obtain their consent. Did Dr. Lee exercise undue influence in order to further his research agenda? As the principal investigator, his salary is likely connected to the success of his obtaining grant support. In Colorado, his actions may be viewed as exploitation of the research subjects for personal gain.

Cultural Considerations

Global Discussion

Canadian Code of Ethics for Psychologists

> Principle I: Respect for the dignity of persons.
>
> *Freedom of consent.*
>
> I.28. Not proceed with any research activity, if consent is given under any condition of . . . undue reward.
>
> I.29. Take all reasonable steps to confirm or re-establish freedom of consent, if consent for service is given under conditions of duress or conditions of extreme need.
>
> *Protections for vulnerable persons.*
>
> I.31. Seek an independent and adequate ethical review of human rights issues and protections for any research involving members of vulnerable groups . . . before making a decision to proceed.
>
> I.32. Not use persons of diminished capacity to give informed consent in research studies, if the research involved may be carried out equally well with persons who have a fuller capacity to give informed consent.

Dr. Lee should not have proceeded with any research because consent by homeless individuals and students was likely given under "undue reward" (I.28). Offering grocery store gift cards to persons without income can be coercive. He is obligated to reestablish consent with his participants (I.29), which he failed to do. Students are "vulnerable persons" if they are being asked to do research by their supervisors or instructors; the statistics linking the numbers of homeless persons with both mental illness and substance addictions place them in the category of "vulnerable person" in many countries, including Canada. In "Protections for vulnerable persons," Dr. Lee is to seek an independent and "adequate" ethical review, which he also failed to do (I.31). By design, Dr. Lee's study seems to target those most vulnerable and in need of his incentive in order to get their consent.

American Moral Values

1. Will the incentive of earning up to $150 a week coerce students and homeless individuals? Will they change their feedback to meet what they think is desired by the company? How is pain to be measured? If there are no physical criteria to accompany self-reporting, is the reporting of pain susceptible to distortion through coercion?
2. How does a gift card for a grocery store affect subjects' diets and overall lifestyle? Will alcohol be more available to these subjects? How will increased usage of the gift cards affect the study? Could this gift card stabilize the amount of food the homeless individuals or students eat, or even the amount of sleep they get, thus undermining the premise of their selection as subjects? Would it undermine the efficacy of the research if subjects changed their eating habits during the study?
3. Could this study be more coercive for homeless subjects than for students? Have they had the exposure to these types of studies that undergraduates have? Does this study differ more sharply from their usual treatment in society? How will this context of reporting pain compare to contexts like hospitals, shelters, or agencies where the level of service can vary widely depending on such reporting? Would it make financial sense for some of them to choose this study over job opportunities? Is their health more likely to suffer for participating? Is carrying around a gift card for this amount dangerous for those living on the street?
4. How does the company's policy of distributing money compare to a university? Does the company understand what universities usually pay students for these types of studies? Are they trying to draw away students from other studies? Will this amount of compensation draw too much attention to the company's project? Will it encourage students' misreporting in order to qualify for the experiments?
5. What is the social value of this study, given the populations involved? Is the variance of pain with nutrition and sleep an important phenomenon to document for the sake of homeless individuals? Could it be worth possible disruptions to homeless subjects' lives to gain more knowledge in this area, especially for those interested in policies pertaining to fighting homelessness?

Ethical Course of Action

Directive per APA Code

The financial inducement of $50 seems excessive for a few seconds of pressure from a blood pressure cuff and answers to a few questions. Further, $50–$150 is enough of an inducement for poor students and homeless individuals as to be coercive. Dr. Lee appears to have violated Standard 8.06.

Except for the biotechnical company paying out some money, it does not appear that the experimental conditions create any harm to the participants, thus upholding Standard 3.04 and Standard A. The distribution of money through a grocery store seems well-intentioned to dictate that subjects spend the money in ways that are good for them. However, the unrestricted nature of the grocery store gift card may enable access to drugs and alcohol. It is questionable how far psychologists' responsibilities extend in carrying out the directives of Standard 3.04. If they extend to how subjects could use the incentive for ill, then Dr. Lee has violated Standard 3.04.

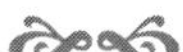

Dictates of One's Own Conscience

If you were Dr. Lee, contemplating how best to structure the financial inducement, which of these might you do?

1. Give cash rewards. Reason that psychologists are to respect people's right to self-determination, Principle E, so subjects should be free to use the financial incentive however they want.
2. Give gift cards to coffee shops where there is no alcohol or drugs besides caffeine being sold.
3. Give subjects a choice of a free night in a local hotel or a gift card worth an equal amount for a bookstore.
4. Give subjects material items like a nutritious three-course meal at a healthy restaurant.
5. Combinations of the above-listed possible courses of action.
6. Or one that is not listed above.

If you were Dr. Lee working in Canada and contemplating how best to structure the financial inducement, what might you do?

1. Keep the inducement level, and use the inducement to request that subjects voluntarily alter their sleep and eating patterns the day before the experiment.
2. Keep the same population as research subjects but use no inducement; just appeal to their goodwill.
3. Keep the same population as research subjects, but use non-monetary equivalent inducements.

STANDARD 8.06: OFFERING INDUCEMENTS FOR RESEARCH PARTICIPATION

. . . (b) When offering professional services as an inducement for research participation, psychologists clarify the nature of the services, as well as the risks, obligations, and limitations.

A CASE FOR STANDARD 8.06 (B): Too Good to Be True

Dr. Walker received a grant from the Veteran's Administration (VA) Hospital to conduct efficacy studies on the use of eye movement desensitization and reprocessing (EMDR) for treatment of combat veterans who report symptoms of post-traumatic stress disorder (PTSD). The research study advertises among and recruits from a population of veterans who are unsuccessful at reintegration into civilian life due to their PTSD symptoms. The research advertisement promises to provide medical and mental health treatment for the subject's family through the medical facilities at the New Center University if the veteran participates in the EMDR efficacy research project. The facility at the New Center University does not require military veterans to have a disability rating in order to receive treatment with the research project. The treatment for the veterans is EMDR.

Issues of Concern

There are two arenas of interest. One is the experimental nature of EMDR; the other is the nature of the inducement. Standard 8.06 requires Dr. Walker to clarify the risks and benefits of EMDR. The treatment technique is controversial, and past studies have reported inconclusive evidence that EMDR is effective (Devilly, 2005; Rubin, 2003; Schubert & Lee, 2009). The inducement is quite lavish. If the university has a full-service hospital, the secondary benefit to the veteran and his or her family could be enormous. Is the incentive for this project so lavish for the target population that it is coercive?

APA Ethics Code

Companion General Principle

Principle A: Beneficence and Nonmaleficence

> Psychologists strive to benefit those with whom they work and take care to do no harm.

Ideally, as stated in Principle A, Dr. Walker's study would be of benefit to the veterans suffering from PTSD. Would it be harmful to have veterans participate in a treatment that, at best, is inconclusively effective?

Companion Ethical Standard(s)

Standard 8.06: Offering Inducements for Research Participation

> (a) Psychologists make reasonable efforts to avoid offering excessive . . . inducements for research participation when such inducements are likely to coerce participation.

Included in unsuccessful reintegration into civilian life are unemployment or underemployment, as well as difficult family relationships. The availability of medical services if the family does not have health insurance through a workplace is invaluable. The inducement is so lavish for those without health insurance that it would most definitely be coercive. Standard 8.06 (a) does not prohibit excessive inducements. It directs Dr. Walker to make efforts to *avoid* use of excessive inducements. Based on the permissible language of Standard 8.06 (a), Dr. Walker is not in violation of this section of the code, but may be in violation of the spirit of Standard 8.06 (a).

Standard 8.02: Informed Consent to Research

> . . . (b) Psychologists conducting intervention research involving the use of experimental treatments clarify to participants at the outset of the research (1) the experimental nature of the treatment [and] . . . (5) compensation for or monetary costs of participating.

Following the directives of Standards 8.02 (b), Dr. Walker would need to tell the veterans what is known about EMDR and its effectiveness in treatment of PTSD. In the already-difficult lives of veterans suffering from PTSD, would including other treatment methods be sufficiently aversive to balance the excessive inducement?

Legal Issues 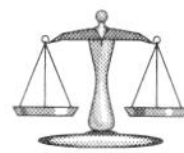

Hawaii

> *Haw. Code R. § 16-98-34 (2010). Unethical Practice of Psychology.*
>
> (e) The psychologist shall respect the integrity and protect the welfare of the person or group with whom the psychologist is working:
>
> (1) The psychologist in . . . education . . . in which conflicts of interest may arise among various parties . . . shall define the nature and direction of the psychologist's loyalties and responsibilities and keep all parties concerned informed of these commitments;
>
> (2) When there is a conflict among professional workers, the psychologist shall be concerned primarily with the welfare of any client involved and only secondarily with the interest of the psychologist's own professional group. . .
>
> (m) The psychologist shall assume obligations for the welfare of the psychologist's research subjects . . .
>
> (1) Only when a problem is of scientific significance and it is not practicable to investigate it in any other way is the psychologist justified in exposing research subjects . . . to physical or emotional stress as part of the investigation;
>
> (3) The psychologist shall seriously consider the possibility of harmful after-effects and avoid them, or remove them as soon as permitted by the design of the experiment.

Indiana

> *868 Ind. Admin. Code 1.1-11-2 (2010). Relationships With Other Professionals.*
>
> (h) A psychologist shall not unjustly exploit persons over whom the psychologist . . . [has] authority such as the following[:] . . .
>
> (4) Research participants.

868 Ind. Admin. Code 1.1-11-4.1 (2010). Relationships Within Professional Practice.

(l) A psychologist shall exercise reasonable care and diligence in the conduct of research and shall utilize generally accepted scientific principles and current professional theory and practice. New or experimental procedures, techniques, and theories shall be utilized only with proper research safeguards, informed consent, and peer review of the procedures or techniques.

The Hawaiian law calls for Dr. Walker to inform the veterans that her primary loyalty is to the funding agency and the research project, and secondarily to the welfare of the veterans. In addition, the lack of adequate disclosure about the possible effects or lack of effects from EMDR treatment also appears to violate the law. The law in Indiana calls for Dr. Walker to determine whether EMDR is a generally accepted practice or an experimental procedure. In light of the earlier controversial treatment outcomes related to this practice, adequate disclosure must occur for Dr. Walker to avoid the taint of engaging in coercive inducement to essentially recruit the veterans to the research project.

Cultural Considerations

Global Discussion

Hong Kong Psychological Society:
Professional Code of Practice

6: Research in psychology.

6.7. A Member must not use a position of authority to exert undue pressure on potential subjects for the purpose of securing their participation in a particular research project. A Member engaged in research shall allow a reasonable opportunity for subjects to withdraw their participation after becoming acquainted with the roles and tasks expected of them.

Hong Kong's code declares that psychologists may not use their position of authority to coerce potential participants into research studies. Although Hong Kong's code is silent on the particular use of rewards or services to induce participation, offering free health care to veterans suffering from PTSD as a function of Dr. Walker's privilege as a psychologist working in a large hospital is in violation of Hong Kong's code for using her authority to apply pressure on these veterans to participate.

American Moral Values

1. Is Dr. Walker's offer of health services to the veterans and their families too coercive for those who suffer from PTSD? Even if it is made clear to the veterans how questionable EMDR is as a treatment for PTSD, would the family benefits alone coerce veterans into participating? What if the EMDR treatment precluded other treatments the veteran would have preferred but for the family health care issue?
2. What characterizes failing to reintegrate into civilian life? If that means not having a job, does that make the offer of health benefits even more coercive? Is a project like Dr. Walker's worth the risks it takes with the lives of this population, given how fragile their situation probably is? Or is this akin to experimental treatments for cancer at the end of life, in that all other approaches to treating PTSD in this population have been unsuccessful?
3. What will be the impact on veterans' families if they come to believe that their own health care depended on the veterans' sustained willingness to obtain treatment for their PTSD? What forms of guilt, recrimination, and resentment could be created, both within the family and between family members and Dr. Walker (or the hospital, the university, the VA, etc.) if the veteran claimed that EMDR treatment is not helpful and wished to withdraw from the study? Does Dr. Walker need to consult with social workers at the hospital who work with families?
4. Will the grant Dr. Walker has received be able to cover the health expenses that might be incurred? What will happen if the money runs out on families who have been promised health care? Does Dr. Walker or the hospital research director need to consult with financial experts to chart out the viability of this offer? Is it better to provide EMDR and health care to families for as long as the money is available, or should the offer be withdrawn before anyone is prematurely cut off?

Ethical Course of Action

Directive per APA Code

To comply with Standard 8.06 (b) and 8.02 (b), Dr. Walker needs to fully explain the controversy around the use of EMDR for treatment of PTSD. If the treatment regimen in combination with the medical support to the family members were helpful, that knowledge would be of great benefit to a population that is most deserving of support. Though the incentive for this study seems sufficiently excessive as to be coercive, Standard 8.02 (b) does not prohibit such incentives.

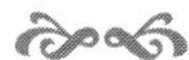

Dictates of One's Own Conscience

If you were the director of the university's medical services, which of these would be your response to Dr. Walker's research?

1. Hope that the grant is sufficient to offset the cost of services the facility will be providing to the subjects and their families.
2. Think that the cause is worthy enough to donate more resources. So you direct the chief grants officer of the medical center to search for other sources to support the cost of delivering services to families of veterans.
3. Think that Dr. Walker is so naïve about finances that this study will be unsustainable in short order.
4. Object that neither Dr. Walker nor the university's grants office thought to consult you on the viability of using such an inducement for the study.
5. Tell the university that the incentive is so excessive that you would need to amend the grant for more funding to support the incentive.
6. Combinations of the above-listed possible courses of action.
7. Or one that is not listed above.

If you were Dr. Walker conducting this project in Hong Kong, which of these might you say to the university's medical director?

1. That you are not using your position of authority to exert pressure on research subjects, but that in fact you are using your position to do for the veterans what every citizen in the country should do in recognition for all that these veterans have given to the country.
2. That you have secured grant money to offset some of the cost to the university medical facility, and now you ask the medical director to use his or her position of authority to better the lives of those veterans who have given their mental health for the country.
3. That you are not exploiting the veterans, because they can withdraw their participation at any time.

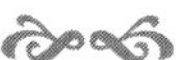

STANDARD 8.07: DECEPTION IN RESEARCH

(a) Psychologists do not conduct a study involving deception unless they have determined that the use of deceptive techniques is justified by the study's significant prospective scientific, educational, or applied value and that effective nondeceptive alternative procedures are not feasible.

A CASE FOR STANDARD 8.07 (A): When Deception Is Never Justified

Dr. Hall is conducting research to determine whether an association exists between suicide and polygamy among transgender couples. After months of advertisement, Dr. Hall is unsuccessful in recruiting subjects for her study. She then revised the recruitment strategy by advertising that she would be studying satisfaction in long-term marital relationships for transgendered individuals.

Jay and Jon responded to the advertisement and agreed to participate. For the marital satisfaction study, they were asked to complete a set of questionnaires, including the Beck Depression Inventory (BDI), the Minnesota Multiphasic Personality Inventory (MMPI), and a sexual history. Following the completion of the questionnaires, they were interviewed by Dr Hall. The interview invited Jay and Jon to discuss their current marital satisfaction and asked whether they had or would consider an open marriage. After the interview, the BDI was readministered. In the post-interview BDI, Jay scored significantly higher on the depression scale with endorsement for suicidal ideation.

On debriefing, Dr. Hall explained that the study actually focused on possible relationships between suicide and polygamy among transgender couples. Jay and Jon were distressed to find out that they had participated in a study that would perpetuate negative stereotypes of transgendered individuals.

Issues of Concern

Deception research tends to create distrust as well as a possibility of distress for participants. Under very special circumstances specified in Standard 8.07, the use of deception in research may be justified. Dr. Hall could argue that her study met the criteria set by Standard 8.07. Dr. Hall must prove the research question is of significant value to justify deception. She could claim that her study would contribute a great deal to suicide prevention in an emerging population. Is her study of scientific value if the research question seems to be based on negative stereotypes of the transgender population?

Under Standard 8.07, Dr. Hall must prove that nondeceptive alternatives are not feasible. She could claim that she had tried nondeceptive advertisements and was unable to recruit any subjects. Inability to recruit subjects is a difficulty faced by many research projects and can be caused by a variety of things. One possible reason Dr. Hall was unsuccessful in recruiting subjects could be that the stereotype was offensive to the population she wished to study, or that there is no scientific value to this research question. Is the inability to recruit subjects a justifiable reason to use deception?

APA Ethics Code

Companion General Principle

Principle B: Fidelity and Responsibility

> Psychologists establish relationships of trust with those with whom they work.

The breach of trust between psychology and society through the use of deception is contrary to Principle B: Fidelity and Responsibility.

Principle C: Integrity

> In situations in which deception may be ethically justifiable to maximize benefits and minimize harm, psychologists have a serious obligation to consider the need for, the possible consequences of, and their responsibility to correct any resulting mistrust or other harmful effects that arise from the use of such techniques.

When psychologists use deception, Principle C suggests that psychologists act to correct any harmful effects. If Dr. Hall were to aspire to enact the value of integrity, she would need to correct the mistrust Jay and Jon now likely have of psychologists.

Principle E: Respect for People's Rights and Dignity

> Psychologists respect the dignity and worth of all people. . . Psychologists are aware of and respect cultural . . . differences, including those based on . . . gender identity . . . culture . . . [and] sexual orientation . . . and consider these factors when working with members of such groups. Psychologists try to eliminate the effect on their work of biases based on those factors, and they do not knowingly participate in or condone activities of others based upon such prejudices.

Does the nature of the research question suggest that Dr. Hall is unaware of her biases? Or does it show respectful inquiry into an understudied population?

Companion Ethical Standard(s)

Standard 2.04: Bases for Scientific and Professional Judgments

> Psychologists' work is based upon established scientific and professional knowledge of the discipline.

Dr. Hall's research question should be embedded in the known literature of the field. Is there anything in the published literature that suggests transgendered couples are not monogamous, or are less monogamous than the general population? Does her work violate Standard 2.04?

Standard 3.01: Unfair Discrimination

> In their work-related activities, psychologists do not engage in unfair discrimination based on . . . [g]ender identity [or] . . . [s]exual orientation.

Does the very nature of Dr. Hall's research question suggest discrimination? Has Dr. Hall violated Standard 3.01?

Standard 5.01: Avoidance of False or Deceptive Statements

> (a) psychologists do not knowingly make public statements that are false . . . [or] deceptive . . . concerning their research.

Her first public recruitment statement was accurate and in compliance with Standard 5.01 (a). Her second public statement was false, and thus in violation of Standard 5.01 (a).

Standard 8.08: Debriefing.

> . . . (c) When psychologists become aware that research procedures have harmed a participant, they take reasonable steps to minimize the harm.

The operationalization of Principle C and directive of Standard 8.08 (c) require that Dr. Hall needs to minimize the harm done by her deception.

Legal Issues 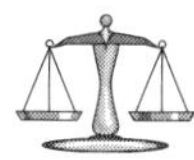

Kansas

Kan. Admin. Regs. § 102-1-1(2010). Definitions.

(b) "Client" or "patient" means a person who meets either of the following criteria:

(1) Is a recipient of direct psychological services within a relationship that is initiated either by mutual consent of the person and a psychologist or according to law.

Kan. Admin. Regs. § 102-1-10a (2010). Unprofessional Conduct.

(e) failing to obtain informed consent, which shall include the following acts:

(1) Failing to obtain and document, in a timely manner, informed consent from the client . . . before the provision of any of these services. . . This informed consent shall include a description of the possible effects of . . . procedures when there are known risks to the client or patient.

(f) ignoring client welfare, which shall include the following acts[:] . . .

(3) engaging in behavior that is abusive or demeaning to a client . . .

(h) misrepresenting the services offered or provided, which shall include the following acts[:] . . .

(4) knowingly engaging in . . . misleading advertising . . .

(n) improperly engaging in research with human subjects, which shall include the following acts:

(1) Failing to consider carefully the possible consequences for human beings participating in the research;

(2) failing to protect each participant from unwarranted . . . mental harm;

(3) failing to ascertain that the consent of the participant is voluntary and informed.

Kentucky

201 Ky. Admin. Regs. 26:145 (2010). Code of Conduct.

Section 1. Definitions.

(6) "Professional service" means all actions of the credential holder in the context of a professional relationship with a client.

(7) "Deception" means, but is not limited to . . .

(b) Preventing another from acquiring information that would affect his or her judgment of a transaction; or

(c) Failing to correct a false impression that the deceiver previously created or reinforced, or that the deceiver knows to be influencing another to whom the person stands in a . . . confidential relationship. . .

(9) "Exploitation" means obtaining or using another person's resources . . . by deception . . . with the intent to deprive the person of those resources.

Section 5. Client Welfare.

(1) Providing explanation of procedures. . . The credential holder shall keep the client fully informed as to the purpose and nature of [a] . . . procedure, and of the client's right to freedom of choice regarding services provided.

Section 6. Welfare of Supervisees and Research Subjects.

(2) Welfare of research subjects. The credential holder shall respect the dignity and protect the welfare of his or her research subjects, and shall comply with all relevant statutes and administrative regulations concerning treatment of research subjects.

Section 8. Representation of Services.

(4) False or misleading information. The credential holder shall not include false or misleading information in a public statement concerning professional services offered.

Both Kansas and Kentucky created laws that apply the standards for clinical relationships to research sub jects. Dr. Hall's reason for the use of deception in advertising her research project violated several of the laws in both jurisdictions by engaging in misrepresentations. At a minimum, in Kansas, Dr. Hall violated the law that calls for carefully considering the harmful consequences of her deception to the research subject or the community of transgendered individuals. In Kentucky, the definitions of deception and exploitation fit the situation of the vignette.

Cultural Considerations

Global Discussion

Singapore Psychological Society:
Code of Professional Ethics

Principle 16. Research Precautions.

1. Only when a problem is of scientific significance and it is not practicable to investigate it in any other way is

> the psychologist justified in exposing research subjects . . . to . . . emotional stress as part of an investigation.
>
> 2. When a reasonable possibility of injurious after-effects exists, research is conducted only when the subjects . . . are fully informed of this possibility and agree to participate nevertheless.
>
> 3. The psychologist seriously considers the possibility of harmful after-effects and avoids them, or removes them as soon as permitted by the design of the experiment.

Singapore's Code charges psychologists to ensure that no research problem that might cause emotional harm or stress is undertaken unless alternative means of investigation are not possible. Deception per se is not mentioned specifically in Singapore's Code, although deception would cause emotional stress. Therefore, under Principle 16.1, Dr. Hall has violated Singapore's Code by exposing her subjects to emotional stress.

Singapore's Code makes no mention of deception in research being allowable. Instead, Singapore mandates that psychologists obtain full consent, particularly if there is reason to believe harmful after-effects will occur. Even if Jon and Jay did give full consent to Dr. Hall's study, they were unaware, until after the study was completed, to what in fact they were consenting. Clearly, Dr. Hall is in violation of 16.2.

Finally, Dr. Hall would need to find some way to "avoid . . . or remove" harmful after-effects of her research (16.3), which will be difficult to do as Jon and Jay are now wary of psychologists in general, and Dr. Hall specifically. Even if studying transgendered couples is deemed scientifically worthwhile, it is likely that her methodology is not supported or justified, and she would need to find other ways to study this topic. In Singapore, Dr. Hall would not be able to recruit, deceive, and collect data from her participants while being in compliance with Singapore's Code.

American Moral Values

1. How has Dr. Hall come to investigate suicide and polygamy as key factors for transgendered couples? Are these variables established in the psychological literature, or is this based on Dr. Hall's thinking alone? Why would she choose these two factors to study? Have there been studies of polygamy and suicide for other kinds of couples? How much of this hypothesis stems from stereotypes?
2. When studying a community with a history of social marginalization, what is the responsibility of the researcher as far as confirming or dispelling stigmas and negative stereotypes? Did Dr. Hall hope to defend the mental health of transgendered couples against popular misconceptions? Does the mere framing of her study in terms of suicide and polygamy implicitly pathologize transgendered relationships?
3. Was Dr. Hall justified in resorting to deception after an initial recruitment failed? Should she have asked herself whether the question of the study was offensive to transgendered couples? Was there a different way to frame her question for recruitment without saying it was "marital satisfaction"? Would the debriefing have been any different with a more general recruiting pitch? Is her question established in the literature, or does it trade on a stereotype?
4. Is the premise of Dr. Hall's method valid in terms of measuring suicidal ideation? Could it have been that Jay was depressed by the stereotypical association of his relationship with polygamy rather than polygamy pure and simple? Has Dr. Hall considered how self-reporting may be affected by the effort to fend off negative portrayals of one's identity?
5. Can Dr. Hall's debriefing process avoid being distressing for transgendered couples? Will couples feel their participation will be used to portray transgendered relationships negatively? Is the research worth the resentment, guilt, and sense of persecution that could come from debriefed subjects? How does a researcher investigate uncomfortable social issues without creating such after-effects?
6. How serious does Dr. Hall believe Jay's suicidal tendencies to be? Is she obliged to advise him to seek treatment? Will she be afraid of how he will portray her study to another therapist? Could she face an ethics inquiry for the distress she is thought to have caused?

Ethical Course of Action

Directive per APA Code

Dr. Hall's reason for the use of deception in advertising her research project does not meet the criteria set in Standard 8.07 (a) that justifies the use of deception. In her use of deception for recruitment, Dr. Hall violated Standards 2.04, 3.01, and 5.01 (a). In her debriefing, she created conditions of distress in her subjects. As directed by Standard 8.08 (c) and acting on the highest ideals of Principle C: Integrity, Dr. Hall would do something to reduce Jay and Jon's distress and correct any misunderstanding.

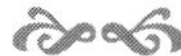

Dictates of One's Own Conscience

If you were Dr. Hall, faced with a research subject's manifestation of suicidal ideation and distress at his or her participation in your study, which of these would you do?

1. Think that your research question is being answered.
2. Give Jay and Jon names of psychologists who provide couples therapy?
3. Refer Jay to the suicide crisis hotline or the hospital emergency room.
4. Ask for clarification as to the nature of Jay and Jon's distress.
5. Realize that your bias and discrimination likely informed your research study and methodology and
   a. apologize to Jay and Jon.
   b. abandon the research.
   c. write an article on the problematic nature of conducting research with this population.
6. Combinations of the above-listed actions.
7. Or one that is not listed above.

If you were Dr. Hall, conducting this research project in Singapore and faced with a research subject's manifestation of suicidal ideation and distress at his participation in your study, which of these would you do?

1. Chances are that you would not be faced with such a situation since the IRB would not approve of the altered design, even if the original design of the study was approved.
2. If you did not seek reapproval for the altered advertisement, but you proceeded without IRB knowledge and approval and found yourself in such a situation, you would immediately stop all study and make amends with Jay and Jon. Amends may include the following:
   a. Apologize to Jay and Jon for the pain you have caused.
   b. Tell Jay and Jon that the project will not proceed any further.
   c. Tell Jay and Jon that you have learned a valuable lesson about your own bias.
   d. Thank Jay and Jon for their generosity in teaching you a lesson.

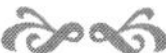

STANDARD 8.07: DECEPTION IN RESEARCH

> . . . (b) Psychologists do not deceive prospective participants about research that is reasonably expected to cause physical pain or severe emotional distress.

A CASE FOR STANDARD 8.07 (B): Taking Unfair Advantage of White Guilt

Dr. Allen is researching the influence of guilt on the amount of giving to multiracial social service agencies. The research design requires the subjects to participate in a multicultural sensitivity training exercise called the "group membership" game. The game is designed to place the subjects in the "White privilege agent" status and is played with the research confederates. After the game is over, the participants are asked to make a financial donation to a charity.

Darlene is recruited through her workplace to participate in this multicultural sensitivity training exercise and agrees to participate in Dr. Allen's project. The study begins with Darlene playing the "group membership" game where the research confederates place Darlene in the most privileged status group. Darlene is then invited to discuss with the group how she feels about the privileges she receives because of her status—namely, that she is a white, college-educated, married professional who was born into a middle-class family. Darlene appears to grow more agitated and defensive as the game progresses. She insists that she is not in the privileged class because she has experienced her own share of discrimination being a female in a professional world. After the multicultural training exercise is finished, Darlene leaves the building by way of a longish hallway. Down this hallway is a desk at which sits a different research confederate who asks Darlene to make a financial donation to the African American Summer Youth Arts Project.

Issues of Concern

Standard 8.07 (a) sets conditions under which the use of deception is justifiable. Section (b) sets the condition under which the use of deception is never justified. Regardless of how valuable the knowledge gained, nothing justifies psychologists inflicting severe emotional distress. Variations of the group membership game are often conducted during multicultural sensitivity trainings. The agitation exhibited and defensiveness expressed by Darlene in this research project may not be anything beyond what she would have experienced in many multicultural training workshops. Does the commonality of the experience allow it to be used in a research project? How much distress is severe? Does Darlene's distress approach the threshold of severe emotional distress?

APA Ethics Code

Companion General Principle

Principle C: Integrity

> In situations in which deception may be ethically justifiable to maximize benefits and minimize harm, psychologists have a serious obligation to consider the need for, the possible consequences of, and their responsibility to correct any resulting mistrust or other harmful effects that arise from the use of such techniques.

Is Dr. Allen justified in using deception? Principle C bases the justification for deception in research on the benefits from the research project. Whether and how much more people will donate to disadvantaged populations if they feel guilty or ashamed of their own privilege status is the research question. Would the findings about this question lead to sufficient benefit to justify any harm? If so, Principle C guides Dr. Allen to feel some obligation to mitigate the negative effects of deception.

Companion Ethical Standard(s)

Standard 3.01: Unfair Discrimination

> In their work-related activities, psychologists do not engage in unfair discrimination based on . . . race, ethnicity, culture [or] . . . socioeconomic status.

The premise of the experiment rests on discrimination and trusts that some will feel bad about their own privileged status. Is the experiment designed to take advantage of Darlene's race (European American), ethnicity (white identified), culture (American), and socioeconomic status (middle class)? If so, is Dr. Allen discriminating against middle-class European Americans?

Standard 8.07: Deception in Research

> (a) Psychologists do not conduct a study involving deception unless they have determined that the use of deceptive techniques is justified by the study's significant prospective scientific, educational, or applied value and that effective nondeceptive alternative procedures are not feasible.

Dr. Allen needs to justify his research design on the grounds that it is not possible to ascertain the influence of guilt on charitable giving without deception and that knowing the direct relationship between guilt and charitable giving is of value to society. Many organizations could and would use such information. However, it may not be true that Dr. Allen would have obtained the same findings by simply asking for a donation after identifying the recipient organization, as many charitable organizations do now. Or could he have deduced the information by examining historical trends in charitable giving?

Standard 8.07: Deception in Research

> . . . (c) Psychologists explain any deception that is an integral feature of the design and conduct of an experiment to participants as early as is feasible, preferably at the conclusion of their participation, but no later than at the conclusion of the data collection, and permit participants to withdraw their data.

Since deception is an integral feature of Dr. Allen's study, he is obligated by Standard 8.07 to explain the true purpose of the experiment to Darlene, preferably after she is beyond the hallway.

Legal Issues 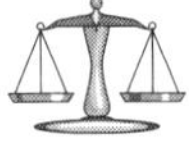

Maryland

> *Md. Code Regs. 10.36.05.02 (2010). Definitions.*
>
> A. In this chapter, the following terms have the meanings indicated.
>
> B. Terms Defined. . .

(2) "Client" means the individual . . . that the psychologist provides . . . with professional services.

Md. Code Regs. 10.36.05.05 (2010). Representation of Services and Fees.

(2) A psychologist may not . . .

(c) Make public statements that contain . . .

(ii) Partial disclosures of relevant facts that misrepresent, mislead, or deceive. . .

B. Informed Consent. When conducting research . . . a psychologist shall . . .

(2) In research, make clear to the client . . .

(c) All aspects of research including any risks and consequences of the research that will reasonably be expected to influence willingness to participate; [and]

(d) The right to withdraw from treatment or research at any time.

Md. Code Regs. 10.36.05.07 (2010). Client Welfare.

A. A psychologist shall:

(1) Take appropriate steps to disclose to all involved parties conflicts of interest that arise, with respect to a psychologist's clients, in a manner that is consistent with applicable confidentiality requirements. . .

B. Exploitation. A psychologist may not:

(1) Exploit or harm . . . research participants.

Michigan

Mich. Admin. Code r. 338.2515 (2010). Prohibited Conduct.

Rule 15. Prohibited conduct includes . . . the following acts or omissions by any individual covered by these rules:

(a) Engaging in harassment or unfair discrimination based on . . . ethnicity, culture, national origin . . . or any basis proscribed by law.

In Maryland and Michigan, Darlene would be considered harmed by her participation in the experiment. Maryland has established a standard that appears to preclude deception in research as the research participants must be alerted to "[a]ll aspects of research including any risks and consequences of the research that will reasonably be expected to influence willingness to participate." Although Michigan does not differentiate between deception in research and any other professional activity engaged in by a psychologist, the design of the study could reasonably be expected to lead participants to feel harassed or unfairly discriminated against.

Cultural Considerations

Global Discussion

New Zealand Psychological Society Code of Ethics

6: Research with humans.

6.2. Psychologists take all possible steps to protect participants from . . . mental discomfort [and] harm. . . If the risk of such consequences exists and the participants give their informed consent to their involvement in the research, all possible steps must be taken to minimise any such risks. Psychologists do not use research procedures if they are likely to cause serious or lasting harm to participants.

New Zealand's code states that if any research procedures, whether they use deception or not, are likely to cause "serious or lasting harm," they cannot be used. Who is the one to determine "serious or lasting harm" in this situation: Dr. Allen, Darlene, the IRB, or some other involved person? If Dr. Allen were white, would he believe that, as he himself would not experience lasting harm from such a procedure, and from being deceived, that his study is methodologically valid, and assume that any participant distress is temporary? If Darlene reports feeling harm and distress from the procedure and the deception used, is that enough to warrant that such methodologies should never be used?

American Moral Values

1. Does Dr. Allen's research cause "severe emotional distress" to subjects? Was the distress Darlene experienced necessary to discover the role of guilt in giving to multiracial agencies? Are there ways to measure guilt without using the group membership game? Is accuracy about guilt more important than avoiding Darlene's level of distress?
2. Is Darlene's experience fairly common for white trainees participating in exercises about race, culture, and class? Is there a difference between putting Darlene through the exercise as a research subject and, for example, a manager on a corporate training retreat?

Is there a level of consent in the work training that Darlene lacks in this research scenario? How would Darlene feel after learning about the deception and the research confederates?

3. How does Dr. Allen view white privilege and Darlene's kind of reaction to a group membership game? Does he feel the game is not severe? Does he in fact believe it is a good, if not fun, experience for all European American people to have, given how white privilege works? Besides his chief goal of evoking guilt in subjects, does Dr. Allen believe that subjects gain valuable insight in exchange for their distress?

4. Will Darlene's mental state after the game shed light on whether guilt leads to giving? Is the group membership game supposed to elicit guilt or replace it with resentment and defensiveness? Does Dr. Allen have a larger social aim in mind with his research? Does he want multiracial agencies to be able to use or avoid guilt in their fund-raising, depending on what effect he finds? Does the deceptive character of the experiment fuel European American suspicions, for example, that crying racism is a way to exploit emotions for material gain?

Ethical Course of Action

Directive per APA Code

The critical question demanded by Standard 8.07 (b) is whether the group membership game inflicted severe emotional distress on Darlene. By the description of Darlene's reaction to the events of the game, it is obvious that she was experiencing emotional distress, and arguably the distress was severe. Even if the study could be justified under Standard 8.07 (a), given the level of Darlene's distress, the experiment probably could not be justified under Standard 8.07 (b).

In addition to inflicting severe emotional distress, it is possible that Dr. Allen's experiment violated Standard 3.01. Under Standard 8.07 (c), Dr. Allen is obligated to fully explain the experiment to Darlene, preferably before she leaves the building.

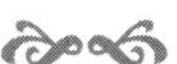

Dictates of One's Own Conscience

If you were Dr. Allen faced with Darlene's severe distress during the experiment, and possibly anger after debriefing, which of these would you do?

1. Try to tell Darlene how her momentary distress may very well benefit many disadvantaged populations.
2. Seeing how distressed Darlene was during the experiment,
   a. stop further work on the project.
   b. admire the elegance of the group membership game.
   c. offer to refer Darlene for further counseling sessions.
3. Combinations of the above-listed actions.
4. Or one that is not listed above.

If you were Dr. Allen working in New Zealand and faced with Darlene's severe distress during the experiment, and possible anger after debriefing, you could protect against causing serious or lasting harm to Darlene by offering free post-experiment counseling sessions should she find herself troubled by her involvement in the study 1 month after the date of experimental participation.

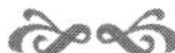

STANDARD 8.07: DECEPTION IN RESEARCH

. . . (c) Psychologists explain any deception that is an integral feature of the design and conduct of an experiment to participants as early as is feasible, preferably at the conclusion of their participation, but no later than at the conclusion of the data collection, and permit participants to withdraw their data.

A CASE FOR STANDARD 8.07 (C): The BBQ—Part II

As previously noted in A Case for Standard 8.03 (1): The BBQ—Part I, the psychology department received several complaints about the social psychology experiment. Dr. Young, chair of the psychology department, asks Professor Garcia whether the students had obtained permission from the institutional review board to conduct this experiment.

Professor Garcia tells Dr. Young that indeed he had sent the proposal of every student to the IRB, and had obtained exemptions from IRB because the research designs were all taking place in public spaces for naturalistic observation. At the urging of Dr. Young and Professor Garcia, Lucille, Clifford, and Jamie posted an e-mail on the all-campus electronic bulletin board explaining the specifics of the social psychology experiment. The students offered the chance for anyone who ate their lunch during the BBQ an option to have their image deleted from the videotape.

Issues of Concern

Previous discussion for Standard 8.03 (1) focused on conditions under which research is exempt from needing subject consent. It was determined that not all commonly used space is public space. The research project designed by Lucille, Clifford, and Jamie violated conditions for exemption to subject consent. The three students now find themselves in a situation where, unintentionally, deception has been used. Standard 8.07 (c) requires that the researcher explain the experiment to the subjects sometime after the subject's participation but before data collection is complete. In addition, subjects are to be given the chance to opt out of the experiment. These conditions were obviously not met. Now Lucille, Clifford, and Jamie have to retroactively explain the experiment to all who participated, which they have done by posting an explanation on a bulletin board. Does a general posting of explanation satisfy the intent of Standard 8.07 (c)? Depending on whether the video has already been shown in the social psychology class, the subjects may or may not have a choice in deleting their images from the video recording.

APA Ethics Code

Companion General Principle

Principle C: Integrity

> In situations in which deception may be ethically justifiable . . . psychologists have a serious obligation to consider the need for, the possible consequences of, and their responsibility to correct any resulting mistrust or other harmful effects that arise from the use of such techniques.

Though the researchers did not realize they were setting up a condition of deception, nonetheless Principle C: Integrity still suggests they would consider their responsibility to correct any negative consequences. Rising to the highest ideals of integrity, Lucille, Clifford, and Jamie should address themselves to those who were videotaped, their fellow classmates, Professor Garcia, and the psychology department. Moreover, if the university were to rise to the highest ideals of integrity, all parties concerned should step up and take responsibility for the inadvertent deception, which includes Professor Garcia and the members of the university's IRB.

Principle E: Respect for People's Rights and Dignity

> Psychologists respect the dignity and worth of all people, and the rights of individuals to privacy.

Do the diners of the small café inside a building with a particular purpose, perhaps unlike those in a large cafeteria or in a shopping mall, have some expectation of privacy? If so, then the nature of the experiment does not respect people's right to privacy by failing to obtain consent for subject participation.

Companion Ethical Standard(s)

Standard 4.07: Use of Confidential Information for Didactic or Other Purposes

> Psychologists do not disclose in . . . public media . . . personally identifiable information concerning their . . . research participants . . . unless . . . (1) they take reasonable steps to disguise the person or organization [and] . . . (2) the person or organization has consented in writing.

Standard 4.07 directs psychologists to respect a research participant's right to privacy in nonpublic space. More likely than not, the reason complaints were made about the BBQ was because, at the heart of it, the research project violated people's right to privacy, Standard 4.07. The necessary condition for showing research participants' images, Standard 3.07 (1), was not met; the necessary condition for breach of research participants' privacy, Standard 4.07 (2), was not met; and since the video recordings were not considered naturalistic observations in public space, the project did not meet the condition for Standard 4.07 (3).

Standard 8.08: Debriefing

> (a) Psychologists provide a prompt opportunity for participants to obtain appropriate information about the nature . . . of the research.

As soon as Professor Garcia, Lucille, Clifford, and Jamie realized that their observations were perhaps not so naturalistic and the café is less then a public place, they were obligated under Standard 8.08 (a) to give participants information about the true nature of the project. Although posting information on a bulletin board may provide information, does this method provide *appropriate* information? What is considered appropriate? Does the method give ample opportunity for participants to ask questions to get the type of information they might consider appropriate, not necessarily the information that Lucille, Clifford, and Jamie considered appropriate?

Legal Issues 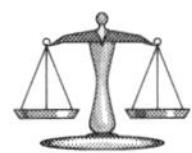

Minnesota

Minn. R. 7200.5400 (2010). Welfare of Students, Supervisees, and Research Subjects.

A psychologist shall protect the welfare of . . . research subjects and shall accord the . . . human research subjects the client rights listed in parts 7200.4700 and 7200.4900.

Minn. R. 7200.4700 (2010). Protecting the privacy of clients.

Subpart 1. In general.

A psychologist shall safeguard the private information obtained in the course of . . . research. With the exceptions listed in subparts 2, 4, 5, 10, and 12, private information is disclosed to others only with the informed written consent of the client.

Minn. R. 7200.4900 (2010). Client welfare.

Subpart 1. Providing explanation of procedures.

A client has the right to have and a psychologist has the responsibility to provide, on request, a nontechnical explanation of the nature and purpose of the psychological procedures to be used. . . The psychologist shall establish procedures to be followed if the explanation is to be provided by another individual under the direction of the psychologist.

Subp. 2. Statement of competence; clients' rights.

A psychologist shall . . . make available as a handout . . . a statement that consumers of psychological services offered by psychologists licensed by the state of Minnesota have the right . . .

F. to privacy as defined by rule and law . . .

I. to be free from exploitation for the benefit or advantage of the psychologist.

Missouri

Mo. Code Regs. Ann. tit. 20, § 2235-5.030 (2010). Ethical Rules of Conduct.

(8) Welfare of Supervisees, Clients, Research Subjects and Students, . . .

(B) Welfare of Clients and Research Subjects. . .

18. Deception and debriefing. The psychologist shall not deceive human participants about the experience of participating in a study. . . Any deceptive aspects of a study shall be explained at the conclusion or earlier.

19. Minimizing invasiveness of data gathering. Interference with the milieu in which data are collected shall be kept to a minimum.

In Minnesota, the BBQ experiment would be in violation of the privacy of those who were eating lunch during the BBQ. The law would suggest no research involving deception is permitted. In Missouri, the BBQ experiment may have satisfied the deception procedures called for by the law before the experiment. However, the IRB, the professor, and the students failed to consider that the conditions of the naturalistic observations would interfere with the milieu. The researchers should have known that the interference would not be kept to a minimum and that invasiveness would arise from the research.

Cultural Considerations

Global Discussion

The Professional Board for Psychology Health Professions Council of South Africa: Ethical Code of Conduct (April 2002)

10.8. Deception in research.

10.8.1. Any other deception that is an integral feature of the design and conduct of an experiment shall be explained to participants as early as is feasible, preferably at the conclusion of their participation, but no later than at the conclusion of the research.

The only obligation under 10.8.1 regarding participants and deception is to explain to the participants the nature of the experiment no later than the conclusion of the research. Seemingly, with the posting of the full experiment's design and purpose to all potential participants prior to any conclusion of the research study,

Professor Garcia and his students are in compliance with this portion of South Africa's Code.

American Moral Values

1. Does the offer of being deleted from the videotape resolve the question of consent raised by this experiment? Could requesting to be deleted bring more attention to one's image than not saying anything at all? Are Lucille, Clifford, and James likely to share the names of those who requested to be deleted, or even those whose images were there to be deleted?
2. How much of the consent issue overlaps with the question of exposure and humiliation? Would department members care about being videotaped if their choice of food was not apparent on the tape? Or is there a principle about invasion of privacy that members want to uphold by requesting to be removed from the tape?
3. Will a request to be removed send unintended secondary messages to students and faculty? Will it be interpreted as a way to undermine the experiment and its political suppositions, or strictly as a matter of consent?
4. Does a community notice safeguard confidentiality, or does it publicize the experiment and its purposes all the more, exacerbating the issue of exposure and food choice vs. principle? Is an announcement offering the chance to be removed from the tape an active enough approach to gaining consent? Does it unfairly put the responsibility for protecting one's confidentiality onto subjects?
5. What does Professor Garcia owe to his three students in terms of handling these kinds of objections? Is he doing his best to make this a teaching opportunity for all his students, perhaps using this as the subject of a lesson? Or would that only compound the problem of publicity noted above? How does Professor Garcia regard his duty to his student researchers and their ambitions in relation to his duties to the rest of the departmental community?

Ethical Course of Action

Directive per APA Code

Standard 8.07 (c) requires that research participants be given an explanation and a chance to withdraw from the experiment once they learn of the deception used in the research. Depending on what exactly is in the e-mail that was posted on the university's electronic bulletin board, the first part of Standard 8.07 (c) may not have been met. Including a general notice in the e-bulletin that individuals may choose to delete their video image may or may not reach all individuals who were captured in the videotape. One cannot be assured that all participants will be reached by the method chosen for notifying research participants. The method does not convey a good faith effort to reach all those who were captured on videotape. To the extent that it falls short of directives in Standard 8.07 (c) and does not approach the aspirations of "serious consideration" espoused in Principle C: Integrity, Lucille, Clifford, and Jamie have not met the requirements of Standard 8.07 (c).

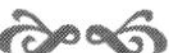

Dictates of One's Own Conscience

If you were Professor Garcia, which of these would you do?

1. Contact the chair of the IRB and ask whether you both went wrong with the original decision to approve Lucille, Clifford, and Jamie's project.
2. Discuss with Dr. Young how to handle the bad press the psychology department might have gotten from the BBQ experiment.
3. Design an in-class exercise to analyze the nature of the complaints regarding the BBQ project?
4. Discuss the design flaws of the BBQ experiment with Lucille, Clifford, and Jamie in private.
5. Ask Lucille, Clifford, and Jamie to present the full project in class and lead a discussion on why complaints were generated.

If you were Lucille, Clifford, or Jamie, would you

1. Ask Professor Garcia why everyone is complaining?
2. Ask to meet with Dr. Young to get a sense of the nature of the complaints?
3. Read Standard 8 of the APA Ethics Code and
   a. identify the participants by watching the video to identify everyone captured in the video by name?
   b. ask Professor Garcia to help you identify everyone who was captured on video?
   c. ask for the identity of those who complained to Dr. Young?
   d. contact the identified participants to schedule individual debriefings and meet with each individually?

4. At a communitywide event conduct a debriefing session and
    a. explain the nature of the project?
    b. apologize for your misjudgment about the nature of the research project?
    c. tell the participants that you have learned a great deal about respect for research participants and will not make the same mistake again?
    d. offer participants the option to have their images deleted from the video?
5. Combinations of the above-listed actions?
6. Or one that is not listed above?

If you were Dr. Young, Professor Garcia, Lucille, Clifford, or Jamie conducting the BBQ study in South Africa, you would know that by alerting potential participants to the deception in the research study before the end of the study, you have satisfied your ethical obligation to the unwitting participants.

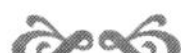

STANDARD 8.08: DEBRIEFING

> (a) Psychologists provide a prompt opportunity for participants to obtain appropriate information about the nature, results, and conclusions of the research, and they take reasonable steps to correct any misconceptions that participants may have of which the psychologists are aware.

A CASE FOR STANDARD 8.08 (A): The BBQ—Part III

As previously described in A Case for Codes 8.03 (1) and 8.07 (c) BBQ vignettes, Lucille, Clifford, and Jamie hosted a BBQ in the building's café, and afterwards posted an e-mail on the e-bulletin board to explain the experiment. Even after the e-bulletin posting, Dr. Young continued to receive complaints. The additional complaints came from the university administration and faculty regarding how the psychology department handled the situation. The complainants thought that the schoolwide e-mail from the students was not a sufficient method for debriefing. To address this complaint, Lucille, Clifford, and Jamie resubmitted their proposal to the IRB and received permission to hold a series of group debriefing sessions. The debriefing sessions were advertised to all members of the school, and they extended an open invitation for anyone affected by the experiment to attend, regardless of whether the individual(s) participated in the actual BBQ. To Lucille, Clifford, and Jamie's surprise and irritation, no one came to the debriefing session.

Issues of Concern

Lucille, Clifford, and Jamie went beyond the requirements for the class project to address further complaints. They wrote another proposal, resubmitted the second proposal to the IRB, advertised the debriefing session, and then actually reserved the time to facilitate the debriefing sessions. They certainly tried to give ample opportunity for participants to obtain appropriate information about the BBQ research project, per Standard 8.08 (a). Had anyone attended the debriefing session, Lucille, Clifford, and Jamie certainly would have corrected any misconceptions that surfaced. Does Standard 8.08 (a) require any other action or activity beyond having offered the debriefing group meeting? It is most likely that Lucille, Clifford, and Jamie might have felt annoyed because no one attended, and might have thought, "You would have come to the meeting if you were so eager to find out about this project. Since no one showed, everyone must have just wanted to complain." Might there be other reasons why no one showed up for the meeting?

APA Ethics Code

Companion General Principle

Principle B: Fidelity and Responsibility

> Psychologists establish relationships of trust with those with whom they work. They are aware of their professional and scientific responsibilities to . . . the specific communities in which they work. . . They are concerned about the ethical compliance of their colleagues' scientific and professional conduct.

Principle B: Fidelity and Responsibility guides psychologists to keep the public's trust by keeping to the professional standards as well as monitoring the behavior of other psychologists. Acting in accordance with the highest ideal of Principle B, Lucille, Clifford, and Jamie would want to repair the broken trust between the psychology department and the other residents of the building in which the café is situated.

Principle C: Integrity

> In situations in which deception may be ethically justifiable to maximize benefits and minimize harm, psychologists have a serious obligation to consider the need for, the possible consequences of, and their responsibility to correct any resulting mistrust or other harmful effects that arise from the use of such techniques.

Even though no one intended to set up a research experiment containing deception, nonetheless one occurred. Principle C: Integrity suggests that psychologists have a responsibility to correct the resulting mistrust.

Companion Ethical Standard(s)

Standard 2.01: Boundaries of Competence

> (a) Psychologists . . . conduct research . . . in areas only within the boundaries of their competence, based on their . . . supervised experience . . . [and] study.

The students in Professor Garcia's class were acquiring the competence to conduct research through engaging in a course of study. The experience was under the direct supervision of Professor Garcia, and then less directly through all the members of the IRB who reviewed this project proposal. To what extent do students hold responsibility for competency when they are engaged in a course of study and their project has been approved by someone else with greater expertise than themselves?

Standard 7.03: Accuracy in Teaching

> (a) Psychologists take reasonable steps to ensure that course syllabi are accurate regarding . . . the nature of course experiences. . . (b) When engaged in teaching or training, psychologists present psychological information accurately.

To a large extent, the university community considers the course-based activities of the student a responsibility of the professor. Could it be argued that the problems generated by the BBQ were a result of Professor Garcia and the faculty members of the IRB not anticipating how Standard 7.03 would arise in the particular research context? If either Professor Garcia or any faculty members of the IRB had been accurate in his or her knowledge of research design in accordance with Standard 7, and had provided accurate information to the students, would they be handling this many complaints?

Standard 3.04: Avoiding Harm

> Psychologists take reasonable steps to avoid harming their . . . students . . . [and] research participants . . . and to minimize harm where it is foreseeable and unavoidable.

The value that underlies Standards 8.01 through 8.09 is the idea of nonmaleficence for the research participants. Standard 3.04 directs Professor Garcia and the three students to minimize harm now that it is unavoidable. The original harm may be with those who were present at the BBQ. Secondary harm seems to have extended to the university community.

Legal Issues 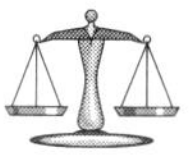

Montana

> *Mont. Admin. R. 24.189.2301 (2009). Representation of Self and Services.*
>
> (1) In representation of self or services, a licensee . . .
>
> (f) shall not use fraud, misrepresentation or deception . . . in conducting any other activity related to the practice of psychology. . .
>
> (3) In regard to representation in the public arena, a licensee or license applicant . . .
>
> (b) shall make reasonable efforts to correct . . . misuse of their work made by others.

> *Mont. Admin. R. 24.189.2305 (2009). Professional Responsibility.*
>
> (2) In regard to respect for others, a licensee:
>
> (a) shall not exploit persons over whom they have . . . evaluative . . . authority such as students . . . [and] research participants.

Nebraska

> *172 Neb. Admin. Code §§ 156-011 (2010). Research With Human Participants.*
>
> A psychologist shall respect the dignity and welfare of human research participants, and shall comply with these regulations governing such psychological research. Unprofessional conduct includes but is not limited to:

011.06 Failure to make reasonable efforts to detect and remove or correct undesirable consequences for the individual participants, including long-term effects.

The licensing boards in both Montana and Nebraska are likely to find that Professor Garcia failed in the post-experiment efforts for debriefing. The deception and misuse of the experimental methodology by the students he supervised required an approach that would remove or correct undesirable consequences that resulted in many other distressed students. To schedule a meeting that no one attended is not a good faith effort at removing or correcting the negative consequences of the effects of the deceptive research.

Cultural Considerations

Global Discussion

Canadian Code of Ethics for Psychologists

Principle II: Responsible caring.

II.23. Debrief research participants in such a way that the participants' knowledge is enhanced and the participants have a sense of contribution to knowledge.

Principle III: Integrity in relationships.

III.26. Debrief research participants as soon as possible after the participants' involvement, if there has been incomplete disclosure or temporary leading of research participants to believe that a research project or some aspect of it has a different purpose.

III.27. Provide research participants, during such debriefing, with a clarification of the nature of the study, seek to remove any misconceptions that might have arisen, and seek to re-establish any trust that might have been lost, assuring the participants that the research procedures were neither arbitrary nor capricious, but necessary for scientifically valid findings.

III.28. Act to re-establish with research participants any trust that might have been lost due to the use of incomplete disclosure or temporarily leading research participants to believe that the research project or some aspect of it had a different purpose.

If this experiment and debriefing session were occurring in a Canadian university, Professor Garcia (and his students) would have a difficult time remaining in compliance with the Canadian Code. The Code speaks of the nature and intent of the debriefing session itself, as well as when it is to occur. Professor Garcia and the students were to have debriefed participants in such a way as to have contributed to knowledge (II.23). In addition, the deceptive research practices they experienced were neither "arbitrary nor capricious," but necessary for valid scientific purposes (III.27). However, the code is silent on how to proceed or do the above when no participants attend the debriefing session. The Canadian code does state, however, that debriefing must occur as soon as possible (III.26) after the experiment has taken place; arguably, a later-than-planned debriefing session is not specifically named in the code, as it is mandated that such post-hoc debriefings do not occur. However, Professor Garcia and his students may be able to achieve some measure of compliance to III.28, which demands that broken trust with research participants be reestablished if it has been breached due to deception or incomplete disclosure; the specifics of how Professor Garcia and the students might go about such repair work is not specified.

American Moral Values

1. Have Lucille, Clifford, and James taken reasonable steps to rectify the problems of consent their initial experiment may have caused? Does their resubmission to their IRB take care of future observations made in the café? Have they addressed the question of singling out subjects by inviting the whole community to discuss the project, and whether they might have been videotaped?
2. Given the lack of participation in the debriefing session, what can the students conclude about the department's attitude toward their experiment? Should they suspect that the community was too sensitive to having their beliefs about food challenged? Was the lack of attendance at the debriefing an act of revenge against their challenging research? How do they see their future in the department, given that this might be a type of freeze-out?
3. Is the lack of attendance at the debriefing session an indication of mistrust? If so, what are the appropriate and reasonable ways to rebuild that trust? Should the three students apologize for the experiment and promise not to engage in this type of deceptive experiment again? Is there a way for them to defend their motives without seeming to begrudge having to concede an error?
4. How should Professor Garcia counsel his students? What responsibility does he bear, as the faculty member overseeing the project, in assuring the community that

he wants to repair trust and increase understanding about this type of experiment? Are the three students being scapegoated? Will faculty expect more projects like this from Professor Garcia's class?

5. What lesson do the three students take from this episode? Will this be more about the content of their experiment and its targeting of psychologists' behavior, or will it be more about consent? Will they pursue their initial idea in a different fashion, or do they need to rethink their motives?

Ethical Course of Action

Directive per APA Code

Standard 8.08 (a) requires Lucille, Clifford, and Jamie to give information promptly and take reasonable steps to correct misconceptions. They can be applauded for going beyond the requirements for the class. Their extra effort is aimed at meeting the requirements of Standard 8.08 (a). Their underlying attitude of appeasing the complainants may have directed the method of debriefing. A public announcement and group meeting do not meet the spirit of Standard 8.08 (a) nor the values in Principles B and C. The public meeting seems cursory and not a reasonable step, as required by Standard 8.08 (a), to minimize harm where it was already unavoidable.

Standard 7.03 directs Professor Garcia to have taken an active role in the supervision of this project. It seems that a teaching moment may have been lost. It does not appear that Professor Garcia engaged in teaching students about their responsibility as researchers toward their research participants and psychologists' reputation in the community, Standard 3.04, 8.01–8.08, and Principles B and C.

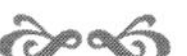

Dictates of One's Own Conscience

If you were at a meeting with Professor Garcia, Lucille, Clifford, and Jamie, finding out about the continued complaints and discussing next steps, what would you advise them?

1. Repair relationships with the Dean?
2. Read, understand, and incorporate all the directives contained in Standards 8.01 through 8.08?
3. Follow the directives of Standard 8.07 as outlined under A Case for Standard 8.07 (c): The BBQ—Part II for identifying and meeting with participants?
4. Focus on repairing the broken trust between the psychology department and the other parts of the university community?
5. Offer a sincere public apology to the residents of the building for the deception in the BBQ experiment?
6. Make a public commitment not to engage in further research involving deception without all of the required safeguards to minimize harm?
7. Use this moment to teach students the harm done by the use of deception?
8. Teach a unit on regret and forgiveness?
9. Combinations of the above-listed actions?
10. Or one that is not listed above?

If you were Professor Garcia and you were teaching in a Canadian University, would you:

1. Require that your students attempt to hold another debriefing session for the whole school community, and add a written statement explaining the scientific contribution the study made to the university and the students?
2. Vow not to conduct "naturalistic" research again without going through a proper informed consent process with participants, including a more timely debriefing process?

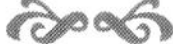

STANDARD 8.08: DEBRIEFING

. . . (b) If scientific or humane values justify delaying or withholding this information, psychologists take reasonable measures to reduce the risk of harm.

A CASE FOR STANDARD 8.08 (B): The Long Tests

The city is under pressure to address its homeless population. Of special interest to the city is the prevalence of mental illness among the homeless and the level of impairment that seems to be prevalent with this particular population. Dr. Hernandez of the Modern School of Psychology in the New Center University received a grant from the city to gather primary data on the city's homeless population. The grant pays for two graduate assistants, Jill and Tommy.

Jill and Tommy go to a homeless shelter to gather data once a week. In exchange for their participation, individuals are given a $50 gift certificate to the local grocery store. Participants are interviewed and administered the Minnesota Multiphasic Personality Inventory (MMPI), Beck Depression Inventory (BDI), Mini-Mental State Examination–2 (MMSE-2), and the Drug Use Screening Inventory–Revised (DUSI-R). At the end of the testing, the participants are told that the tests will be scored within the next week. If they wish to find out the results of their assessments, participants are welcome to call and schedule a feedback session at the school's clinic.

Issues of Concern

The data being collected seem sufficiently comprehensive to answer the city's questions about characteristics of its population in homeless shelters. The results of the study will certainly be of use to the city for the purpose of designing appropriate intervention programs for homeless residents. For the research participants, in addition to the benefit of the $50 gift certificates, could the individual information be of further use to them? Standard 8 does not require individual feedback on assessments. Standard 8.08 (a) directs psychologists to provide information about the nature, results, and conclusions of the research project, not the participant's individual assessment results. Standard 8.08 (b) directs psychologists to reduce risk of harm if information about the nature, results, and conclusions of the research project were to be delayed. Has a significant delay occurred by waiting until the data analyses are complete or the research project is finished? Or is telling the research participants to call for an appointment for results a justifiable delay? Conversely, what responsibility does Dr. Hernandez or the research project have to the individual research participants? Are Dr. Hernandez and the research project obligated to provide assessment results? What responsibility does Dr. Hernandez have to the research participants if the individual assessments resulted in positive findings of neuropsychological damage? What reason would justify either delaying the debriefing or not providing a debriefing to research participants if the assessment findings were positive for psychological or cognitive impairment?

APA Ethics Code

Companion General Principle

Principle A: Beneficence and Nonmaleficence

> Psychologists strive to benefit those with whom they work and take care to do no harm. In their professional actions, psychologists seek to safeguard the welfare and rights of those with whom they interact professionally.

Principle A suggests that psychologists seek to benefit those with whom they work. In the case of the research project, "those with whom they work" are the individuals who are in the homeless shelters. It could be argued that ultimately the results reported to the city would eventually benefit all individuals who find themselves homeless. Does Dr. Hernandez's commitment to benefit those with whom he works extend to those specific individuals who gave of their time to participate in the research? Does part of the commitment to be of benefit include providing individual assessment feedback to the research participants? Or is the monetary remuneration sufficient compensation for a subject's participation?

Principle D: Justice

> Psychologists recognize that fairness and justice entitle all persons to access to and benefit from the contributions of psychology and to equal quality in the processes, procedures, and services being conducted by psychologists.

Principle D imagines Dr. Hernandez providing all of his research participants with equal quality of services. Research participants of a higher socioeconomic status whose lives were sufficiently resourced could easily call the research project office, schedule a feedback session, and get themselves to the appointment on the designated day and time. For such research participants, they would essentially receive a full assessment that is both valuable and expensive. Does Dr. Hernandez's extension of the same offer to individuals who are homeless result in equal quality? The probability of individuals who are struggling to meet basic survival needs being sufficiently resourced to call and then arrive at a designated time and place to receive their assessment results is extremely low.

Does the differential functional result meet the spirit of Principle D: Justice?

Companion Ethical Standard(s)

Standard 3.01: Unfair Discrimination

> In their work-related activities, psychologists do not engage in unfair discrimination based on . . . socioeconomic status.

Standard 3.01 is the operationalization of Principle D: Justice. The same question posed for Principle D applies to Standard 3.01. The same offer for debriefing sessions to individuals of different socioeconomic statuses does not provide the same access. Is Dr. Hernandez's failure to adjust the conditions for debriefing to better match the reality of his research participants a form of discrimination?

Standard 9.10: Explaining Assessment Results

> Psychologists take reasonable steps to ensure that explanations of results are given to the individual or designated representative unless the nature of the relationship precludes provision of an explanation of results . . . and this fact has been clearly explained to the person being assessed in advance.

Dr. Hernandez's activity is a research project. His contact with the individuals in the homeless shelter is not of direct service, providing them with a full battery of assessments. However, the research participants did receive a full battery of assessments. As such, does Standard 9.10 obligate Dr. Hernandez to provide an explanation of assessment results to the individual research participants?

Legal Issues 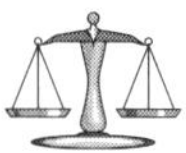

Nevada

> *Nev. Admin. Code § 641.215 (2010). Disclosure to Patient or Legal Representative; Termination of Services; Care of Patients and Research Subjects (NRS 641.100).*
>
> A psychologist . . .
>
> 4. Shall explain clearly to a patient:
>
> (a) The basis and extent of all contemplated services, fees and charges [and] . . .
>
> (c) The prospective benefits to be derived from and the known risks of such services. . .
>
> 13. Shall, in the conduct of psychological research:
>
> (a) Respect the dignity and protect the welfare of his research subjects;
>
> (b) Comply with all relevant laws and regulations concerning the treatment of research subjects;
>
> (c) Fully inform each person who is a prospective subject of research, or his authorized representative, of any danger of serious after-effects before the person is used as a subject; and
>
> (d) Use reasonable efforts to remove any possible harmful after-effects of emotional stress as soon as the design of the research permits.

New Jersey

> *N.J. Admin. Code § 13:42-10.6 (2010). Research*
>
> (a) A licensee shall observe research requirements consistent with accepted standards of practice including, but not limited to, the following[:] . . .
>
> 5. A licensee shall treat research participants ethically and ensure ethical treatment of them by collaborators, assistants, students and employees.

> *N.J. Admin. Code § 13:42-10.13 (2010). Conflicts of Interest; Dual Relationships.*
>
> (d) A licensee shall not enter into any dual relationship. Examples of such dual relationships include, but are not limited to, professional treatment of employees, tenants, students, supervisees, close friends or relatives. Entering into any business relationships or paying or bartering for any services provided by any current client shall also be prohibited.

The research approach does not seem to have violated the laws of either jurisdiction. No overreaching has occurred during the recruitment of the subjects, and debriefing the research subjects is left as an option for the subjects to pursue if they are willing to do so.

Cultural Considerations

Global Discussion

Canadian Code of Ethics for Psychologists

> Principle II: Responsible caring.
>
> II.35. Screen appropriate research participants and select those least likely to be harmed, if more than minimal risk of harm to some research participants is possible.

II.44. Debrief research participants in such a way that any harm caused can be discerned, and act to correct any resultant harm.

The ethics code of Canada does not specify situations or justifications under which a debriefing of research participants may be delayed. Arguably, then, as Canada's code is specific on this point, and demands debriefing "as soon as possible" (III.26), Dr. Hernandez is obligated to provide such debriefings in a timely manner, or risk violation of the letter and intent of these portions of Canada's code. Further, Dr. Hernandez is to debrief his participants well enough that any harm that has been caused can be "discerned," and he must then act to correct any resultant harm (II.44). The difficult issue in this situation is that the likelihood of low numbers of homeless participants being able to attend the debriefing sessions is in and of itself a possible harm. Particularly if Dr. Hernandez was aware in advance of doing the study, or had reasonable cause to suspect that homeless individuals were unlikely to attend debriefing sessions after the fact, he has an obligation and an ethical duty to find a different way to debrief his participants, or he must consider utilizing another subset of this population altogether (II.35). Even if a population of homeless individuals is convenient to use, or there is scientific justification for the research question, and there is potential benefit in developing interventions for homelessness based on such research, Dr. Hernandez is still obligated to select participants who are "least likely to be harmed" (II.35) by his research, rather than select participants with a priori knowledge that they are unlikely to receive assessment results. Any potential benefit to these participants from undergoing extensive assessments can arguably be undermined or outweighed by the risk of very real harm if adverse results of assessments cannot be effectively and expeditiously communicated.

American Moral Values

1. What is the value of the test results for Dr. Hernandez's subjects? Will a week's delay for processing the tests be too long for some of them? What if some subjects are in a critical state in terms of mental health, whether because of medication, suicidal thoughts, hunger, or conflicts on the street? Does Dr. Hernandez have a responsibility to expedite results?

2. How can subjects use these results for their own treatment? Will shelters, agencies, hospitals, or other care providers accept them as authoritative? What will they think of the $50 gift certificate? Will those organizations suspect that it might be used for alcohol and drugs? Should Dr. Hernandez document his research study and its method with written results given back to the subjects? Is it acceptable to have results given orally alone?

3. Has Dr. Hernandez taken sufficient measures to make sure feedback will be given within a week? Is it fair to require subjects to call for an appointment if they do not have access to a phone, or at least an inexpensive phone? Will the shelter facilitate contact between subjects and Dr. Hernandez's team?

4. Could the process of waiting a week or more fuel suspicion of the subjects being exploited or ignored by another health bureaucrat? Does the withholding of information itself create an aura of mistrust around the project?

5. What if homeless individuals are in no position to take specific actions that someone otherwise might on the basis of the results? Does Dr. Hernandez owe them some type of information about local agencies, medical resources, and treatment options?

Ethical Course of Action

Directive per APA Code

Presuming Dr. Hernandez's project was approved by the university's IRB and appropriate informed consent to research was documented for the research participants, all parties concerned would be aware of and in agreement with the arrangements for debriefing.

Standard 8.08 (a) does not direct Dr. Hernandez to provide individual assessment results. Standard 8.08 (b) directs psychologists to reduce risk of harm when information about the research project is to be delayed. Such information would not be available until all data collection was complete, at the earliest. Standard 8.08 is silent on the research project's offer for individual research participants to receive test results. Dr. Hernandez is going beyond the requirements of Standard 8 to make available to individual research participants the results of their assessments, regardless of whether the assessments find psychological or cognitive damage.

It can be a valuable benefit for participants to receive assessment results. Depending on the findings, some of the individuals may have sufficient documentation to be eligible for disability or some other type of support and service. However, the structure of the debriefing sessions does not afford research participants real access to their results. Because access is not equitable, the method of debriefing is discriminatory based on socioeconomic status, and thus in violation of Standard 3.01, unfair discrimination, and the spirit of Principle D: Justice.

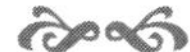

Dictates of One's Own Conscience

If you were a member of the university's IRB, which of these would you say to Dr. Hernandez?

1. Choose different assessment instruments that allow for scoring and feedback on the same visit.
2. Return to the shelter to give feedback to the subjects directly instead of asking them to come back to the clinic. For an incentive, perhaps offer to write up the assessments for each of the subjects for their individual use.
3. Combinations of the above-listed actions.
4. Or one that is not listed above.

If you were a member of the university's IRB located in Canada, which of these would you say to Dr. Hernandez?

1. Choose different assessment instruments that allow for scoring and feedback on the same visit.
2. Find a different means to ensure debriefing will occur with all research participants.

STANDARD 8.08: DEBRIEFING

> . . . (c) When psychologists become aware that research procedures have harmed a participant, they take reasonable steps to minimize the harm.

A CASE FOR STANDARD 8.08 (C): Harm Reduction

Dr. King is a new professor at the Modern School of Psychology in the New Center University. She was hired as a full-time faculty in the Psychodrama Therapy program. Dr. King was also recently appointed to the institutional review board for the university. The IRB is eager to depend upon her expertise in psychodrama therapy, and Dr. King was given a few previously approved projects as part of her orientation to the IRB committee so she could see the types of research projects being sponsored by the university.

One recently approved research project explores the healing experience of reenactment of a traumatic experience. The target population is military veterans with war trauma. The research directive is for the veteran to recall a moment of trauma in his or her military service and depict that moment in a psychodrama human sculpture. The research project claims that no additional harm will come to the participants from this experience because the activity of sculpturing an experience is nondirective about how to express content, and it holds no danger of further traumatizing the participants.

Dr. King is alarmed by the lack of safeguards for retraumatization and the insufficient debriefing protocols built into the design of this research project.

Issues of Concern

Standard 8.08 (a) asks psychologists to conduct debriefing sessions, promptly. When, in the debriefing, a psychologist learns of harm to a research participant directly connected to the research procedure, in accordance with Standard 8.08 (c), the psychologist is to do something to minimize that harm. Dr. King is not the principal investigator for this psychodrama study. She has no direct knowledge based on debriefing that any research participant has been harmed. The study is recently approved, and it is highly probable that the project is either about to get started or is in the data collection phase. Does she need to wait until debriefing for knowledge about harm to surface? Does Dr. King have a responsibility to stop the project based on her belief that the project, as designed, will probably harm some of the research participants? Does the level of her responsibility change based on whether the psychodrama study is a student or a faculty research project? If it is a student project, does Dr. King have a responsibility to review the institutional procedures that allow for student projects to be run without faculty oversight? Or perhaps Dr. King needs to be concerned about the nature and quality of the faculty oversight itself?

APA Ethics Code

Companion General Principle

Principle B: Fidelity and Responsibility

> Psychologists . . . are concerned about the ethical compliance of their colleagues' scientific and professional conduct.

One of the primary functions of the IRB review is to provide a psychologist with feedback from peers. The review and approval by the IRB is a structural procedure that enacts Principle B: Fidelity and Responsibility, where psychologists take on the responsibility of assuring the ethical compliance of other psychologists. Living up to the highest ideal of Principle B, Dr. King is concerned about her colleague's scientific conduct.

Companion Ethical Standard(s)

Standard 2.04: Bases for Scientific and Professional Judgments

> Psychologists' work is based upon established scientific and professional knowledge of the discipline.

Standard 2.04 demands that Dr. King's work on the IRB be based upon established scientific and professional knowledge. This means that Dr. King is required to substantiate her concerns regarding the research design by calling forth established scientific and professional information. Otherwise, what guarantees does the principal investigator of the psychodrama study have that Dr. King is not discriminating against him or her based on any variety of reasons such as race, gender, religion, and so forth?

Standard 3.04: Avoiding Harm

> Psychologists take reasonable steps to avoid harming their . . . research participants . . . and to minimize harm where it is foreseeable and unavoidable.

Standard 3.04 provides the ethical foundation that legitimizes Dr. King's concerns. Based on established scientific and professional knowledge, Dr. King thinks harm is foreseeable and will be inevitable to some participants if the project proceeds as proposed and approved. In such circumstances, Standard 3.04 directs her to take steps to intercede.

Standard 1.04: Informal Resolution of Ethical Violations

> When psychologists believe that there may have been an ethical violation by another psychologist, they attempt to resolve the issue by bringing it to the attention of that individual.

Enacting the principle of responsibility, Standard 1.04 requires that Dr. King attempt to resolve her concerns about the psychodrama study by bringing it up directly with the principal investigator.

Standard 1.05: Reporting Ethical Violations

> If an apparent ethical violation . . . is likely to substantially harm a person . . . and is not appropriate for informal resolution . . . psychologists take further action appropriate to the situation. Such action might include referral to . . . the appropriate institutional authorities.

The IRB is the institutional authority charged with oversight of a researcher's ethical behavior. Does being a member of the IRB make this situation inappropriate for informal resolution per Standard 1.04? Does Dr. King hold a greater burden to enact that part of Principle B cited above?

Standard 7.03: Accuracy in Teaching

> . . . (b) When engaged in teaching or training, psychologists present psychological information accurately.

If the psychodrama research project is conducted by a student, it is most probably being done under the supervision of a faculty member. That faculty member is remiss, and in violation of Standard 7.03 (b), if indeed the probable harm to participants could be predicted based on established scientific and professional knowledge about veterans with war trauma.

Legal Issues 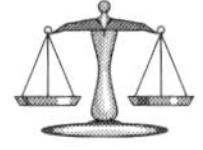

New Mexico

> *N.M. Code R. § 16.22.2.10 (2010). Patient Welfare.*
>
> **J. Avoiding harm.** Psychologists take reasonable steps to avoid harming their . . . research participants . . . and minimize harm where it is foreseeable and unavoidable.

> *N.M. Code R. § 16.22.2.11 (2010). Welfare of Supervisee and Research Subjects.*
>
> **B. Welfare of research subjects.** The psychologist shall respect the dignity and protect the welfare of his research subjects, and shall comply with all relevant statutes and the board's regulations concerning treatment of research subjects.

New York

> *N.Y. Comp. Codes R. & Regs. tit. 8, § 29.1 (2010). General Provisions.*
>
> b. Unprofessional conduct in the practice of any profession licensed . . . shall include:
>
> 1. willful or grossly negligent failure to comply with substantial provisions of . . . regulations governing the practice of the profession.

> *N.Y. Comp. Codes R. & Regs. tit. 8, § 29.12 (2010). Special Provisions for the Profession of Psychology.*
>
> a. Unprofessional conduct in the practice of psychology shall . . . include the following:
>
> 1. in the conduct of psychological research . . . failing to inform prospective research subjects . . . fully of the danger of serious after-effects, if such danger exists, before they are utilized as research subjects.

In both jurisdictions, Dr. King must take reasonable steps to avoid harming the research participants as soon as it becomes apparent that harm is foreseeable. Whether the researcher is a faculty member or student, as an IRB member, Dr. King must act on her knowledge about the foreseeable harmful effects and intervene with the researcher to stop the project. Otherwise, along with the researcher, she likely would be viewed as culpable as well.

Cultural Considerations

Global Discussion

Canadian Code of Ethics for Psychologists

> Principle II: Responsible caring.
>
> II.36. Act to minimize the impact of their research activities on research participants' personalities, or on their . . . mental integrity.
>
> II.42. Be open to the concerns of others about perceptions of harm that they as a psychologist might be causing, stop activities that are causing harm, and not punish or seek punishment for those who raise such concerns in good faith.
>
> II.44. Debrief research participants in such a way that any harm caused can be discerned, and act to correct any resultant harm.

It is likely that this study as designed and approved will harm the "mental integrity" of these veterans (II.36), and Dr. King is obligated to minimize that negative harm. Further, II.42 asks Dr. King, in part, to stop activities that are causing harm, regardless of whether or not she originated them. If Dr. King, as a member of the IRB, allows a research study that she fully believes will likely harm the participants to go forward, she is actively involved in causing harm and needs to take immediate action to stop that harm. If any research subjects have already undergone any portion of the study, Dr. King needs to both "discern . . . and correct" any harm caused by this research (II.44) study, whether it is by offering a different kind of treatment for the war trauma; making sure that informed consent for experimental treatments has been approved, understood, and given freely without coercion; or in some other way seeking to ascertain and resolve the very likely harm that she suspects will be caused by this study.

American Moral Values

1. Does the psychodrama therapy unnecessarily re-traumatize its subjects? Does Dr. King believe it is better to be cautious than to trust the idea that psychodrama is cathartic? Does she have any other knowledge of psychodrama therapy? Could the practice have more to it than the defense she has been given?
2. What bureaucratic steps can Dr. King take within the confines of her position as faculty and IRB member? Does she want to avoid protesting too vehemently on one of her first cases, or does she believe she is doing precisely the job she was hired to do?
3. What kind of reputation does "psychodrama therapy" have on the board and at the school? Does Dr. King have to consider how this case will affect future proposals in psychodrama therapy? Does she feel she need to uphold methodological rigor in order to solidify her place on the board?
4. Is it too late to put a stop to the study? Would stopping the psychodrama exercises before they were completed be even more damaging than letting the subjects finish what they started? How closely should Dr. King work with the project's directors going forward? Do they deserve a chance to respond to her concerns, or is the mental health of the subjects too important to negotiate a solution?
5. What kind of safeguards and debriefing protocol would satisfy Dr. King? Are there ways for this type of exercise to avoid re-traumatization, or does Dr. King believe there is too much of a risk to do the project at all?

6. How much does the religious and cultural background of psychodramas feature into Dr. King's reflections? Does she associate the psychodrama with New Age methods?

Ethical Course of Action

Directive per APA Code

Standard 8.08 (c) obligates psychologists to take steps to minimize harm when psychologists become aware of that harm. The presumption is that, for research projects, such awareness occurs at the moment of debriefing. Dr. King's discovery that the institution has approved a problematic research procedure that she thinks will lead to harm does not occur at the moment of debriefing. Therefore, Standard 8.08 (c) does not apply to her situation at this moment.

Some published literature on veterans and war trauma suggests that recall of the traumatic event may re-trigger the trauma itself. The research design of explicitly directing veterans to recall a traumatic event could then be reasonably expected to re-trigger trauma (Doctor & Shiromoto, 2010; Neuner, Schauer, Karunakara, Klaschik, & Elbert, 2004; Phelps, Forbes, & Creamer, 2008). This satisfies the conditions specified in Standard 2.04: Basis for Scientific and Professional Judgments, and gives Dr. King a basis for her concern.

If the psychodrama study is conducted under the supervision of a faculty member, then Dr. King needs to be concerned with violation of Standard 7.03. Both Standard 3.04: Avoiding Harm, and Principle B call for some type of intervention from Dr. King, based on her well-founded belief that the psychodrama study will harm the research participants. The action required of Dr. King is to first make known her concerns to the principal investigator directly, as specified in Standard 1.04: Informal Resolution of Ethical Violations. As Dr. King is a member of the IRB, this matter falls under Standard 1.05: Reporting Ethical Violations.

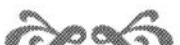

Dictates of One's Own Conscience

If you were Dr. King, being a new junior faculty member reviewing the previous work on the IRB and the research of a more senior faculty member, given your concern that research participants will most likely be harmed if this project proceeds as approved, which of these would you do?

1. Reason that you are inexperienced and should not arrogantly act on your own beliefs, so do nothing.
2. Contact the chair of the IRB to discuss your responsibility in general as a member of the board.
3. Contact the chair of the IRB to discuss your specific concerns about the psychodrama study.
4. Contact the principal investigator to find out more about the status of the project.
5. If the study is already in the data collection phase, ask the principal investigator to send you the debriefing notes.
6. Combinations of the above-listed possible courses of action.
7. Or one that is not listed above.

If you were Dr. King working in Canada, working under the same conditions as described above, which would you do?

1. Contact the chair of the IRB to discuss your concerns about participant harm.
2. Recommend that the IRB approval for the study be rescinded until such a time that the principal investigator is able to provide more justification for the scientific merit of the project and improve upon safeguards for re-traumatization.

STANDARD 8.09: HUMANE CARE AND USE OF ANIMALS IN RESEARCH

(a) Psychologists acquire, care for, use, and dispose of animals in compliance with current federal, state, and local laws and regulations, and with professional standards.

A CASE FOR STANDARD 8.09 (A): The Missing Committee

Erin is a doctoral student submitting her proposal for her dissertation project. She wants to examine whether interactions with dogs reduce the blood pressure of nursing home residents. The project involves weekly visits to five different nursing homes with a team of dog handlers and the use of blood pressure cuffs to measure the resident's blood pressure before and after having contact with the dogs. She has obtained an agreement with Dogs for Care, a service dog–training organization, to provide four dogs and their handlers for weekly visits to four different nursing homes for 10 consecutive weeks. Erin plans to use her own dog to visit the fifth nursing home. The weekly visit includes the handlers measuring a resident's blood pressure at the start of the visit, spending some time with the resident, allowing for individual interactions between the resident and the dog, and then a readministering of the blood pressure measurement. This procedure is then repeated with each resident. Each of the volunteer handlers has agreed to be trained on the proper administration of the blood pressure cuff; five local nursing homes have agreed to have service-dogs-in-training visit their facility.

Erin submits the project to the university's institutional review board. The IRB responds with a reply that indicates it is beyond their purview to review experiments involving animals. The IRB tells Erin that her dissertation should be submitted to an Institutional Animal Care and Use Committee (IACUC). The chair of her dissertation committee tells Erin that the New Center University does not have an IACUC.

Issues of Concern

A university without an IACUC has no capacity to assure that experiments conducted by their students, faculty, and/or staff are in compliance with laws and regulations. Does this mean Erin is unable to conduct her dissertation project as proposed?

Could Erin argue that as her proposed experiment does not acquire, nor care for, the service dogs, her experiment falls outside the authority of Standard 8.09 (a)? In addition, the use of the dogs for the experiment is within the existing use of service dogs, so it does not trigger the need for outside supervision to ensure proper care of the dogs. For these reasons, could Erin argue that Standard 8.09 (a) does not apply, and could the New Center University dispense with IACUC review and allow for an IRB to review the dissertation project?

Could the dissertation committee, however, argue that Erin's proposed experiment requires approval from both the IRB and an IACUC for the use of the dogs?

APA Ethics Code

Companion General Principle

Principle A: Beneficence and Nonmaleficence

> In their professional actions, psychologists seek to safeguard the welfare and rights of . . . animal subjects of research.

Acknowledging that psychologists do engage in research with animal subjects, the guiding principle is to safeguard the welfare of the animals. The value that guides the university, the dissertation committee, and Erin's decision regarding whether to proceed with the experiment as proposed is one of nonmaleficence. The goal is to safeguard the welfare of the dogs.

Companion Ethical Standard(s)

Standard 8.01: Institutional Approval

> When institutional approval is required, psychologists . . . obtain approval prior to conducting the research. They conduct the research in accordance with the approved research protocol.

A relevant question is whether approval is required for the use of the dogs. In addition, missing from the IRB's response is the need for review of the human subjects, which are the nursing home residents who will be interacting with the dogs.

Standard 8.05: Dispensing With Informed Consent for Research

> Psychologists may dispense with informed consent only . . . (1) where research would not reasonably be assumed to create distress or harm and involves . . . (a) the study of normal educational practices, curricula, or classroom management methods conducted in educational settings . . .
>
> (b) only anonymous questionnaires, naturalistic observations, or archival research for which disclosure of responses would not place participants at risk of criminal or civil liability or damage their financial standing, employability, or reputation, and confidentiality is protected; or . . .
>
> (c) the study of factors related to job or organization effectiveness conducted in organizational settings for which there is no risk to participants' employability, and confidentiality is protected or . . . (2) where otherwise permitted by law or federal or institutional regulations.

None of the exceptions to informed consent listed in Standard 8.05 applies to Erin's proposed experiment. In order for Erin to proceed with her proposed dissertation, the institution will have to give her approval. The question is which entity within the university is able to conduct the review and is authorized to grant permission for the study.

Standard 3.10: Informed Consent

(a) When psychologists conduct research . . . they obtain the informed consent of the . . . individuals.

Standard 3.10 indicates that Erin needs to obtain the consent of the nursing home residents. This falls under the sphere of the IRB that has oversight responsibility for human subjects in experiments.

Legal Issues 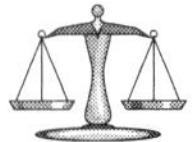

Ohio

Ohio Admin. Code 4732:17-02 (2010). Ethics governing research . . . in which client welfare is directly affected.

(A) Ethical acceptability. In planning a study, the investigator has the personal responsibility to make a careful evaluation of its ethical acceptability, taking into account these principles for research with human beings. . .

(B) Treatment of participants. Responsibility for the establishment and maintenance of acceptable ethical practice in research always remains with the individual investigator. The investigator is also responsible for the ethical treatment of research participants by collaborators . . . all of whom . . . incur parallel obligations.

(C) Full disclosure. Ethical practice requires the investigator to inform the participant of all features of the research that reasonably might be expected to influence willingness to participate. . .

(E) Freedom to decline. Ethical research practice requires the investigator to respect the individual's freedom to decline to participate in research or to discontinue participation at any time. . .

(F) Agreement. Ethically acceptable research begins with the establishment of a clear and fair agreement between the investigator and the research participant that clarifies the responsibilities of each. . .

(G) Risk. The ethical investigator protects participants from physical and mental discomfort, harm, and danger.

Pennsylvania

49 Pa. Code § 41.61 (2010). Code of Ethics

Principle 9. Research with human participants.

(a) The decision to undertake research rests upon a considered judgment by the individual psychologist about how best to contribute to psychological science and to human welfare. Having made the decision to conduct research, the psychologist considers alternative directions in which research energies and resources might be invested. On the basis of this consideration, psychologists carry out their investigations with respect for the people who participate, with concern for their dignity and welfare, and in compliance with Federal and State regulations and professional standards governing the conduct of research with human participants.

Principle 10. Care and use of animals in research.

(b) The acquisition, care, use and disposal of animals are in compliance with current Federal, State or provincial, and local laws and regulations. . .

(d) Psychologists ensure that individuals using animals under their supervision have received explicit instruction in experimental methods and in the care, maintenance, and handling of the species being used. Responsibilities and activities of individuals participating in a research project are consistent with their respective competencies.

Although Ohio is silent about institutional approval, it is quite likely that the licensing board would expect Erin and her doctoral supervisor to follow through with institutional reviews required by the CFR (Code of Federal Regulations), Title 9 (Animals and Animal Products), Chapter 1, Subchapter A—Animal Welfare. Pennsylvania explicitly requires compliance with federal regulations. Both the federal laws (for instance, 9 CFR Ch. I, § 2.131, Handling of Animals) and state laws require that Erin be responsible for how all of the dog handlers are caring for their service dogs while part of this experiment.

Cultural Considerations

Global Discussion

Hong Kong Psychological Society:
Professional Code of Practice

Chapter 6: Research in Psychology

6.1. In planning a psychological experiment, Members shall undertake a careful evaluation of the ethical issues involved. . . [T]he responsibility for ensuring ethical practice in research remains with the principal investigators and cannot be shared. They are also responsible for the ethical treatment of research participants by collaborators . . . all of whom incur similar obligations.

6.8. Research designs using animal subjects should be developed with as much consideration as possible for the welfare of the animals and in accordance with existing ordinances.

It is unclear as to the exact meaning of "in accordance with existing ordinances." This may mean that research proposals are to be vetted by an outside authority, such as an IRB/IACUC or its equivalent. Regardless of existing ordinances, in accord with 6.1, ethical responsibility for all aspects of the research is situated with the principal investigator.

American Moral Values

1. How should Erin classify her experiment's employment of the service dogs? Are the dogs just performing their regular work, with Erin's work being akin to naturalistic observation? Does the blood pressure measurement by the handlers change the nature of their work with the dogs?
2. What do the handlers think of their role in the experiment? Do they consider this experiment to be an alteration of their usual work? Does it threaten the training and expertise they and their dogs usually reflect at a nursing home? Will the interactions between dogs and residents be conducted the way the handlers would have wanted had they not been asked as part of the experiment? If not, would the handlers worry that nursing home residents might get an inaccurate picture of dog visits from this experiment?
3. Can Erin find fault with the university for not having an IACUC already? Is there any moral leverage in suggesting that the university has been irresponsible in its planning and consideration for experiments with animals? Would the IRB be more likely to approve Erin's proposal because of a feeling that the university is at fault for not having an IACUC?
4. What are Erin's alternatives if the IRB does not approve her experiment? Should she fight for an immediate establishment of an IACUC, or does her career development demand a move to another program? Can she convince her IRB to use an IACUC at a competing university? What has the department's policy been regarding experiments with animals? Was she given any indication by her advisor or other faculty that these experiments would be harder to conduct? Does she owe it to the department to wait for an IACUC or another solution?
5. How do the department's faculty members regard Erin's case? Is there some institutional support that the department should give to Erin? What will this mean for future students and applicants, especially those who might hear about Erin's specific case?
6. What will be the effect of this work on the service dog agency? Would the agency want to develop a different relationship with the nursing homes the handlers visited? Does Erin need to make sure they have a way to explain their own purpose and vision to the nursing home, apart from the purposes of Erin's experiment?

Ethical Course of Action

Directive per APA Code

Standard 8.09 (a) directs Erin to comply with regulations and standards of animal care. Standard 8.01 requires Erin to obtain institutional approval for any research. Standard 3.10 (a) requires Erin to obtain subjects' consent to participate in the research, unless her experiment meets the conditions listed in Standard 8.05. Erin's experiment does not meet any of the listed conditions of Standard 8.05.

Therefore, to be in compliance, Erin needs to obtain approval from both the IRB and an IACUC. To sponsor Erin's dissertation, the New Center University has to have both an IRB and an IACUC to review Erin's dissertation. If these conditions are not met, for whatever reason, Erin is not to proceed with her dissertation project as proposed.

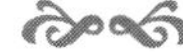

Dictates of One's Own Conscience

If you were Erin, having spent months putting together the project, which of these would you do?

1. Ask the New Center University to establish an IACUC in order to review your proposal.
2. Ask the New Center University to establish a "borrowing" privilege with another university for the use of its IACUC.
3. Ask the IRB to give approval for the portion of the study that involves the nursing home residents.
4. Alter the project to include the use of your own dog only.
5. Ask the chair of your dissertation committee to intervene.
6. Give up on this project and propose something else completely.
7. Combinations of the above-listed actions.
8. Or one that is not listed above.

If you were Erin, studying in a psychology program in Hong Kong, having spent months putting together the project, would you proceed with the dissertation as proposed, but notify your major professor and the chair of your dissertation committee?

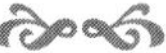

STANDARD 8.09: HUMANE CARE AND USE OF ANIMALS IN RESEARCH

> . . . (b) Psychologists trained in research methods and experienced in the care of laboratory animals supervise all procedures involving animals and are responsible for ensuring appropriate consideration of their comfort, health, and humane treatment.

A CASE FOR STANDARD 8.09 (B): The Helpful Assistant

Dr. Wright is conducting a study examining the effect of environmental noise on cognitive functioning. This study involves observing rats running through a maze for a food reward after differential exposure to duration and intensity of noise. During one of the weekly lab meetings, Dr. Wright remarks that the rats have been running the maze faster than in previous weeks. He invites speculation as to why this might be, to which Lauren, a new graduate lab assistant, says, "It's because on test day and the day before I figured out that not feeding them or filling their water bottles makes them more eager. They'll do anything to get the treats you're handing out."

Issues of Concern

Dr. Wright is responsible for proper care of the animals used in the experiments regardless of who is actually handling the rats. Presumably, the feeding schedule for the rats was designed to ensure that the rats remain in good health. Thus, regardless of who is doing the actual handling of the rats, be it Dr. Wright or Lauren, it is Dr. Wright's responsibility to see to it that the rats are fed the proper amounts at preestablished times. What parameters does he need to establish for lab assistants to properly execute his responsibility? What is his supervisory responsibility for Lauren? Does Dr. Wright have a direct line of supervision to Lauren? What does Dr. Wright need to do, now that he is aware of the change in feeding schedule?

APA Ethics Code

Companion General Principle

Principle A: Beneficence and Nonmaleficence.

> In their professional actions, psychologists seek to safeguard the welfare and rights of . . . animal subjects of research.

The principle that should guide Dr. Wright is one of nonmaleficence. The goal is to safeguard the welfare of the rats under the lab's care.

Companion Ethical Standard(s)

Standard 2.05: Delegation of Work to Others

> Psychologists who delegate work to . . . research . . . assistants . . . take reasonable steps to . . . (2) authorize only those responsibilities that such persons can be expected to perform competently on the basis of their education, training, or experience, either independently or with the level of supervision being provided; and . . . (3) see that such persons perform these services competently.

Presumably, Dr. Wright, or someone in his lab, gave an orientation to Lauren regarding the proper handling and feeding of the rats used in the experiment. However, it appears that Dr. Wright was remiss in following the directives of Standard 2.05 (3).

Legal Issues 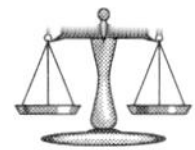

South Carolina

> *S.C. Code Ann. Regs.100-4 (2010). Code of Ethics.*
>
> F. Welfare of supervisees and research subjects. . .
>
> (2) Welfare of research subjects. The psychologist shall . . . protect the welfare of his/her research subjects and shall comply with all relevant statutes and administrative rules concerning treatment of research subjects. . .
>
> L. Aiding illegal practice. . .
>
> (2) Delegating professional authority. A psychologist shall not delegate responsibilities to a person not

appropriately credentialed or otherwise appropriately qualified to provide such services.

(3) Providing supervision. A psychologist shall exercise appropriate supervision over supervisees, as set forth in the rules and regulations of the Board.

Texas

22 Tex. Admin. Code § 465.19 (2010). Teaching.

(b) Relationships with students and trainees. . .

(3) Licensees establish an appropriate process for providing feedback to students and trainees.

(4) Licensees do not permit students or trainees to provide services that they are not competent to perform.

22 Tex. Admin. Code § 465.20 (2010). Research.

(a) Conducting research. . .

(2) Licensees shall conduct all research involving animals in a humane manner which minimizes the discomfort . . . of animal subjects. A procedure subjecting animals to . . . privation is used only when an alternative procedure is unavailable and the goal is justified by its prospective scientific, education or applied value.

South Carolina law does not appear to distinguish between human and nonhuman research subjects. In both jurisdictions, Dr. Wright would need to protect the welfare of the rats, which would include feeding them properly. In Texas, Dr. Wright would likely be found to have failed in his supervision of Lauren.

Cultural Considerations

Global Discussion

The Professional Board for Psychology Health Professions Council of South Africa: Ethical Code of Professional Conduct. (April 2002)

10.8. Care and use of animals in research.

Psychologists who conduct research involving animals shall treat them humanely and according to international standards.

South Africa is nonspecific in the operationalization of "humane" treatment and "international standards." Other codes of ethics are similarly nonspecific with regard to how animal subjects shall be treated. Presumably, withholding food and water from animal subjects can be considered "inhumane" by most standards, and likely would not meet the letter or intent of the South African Code.

American Moral Values

1. Does Dr. Wright hold Lauren responsible for withholding food and water from the rats? Did he give sufficiently clear directions when he trained her? Did she think that getting the rats to perform was the goal of the study? Is this an understandable mistake, or does Dr. Wright conclude the Lauren can no longer be trusted with the rats?
2. How can Dr. Wright train Lauren or a future lab assistant not to change things like food and water consumption? Should he spell out what must be kept the same in caring for the rats?
3. Does Dr. Wright hold himself responsible for delegating this work to begin with? Is it too much for one researcher to carry out? Does he have too many responsibilities to execute the experiment himself?
4. What will Dr. Wright do with the rats he has been testing? Have they been compromised as test subjects? Will he have to get rid of them?
5. Are there colleagues in the lab that will hold Dr. Wright responsible? To whom should he report what has happened in the experiment? Does he need to warn colleagues about Lauren as a potential hire? Does he just need to share his mistake in training an assistant?

Ethical Course of Action

Directive per APA Code

As in all experiments, Dr. Wright surely has set various parameters for his experiment. The feeding schedule for the rats is probably one of the set parameters. Standard 8.09 (b) directs Dr. Wright to supervise Lauren on handling of the rats with due consideration for the needs of the experiment as well as the comfort, health, and humane treatment of the rats.

Dr. Wright's lack of training and monitoring to assure that Lauren was competent to handle the care of the rats before he delegated the work to Lauren is a violation of Standard 2.05 (2). Dr. Wright's lack of proper supervision of Lauren to have prevented the alteration of the feeding schedule is a violation of Standard 8.09 (b). Now that he knows Lauren has not been feeding the rats properly, Standard 2.05 (3) directs Dr. Wright to assure that the rats are fed properly, and that Lauren is trained and monitored better.

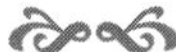

Dictates of One's Own Conscience

If you were Dr. Wright, faced with such a revelation from Lauren, which of these would you do?

1. Ask Lauren why she thought to take it upon herself to alter the feeding schedule, regardless of the rats' performance.
2. Have Lauren document the exact feeding schedule she has been performing.
3. Reprimand Lauren for deviating from protocol.
4. Consult with the staff veterinarian as to the needs of the rats, now that the altered feeding schedule is known.
5. Delete the data from those experiments with the altered feeding schedule.
6. Delete all data for the current set of rats.
7. Restart the whole experiment using all new animals.
8. Combinations of the above-listed actions.
9. Or one that is not listed above.

If you were Dr. Wright, working in South Africa, and were faced with such a revelation from Lauren, would you

1. Consult with the staff veterinarian as to the needs of the rats, now that the altered feeding schedule is known?
2. Delete the data from those experiments with the altered feeding schedule?
3. Delete all data for the current set of rats?
4. Restart the whole experiment using all new animals?

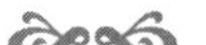

STANDARD 8.09: HUMANE CARE AND USE OF ANIMALS IN RESEARCH

> . . . (c) Psychologists ensure that all individuals under their supervision who are using animals have received instruction in research methods and in the care, maintenance, and handling of the species being used, to the extent appropriate to their role.

A CASE FOR STANDARD 8.09 (C): The Pet Dog

Holly is an undergraduate research assistant new to Dr. Lopez's study team. Dr. Lopez's lab consists of a graduate student, a postdoctoral fellow, Dr. Lopez, and now Holly. Dr. Lopez is using dogs to conduct studies on the alleviation of learned helplessness. Dr. Hill, the postdoctoral fellow, is charged with doing the orientation for undergraduate assistants.

Holly loves dogs and wants to get her own dog but can't because she lives in a residence hall. She was eager to get into a study that gives her an opportunity to interact with dogs. During the course of the semester, Holly gets attached to one of the dogs used in the experiment. Gradually, she starts delaying the return of the dog after the experiment. By the end of the semester, Holly is in the habit of retrieving this dog when she comes into the lab and returning him when she leaves the lab.

Holly goes home during winter break. When she returns, Dr. Lopez pulls her aside and says, "What did you do to the dogs, that little one especially? He cried all night and day the whole time you were gone; he wouldn't eat or sleep. He also wouldn't cooperate with the study, so I had to replace him with another dog. What exactly were you doing with that dog?"

Issues of Concern

Standard 8.09 (c) directs psychologists to make sure their supervisees are properly trained in research methods and in animal care. Though Dr. Lopez is the psychologist heading the lab, there are two psychologists working in the lab. Dr. Hill, the postdoctoral fellow, is as bound to comply with Standard 8.09 (c) as is Dr. Lopez. Per Standard 8.09 (c), Dr. Lopez is to make sure that Dr. Hill has been instructed both in the research methods and in proper animal care. Dr. Hill, in turn, is to make sure that Holly gets proper instruction on research methods and animal care.

Did Holly know she was altering the research protocol? Was Holly aware of the possible impact her loving attention was having on this one dog? How was it that she established such a bond with one research animal?

APA Ethics Code

Companion General Principle

Principle A: Beneficence and Nonmaleficence

> In their professional actions, psychologists seek to safeguard the welfare . . . of animal subjects of research.

Presumably, Dr. Hill articulated the principle of nonmaleficence when he did the orientation for Holly.

Companion Ethical Standard(s)

Standard 2.01: Boundaries of Competence

> (a) Psychologists . . . conduct research . . . in areas only within the boundaries of their competence, based on their education, training, supervised experience, consultation, study, or professional experience.

Dr. Lopez is presumably competent to conduct experiments with animals based on her education, training, experience, and professional experience. Dr. Hill is presumably competent to work in Dr. Lopez's lab based on his prior education and training, and current supervision from Dr. Lopez. Holly is not competent based on education or prior training, and would not be expected to be competent to work independently in Dr. Lopez's lab.

Standard 2.05: Delegation of Work to Others

> Psychologists who delegate work to . . . research . . . assistants . . . take reasonable steps to . . . (2) authorize only those responsibilities that such persons can be expected to perform competently . . . with the level of supervision being provided; and (3) see that such persons perform these services competently.

There are several layers of delegation in this situation. Dr. Lopez delegated the orientation, training, and possibly the supervision of the undergraduate assistant to Dr. Hill. Dr. Hill delegated the handling of the dogs before and after the experiment to Holly. Dr. Hill was to ensure that Holly was competent to care for the dogs. Dr. Lopez was to ensure that Dr. Hill was competent to supervise Holly.

Standard 8.09: Humane Care and Use of Animals in Research

> . . . (b) Psychologists trained in research methods and experienced in the care of laboratory animals supervise all procedures involving animals and are responsible for ensuring appropriate consideration of their comfort, health, and humane treatment.

Presumably, a postdoctoral fellow is both trained in research methods and experienced in caring for the animals. Per Standard 8.09 (b) Dr. Hill is to supervise all procedures involving the dogs. This includes when experimental dogs are checked in and out of the lab. Dr. Hill is in violation of Standard 8.09 (b) by allowing Holly to keep one dog in excess of needed time to run the experiment.

Standard 7.06: Assessing Student and Supervisee Performance

> . . . (b) Psychologists evaluate . . . supervisees on the basis of their actual performance on relevant and established program requirements.

Based on a chain of command, it is Dr. Hill's responsibility, per Standard 7.06 (b), to evaluate Holly. Also, it is Dr. Lopez's responsibility to evaluate Dr. Hill. It is unclear whether the university has established requirements for postdoctoral fellows or undergraduate lab assistants if their work is outside of an established program.

Legal Issues 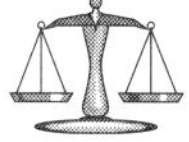

Virginia

> *18 Va. Admin. Code § 125-20-150 (2010). Standards of Practice.*
>
> B. Persons licensed by the board shall:
>
> 1. Provide and supervise only those services . . . for which they are qualified by training and appropriate experience. Delegate to their . . . supervisees . . . and research

> assistants only those responsibilities such persons can be expected to perform competently... Take ongoing steps to maintain competence in the skills they use...
>
> 5. Avoid harming . . . students . . . and minimize harm when it is foreseeable and unavoidable. Not exploit or mislead people for whom they provide professional services. Be alert to and guard against misuse of influence.

Washington

> *Wash. Admin. Code § 246-924-361 (2009). Guidelines for the Employment and/or Supervision of Auxiliary Staff.*
>
> (3) Responsibilities of the supervisor: . . . The supervisor is responsible for assuring that appropriate supervision is available or present at all times...
>
> (4) Conduct of supervision: . . . In the case of auxiliary staff providing psychological services, a detailed job description shall be developed and a contract for supervision prepared.
>
> (5) Conduct of services that may be provided by auxiliary staff: Procedures to be carried out by the auxiliary staff shall be planned in consultation with the supervisor.

In both Virginia and Washington, the laws place the responsibility for Holly's job performance on the supervisor. In this lab, both Dr. Lopez and Dr. Hill would be viewed as responsible for training, supervising, and evaluating Holly. Even though Dr. Lopez had the direct responsibility to supervise Dr. Hill, Dr. Lopez also would be held responsible for Dr. Hill's poor training, supervision, and evaluation of Holly because of his inadequate supervision of Dr. Hill. Dr. Hill in turn would be held responsible for his poor training, supervision, and evaluation of Holly.

Cultural Considerations

Global Discussion

Singapore Psychological Society:
Code of Professional Ethics

> Principle 16. Research precautions.
>
> The psychologists assume obligations for the welfare of their research subjects, both animal and human.
>
> 4. A psychologist using animals in research adheres to the provisions of the Rules and Regulations of the Singapore Society for the Prevention of Cruelty to Animals.

If Dr. Hill, Dr. Lopez, and Holly were in Singapore, Drs. Lopez and Hill would be charged with the welfare of the dogs. Singapore's Code is one of the only extant codes translated into English that places animal and human subjects on a similar level of obligation. It would seem that unless Holly's conduct with the dogs, in particular the one dog she has most closely bonded with, can be seen as a violation of the society's Rules and Regulations, none of the psychologists or students in this vignette would be found in violation of Singapore's Code.

American Moral Values

1. Did Dr. Hill and Dr. Lopez adequately train Holly to know that bonding was to be avoided, or even that bonding would occur if she spent too much time with one dog? Do they view Holly's actions as thoughtless or deliberately defiant? Can Holly be better trained and continue in the lab, perhaps after some form of punishment? Or has Holly shown she cannot be trusted in the lab?
2. Should Dr. Hill have noticed the dog was gone? Should there be more systematic monitoring and record keeping to prevent this type of action? Was this a failure of Dr. Lopez to train Dr. Hill in supervision? Can he be trusted to supervise work with animals more closely?
3. What are Holly's views about the use of dogs in the experiment? Was her interaction with a single dog an implicit protest against what she perceived as an impersonal or unemotional relationship with these dogs? How should her own love for dogs and desire to own one affect Dr. Hill and Dr. Lopez's judgment of how to proceed? Should she be removed from lab work that involves animals?
4. Does Holly's relationship with the dog offer Dr. Hill and Dr. Lopez a reason to reconsider how the dogs are being used? Was Holly's repeated work with one dog a form of abuse, given that Holly would never be able to continue it long term? Is Holly alone culpable for that situation, or is it too much to ask undergraduates who like animals to carry out these experiments without such emotional connections developing?
5. How does the issue of learned helplessness affect the expectations for interactions with the dog? Would Dr. Lopez mind as much if Holly's interactions did not affect the measurement of learned helplessness? Or is there a strict line between personal and professional,

or between scientist and animal lover, that Holly should not have crossed no matter what the dogs were being used for?

6. How will Dr. Lopez's decision affect relations between the lab and other faculty and students? Does she need to enforce high standards and expectations? Will she be seen as callous toward animal welfare? Does she need to develop a more supportive training regimen for students who want to work in the lab?

Ethical Course of Action

Directive per APA Code

Standard 8.09 (c) directs Dr. Lopez to assure that both Dr. Hill and Holly receive training in research methods and care of animals. Dr. Lopez should be able to safely assume that Dr. Hill is competent to work somewhat independently in the lab, per Standard 2.01 (a), based on his education, his training, and his current supervision. Thus, Dr. Lopez appropriately delegates responsibility to Dr. Hill, per Standard 2.05 (2). Holly, an undergraduate assistant, is presumed not to be competent, and thus delegation of any work would require instruction and ongoing supervision, per Standards 2.05 (3) and 8.09 (b).

It appears that Dr. Lopez has already taken care of the problem in relation to the research. Standard 7.06 (b) calls into question the breach in research protocol, and Dr. Lopez and Dr. Hill's responsibility to evaluate Holly, and Dr. Lopez's responsibility to evaluate Dr. Hill. Especially in light of the breach of research protocol, though not of animal care, Dr. Lopez and Dr. Hill must decide to fire Holly or retrain and supervise her properly for the work she is assigned.

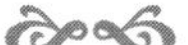

Dictates of One's Own Conscience

If you were Dr. Hill, faced with the discovery of a breach of research protocol, which of these would you do?

1. Defend Holly to Dr. Lopez on the grounds that the dog has been receiving excellent care.
2. Send Holly for further instruction on research methods and the importance of following protocol.
3. Give Holly a verbal reprimand for breach of research protocol.
4. Dismiss Holly from the lab.
5. Write an incident letter to Holly's academic advisor.

If you were Holly, faced with questions from Dr. Lopez, would you

1. Defend yourself on the grounds that you were taking good care of the dog?
2. Accuse Dr. Hill of not telling you that you could not keep the dogs out for longer than required for just running the experiment?

If you were Dr. Lopez, besides changing the dog, what else might you do?

1. Reprimand Dr. Hill for improperly training and supervising Holly?
2. Reprimand Holly for breaching research protocol?
3. Send Dr. Hill for supervisory training?
4. Send Holly for further training in research methods and animal care?
5. Combinations of the above-listed actions?
6. Or one that is not listed above?

If Dr. Lopez's lab was in Singapore, and you were Dr. Hill, faced with the discovery of a breach of research protocol, which of these actions would you choose?

1. Send Holly for further instruction on research methods and the importance of following protocol?
2. Commend Holly for humane treatment of animals, and give Holly a verbal reprimand for breach of research protocol?
3. Remind Holly that she needs to discuss any changes in protocol with you before she makes any changes?
4. Discuss with Dr. Lopez how best to use the experimental data, now that the altered condition for handling of the dog is known.

If you were Holly in Dr. Lopez's lab in Singapore, faced with questions from Dr. Lopez, would you

1. Apologize for your ignorance, claiming undue influence in your attachment to the dog?
2. Ask for forgiveness?

If you were Dr. Lopez working in Singapore, besides changing the dog, what else might you do?

1. Reprimand Dr. Hill for improperly training, evaluating, and supervising Holly?
2. Reprimand Holly for breaching research protocol?
3. Send Dr. Hill for supervisory training?
4. Send Holly for further training in research methods and animal care?
5. Combinations of the above-listed actions?
6. Or one that is not listed above?

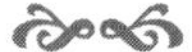

STANDARD 8.09: HUMANE CARE AND USE OF ANIMALS IN RESEARCH

> . . . (d) Psychologists make reasonable efforts to minimize the discomfort, infection, illness, and pain of animal subjects.

A CASE FOR STANDARD 8.09 (D): Pilfering Medication

Dr. Chapman is studying the effects of stress on the body's immune system. The study involves exposing guinea pigs to various noxious noises, then measuring blood cortisol levels and healing time for lesions. The experiment calls for an introduction of a loud noise, followed by taking a sample of blood, and surgically making a 1-inch cut in various places on the body. The guinea pig is bandaged, medicated with morphine, and given extra fluids after the surgical lesions are made.

Cathy, an undergraduate student, has proven herself to be an excellent assistant. In the course of her tenure in Dr. Chapman's lab, she has been given increasing levels of responsibility. She is to run the experiment once a week and check on the guinea pig's wound daily. Soon after being given the responsibility of running the experiment, Cathy begins to give the injections of morphine and make the lesions. Cathy realizes that she could inject the guinea pigs with saline solution and keep the morphine for her own later use.

During semester break, Cathy and all other student assistants are out of the lab. Dr. Chapman is in town and decides to run the experiment himself. He gives the shots and notices that healing times and cortisol levels are so drastically different that he runs the experiment again for the duration of the semester break. Concurrently, he receives the university's statement for requisition funds and notices excessive charges for saline solution.

When the students return from break, Dr. Chapman asks Cathy about the supply use and whether she has any idea as to changes in conditions for the guinea pig that might account for the changes in recovery time.

Issues of Concern

In accordance with Standard 8.09 (d), morphine is used to minimize the pain associated with surgical wounds. Like in A Case for Standard 8.09 (c): The Pet Dog, this could be a case of improper supervision. Even if Dr. Chapman had been in the room at all times when Cathy was performing the experiment, it is doubtful that Dr. Chapman could have noticed or discovered the exchanges of saline solution for morphine. Should he have noticed the increase in saline solution sooner? Was it possible that Dr. Chapman might have noticed changes in Cathy's behavior if she was abusing opiates or becoming addicted?

Of issue for this vignette is Cathy's attitude toward the treatment of animals versus treatment of humans. Would Cathy have made the same exchange of medication if she were making incisions on humans?

APA Ethics Code

Companion General Principle

Principle A: Beneficence and Nonmaleficence

> In their professional actions, psychologists seek to safeguard the welfare . . . of animal subjects of research.

Is it possible to provide the appropriate safeguards when the researcher or the researcher's assistants are actively abusing mind-altering substances?

Companion Ethical Standard(s)

Standard 2.04: Informal Resolution of Ethical Violations

> When psychologists believe that there may have been an ethical violation by another psychologist, they attempt to resolve the issue by bringing it to the attention of that individual.

If Dr. Chapman was knowledgeable and competent in the diagnosis and treatment of drug abuse, then he as a result would/might have noticed Cathy's behavior to be similar to those who were drug abusive. Altering the experimental procedure for the purpose of procuring mind-altering substances for her own personal consumption is evidence of unethical behavior defined by Standard 2.06. Standard 1.04 obligates Dr. Chapman to discuss the unethical behavior with Cathy.

Standard 1.05 Delegation of Work to Others

> Psychologists who delegate work to . . . research . . . assistants . . . take reasonable steps to . . . (3) see that such persons perform these services competently.

Based on the results of how the experiment was altered and how Cathy was not following experimental procedure, Dr. Chapman must not have provided an appropriate level of supervision, and thus was in violation of Standard 2.05. However, if Cathy was logging in all of the experimental procedures, it is doubtful that Dr. Chapman would have been able to identify that Cathy had altered the experimental procedure. This situation may be one that points to the inherent difficulties of delegating work to employees and assistants.

Standard 2.06: Personal Problems and Conflicts

> (a) Psychologists refrain from initiating an activity when they know or should know that there is a substantial likelihood that their personal problems will prevent them from performing their work-related activities in a competent manner. (b) When psychologists become aware of personal problems that may interfere with their performing work-related duties adequately, they take appropriate measures, such as obtaining professional consultation or assistance, and determine whether they should limit, suspend, or terminate their work-related duties.

Though the APA Ethics Code does not apply to Cathy since she is not a psychologist, but instead an undergraduate student, the standard provides guidance about how Dr. Chapman should treat Cathy's drug abuse.

Standard 3.06: Conflict of Interest

> Psychologists refrain from taking on a professional role when personal . . . interests . . . could reasonably be expected to (1) impair their objectivity, competence, or effectiveness in performing their functions as psychologists or (2) expose the person or organization with whom the professional relationship exists to harm or exploitation.

Again, though the APA Ethics Code does not apply to Cathy, Cathy's access to prescriptive opiates and her use of the morphine were clear conflicts of interest and in violation of Standard 3.06.

Legal Issues 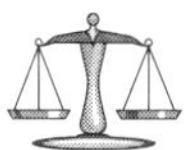

California

> *Cal. Code Regs. tit. 16, § 1387.1 (West 2010). Qualifications and Responsibilities of the Primary Supervisors.*
>
> (d) Primary supervisors shall be responsible for ensuring compliance at all times by the trainee. . .
>
> (e) Primary supervisors shall be responsible for ensuring that all . . . record keeping is conducted in compliance with the Ethical Principles and Code of Conduct of the American Psychological Association. . .
>
> (h) Primary supervisors shall be responsible for monitoring the performance and professional development of the trainee.

Colorado

> *Colo. Rev. Stat. Ann. § 12-43-222 (West 2010). Prohibited Activities—Related Provisions.*
>
> (e) Is habitually intemperate or excessively uses any habit-forming drug or is a habitual user of any controlled substance . . . which renders him or her unfit to practice pursuant to part 3, 4, 5, 6, 7, or 8 of this article. . .
>
> (n) Has failed to render adequate professional supervision of persons practicing pursuant to this article under such person's supervision according to generally accepted standards of practice. . .
>
> (u) Has falsified or repeatedly made incorrect essential entries.

Dr. Chapman failed to monitor the performance of the trainee. The welfare of the animals was hurt as a result of his poor monitoring and minimal supervision of Cathy. Expert witnesses would testify as to whether the use of the highly addictive substance of morphine should have been controlled and monitored better by Dr. Chapman. In all likelihood, experts would be found to testify that Dr. Chapman violated the laws regarding appropriate supervision in this fact scenario.

Cultural Considerations

Global Discussion

Canadian Code of Ethics for Psychologists

> Principle II: Responsible caring.
>
> II.45. Not use animals in their research unless there is a reasonable expectation that the research will increase understanding of the structures and processes underlying behaviour, or increase understanding of the particular animal species used in the study, or result eventually in benefits to the health and welfare of humans or other animals.
>
> II.46. Use a procedure subjecting animals to pain, stress, or privation only if an alternative procedure is unavailable and the goal is justified by its prospective scientific, educational, or applied value.
>
> II.47. Make every effort to minimize the discomfort, illness, and pain of animals. This would include performing surgical procedures only under appropriate anaesthesia, using techniques to avoid infection and minimize pain during and after surgery and, if disposing of experimental animals is carried out at the termination of the study, doing so in a humane way.

If Dr. Chapman was performing this experiment in Canada, and had received permission from the governing body for animal experimentation, then he likely would not be in violation of II.45, as he would have outlined in his research proposal the justification for performing surgery on his animal subjects without anesthesia. Under the same justification, he would also likely not be in violation of II.46, if he could prove that an "alternative procedure" is unavailable, and his possible research findings justify his actions. However, as this research study has been designed, the probable result of Dr. Chapman proposal is that it would not be approved under the demands of II.47, which states in part that Dr. Chapman would need to "perform . . . surgical procedures only under appropriate anaesthesia," which Dr. Chapman study design does not call for. Therefore, this situation would be unlikely to occur in Canada, as Dr. Chapman original study design would not be allowed by the provincial governing body that oversees the welfare and treatment of nonhuman animal subjects.

American Moral Values

1. How does Dr. Chapman analyze Cathy's action and its implications? Did Cathy show herself callous or even cruel toward the guinea pigs? Did she have any concern for the pain they were suffering? If not, should Cathy be allowed to work in a lab again, especially with work involving animals?
2. In terms of research, did Cathy understand how her use of saline solution would affect the results of the experiment? Did she understand the purpose of the experiment? Does this render her unfit to work in experimental conditions?
3. Did Cathy steal the morphine for her personal use, or for the use of someone she knew? Does Dr. Chapman need to inquire about an addiction before deciding how Cathy's case should be handled? Or could she have stolen morphine to sell? What would the use of morphine for personal profit mean for addressing Cathy's action? Would it justify expulsion?
4. How does Dr. Chapman assess his own responsibility for Cathy's work? Did he instruct her about the nature of the experiment, the need for each step in terms of gathering of data, and specifically the importance of the morphine? Did he screen her adequately in terms of her experience, understanding of the work, and so on?
5. Should Dr. Chapman have established better supervision procedures, whether by him or others working in the lab? Is the presence of morphine too tempting to entrust to undergraduate research assistants? Should there have been specific screening and training for those working with that drug in their experiments?
6. Did Dr. Chapman follow existing lab policy in his work with Cathy? Should he be disciplined by the university for not providing needed supervision? Should the lab as an institution revise its policies to prevent these kinds of situations, whether greater oversight or stricter screening? Should Cathy, or even Dr. Chapman, be considered a regrettable bad apple and not a symptom of a general problem in the lab? Is this case enough of a reason to make doing lab work more complicated through safeguards? Would stricter policies hamper the amount of research conducted in the lab?

Ethical Course of Action

Directive per APA Code

Per 8.09 (d) directives, Dr. Chapman has put in place more than adequate procedures to minimize the discomfort of his laboratory animals. It may be unreasonable to expect that any supervisor be omnipresent and could monitor for all infractions of his or her employees. For this situation, Standard 2.05 and Standard 1.04 apply once Dr. Chapman discovers Cathy's breaches of experimental protocol and her morphine abuse. As directed by Standards 2.05 and 1.04, Dr. Chapman would need to discuss the problem with Cathy and remove her from access to the morphine.

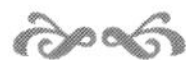

Dictates of One's Own Conscience

If you were Dr. Chapman, asking Cathy about apparent differences in experimental results and the bill from the university's procurement office, which of these might you expect and what might you do?

1. Expect Cathy to be defensive and possibly less than absolutely truthful.
2. Ask others in the lab the same set of questions to see if anyone noticed any unusual occurrences.
3. If Cathy is forthcoming about her use of morphine,
   a. refer her to the university counseling center for evaluation and treatment.
   b. suspend her as your lab assistant.
   c. recommend that she seek a position within the university that does not afford her access to prescription drugs.
4. Combinations of the above-listed actions.
5. Or one that is not listed above.

STANDARD 8.09: HUMANE CARE AND USE OF ANIMALS IN RESEARCH

> . . . (e) Psychologists use a procedure subjecting animals to pain, stress, or privation only when an alternative procedure is unavailable and the goal is justified by its prospective scientific, educational, or applied value.

A CASE FOR STANDARD 8.09 (E): Collateral Damage?

Dr. Green, a civilian psychologist and a contractor with the U.S. Department of Defense, heads a study on the effects of pain on higher levels of cognitive functioning. The aim of this study is to determine the average level of cognitive functioning under any given level of pain. It is hoped that such information may better inform the military regarding the impact of physical pain on problem solving and the extraction of strategic information. The experiment involves the use of chimpanzees that have been trained to carry out complex intelligence tasks. The chimpanzees are stabilized in a vise-like instrument, which applies graduated increases of pressure to arm bones while their functioning is observed under different levels of inflicted pain, ranging from mild sustained pressure to complete fracture of the arm bones. At the end of the experiment, the chimpanzees are euthanized.

Dr. Adams is a military psychologist who began his military career as an enlisted Navy SEAL. He was in combat situations before earning his psychology degree through the military education program. He is a recent addition to the pain and cognition chimpanzee study. He files a complaint with the IACUC contesting that the experimental conditions do not simulate any active combat conditions, and thus the study is of poor design. He also contends that the euthanization of the chimpanzees is unnecessary and inhumane. Instead, he recommends that the injured chimpanzees be rehabilitated back to health and returned to the laboratories.

Issues of Concern

Standard 8.09 (e) demands that if an animal is to be subjected to pain or stress, then the psychologist must first prove that an alternative procedure is unavailable to glean the information sought by the experiment. In addition, Standard 8.09 (e) demands that the information gained from the experiment must be of sufficient value to justify the pain inflicted.

Dr. Adams questions the worth of this experiment on both of these grounds. Dr. Adams does not think the information gained from the experiment would generalize to human combat conditions. The experiment appears to generate no valuable scientific, educational, or applied information. In addition, Dr. Adams suggests that there is at least one viable alternative procedure where the chimpanzees do not have to be euthanized. If Dr. Adams is correct in his assessment of the experiment, then Dr. Green is in violation of the conditions for Standard 8.09 (e).

APA Ethics Code

Companion General Principle

Principle A: Beneficence and Nonmaleficence

> In their professional actions, psychologists seek to safeguard the . . . welfare of animal subjects of research.

Dr. Green would certainly want to know of Dr. Adams's thoughts and ideas for alterations to the experimental procedure if the project were to enact Principle A and safeguard the welfare of the chimpanzees.

Companion Ethical Standard(s)

Standard 1.04: Informal Resolution of Ethical Violations

> When psychologists believe that there may have been an ethical violation by another psychologist, they attempt to resolve the issue by bringing it to the attention of that individual.

It appears that Dr. Adams thinks Dr. Green is in violation of Standard 8.09 (e). Under such circumstances, Standard 1.04 directs Dr. Adams to first approach Dr. Green to attempt some type of resolution that addresses Dr. Adams's concerns. It does not appear that Dr. Adams attempted an informal resolution.

Standard 1.05: Reporting Ethical Violations

> If an apparent ethical violation has substantially harmed . . . a person or organization and is not appropriate for informal resolution . . . or is not resolved properly in that fashion, psychologists take further action appropriate to the situation. Such action might include referral to . . . appropriate institutional authorities.

Standard 1.05 directs Dr. Adams to take action beyond informal resolution under three conditions. The first condition is if Dr. Adams thinks the violation has substantially harmed a person or an organization. The death of chimpanzees, not being human or an organization, does not meet the first condition for reporting ethical violations.

The second condition is if the situation is not appropriate for informal resolution because by approaching the offending psychologist, confidentiality would be compromised. Chimpanzees are not included in the category of being that holds the privilege of confidentiality. The situation does not meet the condition for reporting ethical violations.

The third condition is that informal resolution has already failed. Dr. Adams does not appear to have attempted informal resolution. Thus, the third condition for reporting ethical violation is not met either.

Egregious as it seems, the death of chimpanzees does not come up to the standard for reporting ethical violations without first attempting information resolution. Dr. Adams is in violation of Standard 1.05.

Standard 2.01: Boundaries of Competence

> (a) Psychologists . . . conduct research . . . in areas only within the boundaries of their competence, based on their education, training, supervised experience, consultation, study, or professional experience.

Standard 2.01 requires that Drs. Green and Adams be competent to conduct research both in the content area of cognitive functioning under conditions of physical pain and in generalizability of chimpanzee behavior to human conditions. In the absence of knowledge about the basis of Dr. Green's credentials, it appears that Dr. Adams has a claim to competence in the area of study based on his training and professional experience. Therefore, it appears that Dr. Adams holds sufficient knowledge to legitimately question Dr. Green's experimental design.

Standard 3.06: Conflict of Interest

> Psychologists refrain from taking on a professional role when personal, scientific, professional, legal, financial, or other interests or relationships could reasonably be expected to . . . (1) impair their objectivity, competence, or effectiveness in performing their functions as psychologists or . . . (2) expose the person or organization with whom the professional relationship exists to harm or exploitation.

Dr. Adams's reporting of Dr. Green directly to IACUC without an attempt at informal resolution as directed by Standard 1.04 suggests the possibility of an ulterior motive on Dr. Adams's part. In the absence of further knowledge about Dr. Green's and Dr. Adams's relationship or their professional credentials, it is impossible to determine whether or not Dr. Adams's course of action was motivated by something less than noble.

Legal Issues 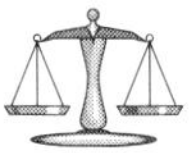

Missouri

Mo. Code Regs. Ann. tit. 20, § 2235-5.030 (2010). Ethical Rules of Conduct.

(8) Welfare of Supervisees, Clients, Research Subjects, and Students. . .

(B) Welfare of Clients and Research Subjects. . .

15. Research planning. In planning a study, the psychologist shall carefully evaluate ethical acceptability. . .

16. Animal subjects' welfare. When working with animal subjects, the psychologist shall ensure that the animals will be treated humanely. The psychologist shall only inflict . . . pain when the objectives of the research cannot be achieved by other methods. Any procedures that do inflict pain . . . must be strongly justified by their prospective scientific, educational, or applied value. . .

(15) Resolving Issues.

(A) Reporting of Violations to Committee.

The psychologist who has knowledge . . . that there has been a violation of the statutes or rules of the committee shall inform the committee in writing.

Pennsylvania

49 Pa. Code § 41.61 (2010). Code of Ethics.

Principle 2. Competency.

(b) . . . When a psychologist . . . violates ethical standards, psychologists who know first hand of these activities attempt to rectify the situation. When such a situation cannot be dealt with informally, it is called to the attention of the Board.

Principle 10. Care and use of animals in research.

(a) . . . the investigator ensures the welfare of animals and treats them humanely.

(b) The . . . use and disposal of animals are in compliance with current Federal . . . laws and regulations.

(e) Psychologists make every effort to minimize . . . pain of animals. A procedure subjecting animals to pain . . . is used only when an alternative procedure is unavailable and the goal is justified by its prospective . . . applied value.

(f) When it is appropriate that the animal's life be terminated, it is done rapidly and painlessly.

In both jurisdictions, Dr. Green engaged in multiple violations of the laws regulating animal research. Under Missouri law, Dr. Adams is to file a formal written complaint with the committee (Missouri's licensing board). In Pennsylvania, Dr. Adams must attempt to rectify the situation first before filing a complaint with the licensing board.

Cultural Considerations

Global Discussion

Code of Ethics for the Psychologist: Spain

> ***Article 7.*** Psychologists must not . . . contribute to any practices that may violate individual liberty or physical or psychological integrity. . . They must never participate in any way, nor as researchers . . . on the practice of torture, or any other cruel, inhuman and degrading practices . . . regardless of . . . the information that might be obtainable from them. . .
>
> ***Article 24.*** Psychologists must refuse to provide their services whenever they are certain that these will be . . . used against the legitimate interests of individuals, groups, institutions or communities.
>
> ***Article 38.*** Experiments with animals must also avoid or minimize suffering, harm and discomfort that is not absolutely necessary and justified by goals of recognised scientific and human worth. . . [P]ersonnel directly involved in research with animals must follow the procedures for . . . elimination of animals by euthanasia. . .

This experiment violates Article 38 by failing to "avoid or minimize suffering [or] harm . . . that is not absolutely necessary and justified." The overarching concern and the most problematic violations of the code, however, have to do with the implicit nature and purpose of the research itself. If the experiment is to determine how to better extract information from prisoners of war who are exposed to painful stimuli (i.e., who is tortured) or to know how captured soldiers will likely respond to pain, then the intent and purpose of the research is in violation of Articles 7 and 24 of the Spanish code. Article 24 requires that psychologists not allow their services to be used by those who will "misuse them" against "the interests of . . . individuals." Attempting to discover techniques that can be used to extract information forcibly would qualify as torture, which in Article 7 is condemned most strongly. To participate directly in the maltreatment of others, the Spanish code points out, is to not only violate the ethics code of psychologists, but it is also to commit the gravest of crimes against humanity. Both Drs. Green and Adams would likely be found to be in violation of the letter and intent of these articles of the Spanish code.

American Moral Values

1. What are the scholarly and social benefits of this kind of pain research? Are there any larger causes that Dr. Adams would find worth supporting through this research? Does Dr. Adams believe other psychologists could ethically pursue this research?
2. Could this study help conditions of people expected to work or serve in pain? Could it be an important contribution to safety standards in the workplace? What evidence is there that such research will yield those beneficial results?
3. Does Dr. Adams suspect this could be used for purposes beyond problem solving, for example, pain tolerance during torture? Do examples of governments using torture, for example, to combat terrorism, make him more careful about what work he would agree to support?
4. How does Dr. Adams think about animals, consciousness, and pain? Does a chimp's intelligence level make their treatment in the study close to the torture of human beings than inflicting pain on other animals? Does pain increase when it involves psychological and physiological responses?
5. What will this type of pain procedure do to the psychologists carrying it out? Will it deaden their sensitivity to and sympathy for suffering? Will they have to dissociate emotionally from the work, and will that be sustainable or advisable?
6. Should Dr. Adams work with animal rights groups to expose this experiment? Would that jeopardize his career? At what point does one have to join extra-academic organizations to lobby against an objectionable form of animal testing?
7. Are there viable ways to conduct such research without this manner of inflicting and measuring pain?

Ethical Course of Action

Directive per APA Code

If Dr. Adams's charges are valid, then Dr. Green is in violation of Standard 8.09 (e) for unnecessarily inflicting pain and causing the death of research animals. If Dr. Adams suspects that the experiment violates any part of the ethics code, and specifically violates Standard 8.09 (e), he is to approach Dr. Green directly as dictated by Standard 1.04. In the absence of an attempt at informal resolution, Dr. Adams' behavior is suspect and open to speculations about conflict of interest.

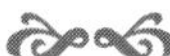

Dictates of One's Own Conscience

If you were Dr. Green and you received a notice from IACUC that Dr. Adams has lodged a complaint, and to suspend operations pending further examination of the experimental design, what would you do?

1. Stop further experiment immediately?
2. Make further inquiry with IACUC to discover the exact nature of the complaint?
3. Approach Dr. Adams to find out the exact nature of his complaints?
4. Combinations of the above-listed actions?
5. Or one that is not listed above?

If you were Dr. Adams working in Spain, which of these might you do?

1. Engage in sufficient disclosure about the situation so that permission would probably not have been granted for such an experiment with the chimpanzees.
2. If for some reason you took the job without knowledge of the exact nature of Dr. Green's experiments, then immediately voice your concern to Dr. Green, stop work, and report Dr. Green and the lab to the IACUC.

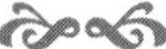

STANDARD 8.09: HUMANE CARE AND USE OF ANIMALS IN RESEARCH

. . . (f) Psychologists perform surgical procedures under appropriate anesthesia and follow techniques to avoid infection and minimize pain during and after surgery.

A CASE FOR STANDARD 8.09 (F): The Whistle-Blower

Dr. Baker's lab is studying the rate of nerve degeneration post spinal cord injury. In this experiment, cats are exposed to a sudden-impact injury, similar to those experienced in car accidents. The cats are decapitated at a set time interval after injury for postmortem microscopic examination of nerve tissues. To retain the integrity of the cells, the cats are not given anesthesia at the time of decapitation. Dr. Baker trains Sally, a graduate lab assistant, to run the experiment, including the proper surgical procedure for decapitation without anesthesia.

In the last few weeks, Dr. Baker notices that the condition of the nerve cells has changed and asks Sally if there have been any changes in the care of the cats in the surgical procedures or in the post-surgical extraction of the nerve cells. Sally says yes, that she has started to administer anesthesia prior to decapitation. Sally contends that decapitation without the use of anesthesia is unnecessarily cruel, and its use does not violate the integrity of the study. She began to engage in the procedural change only after filing a complaint with the National Institutes of Health (NIH), their granting organization, and the university's IACUC.

Issues of Concern

Presumably, Dr. Baker received authorization from the IACUC to forego the use of anesthesia. For the IACUC to authorize a deviation from standard procedure that complies with Standard 8.09 (f), Dr. Baker must have had a very compelling argument. Was Sally ignorant of the reasons for these specific experimental procedures? Regardless of whether she was in agreement with the rationale that justified withholding anesthesia, was Sally justified in changing the experimental procedures without appropriate notification to Dr. Baker and anyone else who might be conducting research based on their experiment?

APA Ethics Code

Companion General Principle

Principle A: Beneficence and Nonmaleficence

> In their professional actions, psychologists seek to safeguard . . . the welfare of animal subjects of research.

Principle A: Beneficence and Nonmaleficence is most likely the underlying value for Sally's actions. Principle A calls for psychologists to engage in examination and reflection regarding the question of whether it is necessary to inflict pain by withholding anesthesia during surgery.

Companion Ethical Standard(s)

Standard 1.03: Conflicts Between Ethics and Organizational Demands

> If the demands of an organization . . . for whom they are working are in conflict with this Ethics Code, psychologists clarify the nature of the conflict, make known their commitment to the Ethics Code, and take reasonable steps to resolve the conflict consistent with the General Principles and Ethical Standards of the Ethics Code.

Sally obviously had a conflict with Dr. Baker's demand for surgical procedures without anesthesia. If Sally is a psychology graduate student, then she is bound by Standard 1.03 to make known her conflict. Her submitting of a complaint to the university IACUC is one way to clarify her conflict and make known her objections. She then proceeded to take steps to resolve her conflict in a way that was consistent with Principle A and Standard 1.03.

Standard 1.04: Informal Resolution of Ethical Violations

> When psychologists believe that there may have been an ethical violation by another psychologist, they attempt to resolve the issue by bringing it to the attention of that individual, if an informal resolution appears appropriate.

As directed by Standard 1.04, Sally needed to have discussed her conflict with Dr. Baker first and attempted to come to some type of resolution that would uphold Standard 8.09. Her failure to do so means that she is in violation of Standard 1.04.

Standard 1.05: Reporting Ethical Violations

> If an apparent ethical violation has substantially harmed . . . a person [and] . . . is not appropriate for informal resolution . . . or is not resolved properly in that fashion, psychologists take further action appropriate to the situation. Such action might include referral to . . . the appropriate institutional authorities.

Regardless of whether Sally thought Dr. Baker's experimental protocol did or did not protect the welfare of the cats, Standard 1.05 does not give her justification to submit a complaint to the IACUC nor to change experimental protocols. Standard 1.05 only applies to situations where humans are or may be harmed. Standard 1.05 does not apply to nonhuman animals.

Standard 6.01: Documentation of Professional and Scientific Work and Maintenance of Records

> Psychologists create . . . records and data relating to their . . . scientific work in order to . . . (2) allow for replication of research design and analyses, (3) [and] meet institutional requirements . . .

For Dr. Baker not to know that an experimental protocol had been changed, he was either remiss in not keeping up with reading the lab logs, or Sally was remiss in not making accurate entry into the logs.

Legal Issues 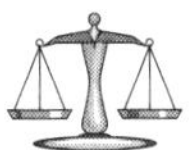

South Carolina

> *S.C. Code Ann. Regs.100-4 (2010). Code of Ethics.*
>
> K. Violations of law.
>
> (1) Violation of applicable statutes. The psychologist shall not violate any applicable statute or administrative rule regulating the practice of psychology. . .
>
> L. Aiding illegal practice. . .
>
> (4) Reporting of violations to Board. The psychologist who has substantial reason to believe that there has been a violation of the statutes or rules of the Board shall so inform the Board in writing on forms provided by the Board. . .
>
> Appendix B
>
> Principle 10: Care and Use of Animals
>
> d. Psychologists make every effort to minimize . . . pain of animals. A procedure subjecting animals to pain . . . is used only when an alternative procedure is unavailable and the goal is justified by its prospective . . . applied value. Surgical procedures are performed under appropriate anesthesia. . .
>
> e. When it is appropriate that the animal's life be terminated, it is done rapidly and painlessly.

Texas

> *22 Tex. Admin. Code § 465.13 (2010). Personal Problems, Conflicts and Dual Relationships*
>
> (a) In General. . .
>
> (5) Licensees withdraw from any professional relationship that conflicts, or comes into conflict with, their ability to comply with Board rules relating to other existing professional relationships.
>
> *22 Tex. Admin. Code § 465.20 (2010). Research.*
>
> (a) Conducting Research. . .
>
> (2) Licensees shall conduct all research involving animals in a humane manner which minimizes the . . . pain of animal subjects. A procedure subjecting animals to pain . . . is used only when an alternative procedure is unavailable and the goal is justified by its prospective . . . applied value.

In both jurisdictions, the research protocol created unnecessary pain and violated the laws. In South Carolina, Sally should have informed the licensing board about Dr. Baker's research protocol that violated the laws. In Texas, she is instructed by the law to withdraw from her professional relationship with Dr. Baker.

Cultural Considerations

Global Discussion

Canadian Code of Ethics for Psychologists

> Principle II: Responsible caring.
>
> II.45. Not use animals in their research unless there is a reasonable expectation that the research will increase understanding of the structures and processes underlying behaviour. . .
>
> II.46. Use a procedure subjecting animals to pain . . . only if an alternative procedure is unavailable and the goal is justified by its prospective . . . applied value.
>
> II.47. Make every effort to minimize the . . . pain of animals. This would include performing surgical procedures only under appropriate anaesthesia . . . and, if disposing of experimental animals is carried out at the termination of the study, doing so in a humane way.

If Dr. Baker received permission from the governing body for animal experimentation, then he likely would not be in violation of II.45, as he would likely have outlined in his research proposal the justification for performing surgery on the animal subjects without anesthesia. Under the same justification, he would also likely not be in violation of II.46 if he could prove that an "alternative procedure" is unavailable, and his likely research findings justify his actions. However, as this research study has been designed, the likely result of Dr. Baker's proposal is that it would not be approved under the demands of II.47, which states in part that Dr. Baker would need to "perform . . . surgical procedures only under appropriate anaesthesia," which Dr. Baker's study design does not call for. Therefore, this situation would be unlikely to occur in Canada. The provincial governing body that oversees the welfare and treatment of nonhuman animal subjects would not allow Dr. Baker's original study design.

American Moral Values

1. Was using anesthesia the best way for Sally to fight against the method of decapitation Dr. Baker had instructed her to use? Did she believe he was wrong to think anesthesia would affect nerve cells? Or did she think that the collection of data from the nerve cells was less important than sparing the cats pain? If Dr. Baker now cannot use any data from the anesthetized cats, were the cats' lives wasted? Did Sally prevent those cats from helping to rehabilitate victims of spinal cord injury?

2. What reasons did Sally have for going against Dr. Baker's orders in this fashion? Why did she not refuse to work on the experiment any longer, or at least until her complaint was settled by the IACUC? Did she believe the lab had betrayed her by making her perform Dr. Baker's method, but that she was owed the money agreed upon for her work? Did she think she would not get caught, and that she would not risk Dr. Baker's criticism or punishment as her boss?

3. How does Dr. Baker interpret Sally's action with respect to his work and himself as a person? Are her action and complaint an accusation? Does he need to defend himself for the sake of his career or family? Or was it understandable that Sally balked at the decapitation method? Does he feel she was afraid to tell him about the anesthesia, or was she lying to him so that the animals would continue to receive anesthesia?

4. Did Dr. Baker adequately explain to Sally the experiment's purposes and the reasons for not using anesthesia? Had she given any signs of consent to such an explanation, if it occurred? Does Dr. Baker need to rethink how he explains the experiment to other lab assistants?

5. Presumably, Dr. Baker obtained IACUC approval for the experiment. Did Sally know about this approval? Does Sally have testimony about how the cats suffer that might change the IACUC's decision? Does Dr. Baker need to develop a stronger justification for the experiment?

6. How much is Dr. Baker responsible for the effect of his experiments on the development of spinal cord injury research? What will happen if the university community, or the public at large, learns of this complaint? Will this hamper further efforts along these lines? What are his views of the social good to be accomplished by this research? To what degree does he believe that animals' pain is a limiting factor for researching treatments for humans? Should he share those views honestly, or should he try to "spin" a PR-friendly defense for the sake of this medical cause?

Ethical Course of Action

Directive per APA Code

Standard 8.09 (f) calls for appropriate use of anesthesia when surgical procedures are involved in the experiment. Decapitation of cats is a surgical procedure. Thus, under normal laboratory procedures, Sally would have been administering anesthesia before conducting any surgical procedure. If there were no compelling reason to justify withholding anesthesia, it was appropriate for Sally to make known her commitment to Standard 8.09 (f). It is questionable whether single-handedly changing experimental protocol without consultation or notification to Dr. Baker would be deemed taking "reasonable steps" toward resolution, per Standard 1.03. At a minimum, Sally needed to attempt an informal resolution, per Standard 1.04, by bringing her concerns directly to Dr. Baker. Based on the directives of Standard 1.04 or 1.05, Sally was not justified to have submitted a complaint to the IACUC and to change experimental protocols without consultation or the failure of informal resolution.

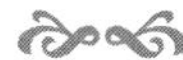

Dictates of One's Own Conscience

If you were Dr. Baker, having discovered that Sally has changed experimental protocol without authorization, which of these would you do?

1. Have a long conversation with her to understand her rationale for taking the course of action she did.

2. Write a letter of reprimand.

3. Contact Human Resources to start procedures for dismissal.
4. Contact anyone else who is conducting research based on the cell slides.
5. Withdraw all cell samples from the date of change in protocol.
6. Note the change in experiment protocol for effective slides.

If you were Sally, thinking that you will be reprimanded for withholding anesthesia, which of these actions would you take?

1. Visit the union office to seek advice about how to protect yourself from possible retaliation from Dr. Baker.
2. Contact local and national animal protection agencies in order to expose the animal cruelty in Dr. Baker's lab.
3. Retain an attorney to protect yourself from retaliation for blowing the whistle on Dr. Baker for animal cruelty and the university IACUC for authorizing animal cruelty.
4. Combinations of the above-listed actions.
5. Or one that is not listed above.

If you were Dr. Baker or Sally working in a lab in Canada, it is very unlikely that you would find yourself in this situation since the experiment as designed would likely never have received institutional approval.

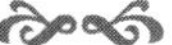

STANDARD 8.09: HUMANE CARE AND USE OF ANIMALS IN RESEARCH

> . . . (g) When it is appropriate that an animal's life be terminated, psychologists proceed rapidly, with an effort to minimize pain and in accordance with accepted procedures.

A CASE FOR STANDARD 8.09 (G): To Eat or Not to Eat

Dr. Gonzalez's study has come to an end. The rabbits used in the study are no longer needed, and they cannot be used for other experiments. Per lab protocol, Dr. Gonzalez instructs Regina, his lab assistant, to euthanize the remaining rabbits.

Dr. Gonzalez's laboratory at New State University is in a town located in an idyllic rural farming area. Regina is a single mother from a neighboring farm who has recently started at the university. She considers herself lucky to have such a high-paying part-time job with the local university. Her first assignment is in Dr. Gonzalez's lab. Regina thinks Dr. Gonzalez, like all of the doctors at the university, has an overly sentimental view of animals. When Regina was told to euthanize the rabbits, she reasoned that since the rabbits had not received any medications or chemicals, they were good for butchering. She decides that killing the rabbits and cremating their remains is a waste, especially when she has hungry children at home. Regina loads the rabbits into a cardboard box, takes them home, and raises the rabbits on her farm, allowing them to live their normal lives, until she uses them for a nice rabbit stew.

Issues of Concern

Dr. Gonzalez was to assure that when the rabbits were terminated at the end of the experiment, it was done rapidly with minimal pain to the rabbits. Presuming that Dr. Gonzalez had trained Regina in appropriate methods of terminating the rabbits' lives, he would have no reason to believe Regina would not carry out proper protocol or his direct orders. Does Dr. Gonzalez's responsibility extend to having to personally ensure that Regina has carried out the order to terminate the rabbits' lives?

From the university's perspective, it is an extra expense to keep the rabbits around once the experiment is over and they are not needed for any other research. Does it affect the university financially for Regina to take the rabbits home or to terminate their lives? Either way, the university no longer bears any financial burden for the upkeep of the rabbits.

APA Ethics Code

Companion General Principle

Principle A: Beneficence and Nonmaleficence

> In their professional actions, psychologists seek to safeguard the welfare . . . of animal subjects of research.

Principle A would guide Dr. Gonzalez to make sure that the research animals do not suffer under his care. Dr. Gonzalez would need to ask himself whether it is more humane to euthanize laboratory animals once they are no longer needed for experiments or to retain them in the university's animal facility until they come to a natural death.

Companion Ethical Standard(s)

Standard 2.05: Delegation of Work to Others

> Psychologists who delegate work to employees . . . take reasonable steps to . . . (1) avoid delegating such work to persons who have a multiple relationship with those being served that would likely lead to exploitation or loss of objectivity[,] . . . (2) authorize only those responsibilities that such persons can be expected to perform competently on the basis of their . . . training . . . with the level of supervision being provided; and . . . (3) see that such persons perform these services competently.

Presumably, Dr. Gonzalez followed the dictates of Standard 2.05 and only assigned work that he had trained Regina to perform in the lab. Standard 2.05 (3) directs Dr. Gonzalez to see to it that Regina is doing her job competently. At question here is the level of oversight deemed to be adequate in order to meet the requirements of Standard 2.05 (3). Is it a more competent move to decide for the rabbits to be adopted out at the end of their use in the experiments? Is it more reasonable to simply order the rabbits to be euthanized than to look for adoption homes for them?

Standard 3.06: Conflict of Interest

> Psychologists refrain from taking on a professional role when personal[,] . . . financial[,] . . . or other interests or relationships could reasonably be expected to (1) impair their objectivity . . . in performing their functions as psychologists.

With her attitude toward animals, it was probably not a good idea for Regina to take on work with laboratory animals. Since Regina is not a psychologist, she cannot be in violation of Standard 3.06. However, if Dr. Gonzalez had some awareness of the prevailing attitude toward animals held by farmers, was he in violation of Standard 3.06 for hiring a farmer into his animal lab?

Legal Issues 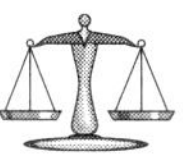

Virginia

> *18 Va. Admin. Code § 125-20-150 (2010). Standards of Practice.*
>
> B. Persons licensed by the board shall:
>
> *1. . . Delegate to their employees . . . only those responsibilities such persons can be expected to perform competently by . . . training and experience.*

Washington

> *Wash. Admin. Code § 246-924-361 (2009). Guidelines for the Employment and/or Supervision of Auxiliary Staff.*
>
> (3) Responsibilities of the supervisor: The supervisor accepts full legal and professional responsibility for all services that may be rendered by the auxiliary staff. . . The supervisor is responsible for assuring that appropriate supervision is available or present at all times.

In both Virginia and Washington, no law exists that would find the research protocol was structured illegally. If charges were brought for violating the protocol, the likely interpretation of the laws would be to place the responsibility for Regina's job performance on Dr. Gonzalez, the supervisor.

Cultural Considerations

Global Discussion

Canadian Code of Ethics for Psychologists

> Principle II: Responsible caring.
>
> II.47. Make every effort to minimize the discomfort . . . of animals . . . if . . . disposing of experimental animals is carried out at the termination of the study, doing so in a humane way.
>
> II.49. Encourage others . . . to care responsibly.
>
> II.50. Assume overall responsibility for the . . . activities of their . . . employees . . . with regard to the Principle of Responsible Caring, all of whom, however, incur similar obligations.

It is unclear whether Dr. Gonzalez is in violation of Article II.47. At issue is what is defined as humane and by whom. Regina's method of killing the rabbits is as humane as whatever protocol she was going to perform in the lab, freeing the rabbits from confinement and allowing them to live their final days in an outside setting with fresh air, proper food and water, and socialization with other rabbits is far more humane than ending their days in a cage and awaiting death. Per II.50, Dr. Gonzalez is responsible for encouraging Regina to care responsibly for her animal charges, which she has done. He also assumes responsibility for the activities of those he supervises; therefore, if Regina's activities with the rabbits are in violation of laboratory procedure, university research protocol, or the parameters set in his proposed study design, the responsibility for resolving this violation lies with Dr. Gonzalez, not Regina.

American Moral Values

1. What objections will Dr. Gonzalez have to Regina's action? Of what importance is it that Regina directly disobeyed a directive from her boss? Can Dr. Gonzalez trust Regina with other decisions? Does Dr. Gonzalez believe that Regina was reckless in not following lab protocol for euthanizing the rabbits? Does he believe Regina was cruel to the rabbits relative to how they would have been euthanized? Does Dr. Gonzalez believe this sets a bad precedent for other lab assistants, who might get ideas about how to take home or sell lab animals for pets?
2. What is the purpose of the lab protocol? Is it to ensure that the pets will not suffer anymore than they already have in experiments? How is the value of avoiding pain balanced against a respect for and protection of life? Could Regina argue that the rabbits had a longer and happier existence coming home with her than they would have had otherwise? Is it more important for animals to live longer than to stop suffering? Which is worth risking at the expense of the other? Is Dr. Gonzalez responsible for making sure the rabbits are treated humanely after leaving the lab?
3. What are the cultural and class differences at work between Dr. Gonzalez and Regina? Should Regina have raised the issue with Dr. Gonzalez before taking the rabbits home? Should Dr. Gonzalez be accommodating to Regina, given her views that the rabbits should not be wasted? Should he think about alternative means for lab animals to be cared for after the experiments, including being cared for humanely and then killed for meat? Could Dr. Gonzalez go further and suggest the rabbits go to a petting zoo to live even longer?
4. How far does Dr. Gonzalez wish to push for changes in protocol? How will this affect his relationship with other faculty and students doing lab work? Will new options disrupt a stable protocol that protects against wanton and unusual acts being taken with animals?
5. Are there experiments where animals could carry harmful diseases or behaviors to the outside world? Does euthanasia ensure that those will not become a public health concern?

Ethical Course of Action

Directive per APA Code

It is appropriate that the animals be treated humanely when they are no longer needed for further experiments. One option for humane treatment is a quick and painless death, per Standard 8.09 (g). It is unclear whether Dr. Gonzalez had the option to give the rabbits up for pet adoption. Since he did not opt for adoption, it is his responsibility to see that Regina knew how to terminate the rabbits' lives, per Standard 8.09 (c) and Standard 2.05 (2). Further, it was Dr. Gonzalez's job to make sure that Regina carried out his orders, per Standard 2.05 (3).

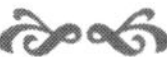

Dictates of One's Own Conscience

If you were Dr. Gonzalez and you heard from the other lab assistants that Regina took the rabbits home for butchering, which of these would you do?

1. Dismiss the matter, thinking that what Regina did was in line with what all of the farmers do when any of them starts working in the university animal labs.
2. Ask Regina what happened to the rabbits the next time you see her.
3. Talk to Regina about the importance of following experimental protocol, regardless of whether she disagrees with how the animals are being handled.
4. Talk to Regina about how to appropriately change experimental protocol if she wants to take the rabbits home in the future.
5. Tell Regina that what she did with the rabbits was okay this time because it did not affect the research experiment, but that she is not to alter any protocols in the future.

6. Tell Regina that you are happy about the rabbits getting a good long life, but that it is extremely egregious to violate research protocol and that you are putting her on probation.
7. Combinations of the above-listed actions.
8. Or one that is not listed above.

If you were Dr. Gonzalez working in Canada and found out that Regina has been taking the animals home with her, would you talk to Regina about how to appropriately change the experimental protocol if she wants to take the rabbits home in the future?

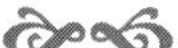

STANDARD 8.10: REPORTING RESEARCH RESULTS

(a) Psychologists do not fabricate data.

A CASE FOR STANDARD 8.10 (A): The Whole Picture

Erica knew she wanted to study anorexia since she started graduate school. She takes the opportunity to write all of her courses' assigned papers on the topic of anorexia. She has also conducted several small survey studies on anorexia in her research courses. She is finally starting her dissertation. Armed with her review of literature and various surveys that she has done over her graduate school career, she goes into her first meeting with the chair of her dissertation committee, Dr. Nelson.

Erica proposes that for her dissertation, she will combine the three different surveys she has already done into one big survey. In this manner, her data collection would be complete, and she could then proceed to the analysis phase of her dissertation.

Issues of Concern

The various surveys conducted throughout her graduate school career may or may not have anything in common besides the topic of anorexia. Depending on the design of the survey and the subjects surveyed, Erica may or may not have experiments that can be collapsed. If she has the raw data from all of her surveys, could she comingle the information and proceed as if it was one study?

APA Ethical Code

Companion General Principle

Principle C: Integrity

> Psychologists seek to promote accuracy . . . and truthfulness . . . in the science . . . [or] teaching . . . of psychology. In these activities, psychologists do not . . . cheat, or engage in . . . intentional misrepresentation of fact.

The goal is for psychologists, and those in training, to be accurate and truthful in such a manner that misrepresentation of fact does not occur. The focus for Dr. Nelson, the chair of the dissertation committee, is to provide sufficient monitoring so that Erica's work is accurate and truthful. Erica is to aim for accuracy and truthfulness in all of her work. If the data is comingled, how could she accurately depict the data so that the full scope of the experiment is truthfully represented?

Companion Ethical Standard(s)

Standard 7.06: Assessing Student and Supervisee Performance

> (a) In academic . . . relationships, psychologists establish a timely and specific process for providing feedback to students.

Standard 7.06 (a) would direct Dr. Nelson to give Erica feedback in a timely manner so that Erica does not pursue a path that will ultimately be a waste of time.

Standard 2.04: Bases for Scientific and Professional Judgments

> Psychologists' work is based upon established scientific and professional knowledge of the discipline.

Erica, being a student, is learning the existing body of professional knowledge. Dr. Nelson has the responsibility to ensure that Erica's dissertation is based on sound research methods.

Standard 6.01: Documentation of Professional and Scientific Work and Maintenance of Records

> Psychologists create, and . . . maintain[,] . . . store, retain, and dispose of[,] . . . data relating to their . . . scientific work in order to . . . (2) allow for replication of research design and analyses.

If Erica has retained all of her data, Dr. Nelson could help Erica review the parameters of her previous surveys to determine whether a meta-analysis is an appropriate method for re-approaching the data from the previous surveys. Such an approach presumes that Erica conducted the surveys without participation from other classmates and that she is the sole owner of the data.

Legal Issues 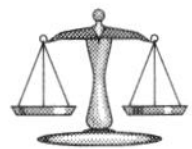

California

Cal. Code Regs. tit. 16, § 1387.1 (West 2010). Qualifications and Responsibilities of the Primary Supervisors.

(d) Primary supervisors shall be responsible for ensuring compliance at all times by the trainee with the provisions of the Psychology Licensing Law and the regulations adopted pursuant to these laws. . .

(h) Primary supervisors shall be responsible for monitoring the performance and professional development of the trainee.

Cal. Bus. & Prof. Code § 2960 (West 2010). Causes for Disciplinary Action.

Unprofessional conduct shall include, but not be limited to . . .

(n) The commission of any dishonest, corrupt, or fraudulent act.

Colorado

Colo. Rev. Stat. Ann. § 12-43-222. (West 2010) Prohibited Activities—Related Provisions.

(g) Has acted or failed to act in a manner that does not meet the generally accepted standards of the professional discipline under which such person practices. . .

(n) Has failed to render adequate professional supervision of persons practicing pursuant to this article under such person's supervision according to generally accepted standards of practice.

In both jurisdictions, no laws would be broken as long as Erica, under Dr. Nelson's supervision, concretely establishes how the data were collected, the approach did not violate the doctoral program's requirements for originality, and nothing was hidden from the readers of the dissertation. Otherwise, Erica may be viewed as having committed fraud, and Dr. Nelson would have failed to provide adequate supervision.

Cultural Considerations

Global Discussion

Singapore Psychological Society:
Code of Professional Ethics

Principle 1. Responsibility.

1. . . . research is planned in such a way as to minimise the possibility that findings will be misleading; and the psychologist publishes full reports of such works, never discarding without explanation data which may modify the interpretation of results.

If the findings are in some way altered by collapsing the three studies into one, rather than doing an entirely new study, Erica could be putting forth results that might then be misleading. It would probably fall on Dr. Nelson, as the chair of the committee, the license holder of record, and the person charged with inducting Erica into the professional role of a psychologist, to ensure that Erica's study meets the intent of Principle 1: Responsibility.

American Moral Values

1. Is it methodologically honest to present these surveys as a unified collection of data? Could the surveys have had some of the same people as subjects? Is it a problem that they were done over separate stretches of time? Could one publish these surveys with acceptable transparency to the reader and maintain the integrity of each survey's data?
2. Does Erica have an exclusive right to this data? Did she work with other students on these surveys as a class project?
3. What obstacles does Erica face in conducting an original survey for her dissertation research? Is she proposing using the previous surveys due to a lack of financial or career support? Could the department do more to assist her with an original project?
4. What does Dr. Nelson need to require of Erica as her advisor and mentor? Are there scholarly values concerning originality and transparency that Dr. Nelson needs to convey? Could Dr. Nelson help Erica think of other ways to use these earlier surveys (separate articles, etc.)?

5. What kind of example would this type of dissertation set for students? Could it lead to more pre-dissertation pieces for classes? Would that harm the course of scholarly development, or would it be commendably ambitious for a contemporary academic job market?

6. Is anorexia in urgent need of more published material? Does anorexia's social relevance bear on the way Erica's project should be treated? How much should social relevance and the public good determine the standards for data collection and publication? Are there sufficient nonacademic ways to get important data to society at large?

Ethical Course of Action

Directive per APA Code

It is Dr. Nelson's responsibility to guide Erica in this dissertation project, per Standard 7.06 (a). Part of the guidance is to assure that Erica's work is based on sound research methods, per Standard 2.04. If Erica has kept accurate records of her previous work, per Standard 6.01 (2), then Erica, with the help of Dr. Nelson, could determine how best to use the information for her dissertation project. For Erica to comingle her data from several previous surveys would be a violation of Standard 8.10 (a) if the design of the dissertation did not detail this approach. Otherwise, potential readers may be deceived by the unarticulated approach, and such an approach may be viewed as a fabrication.

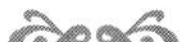

Dictates of One's Own Conscience

If you were Dr. Nelson, listening to Erica, what would you say to her?

1. Ask Erica for her rationale, other than convenience, as to why she wants to combine the surveys?

2. Pose the possibility that combining the surveys is in violation of Standard 8.10 (a) and ask Erica to come up with the reasons why she thinks she would not be fabricating data?

3. Ask to see all of her raw data to help decide how best to proceed?

4. Combinations of the above-listed actions?

5. Or one that is not listed above?

If Dr. Nelson was working with Erica in Singapore, the above-listed options would still apply, as the responsibilities of faculty for students' work are not substantially different from those listed by the APA Ethics Code.

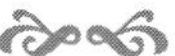

STANDARD 8.10: REPORTING RESEARCH RESULTS

> . . . (b) If psychologists discover significant errors in their published data, they take reasonable steps to correct such errors in a correction, retraction, erratum, or other appropriate publication means.

A CASE FOR STANDARD 8.10 (B): The Unpublished Data set

Dr. Carter's dissertation is a meta-analysis on studies of autism. To increase the strength of the study, Dr. Carter contacted some already-published authors for any unpublished studies. Dr. Mitchell sent him two studies that had shown no effect and were unpublished. With Dr. Mitchell's permission, Dr. Carter included the unpublished studies from Dr. Mitchell in his dissertation. The dissertation was defended, and Dr. Carter was duly graduated.

A few months after graduation, Dr. Mitchell contacted Dr. Carter. After sending her unpublished data to him she had decided to take a second look at the data set and discovered that there was a mistake in her analysis. Dr. Mitchell tells Dr. Carter that he should not use the analysis she sent him from one of the studies. In fact, the new analysis shows that a treatment effect occurred in the study. Dr. Carter contacts the library of his university and discovers that the dissertation has already been published in *Dissertation Abstracts.*

Issues of Concern

Standard 8.10 directs psychologists to correct any mistakes in published works. Dr. Mitchell took steps to correct a mistake, even though her work was not published. Dr. Carter's work is, however, published. The entry of one's dissertation into the *Dissertation Abstracts* makes the work available to the public. Standard 8.10 (a) directs Dr. Carter to take reasonable steps for corrections. What types of activity are considered reasonable effort? What activities might be deemed appropriate publication means?

APA Ethics Code

Companion General Principle

Principle C: Integrity

> Psychologists seek to promote accuracy . . . in the science, teaching, and practice of psychology. In these activities, psychologists do not . . . engage in . . . intentional misrepresentation of fact.

While Dr. Carter has not engaged in anything that may be considered as intentional misrepresentation, his published dissertation is not accurate. Striving for Principle C: Integrity, Dr. Carter would wish to be accurate.

Companion Ethical Standard(s)

Standard 5.01: Avoidance of False or Deceptive Statements

> (a) Public statements include . . . published materials. Psychologists do not knowingly make public statements that are false . . . concerning their research.

Dr. Carter, unbeknownst to him, has made a false public statement and thus violated Standard 5.01 (a).

Standard 1.01: Misuse of Psychologists' Work

> If psychologists learn of . . . misrepresentation of their work, they take reasonable steps to correct or minimize the . . . misrepresentation.

Not knowing who might make use of the information in his dissertation, Standard 1.01 directs Dr. Carter to take reasonable steps to correct the dissertation.

Legal Issues 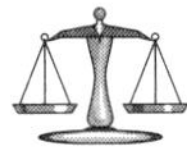

Florida

> *Florida Statute 490.009 (2010). Discipline.*
>
> (1) The following acts constitute grounds for denial of a license or disciplinary action, as specified in s. 456.072(2)[:] . . .
>
> (l) Making . . . untrue, or fraudulent representations in the practice of any profession licensed under this chapter. . .
>
> (r) Failing to meet the minimum standards of performance in professional activities when measured against generally prevailing peer performance.

Hawaii

> *Haw. Code R. § 16-98-34 (2010). Unethical Practice of Psychology.*
>
> (1) Psychologists who interpret the science of psychology . . . have an obligation to report fairly and accurately[;] . . . misrepresentation shall be avoided.

As long as Dr. Carter attempts to correct the erroneous findings that were published, he would not violate the laws of either jurisdiction.

Cultural Considerations

Global Discussion

The New Zealand Psychological Society Code of Ethics

> 8: Publication and public statements.
>
> 8.4. Where incorrect . . . reports have been given in reference to the work of a psychologist, all reasonable steps are taken to correct the error.

Dr. Carter must make "all reasonable" effort to correct the errors that are now, inadvertently and through no fault of his, a part of his published dissertation. How he does that, or what may constitute "reasonable," are specific details on which New Zealand's code is silent. Nonetheless, Dr. Carter is charged with correcting the errors in his dissertation.

American Moral Values

1. Does Dr. Carter's dissertation depend on Dr. Mitchell's data? Does the retraction of her analysis threaten the core of his argument? How much does his use of her mistaken analysis undermine his project?
2. Now that the dissertation is published in *Dissertation Abstracts,* what steps can Dr. Carter take to prevent its readers from being misled about his project? Is there an addendum that could be promptly added?
3. Does Dr. Carter owe his dissertation committee, department, and university any kind of retraction? Would they need to be aware of the addendum he might make? Does it make a difference *when* Dr. Mitchell discovered her error? What if she had discovered it 20 years after Dr. Carter had graduated? Would it still make sense to contact the committee, department, and university to consider action about it?

4. Did Dr. Carter examine unpublished data with due diligence? Was it Dr. Mitchell's responsibility to check her analysis? Was Dr. Carter acting within standard scholarly practice to incorporate Dr. Mitchell's findings without going back over her analysis?

Ethical Course of Action

Directive per APA Code

Standard 8.10 (b) calls for Dr. Carter to take reasonable steps to correct his published dissertation. Making these corrections would accomplish the accuracy suggested in Principle C: Integrity; comply with Standard 5.01: Avoidance of false statements; and guard against anyone misusing his work, as outlined in Standard 1.01. If Dr. Carter had published in a journal, he would most probably submit a correction to be included in any subsequent publication of the same journal. Under the circumstances, many options are open to Dr. Carter. However, one option that is precluded is for Dr. Mitchell not to attempt to correct the accuracy of what has been published.

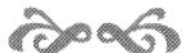

Dictates of One's Own Conscience

If you were Dr. Carter, having defended your dissertation and graduated already, receiving notice from Dr. Mitchell, which of these would you do with the information?

1. Reanalyze everything, and see if the corrected information from Dr. Mitchell makes any difference to your results.
2. Submit an addendum to *Dissertation Abstracts* explaining the problem and recommend that no one use your dissertation.
3. Contact the chair of your dissertation committee to let him or her know of the problem and ask for further direction.
4. Contact the chair of your department to let him or her know of the problem and ask for further direction.
5. Contact the university, chair of the department, and chair of your dissertation committee to retract your full dissertation.
6. Combinations of the above-listed actions.
7. Or one that is not listed above.

If you were Dr. Carter who earned his graduate psychology degree from a program in New Zealand, the above-listed options would still apply since the responsibility of making corrections to published works is not substantially different from that listed by the APA Ethics Code.

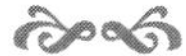

STANDARD 8.11: PLAGIARISM

Psychologists do not present portions of another's work or data as their own, even if the other work or data source is cited occasionally.

A CASE FOR STANDARD 8.11: Who Copied Whom?

Leo and Dolores have formed a close supportive bond since the first days of their studies at the Modern School of Psychology in the New Center University. They have taken most of their courses together and helped support each other through their many assignments. They have chosen very different topics for their dissertations, but both have chosen to use the same research method. It is not uncommon for Leo and Dolores to engage in many hours of discussion on their research projects, to read each other's documents and give feedback/critique. At one point, Dolores asks Leo if she could use some of his wording in the methods section in her dissertation write-up. After such long association and mutual support, and not thinking a few sentences in a document as large as a dissertation would be of significant impact, Leo says yes. Dolores passes her defense and lavishly praises Leo in the acknowledgments section of her dissertation.

A month after Dolores's defense, Leo submits his dissertation to Dr. Perez, chair of his dissertation committee. Leo receives an invitation to meet with Dr. Roberts, chair of the psychology program, concerning his dissertation. At his meeting, Dr. Roberts notifies Leo that the program is proceeding with dismissal based on charges of plagiarism. As evidence, Dr. Roberts points to complete parallel organization of his methods section and one paragraph being a verbatim duplication of the methods section in Dolores's dissertation document. Leo claims that he did not copy Dolores, but that Dolores had copied his work.

Issues of Concern

Standard 8.11 prohibits liberal use of another person's work, regardless of whether the source is acknowledged. This means that neither Delores nor Leo is to use each other's work as liberally as they apparently have in the methods section of the manuscript. One month's time between submission of documents does not seem to be sufficient to definitely say Leo was the person who plagiarized Dolores. In the long run, is it possible to say who copied whom if Dolores and Leo had been continuously discussing the ideas in their writing? Does Dolores's acknowledgment of Leo's support give credence to his not being guilty of plagiarism? If neither Dolores nor Leo were guilty of plagiarism, how might Leo proceed to prove that he did not copy Dolores's work, or that Dolores had asked permission from him to use some of his writing in her dissertation?

APA Ethics Code

Companion General Principle

Principle C: Integrity

> Psychologists seek to promote . . . honesty . . . and truthfulness in the science . . . of psychology. In these activities psychologists do not . . . cheat.

It is not possible to have word-for-word duplication of one full paragraph without one person copying the other. The value of Principle C: Integrity would prohibit cheating by copying someone else's work. Even if the copying were not intentional, the spirit of intellectual property would suggest to both Dolores and Leo that they need to keep meticulous track of their sources.

Companion Ethical Standard(s)

Standard 6.01: Documentation of Professional and Scientific Work and Maintenance of Records

> Psychologists create . . . [and] maintain . . . data relating to their . . . scientific work in order to . . . (2) allow for replication of research design and analyses . . . [and] (5) ensure compliance with law.

One's dissertation is scientific work. Standard 6.01 requires that psychologists create a record of that work. To meet the requirements of Standard 6.01, Leo and Dolores would each have kept careful records of their research. Does part of the record include progressive drafts of one's manuscript? Is it possible for Leo to recreate the progression of this writing so as to provide some evidence that the paragraph in question was written in one of his numerous drafts?

Standard 7.06: Assessing Student and Supervisee Performance

> . . . (b) Psychologists evaluate students . . . on the basis of their actual performance on relevant and established program requirements.

Certainly a standard academic requirement is integrity of one's work and absence of plagiarism. The faculty was following the directives of Standard 7.06 (b) when they acted on evidence of plagiarism in Leo's dissertation.

Legal Issues 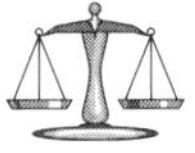

Indiana

> *868 Ind. Admin. Code 1.1-11-4.1 (2010). Relationships Within Professional Practice.*
>
> (l) A psychologist shall exercise reasonable care and diligence in the conduct of research.

Kansas

> *Kan. Admin. Regs. § 102-1-10a (2010). Unprofessional Conduct.*
>
> (a) Practicing psychology in an incompetent manner, which shall include the following acts[:] . . .
>
> (2) performing professional services that are inconsistent with the licensee's education, training, or experience; and . . .
>
> (h) misrepresenting the services offered or provided, which shall include the following acts[:] . . .
>
> (5) taking credit for work not personally performed.

In both jurisdictions, Dolores and Leo would likely be found to have violated the law. In Indiana, they are likely to be found to have failed to follow generally acceptable research practices. In Kansas, Leo would be found to have engaged in a professional service that permitted Dolores to take credit for work she did not perform. Both would likely be found guilty of breaking the law.

Cultural Considerations

Global Discussion

Canadian Code of Ethics for Psychologists

> Principle III: Integrity in relationships.
>
> III.1. Not knowingly participate in, condone, or be associated with dishonesty.
>
> III.7. Take credit only for the work and ideas that they have actually done or generated, and give credit for work done or ideas contributed by others (including students), in proportion to their contribution.

Both Dolores and Leo are in violation of this portion of Canada's code, and both are responsible for the outcome and the decision of their school. When Leo allowed Dolores to use his finished dissertation draft, he violated III 1. by "knowingly" condoning dishonesty, fraud, or misrepresentation. When Dolores copied Leo's work onto her own, even though she thanked him in her acknowledgments section, she became guilty of misrepresentation, even with Leo's permission to do so. Dolores also violated III.7 when she did not disclose that a paragraph of her methods section was, in fact, written by Leo, not by her.

American Moral Values

1. Do Dr. Roberts and Dr. Perez believe it is only fair to investigate Leo's countercharge of plagiarism? Even if Leo is correct, do they believe he should have been more careful with his dissertation materials? Do they believe that friendships between students should not be allowed to interfere with the integrity of one's work?

2. What would be the fairest way to proceed in investigating this issue? Should Dolores first be confronted with the situation and asked if she plagiarized? What will be the consequences for her career if she admits to plagiarism? What will happen if she pleads ignorance or claims that Leo must have plagiarized her? Should Dolores be required to submit her documents and notes to compare with Leo's?

3. If Leo's story checks out, should he and Dolores both be punished for his initial agreement to let Dolores borrow some of his wording for her methods section?

4. What will happen with Leo and Dolores's respective careers moving forward? Will the university allow one to graduate but not the other? Will the department write recommendations for one or both? Will the department and the university try to defuse any harm this case might cause to the two students' reputations? What kind of message does the department need to send to present and future students?

5. Was Leo and Dolores's partnership ever noted in the department before this point? Has it been an accepted practice for students to collaborate so closely? Were there ever any discussions about how writing papers in close collaboration could cross the line into plagiarism of one another's work? Does the department need to warn present and future students about how to set limits in one's collaborative relationships?

Ethical Course of Action

Directive per APA Code

Leo is in violation of Standard 8.11 because his was the second submission, regardless of whether Delores copied his work or not. Leo counter-claimed that Dolores was the one who plagiarized. The faculty appropriately acted in compliance with Standard 7.06 (b).

In the best of all possible worlds, with all psychologists meeting the aspirational Principle C: Fidelity and Responsibility, perhaps neither Dolores nor Leo had plagiarized, but merely kept sloppy notes. If Dolores and Leo had collaborated very closely and developed their ideas in tandem, Leo may be able to provide evidence of the evolution of his work if he meticulously followed the directive of Standard 6.01.

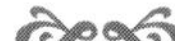

Dictates of One's Own Conscience

If you were Leo, what evidence might you produce to defend yourself against the charge of plagiarism?

1. Turn over your computer to have all drafts of your manuscript time stamped.
2. Produce all of your various drafts to give time-stamped evidence of when you wrote the paragraph in question.
3. Ask Dolores to do the same with her computer.
4. Ask Dolores to have a joint meeting with Drs. Perez and Roberts; perhaps include the chair of Dolores's dissertation committee.

If you were Drs. Roberts or Perez, faced with Leo's claim that Dolores took his work, which of these actions would you take?

1. Refer the matter to the university's student grievance committee.
2. Meet individually with Dolores and Leo.
3. Request that both Dolores and Leo turn over their computers for university-sponsored independent analysis of the various drafts of their dissertations.
4. Hold a special meeting of the full faculty to deliberate on the matter after a forensic document specialist has analyzed Leo and Dolores's computers.
5. Consult with a university attorney as to how best to proceed.
6. Seek information about what is known of the character of each student prior to dissertation submission.
7. Combinations of the above-listed actions.
8. Or one that is not listed above.

If you were Drs. Roberts or Perez, faced with a possible situation of plagiarism, and you hear Leo's claim that Dolores took his work, which of these would you do?

1. First rescind the award of a doctorate degree to Dolores.
2. Request that both Dolores and Leo turn over their computers for university-sponsored independent analyses of the various drafts of their dissertations.
3. Hold a special meeting of the full faculty to deliberate on the matter after a forensic document specialist has analyzed Leos and Dolores' computers.

STANDARD 8.12: PUBLICATION CREDIT

> (a) Psychologists take responsibility and credit, including authorship credit, only for work they have actually performed or to which they have substantially contributed.

A CASE FOR STANDARD 8.12 (A): Research Individuation—Part I

Michael works as a graduate assistant to Dr. Turner. As part of his duties, Michael is involved with Dr. Turner's research on multicultural competency training. Subsequently, he has been assigned to interview students who participated in Dr. Turner's Multicultural Training course. Michael is interested in a particular aspect of the training that is not under consideration in Dr. Turner's study. He therefore requests and obtains permission from Dr. Turner to insert one extra question in the interview protocol. Michael conducts the interviews and transcribes the responses to Dr. Turner's interview questions, and under Dr. Turner's supervision, analyzes the qualitative data.

Michael decides to use the interview responses from his one question for his dissertation. On his own time, independent of any time working for Dr. Turner, Michael transcribes, analyzes, and writes his dissertation. Simultaneously, Michael writes an article for publication based on the information obtained from that one question. He asks Dr. Turner to review his article before submission to a journal. Dr. Turner returns the paper with minimal edits and puts her own name on the article as first author. Dr. Turner informs Michael that the content of the article came out of her research project; thus, by rights, she is first author for any publication.

Issues of Concern

Standard 8.12 (a) requires that authorship for publication is claimed only if one has either done the work or in some other way substantially contributed to the work. Surely Dr. Turner cannot make claim of first authorship based on work actually performed. Dr. Turner could argue that she was the person who developed the research design, and Michael's data collection was done while under her employment. Is it understandable for Dr. Turner to claim first authorship based on substantial contribution? What amounts to substantial contribution?

APA Ethics Code

Companion General Principle

Principle C: Integrity

> Psychologists seek to promote accuracy, honesty, and truthfulness in the science . . . [and] teaching . . . of psychology. In these activities, psychologists do not steal.

Principle C: Integrity suggests psychologists accurately attribute work to appropriate persons. In this situation, is it Michael who is dishonest as to the context of his data? Or is it Dr. Turner who is dishonest about how much of her own work was put into the article?

Companion Ethical Standard(s)

Standard 3.08: Exploitative Relationships

> Psychologists do not exploit persons over whom they have . . . evaluative . . . authority such as . . . students.

Michael is the person who thought of his own dissertation question and who put in the time to conduct the interviews, to transcribe the recordings, to analyze the transcripts, and to write the article. Based on these activities, is Dr. Turner's claim to first authorship one that is purely based on her position as someone with evaluative authority over Michael? Has Dr. Turner exploited Michael?

Standard 1.04: Informal Resolution of Ethical Violations

> When psychologists believe that there may have been an ethical violation by another psychologist, they attempt to resolve the issue by bringing it to the attention of that individual.

Having both Dr. Turner and Michael claiming first authorship, at a minimum, is a conflict. Michael might experience Dr. Turner's claiming first authorship as taking unfair advantage of him as a student. If so, the situation would fall under Standard 1.04 for method of resolution.

Legal Issues 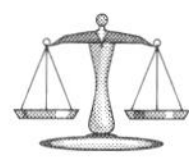

Kentucky

> *201 Ky. Admin. Regs. 26:145 (2010). Code of Conduct.*
>
> Section 1. Definitions.
>
> (6) "Professional service" means all actions of the credential holder in the context of a professional relationship. . .
>
> (9) "Exploitation" means obtaining or using another person's resources . . . by deception, intimidation, or similar means, with the intent to deprive the person of those resources. . .
>
> Section 8. Representation of Services.
>
> (4) False or misleading information. The credential holder shall not include false or misleading information in a public statement concerning professional services offered.
>
> (5) Misrepresentation of . . . products. The credential holder shall not associate with or permit his or her name to be used in connection with a . . . product in a way which misrepresents . . .
>
> (c) The nature of his or her association with the . . . product.

Maryland

> *Md. Code Regs. 10.36.05.05 (2010). Representation of Services and Fees.*
>
> (2) A psychologist may not . . .
>
> (c) Make public statements that contain:
>
> (i) . . . misleading, or deceptive statements;
>
> (ii) Partial disclosures of relevant facts that misrepresent, mislead, or deceive.
>
> *Md. Code Regs. 10.36.05.07 (2010). Client Welfare.*
>
> B. Exploitation. A psychologist may not:
>
> (1) Exploit . . . students . . . [or]
>
> (3) Exploit the trust and dependency of . . . students . . . and subordinates.

Dr. Turner would have violated the law in both Kentucky and Maryland for misrepresenting her contribution to the project and exploiting Michael by insisting that she take first authorship of the paper. In Kentucky, Michael would violate the law if he allowed the misrepresentation to occur.

Cultural Considerations

Global Discussion

Code of Ethics: Netherlands

> Principle III: Integrity.
>
> III.1.2. Honesty.
>
> III.1.2.1 Avoidance of deception.
>
> The psychologist refrains from any form of deception in his professional conduct.
>
> III.1.2.2 Avoidance of misuse of . . . authority. . .
>
> The psychologist does not misuse . . . the authority that stems from his . . . professional status.
>
> III.1.2.7 Mention of source.

> In presenting scientific . . . work . . . the psychologists adequately refers to his sources, insofar the results or the ideas aren't the results of his own professional activities.

Dr. Turner is engaging in deception by claiming first authorship for Michael's article, even though it was based in large part upon her own research. Also, Dr. Turner misused her authority by demanding that she be listed as first author on Michael's study; would she make the same demand of another psychologist who was not a subordinate? Finally, III.1.2.7 asks that Michael correctly cite and credit Dr. Turner as the source of the original idea from which his research evolved, and to clearly delineate the portion of the work that is his own versus that of Dr. Turner.

American Moral Values

1. What are the competing claims for primary authorship that Dr. Turner and Michael can make? Is Dr. Turner, as the principal investigator of her project, the rightful primary author of any article that stems from her research interviews? Does Michael's original question, appended to the interviews, constitute an independent piece of research that he transcribed, analyzed, and wrote up?
2. How should Michael handle this conflict? Does Dr. Turner have too much power over him for him to confront her as a colleague? Should he be grateful that she allowed him to write up his dissertation on the basis of a question appended to her interviews? Or is she taking advantage of his independent work to gain publishing credit?
3. How much does Michael owe Dr. Turner for the thinking and methodology that he drew upon to arrive at his question? Was his idea parasitic upon the research into multicultural training he performed for Dr. Turner? Did she give him the theoretical framework for testing such training? Is that any different from other scholars who use their mentor's work as a springboard for their original ideas? Or does the fact that Michael used Dr. Turner's research project as a vehicle for his question undermine his independence?
4. Should Dr. Turner give Michael more credit for his question, especially given that he conducted the interviews in which the question was asked? How does she regard the "content" of the article? Is the multicultural training course she teaches what anchors Michael's analysis? What part of his article did she herself write, if any? In what cases should primary authors be able to have such a removed role from writing the actual text?

Ethical Course of Action

Directive per APA Code

Dr. Turner could claim substantial contribution based on being the research study's principal investigator (PI); Michael could claim actual work performed as well as substantial contribution. Standard 8.12: Publication Credit requires that Dr. Turner and Michael come to an agreement about what is substantial contribution and what is actual work performed. Based on the role Dr. Turner holds as faculty with evaluative authority over Michael, making the demand that she be first author appears to be exploitative per Standard 3.08.

Dictates of One's Own Conscience

If you were Michael, which of these would you do?

1. Acknowledge Dr. Turner's authority as PI and thus accept her claim of first authorship.
2. Acknowledge Dr. Turner's authority as PI, decide not to challenge her directly, and move to not submit the article for publication.
3. Acknowledge Dr. Turner's authority as PI, and seek consultation from faculty independent of your university.
4. Challenge Dr. Turner's claim for first authorship as exploitative.
5. Taking the directive of Standard 1.04, ask to talk to Dr. Turner about your differences of opinion.
6. Combinations of the above-listed actions.
7. Or one that is not listed above.

If you were Michael in a graduate program in the Netherlands, what would you do?

1. Acknowledge improper crediting of Dr. Turner's contributions to the article written?
2. Discuss with Dr. Turner how best to acknowledge her contribution to your article, short of first authorship; perhaps as second author?

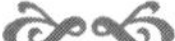

STANDARD 8.12: PUBLICATION CREDIT

> . . . (b) Principal authorship and other publication credits accurately reflect the relative scientific or professional contributions of the individuals involved, regardless of their relative status. Mere possession of an institutional position, such as department chair, does not justify authorship credit. Minor contributions to the research or to the writing for publications are acknowledged appropriately, such as in footnotes or in an introductory statement.

A CASE FOR STANDARD 8.12 (B): When Status Hides Contribution

Gordon is interested in the use of meditation in cancer treatments. Gordon hopes to select some aspect of meditation or cancer treatment for his dissertation, and he reasons that Asian Americans are a good community in which to explore meditation since the practice is congruent with their heritage. Gordon asks Dr. Phillips to sponsor his independent study because she is the one faculty of color in the New School of Psychology and is believed to have connections and access to minority communities.

Dr. Phillips agrees to mentor Gordon for this independent study if Gordon produces (1) a paper based on an extensive review of the published literature on medical use of meditation, and (2) a paper of publication quality for journal submission. Gordon turns in a paper to Dr. Phillips after what he thinks is a great deal of work. Dr. Phillips notes good base data but tells Gordon that his draft needs extensive revision in framing the study and in interpretation of the results. Gordon attempts a revision without substantial improvement. Dr. Phillips makes extensive revision and gives it back to Gordon. She also has declared herself the first author.

Issues of Concern

Standard 8.12 (b) directs psychologists to claim authorship when there is actual evidence of contribution, regardless of institutional status. Dr. Phillips holds the position of faculty, which is of higher status than that of Gordon as a student. Standard 8.12 (b) prohibits Dr. Phillips's claim of first authorship on the grounds of her faculty status alone. Does Dr. Phillips's work in revision of the paper justify first authorship? How much work would a person of higher status need to contribute in order to avoid the accusation of exploitation? Would Gordon feel exploited by Dr. Phillips no matter how much work Dr. Phillips puts into the paper or how much the paper is revised by her?

APA Ethics Code

Companion General Principle

Principle B: Fidelity and Responsibility

> Psychologists . . . clarify their professional roles and obligations . . . and seek to manage conflicts of interest that could lead to exploitation.

Keeping to her professional role of teaching Gordon is what Principle B suggests Dr. Phillips would do. For Dr. Phillips, the conflicting interest would be between remaining faithful to her role as a teacher and addressing professional pressures for publication.

Principle C: Integrity.

> Psychologists seek to promote . . . honesty, . . . in . . . teaching. . . of psychology. In these activities, psychologists do not steal.

Gordon would wish for Dr. Phillips to act with honesty about the amount of contribution she actually made to the paper. For Gordon, the difficulty is in challenging the authority of a professor or being left to perhaps feel exploited.

Companion Ethical Standard(s)

Standard 3.06: Conflict of Interest

> Psychologists refrain from taking on a professional role when . . . professional . . . interests . . . could reasonably be expected to . . . (2) expose the person . . . with whom the professional relationship exists to . . . exploitation.

Standard 3.06 requires Dr. Phillips not to mentor Gordon if such a relationship could lead to exploiting Gordon. Dr. Phillips made the condition for Gordon producing a publishable paper. Could she have avoided this difficult situation by following the directives of Standard 3.06 and by declining to ask for a publishable-quality paper, or deciding not to put in the extra effort when Gordon's work was not of publishable quality?

Standard 3.08: Exploitative Relationships

> Psychologists do not exploit persons over whom they have . . . evaluative . . . authority[,] such as . . . students.

Listing herself as first author on a student's paper certainly appears exploitative. Was there any way for Dr. Phillips to comply with Standard 3.08?

Legal Issues 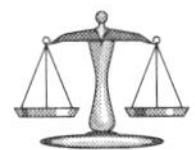

Michigan

> *Mich. Admin. Code r. 338.2515 (2010). Prohibited Conduct.*
>
> Rule 15. Prohibited conduct includes, but is not limited to, the following acts or omissions by any individual covered by these rules[:] . . .
>
> (c) Taking on a professional role when . . . professional . . . relationships could impair the exercise of professional discretion or make the interests of a . . . student secondary to those of the licensee.

Minnesota

> *Minn. R. 7200.5400 (2010). Welfare of Students, Supervisees, and Research Subjects.*
>
> A psychologist shall protect the welfare of psychology students . . . and shall accord the students . . . the client rights listed in parts 7200.4700 and 7200.4900.
>
> *Minn. R. 7200.4900 (2010) Client Welfare.*
>
> **Subp. 7a.** Exploitation of client.
>
> A psychologist must not exploit in any manner the professional relationship with a client for the psychologist's . . . personal advantage or benefit.
>
> **Subp. 11.** Communicating complaints to psychologist or board.
>
> A psychologist informed of conduct of another psychologist which appears to be in violation of any rule of conduct.

Unless the contribution of Dr. Phillips is greater than Gordon's, Dr. Phillips has broken the laws of both jurisdictions by exploiting Gordon.

Cultural Considerations

Global Discussion

Singapore Psychological Society:
Code of Professional Ethics

> Principle 17. Publication credit.
>
> Credit is assigned to those who have contributed to a publication, in proportion to their contributions, and only to these.
>
> 1. Major contributions of a professional character, made by several persons to a common project, are recognised by joint authorship. The experimenter or author who has made the principal contribution to a publication is identified as the first author.
>
> 2. Minor contributions of a professional character, extensive clerical or similar non-professional assistance, and other minor contributions are acknowledged in footnotes or in an introductory statement.

Dr. Phillips's status as a member of faculty or as Gordon's instructor should have nothing to do with how much credit she would receive for her work on Gordon's paper. If Dr. Phillips's self-assignation of first authorship were based more upon her position than the proportion of her work, then she would be in violation of Singapore's code. She would likely also violate the intent of 17.1 by not suggesting "joint authorship."

American Moral Values

1. How did Dr. Phillips assess Gordon's judgment of meditation as "congruent" with Asian Americans? How well does Gordon know Asian American culture and history? Was this part of what hurt his framing and interpretation of results? Was Dr. Phillips's revision a way of showing Gordon what he was missing in his initial takes on meditation and Asian American subjects? If so, was there a better way to make that point?
2. What kind of access does Gordon believe Dr. Phillips has to communities of color? Does Dr. Phillips feel she is set up to be the go-to faculty member for researching communities of color? Does Dr. Phillips need to defend her time more carefully as the only faculty member of color in the department? Was this draft a way of sending a message to Gordon and other students about the expertise needed to research issues with communities of color? What kind of a message

would be sent by Dr. Phillips's revision, where base data is reframed and interpreted by Dr. Phillips as first author? How will this go over with the rest of the department?

3. What was the reason behind editing Gordon's paper and Dr. Phillips putting herself as first author? Was it justified by his first revision not showing much improvement? Should Dr. Phillips have told Gordon beforehand that this was what she was going to do with his piece? Now that she has completed the work, does this put Gordon in too difficult a position to tell her he does not want it published? Is Dr. Phillips abusing her power as a faculty member to get Gordon to publish his base data? Is Gordon's independent study dependent on his agreeing to her arrangement? Should Dr. Phillips pass Gordon for the independent study but offer this secondary author status as a separate consideration?

4. Does Gordon still have a chance to publish something on his own with his data, given enough revisions? Is Dr. Phillips proposing to Gordon that if his data are to be published, they will have to match the kind of quality she has shown through her framing and interpretation? Or has Dr. Phillips basically forced the data to be published her way, since any subsequent revision Gordon did would be difficult to complete without some influence from Dr. Phillips's current draft?

Ethical Course of Action

Directive per APA Code and State Law

Standard 8.12 (b): Publication Credit calls for an evaluative judgment on the relative worth of Dr. Phillips's work versus Gordon's work. To comply with Standard 8.12 (b), Dr. Phillips needs to have made a greater contribution to the paper than Gordon. Unless Dr. Phillips's contribution is unequivocally greater than Gordon's, she is vulnerable to charges of self-interest, violating Standard 3.06, and exploitation, violating Standard 3.08.

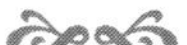

Dictates of One's Own Conscience

If you were Dr. Phillips, faced with a student paper that is less than acceptable quality for publication, which of these would you do?

1. Give him feedback at the level of a term paper.
2. Recommend that he not submit for publication.
3. Return his paper with a requirement for him to rewrite.
4. Tell Gordon that you are only willing to put in the necessary work in revising the paper if you are named first author.

If you were Gordon, faced with this returned paper from Dr. Phillips, which action would you take?

1. See the extent of the revisions and deem her contribution is worthy of first authorship.
2. Thank her for the opportunity to be second author, and submit the paper for publication.
3. Make an appointment to talk to Dr. Phillips about the changes.
4. Ask Dr. Phillips to submit your grade for the independent study, and have no further interactions with Dr. Phillips.
5. Challenge Dr. Phillips on the grounds of Standard 8.12 (b).
6. Combinations of the above-listed actions.
7. Or one that is not listed above.

If you were either Dr. Phillips or Gordon in a graduate program in Singapore, what would you do?

1. Review Gordon's paper at the level of a term paper only?
2. Thank Dr. Phillips for her contribution by offering her second authorship, and ask for permission to submit the paper for publication?

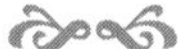

STANDARD 8.12: PUBLICATION CREDIT

. . . (c) Except under exceptional circumstances, a student is listed as principal author on any multiple-authored article that is substantially based on the student's doctoral dissertation. Faculty advisors discuss publication credit with students as early as feasible and throughout the research and publication process as appropriate.

A CASE FOR STANDARD 8.12 (C): Research Individuation— Part II

In A Case for Standard 8.12 (a): Research Individuation—Part I, Michael is faced with Dr. Turner's placement of her own name on his article as first author on the grounds that the content of the article came out of her research project. She thought by rights that she should be first author for any such publication.

Michael responds with objections to Dr. Turner's claim of first authorship. As evidence for the legitimacy of *his* claim to first authorship, Michael reminds Dr. Turner that (1) his dissertation is derived from the analysis of one question from Dr. Turner's data; (2) the one question was devised by Michael and was not originally in Dr. Turner's interview questions; (3) Dr. Turner had given her permission to use data from the existing data set; (4) Dr. Turner has not been involved in his dissertation; and finally, (5) contrary to Standard 8.12 (c), no exceptional circumstances existed to justify her claim to first authorship.

Issues of Concern

Standard 8.12 (c) requires faculty to discuss publication credit early and often. Whatever arrangements were made between Dr. Turner and Michael, it appears that Dr. Turner's actions came as a surprise, eliciting a very strong objection from Michael. Dr. Turner appears to base her claim on ownership of the data as principal investigator. Michael's claim is based on his dissertation. Standard 8.12 (c) permits, under exceptional circumstances, the publication credit to be given to someone other than Michael. What circumstance would qualify as exceptional? Does ownership of a data set qualify as an exceptional circumstance?

APA Ethics Code

Companion General Principle

Principle B: Fidelity and Responsibility

> Psychologists uphold professional standards of conduct, clarify their professional roles and obligations[,] . . . and seek to manage conflicts of interest that could lead to exploitation.

Principle B directs Dr. Turner's attention to circumstances that could lead to exploitation of a student. What possible professional role could allow Dr. Turner to unequivocally make a first author publication claim based on Michael's dissertation?

Companion Ethical Standard(s)

Standard 3.08: Exploitative Relationships

> Psychologists do not exploit persons over whom they have . . . authority such as . . . students.

Standard 3.08 is the companion to Principle B: Fidelity and Responsibility. Standard 3.08 takes an unequivocal stance against exploiting a subordinate. Viewed exclusively from the perspective of role status, it appears that Dr. Turner was in violation of Standard 3.08 when she made claims for any publication credit.

Legal Issues 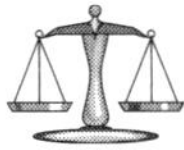

Missouri

> *Mo. Code Regs. Ann. tit. 20, § 2235-5.030 (2010). Ethical Rules of Conduct.*
>
> (8) Welfare of Supervisees, Clients, Research Subjects, and Students.
>
> (A) Welfare of Supervisees and Students.
>
> The psychologist shall not . . . exploit a . . . student in any way. . . The psychologist as a teacher shall recognize that the primary obligation is to help others acquire knowledge and skill.

Montana

> *Mont. Admin. R. 24.189.2309 (2009). Professional Responsibility.*
>
> (2) In regard to respect for others, a licensee:
>
> (a) shall not exploit persons over whom they have . . . authority such as students.

In both jurisdictions, Dr. Turner would be viewed as having violated the laws in her exploitation of Michael. Neither jurisdiction permits exploitation of a student for publication credit because of a claim of exceptional circumstances.

Cultural Considerations

Global Discussion

Canadian Code of Ethics for Psychologists

> Principle III: Integrity in relationships.
>
> *Accuracy/honesty.*
>
> III.7. Take credit only for the work and ideas that they have actually done or generated, and give credit for work done or ideas contributed by others (including students), in proportion to their contribution.

Dr. Turner could argue that she deserves credit for the ideas and original work that led to Michael's dissertation. Dr. Turner's claim to authorship supposes that she has generated the research idea that rightly belongs to Michael. The Canadian code specifies that credit belongs to those who have generated both the work and the ideas, and that it would be dishonest for a faculty member to take undue credit for a student's work. Dr. Turner would be found in violation of this portion of Canada's code. Michael would be correct, however, in naming Dr. Turner's contribution to his dissertation idea, and his article, and disclosing the extent to which her work was the genesis and the springboard for his own.

American Moral Values

1. If work stemming from a dissertation were presumed to have the student as first author, how would Dr. Turner claim exceptional circumstances? Is the fact that Michael's interviews were conducted as part of hers such a circumstance? What makes his original question depend on the content of the whole interview? How interrelated does the question have to be with the rest of the interview for Michael to be able to claim primary authorship of a resulting article?
2. How does Dr. Turner explain her permission for Michael to use the data he gathered from the interviews? Did she think he would just use the data for his dissertation? Was it reasonable to think that he would not try to publish an article on the basis of this research as well?
3. Did Dr. Turner discuss authorship in the timely manner suggested by this standard? Should she have anticipated that he would write an article, and should she have informed him straightaway that she would be the primary author of any article that came from the data? Should she have discussed the issue of publication with Michael before putting her name on a revision of his paper? Was this gesture an attempt at intimidation?
4. Is Michael at a point where he would consider complaining to the department or the university? Would he be willing at this point to risk irreparable harm to his relationship with Dr. Turner?

Ethical Course of Action

Directive per APA Code

A student's dissertation is a substantial amount of work done under the scrutiny of dissertation committee members. The dissertation is protected intellectual property that is attached to the student. Standard 8.12 recognizes the significance of the work by designating the student as the principal author. The exception to this directive is when there are unusual circumstances. Michael seems to have done a thorough job in articulating all the reasons why Dr. Turner does not have a claim for exceptional circumstances that would allow her to make any claims for publication credits, let alone first authorship. In light of Michael's explanations, it appears that Dr. Turner is in violation of Standard 3.08: Exploitative Relationships.

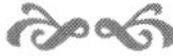

Dictates of One's Own Conscience

If you were Dr. Turner in receipt of Michael's list of objections, which of these would you do?

1. Consult with a colleague to help you determine the legitimacy of Michael's objections.
2. Comment that Michael seems rather touchy and wonder whether he has gotten uppity since graduation.
3. Acknowledge the legitimacy of his objections and apologize.
4. Be taken aback at how you have lost sight of your own integrity.
5. Note that this was done to you, and know these kinds of authorship claims occur all the time in academic settings.
6. Combinations of the above-listed actions.
7. Or one that is not listed above.

If Michael and you, as a professor, were working in Canada, and you were in receipt of Michael's list of objections, what would you do?

1. Negotiate with Michael as an equal?
2. File a complaint with the university and the College of Psychologists (the provincial name for a licensing board)?

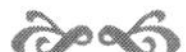

STANDARD 8.13: DUPLICATE PUBLICATION OF DATA

> Psychologists do not publish, as original data, data that have been previously published. This does not preclude republishing data when they are accompanied by proper acknowledgment.

A CASE FOR STANDARD 8.13: The Forever Review Process

Dr. Campbell's primary area of research is in program evaluation. She has developed a model of evaluating psychology training programs that is competency based. Dr. Campbell, in collaboration with Dean, a graduate assistant, was engaged in two related writing projects based on the competency-based evaluation model. One writing project was a small book with a detailed explication of the method; the other was a journal article reporting on the evaluation of the training program at the Modern School of Psychology in the New Center University. Given that the book was very small, the project was on a short timeline with the publisher. The journal article, though written and submitted, had not been accepted for publication. Therefore, Dr. Campbell could not reference the article in her book. Instead of referencing the journal article, Dr. Campbell had to use the same information as that used in the article when she wrote her book.

After several rounds of revisions, the journal article was finally published, but this was after the book had already gone to press.

Issues of Concern

Following the directive of Standard 8.13 means that a psychologist avoids the phenomenon of multiple articles by the same author based on the same set of data. Due to awkward timing of the publication process, Dr. Campbell did not reference herself, as directed in Standard 8.13, but instead replicated the same data from the same study in two different publications. Was there any way for Dr. Campbell to have avoided the resultant violation of Standard 8.13?

APA Ethics Code

Companion General Principle

Principle C: Integrity

> Psychologists seek to promote . . . honesty [and] and truthfulness in the science . . . of psychology. In these activities, psychologists do not . . . engage in . . . intentional misrepresentation of fact.

Principle C: Integrity would have all psychologists be honest and truthful under all circumstances. If psychologists cannot be honest and truthful, they are at a minimum at least not to intentionally misrepresent facts. Publications are original works; when data is duplicated in two different published works, it misrepresents the work as original in both publications.

Companion Ethical Standard(s)

Standard 5.01: Avoidance of False or Deceptive Statements

> (a) Public statements include . . . published materials. Psychologists do not knowingly make public statements that are . . . fraudulent concerning their research.

The enforceable aspect of Principle C: Integrity is Standard 5.01 (a). Standard 5.01 (a) requires psychologists not to be fraudulent. Replicating the same data under two different publications, without referencing the other publication, fraudulently represents each of the publications as original. Albeit unintentionally, did Dr. Campbell knowingly allow for both publications to go forward without duly referencing the other publication.

Legal Issues 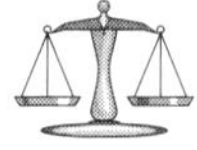

Nevada

> *NAC 641.239 Misrepresentation of . . . Psychological Findings. (NRS 641.100).*
>
> 6. A psychologist shall not distort . . . [or] misuse . . . any psychological finding, and shall attempt to prevent . . . the

distortion . . . [or] misuse . . . of any psychological finding by any institution of which he is an employee.

New Jersey

N.J. Admin. Code § 13:42-10.6 (2010). Research.

(a) A licensee shall observe research requirements consistent with accepted standards of practice including, but not limited to, the following:

1. A licensee shall minimize the possibility that research findings will be misleading and shall not knowingly publish misleading . . . findings;

2. A licensee shall provide thorough discussion of the limitations of the published data.

Dr. Campbell misrepresented the findings in both publications by not conveying that one data set was drawn upon. Certainly, a discussion about one data set being used for both publications is a limitation that was not addressed.

Cultural Considerations

Global Discussion

Canadian Code of Ethics for Psychologists

Principle III: Integrity in relationships.

III.19. . . . [P]resent . . . and discuss research in a way that is consistent with a commitment to honest, open inquiry, and . . . clear communication of any research aims . . . that might affect or appear to affect the research.

Canada's code demands in III.19 that all research be carried out with honesty, transparency, and clarity. Dr. Campbell knowingly misrepresented both publications with one data set as original; she could be found in violation of III.19.

American Moral Values

1. What is the value behind this standard of original research? Is it meant to maintain a scholarly standard of original work for publication? Does it maintain research discipline? Is Dr. Campbell supposed to wait for the journal article to be published before publishing her book, or should she withdraw her article until the book is finished? Would either of those options prevent the scholarly community from being deceived?

2. Did Dr. Campbell have a way to avoid presenting the same data as original in two separate publications? Is it a common and understandable occurrence for journal articles and books to be on conflicting publishing schedules? Did Dr. Campbell have any help from colleagues or her publishers with how to manage this kind of problem?

3. Does Dr. Campbell have a good relationship with her press and the journal? Would it be out of line or unprofessional to pressure the journal to help resolve the question of publishing the article? Does she need to delay the book's publication?

4. Does Dr. Campbell fear for her reputation if other scholars wonder about her citations? Would her publications be seen as unnecessarily close in timing? Would it be attributed to seeking tenure, or laziness, or would it be seen as an understandable problem? Is there a form of acknowledgment in the book that could be transparent about the conflict?

Ethical Course of Action

Directive per APA Code

Once published, the work stands on its own without caveat. Dr. Campbell now has two different publications with the same data without proper acknowledgment of each other. Regardless of how understandable or seemingly unavoidable, Dr. Campbell is in violation of Standard 8.13.

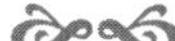

Dictates of One's Own Conscience

If you were Dr. Campbell, knowing the directive of Standard 8.13, which of these would you do?

1. Claim you did not knowingly duplicate the data, as allowable under Standard 5.01 (a).

2. Try to stop the press for the book so you could insert a reference to the journal article.

3. Try to revise the journal article to reference the book.

4. Resend the journal article giving duplication of data as the reason.

5. Combinations of the above-listed actions.

6. Or one that is not listed above.

If you were Dr. Campbell working in Canada, the above-listed options would still apply since the guideline for publication of original data is not substantially different from that listed by the APA Ethics Code.

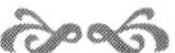

STANDARD 8.14: SHARING RESEARCH DATA FOR VERIFICATION

> (a) After research results are published, psychologists do not withhold the data on which their conclusions are based from other competent professionals who seek to verify the substantive claims through reanalysis and who intend to use such data only for that purpose, provided that the confidentiality of the participants can be protected and unless legal rights concerning proprietary data preclude their release. This does not preclude psychologists from requiring that such individuals or groups be responsible for costs associated with the provision of such information.

A CASE FOR STANDARD 8.14 (A): Research Individuation— Part III

In A Case for Codes 8.12 (a) and 8.12 (c), Michael defends his work against encroachment from Dr. Turner. Dr. Turner is not yet ready to publish because she is using a larger set of data as well as her whole course design. So Michael's dissertation is the first publication based off of Dr. Turner's project.

Yvonne contacts Michael while authorship between Michael and Dr. Turner is being contested. Yvonne, a graduate assistant for Dr. Sanchez at the Midwest School of Professional Psychology, has been charged by Dr. Sanchez to look for new ideas and approaches to designing multicultural courses, including looking through the *Dissertation Abstracts.* Yvonne says that Dr. Sanchez is intrigued with Michael's theories. He would like to determine if the theory is applicable and could be used for the multicultural course at the Midwest School of Professional Psychology. Dr. Sanchez is asking for the data to review the work in order to find out if it is applicable. To this request, Michael replies that (1) he only used a small part of the data set; (2) the larger portion of the data set, including pedagogical methods, belongs to Dr. Turner; (3) Dr. Turner has not given him permission to release the data set; and (4) his analysis was based on established grounded theory. Grounded theory considers all information, regardless of source, as data. Thus, Michael could not replicate all of the disparate threads of information that influenced his thinking as he was writing his dissertation.

Issues of Concern

Dissertation Abstracts is in the public domain. Thus, Michael's dissertation is within the province of Standard 8.14 (a) as published research results. Standard 8.14 (a) requires that Michael release his data to anyone who requests it. The conditions under which he may refuse release are the following: if the data are to be used for verification of the research results, if the release would compromise confidentiality of research participants, or if the data legally belong to someone else. One of the reasons Michael gives Yvonne for not releasing his data is the claim that the data are someone else's property. Could Michael reasonably deny the release based on the fact that Dr. Sanchez is not using the data to verify results, but rather to develop a different application?

APA Ethics Code

Companion General Principle

Principle B: Fidelity and Responsibility

> Psychologists . . . are aware of their . . . scientific responsibilities to society and to the specific communities in which they work.

One scientific responsibility is to make available their work for the purpose of verification and duplication. To meet the highest aspirational values of responsibility would be for Michael to have his research data available for examination.

Companion Ethical Standard(s)

Standard 6.01: Documentation of Professional and Scientific Work and Maintenance of Records

> Psychologists create, and to the extent the records are under their control, maintain, disseminate, store, retain, and dispose of . . . data relating to their . . . scientific work in order to . . . (2) allow for replication of research design and analyses.

As explicitly stated in Standard 6.01 (2), Michael is required to disseminate his stored research data. At a minimum, Michael is to have created data from his research. Does his claim that research methodology precludes the creation of, and therefore the ability to disseminate, his research data stand up to scientific scrutiny, and thereby release him of his obligations under Standard 8.10?

Standard 8.10: Reporting Research Results

> (a) Psychologists do not fabricate data.

If a scientist is unable to produce his or her research data, how is it possible to verify that the results are real and not fabricated? For Michael to claim his research methodologies preclude the creation of research data appears to be an excuse that leads to a violation of Standard 8.10.

Legal Issues 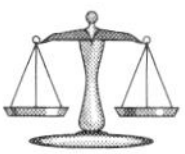

New Mexico

> *N.M. Code R. § 16.22.2.13 (2010). Disclosure and Misrepresentation of Services.*
>
> **A. Definition of public statements.** Public statements include but are not limited to . . . printed matter. . .
>
> F. Promotion of psychological services and products.
>
> (1) The psychologist shall offer his/her . . . publications in an accurate and truthful manner. . . The psychologist shall be guided by the primary obligation to aid the public in forming their own informed judgments, opinions, and choices.

New York

> *N.Y. Comp. Codes R. & Regs. tit. 8, § 29.1 (2010). General Provisions.*
>
> b. Unprofessional conduct in the practice of any profession licensed . . . shall include:
>
> 1. willful or grossly negligent failure to comply with substantial provisions of Federal, State or local laws, rules or regulations governing the practice of the profession.

It only appears that Michael's failure to release his data set to Dr. Sanchez violates the law in New Mexico. New York does not appear to have any specific law, rule, or regulation that directs Michael to release his data set to a colleague who makes a reasonable request to review the data set.

Cultural Considerations

Global Discussion

Canadian Code of Ethics for Psychologists

> Principle III: Integrity in relationships.
>
> III.21. Encourage and not interfere with the free and open exchange of psychological knowledge . . . between . . . colleagues. . .
>
> Principle IV: Responsibility to society.
>
> *Development of knowledge.*
>
> IV.1. Contribute to the discipline of psychology . . . through free . . . transmission . . . and expression of knowledge and ideas, unless such activities conflict with other basic ethical requirements.
>
> IV.2. Not interfere with . . . free . . . transmission . . . of knowledge and ideas that do not conflict with other basic ethical requirements.

Canada's code demands that one "not interfere" with the open and free exchange of information. If Michael's release of his data set could conflict with other requirements under Canada's code, then he could refuse Dr. Sanchez's request without being in violation of IV.2. Otherwise, to refuse a request to release the data set behind his research study violates Canada's code.

American Moral Values

1. How does Dr. Sanchez assess Michael's reasons for refusal? Is it enough that the data set from which Michael drew is not his to release? What is the small part Michael used, and how does it relate to the rest of the research data? If the data are not Michael's, does Dr. Sanchez begin to wonder if Michael's theory is originally his?
2. Does the issue of proprietary rights indicate to Dr. Sanchez a conflict between Michael and Dr. Turner? Should Dr. Sanchez contact Dr. Turner about the data? Would this threaten his relationship with Michael? How does Dr. Sanchez believe his course will receive the most assistance? Is he concerned with having these two as colleagues in the future?
3. What does it mean to Dr. Sanchez that Michael claims to have worked from "grounded theory"? Does this

compound the problem of having only used a small part of the data set belonging to Dr. Turner? Should Dr. Sanchez hold off on soliciting Michael for information about "his" theories until he sees Dr. Turner's data set?

4. Should Michael have been more specific with Dr. Sanchez about the circumstances of his work with Dr. Turner? Given that Dr. Sanchez is working on a course in multicultural training, should Michael have been open about the course Dr. Turner taught and the interviews used to assess that course? How much of Michael's use of "grounded theory" relies upon Dr. Turner's work on multicultural training? Would acknowledging such debts to Dr. Sanchez establish Michael's good faith as a scholar, at the expense of getting as much credit from Dr. Sanchez as he might have otherwise? Would it show Dr. Sanchez that he can rise above dispute over authorship?

Ethical Course of Action

Directive per APA Code

Standard 8.14 (a) requires that Michael release his research data for the purpose of verification unless such release violates confidentiality of subjects or proprietary information. Michael gives two reasons for not releasing his research data: No data were created, and parts of the data belong to someone else. As the requested data belong to Dr. Turner, their release by Michael would, in fact, violate the protection of proprietary information; to refuse the request would be in compliance with Standard 8.14 (a). The claim that the research data were not created denies Michael's scientific responsibility, Principle B, and thus violates the dictates of Standard 6.01 (2) and interferes with the scientific community's necessary ability to assure his results are not fabricated, Standard 8.10.

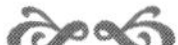

Dictates of One's Own Conscience

If you were Dr. Sanchez in receipt of a denial for research data from Michael with his stated reasons, which of these would you do?

1. Figure this was one more dead end and do nothing.
2. Contact Dr. Turner for the data.
3. Mention to Dr. Turner the denial from Michael and see what she says.
4. Write back to Michael advising him to alter his results if his research method precluded the creation of research data.
5. Make a mental note about Michael in case you run into him in the future.
6. Combinations of the above-listed actions.
7. Or one that is not listed above.

If Dr. Sanchez and Michael were in Canada, the above-listed options would still apply since the guideline for research data is not substantially different from that listed by the APA Ethics Code.

STANDARD 8.14: SHARING RESEARCH DATA FOR VERIFICATION

> . . . (b) Psychologists who request data from other psychologists to verify the substantive claims through reanalysis may use shared data only for the declared purpose. Requesting psychologists obtain prior written agreement for all other uses of the data.

A CASE FOR STANDARD 8.14 (B): Alternative Conclusions

Dr. Parker, an active duty military psychologist, is charged with the psychological treatment of soldiers evacuated from parts of the Middle East. Curious about how his counterparts in other units are handling the treatment demands, Dr. Parker conducts a survey of active duty psychologists. The survey asks whether psychologists have the necessary resources to provide psychological treatment. Not surprisingly, the survey indicated a lack of sufficient resources. Surprisingly, the survey also generated unsolicited comments from psychologists on the deleterious effects of a military culture on mental health.

Dr. Parker submits a request for more personnel resources in combat zones and cites the results of his study as evidence of need. Dr. Parker's report also includes findings about the deleterious effects of military culture on mental health. A short time later, General Evans's office contacts Dr. Parker with a request to obtain his survey data. The primary reason given for General Evans's request is to verify the evidence of need. Dr. Parker supplies General Evans's office with all data from his survey study.

Some time later, General Evans's office issues a report that cites that the conclusions were based on Dr. Parker's survey. However, the report released by General Evans arrives at a very different set of results and excludes any mention of findings based on the unsolicited comments.

Issues of Concern

Standard 8.14 (b) states that psychologists may use shared data, but only for declared purposes. General Evans's declared purpose was to verify Dr. Parker's conclusions for increased supply needs, which he did do. However, in addition, General Evans used the survey data for a very different purpose. If General Evans had been a psychologist, he would be in violation of Standard 8.14 (b). However, General Evans is not a psychologist and is therefore not bound by Standard 8.14 (b). Should Dr. Parker have released the raw data to General Evans? Could Dr. Parker have refused the release of raw data?

APA Ethics Code

Companion General Principle

Principle D: Justice.

> Psychologists recognize that fairness and justice entitle all persons to access to and benefit from the contributions of psychology and to equal quality in the processes, procedures, and services being conducted by psychologists.

It is probably the principle of justice that motivated Dr. Parker to conduct the survey and to act on the results of the survey. Principle D: Justice directs psychologists to provide equal access to all military personnel who are in need. It appears that Dr. Parker was enacting the value in Principle D when he sent in the request for increased resources based on the survey results.

Companion Ethical Standard(s)

Standard 1.01: Misuse of Psychologists' Work

> If psychologists learn of misuse or misrepresentation of their work, they take reasonable steps to correct or minimize the misuse or misrepresentation.

Dr. Parker learns of General Evans's misuse of his work when he reads the different results reported by General Evans. Once having learned of the misrepresentation of the survey results, per Standard 1.01, Dr. Parker is to take reasonable steps to correct the misrepresentation. What might those reasonable steps be for Dr. Parker?

Standard 1.03, Conflicts Between Ethics and Organizational Demands

> If the demands of an organization . . . for whom they are working are in conflict with this Ethics Code, psychologists clarify the nature of the conflict, make known their commitment to the Ethics Code, and take reasonable steps to resolve the conflict consistent with the General Principles and Ethical Standards of the Ethics Code.

Learning that General Evans has misused his work, Dr. Parker is now in the awkward position of having two conflicting demands—one to speak up about the misuse of his research and to correct the misinformation from General Evans's report, and the other to uphold the decision of a commanding general.

Legal Issues 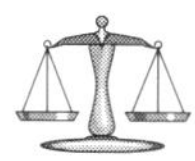

Ohio

> *Ohio Admin. Code 4732:17-01 (2010). General rules of professional conduct pursuant to section 4732.17 of the Revised Code.*
>
> (B) Negligence . . .
>
> (3) Misrepresentation of affiliations. The psychologist . . . shall not misrepresent directly or by implication . . . the . . . characteristics of institutions and organizations with which the psychologist is associated. . .
>
> (d) A psychologist . . . shall not associate with or permit his/her name to be used in connection with any services or products in such a way as to misrepresent them.

Pennsylvania

> *49 Pa. Code § 41.61 (2010). Code of Ethics.*
>
> Principle 1. Responsibility.
>
> (b) As scientists, psychologists accept responsibility for the selection of their research topics and the methods used in investigation, analysis and reporting. They plan

> their research in ways to minimize the possibility that their findings will be misleading. . .
>
> (c) Psychologists clarify in advance with appropriate persons . . . the expectations for sharing and utilizing research data. They avoid relationships that may . . . create a conflict of interest.
>
> (d) Psychologists have the responsibility to attempt to prevent distortion, misuse or suppression of psychological findings by the institution or agency of which they are employees.
>
> (e) As members of governmental or other organizational bodies, psychologists remain accountable as individuals to the highest standards of their profession.

The laws of both jurisdictions call for Dr. Parker to correct General Evans's report that distorted the data that Dr. Parker provided. Although the laws in Ohio are not constructed as specifically as the laws in Pennsylvania, psychologists will be held to high standards in protecting others from irresponsible acts.

Cultural Considerations

Global Discussion

Code of Ethics for the Psychologist: Spain

> ***Article 24.*** Psychologists must refuse to provide their services whenever they are certain that these will be misused or used against the legitimate interests of individuals, groups . . . or communities.
>
> ***Article 4.*** Psychologists must reject any kind of impediment or hindrance to their professional independence and to the legitimate practice of their profession, within the frame of rights and duties outlined in this Code.

Dr. Parker is mandated to refuse to provide that service (in this case, his research data) to General Evans once it becomes evident that General Evans will or has misused information in Dr. Parker's report. As Dr. Parker was not aware in advance of General Evans's report, that he would misuse the information or not include relevant information, Dr. Parker has unwittingly violated Spain's code. Dr. Parker's actions must now be informed by Article 4. At issue is whether Dr. Parker's duty as a psychologist outweighs or obligates his actions more than his position in the military. Spain's code says that if Dr. Parker's capacity to act in accordance with the practices of the code of ethics is somehow impeded, Dr. Parker must reject such impediment and move to act in accordance with the code. This may mean making known to General Evans his duties as a psychologist; attempting to have the full contents of the survey released publicly; having direct conversations with General Evans to resolve this matter; or, barring successful informal resolution, attempting to go up the chain of command to resolve the matter with whoever supervises General Evans.

American Moral Values

1. How does Dr. Parker view his obligation to the military when set against the code for psychologists? Can he resolve competing loyalties? Is there a way to appeal to this standard of releasing data and get the backing of higher military authorities? Now that the data has already been released, what would Dr. Parker want to happen going forward?
2. Did the general act in bad faith by claiming his conclusions were supported by Dr. Parker's report? Did General Evans look at the comments and just disregard them? Was there another way to interpret the data as not verifying the need Dr. Parker requested? Was there a reason to write off the unsolicited comments, for example, to see them as emotional venting during stressful work?
3. Should Dr. Parker have expected General Evans to force the data to support the conclusion he wanted? Was he in a position within the military headquarters to release the data only on the condition he could preview General Evans's report? Should he have refused from the start to release the data, arguing that the general's staff was not trained sufficiently to read the data?
4. Is Dr. Parker afraid of what his colleagues will think of him now that the data are being used in this manner? Will his reputation suffer for this among psychologists? Will it improve within military circles?
5. What does Dr. Parker owe to the psychologists who participated in the study? Does he need to apologize for how their input was used or not used? Do they need to fear for their confidentiality if their comments offended the general and his staff? Should he have removed the comments, or did he owe it to his colleagues to have their voices heard? Does Dr. Parker have any way to protect their confidentiality beyond what he has done thus far?
6. Is Dr. Parker's main concern with the lack of mental health resources for soldiers, or with the military

culture itself? What is the purpose of including a critique of military culture in a report like this? Could this be seen as gratuitous criticism that was out of place in this kind of report?

7. Should the other military psychologists have known what could have been done with these data? Was it common knowledge that generals would only seek and use data to support their conclusions? Are they responsible for any consequences arising from their comments?

8. Should Dr. Parker resign as a protest against the general's report? Would that serve his purposes? Would it defend the integrity of his work, or would it cast doubt on his conclusions? Would the military be free to disparage his work if he left?

9. Should Dr. Parker go public about how his report was handled? Would that cause more damage than it was worth? Would he be going forth as a psychologist or more as a citizen fighting for the specific cause of mental health for soldiers? How would his actions affect the public's opinion of psychologists?

Ethical Course of Action

Directive per APA Code

Dr. Parker is directed to share his research data from two directions, one a commanding authority, and the other being Standard 8.14: Sharing Research Data for Verification. Standard 8.14 (b) pertains only to psychologists who request data from other psychologists. Dr. Parker is not in violation of Standard 8.14 (b) if he declined to release the survey data. Alternatively, as specified in the second sentence of Standard 8.14 (b), Dr. Parker probably should have requested a written statement about General Evans's intended use of the research data.

Now that Dr. Parker has seen the report issued from General Evans's office based on his research data, Standard 1.01: Misuse of Psychologists' Work obligates him to take some type of action to correct the misrepresentation of his research. Hopefully, resolution of the matter is achieved quickly and to Dr. Parker's satisfaction. However, if not, then Dr. Parker is further required, by Standard 1.03: Conflicts Between Ethics and Organizational Demands to take reasonable steps to resolve the conflict consistent with the general principles and ethical standards of the ethics code.

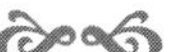

Dictates of One's Own Conscience

If you were Dr. Parker, after reading the report from General Evans, which of these would you do?

1. Take a long walk to calm down.
2. Consult with a colleague to see how other psychologists understand General Evans's report.
3. Contact General Evans's office to follow up on the request for additional resources.
4. Contact General Evans's office to find out who reanalyzed and wrote the report. Make an appointment with that person.
5. Make an appointment to speak to General Evans about his report.
6. Write a letter to General Evans's office voicing your concern per Standard 1.01.
7. Combinations of the above-listed actions.
8. Or one that is not listed above.

If you were Dr. Parker working as a psychologist in the Spanish military, after reading the report from General Evans, which of these actions would you take?

1. Contact General Evans's office to follow up on the request for additional resources.
2. Contact General Evans's office to find out who reanalyzed and wrote the report. Make an appointment with that person and talk about correcting the distortions.
3. Make an appointment to speak to General Evans about his report and talk about correcting the distortions.
4. Write a letter to General Evans's office voicing your concern per Standard 1.01.
5. If the above steps do not resolve the matter, let your concerns be known up the chain of command in the military.
6. If no resolution occurs, publicly publish a correction to General Evans's report based on your data to correct the distortions.

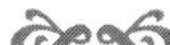

STANDARD 8.15: REVIEWERS

> Psychologists who review material submitted for presentation, publication, grant, or research proposal review respect the confidentiality of and the proprietary rights in such information of those who submitted it.

A CASE FOR STANDARD 8.15: I Can Do It Myself

The Department of Corrections (DOC) has released a request for proposals to provide intervention programs aimed at reducing violence inside correctional facilities. Dr. Edwards works part-time at DOC headquarters and half-time at one of the correctional facilities as a staff psychologist. His job at DOC headquarters includes responsibility for the development of new programs in the correctional facilities. He sits on the review committee for the proposals. One of the submitted proposals pertains to providing workshops on nonviolent communication, followed by mindfulness meditation practice.

Dr. Edwards is intrigued with the study design for meditation and nonviolent communication. Coincidentally, Dr. Edwards is already trained in nonviolent communication and has spent a large portion of time engaged in the practice of meditation. When the governor puts a hold on all new spending for the next fiscal year due to projected budget shortfalls, the DOC stops the review process and cancels all planned new programs. Disappointed that the nonviolent communication and meditation program will not be funded, Dr. Edwards proposes to his supervisor at DOC headquarters that he, with select volunteers, could and would put on this program.

Issues of Concern

Standard 8.15 pertains to Dr. Edwards's work on the review committee for grant proposals. Dr. Edwards is exposed to the design of the nonviolent communication and meditation program through his status as a reviewer for proposals. He comprehends the content of the program based on his own independent training. He sees how the design can be implemented based on his dual role as staff psychologist and headquarters staff member. Faced with the budget shortfall that prohibits the implementation of what Dr. Edwards considers to be a worthy program, it might be understandable that Dr. Edwards would wish to figure out a way to deliver the services to the inmates of the correctional facility. Nonetheless, has Dr. Edwards violated Standard 8.15 and betrayed the proprietary rights of those who submitted their program proposal?

APA Ethics Code

Companion General Principle

Principle B: Fidelity and Responsibility

> Psychologists . . . seek to manage conflicts of interest that could lead to exploitation. . . Psychologists consult with . . . other professionals and institutions to the extent needed to serve the best interests of those with whom they work.

Hopefully, the DOC and Dr. Edwards can be guided by Principle B to consult with organizations that submitted proposals to manage any conflict that might arise from the state's budget shortfall. In the consultation, should the DOC mention its commitment to provide services to the inmates, regardless of whether such services are delivered through their own personnel or through a grant?

Principle C: Integrity

> Psychologists seek to promote . . . honesty . . . in the practice of psychology. In these activities psychologists do not steal, cheat . . . or engage in subterfuge. Psychologists strive to . . . avoid unwise . . . commitments.

There are many gray areas that emerge in situations within the practice of psychology. Given the serendipitous circumstances of the budget freeze and Dr. Edwards's competencies, does his proposal of an intervention program constitute a form of stealing or subterfuge?

Companion Ethical Standard(s)

Standard 3.06: Conflict of Interest

> Psychologists refrain from taking on a professional role when personal[,] . . . professional, legal, financial, or other interests or relationships could reasonably be expected to . . . (2) expose the person or organization with whom the professional relationship exists to harm.

The conflict is between Principle C: Integrity and perhaps Principle A: Beneficence and Nonmaleficence—between respecting the proprietary rights of the grant proposal submitters and the wish to provide a service that could benefit inmates. On a more personal level, Dr. Edwards may have private reasons for wanting to advance his career at the cost of respecting another's proprietary rights.

Standard 8.11 Plagiarism

> Psychologists do not present portions of another's work or data as their own, even if the other work or data source is cited occasionally.

Neither nonviolent communication nor meditation belongs to any one organization. Could the use of these treatment interventions that are in the public domain be considered plagiarism if the DOC or Dr. Edwards acknowledges that some of the interventions are generated from proposals submitted for the now-defunct grant?

Legal Issues 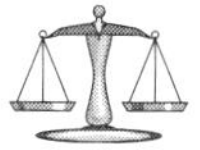

South Carolina

> *S.C. Code Ann. Regs.100-4 (2010). Code of Ethics.*
>
> H. Representation of services. . .
>
> (5) Misrepresentation of services or products. The psychologist shall not associate with or permit his/her name to be used in connection with any services or products in such a way as to misrepresent . . .
>
> (b) The degree of his/her responsibility for the services or products; or
>
> (c) The nature of his/her association with the services or products. . .
>
> K. Violations of law.
>
> (1) Violation of applicable statutes. The psychologist shall not violate any applicable statute or administrative rule regulating the practice of psychology.

Texas

> *22 Tex. Admin. Code § 465.20 (2010). Research.*
>
> (b) Research results. . .
>
> (3) Licensees do not present substantial portions or elements of another individual's research work or data as their own.
>
> (4) Licensees take responsibility and credit, including authorship credit, only for work they have actually performed or to which they have contributed.

In both jurisdictions, Dr. Edwards would violate the laws for running a clinical protocol that he learned about as a reviewer but then used without attribution or permission once the funding for the research team was cut.

Cultural Considerations

Global Discussion

Canadian Code of Ethics for Psychologists

> Principle III: Integrity in relationships.
>
> *Accuracy/honesty.*
>
> III.1. Not knowingly participate in, condone, or be associated with dishonesty, fraud, or misrepresentation.
>
> *Avoidance of conflict of interest.*
>
> III.31. Not exploit any relationship established as a psychologist to further personal . . . or business interests at the expense of the best interests of their clients. . . This includes, but is not limited to . . . using the resources of one's employing institution for purposes not agreed to.

Dr. Edwards is in violation of Article III.1, which demands that he not knowingly participate in or condone dishonesty or fraud. Willfully passing off the ideas of another, regardless of intended or hoped-for positive benefits to the incarcerated members of the prison, is dishonest and fraudulent. Further, Dr. Edwards can also be found in violation of III.31. Dr. Edwards is "using the resources of one's employing institution for purposes not agreed to," by performing the meditation and nonviolent communication program himself. Although his intention is to benefit the prisoners, he is exploiting his position and proprietary knowledge of the submitted confidential proposals for his own gain, and he is using the research proposal submitted to the DOC, his employer, in ways that would clearly not be for the intended purpose.

American Moral Values

1. Is Dr. Edwards being fair to the proposal authors if he goes ahead with a program inspired by the proposal's ideas? Is this a violation of their proprietary rights?

As the person responsible for new program development, how would this action differ from borrowing an idea from an article or scholarly presentation about such an approach? How original does a program have to be, and is there a different standard when it comes to taking material from an actual proposal to one's own department? Would Dr. Edwards be taking advantage of a private proposal instead of a publicly available article?

2. How does Dr. Edwards weigh the circumstances of budget freeze/cuts? Does this proposal have any chance of being accepted and implemented by the DOC in coming years? Would Dr. Edwards's adaptation be the only chance for the program to be executed for the foreseeable future? How important is it to help the inmates and the overall state prison system right now?

3. Does Dr. Edwards have an accurate self-assessment of his training and abilities to implement a program in meditation and nonviolence? What are the risks of badly implementing a program from a proposal sketch alone? Could he harm the cause of these approaches if he performs badly? Should he consult other experts in these interventions? Should he consult the proposal authors, at the risk of their objection to his using their proposal?

4. Could Dr. Edwards's actions create an example for other state governments? Is it unethical to solicit proposals and then adopt an "in-house" version while claiming budget difficulties?

Ethical Course of Action

Directive per APA Code

In his work as a reviewer of grant applications, per Standard 8.15: Reviewers, Dr. Edwards is to respect the proprietary rights of proposal submitters. The ideas and techniques of nonviolent communication and meditation are generally widely known and not proprietary. The implementation strategy outlined in the proposal, however, may be unique and proprietary. If Dr. Edwards, in his work as a staff psychologist, introduced the knowledge of and provided workshops on nonviolent communication and/or meditation, no proprietary infringement would occur. Thus, Dr. Edwards would not be in violation of Standard 8.15. However, if Dr. Edwards's proposal is in large part based on knowledge gained from the grant application, he would then be in violation of Standard 8.15.

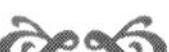

Dictates of One's Own Conscience

If you were Dr. Edwards's supervisor at DOC, listening to Dr. Edwards's ideas, which of these would you do?

1. Tell Dr. Edwards that what he does as a staff psychologist is under the purview of his supervisor at the correctional institution.
2. Dislike the ideas of nonviolent communication and do not believe in meditation, so say no to Dr. Edwards.
3. Think this is an example of plagiarism and refuse Dr. Edwards's ideas.
4. Like the idea of nonviolent communication for inmates, so say yes to Dr. Edwards.
5. Be unsure if introducing nonviolent communication workshops and meditation so close to a review of grant proposals exposes the DOC to charges of plagiarism, so refer the question to the state's attorney general's office?
6. Combinations of the above-listed actions.
7. Or one that is not listed above.

If you were Dr. Edwards's supervisor and both of you were working in Canada, listening to Dr. Edwards's ideas, you might tell Dr. Edwards that regardless of what you think of meditation or nonviolent communication, starting such a program at this moment would give the appearance of plagiarism. Therefore, he should not start the program at this time unless he obtained permission from the author of the research protocol to proceed.

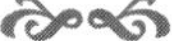

CHAPTER 9

Assessment

Ethical Standard 9

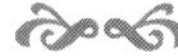

CHAPTER OUTLINE

- Standard 9.01: Bases for Assessments
- Standard 9.02: Use of Assessments
- Standard 9.03: Informed Consent in Assessments
- Standard 9.04: Release of Test Data
- Standard 9.05: Test Construction
- Standard 9.06: Interpreting Assessment Results
- Standard 9.07: Assessment by Unqualified Persons
- Standard 9.08: Obsolete Tests and Outdated Test Results
- Standard 9.09: Test Scoring and Interpretation Services
- Standard 9.10: Explaining Assessment Results
- Standard 9.11: Maintaining Test Security

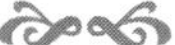

STANDARD 9.01: BASES FOR ASSESSMENTS

(a) Psychologists base the opinions contained in their recommendations, reports, and diagnostic or evaluative statements, including forensic testimony, on information and techniques sufficient to substantiate their findings.

A CASE FOR STANDARD 9.01 (A): It's Just a Letter!

Roberto, a motor vehicles department clerk, has been in treatment for about 3 months with Dr. Freeman for depression. Roberto comes in today asking Dr. Freeman for a letter to attest to the fact that it is safe for him to return to work. He was put on unpaid administrative leave 2 days ago in response to an incident at work. He reported that he lost his temper and yelled at Ethel, a female coworker who holds a similar job in another office. This incident occurred at a meeting of the company's Diversity Committee and has resulted in the requirement that Roberto have a psychological evaluation. Roberto notes that he does not agree with the common practice of assigning racial and ethnic minorities to work on diversity issues. However, some months ago, against Roberto's own recommendation to his superiors, the company assigned him to their Diversity Committee. At this particular meeting in which he lost his temper, Ethel claimed she was not racist and there was no racism in the workplace. Rather, she believed the committee should work on the issue of homophobia because Roberto is discriminatory toward gays and lesbians.

Issues of Concern

Dr. Freeman is and has been Roberto's treating psychologist. It is not uncommon for clients to request correspondence from their doctors for a variety of reasons. In this case, Roberto is requesting a letter from his treating psychologist to allow him to return to work. Standard 9.01 (a) requires that Dr. Freeman have sufficient information to substantiate whatever he writes in this letter.

An issue under consideration for Dr. Freeman is whether or not a "letter" constitutes a "psychological evaluation." For instance, would writing a letter summarizing Roberto's treatment to date be sufficient for Roberto to return to work? Also, does Dr. Freeman have sufficient information to render an opinion regarding the likelihood that Roberto will lose his temper again?

APA Ethics Code

Companion General Principle

Principle B: Fidelity and Responsibility

> Psychologists establish relationships of trust with those with whom they work. They are aware of their professional . . . responsibilities to society. . . Psychologists uphold professional standards of conduct . . . [and] clarify their professional roles and obligations.

The first sentence of Principle B focuses on Dr. Freeman maintaining trust with Roberto. Trust can be broken in many different ways, and one way Dr. Freeman could betray Roberto's trust is to violate confidentiality. In this situation, sufficient discussion would need to occur between Dr. Freeman and Roberto to highlight for Roberto the possible foreseeable ramifications of having his treating psychologist write a letter to his place of work.

Principle B calls a psychologist's attention to those people who may not be in the treatment room with the psychologist, but who may nonetheless be directly affected. Dr. Freeman, in consideration of Roberto's request, must also take into account the possible immediate effects such a letter might have on Ethel and other members of the company's Diversity Committee.

Principle B also directs Dr. Freeman's focus toward the consideration of issues regarding professional conduct, roles, and obligations. This means Dr. Freeman needs to know what professional standards exist in regard to writing a letter versus conducting a psychological evaluation, and whether his jurisdiction views such a practice as a form of a multiple relationship.

Principle E: Respect for People's Rights and Dignity.

> Psychologists respect the dignity and worth of all people, and the rights of individuals to privacy, confidentiality, and self-determination.

Principle E calls Dr. Freeman's attention to the special need of ensuring Roberto is informed of all possible and foreseeable ramifications that accompany writing the letter he is requesting. For instance, writing a letter such as this entails a break in confidentiality. Before confidentiality is broken, Dr. Freeman might have Roberto consider the effects of his workplace knowing that he is in treatment and that some of the details about his treatment will become known by his supervisor and possibly others within the business. The information Roberto gave to Dr. Freeman was for the purpose of treatment under the assumption of privacy. Individuals usually filter the type of information given depending on the purpose of the disclosure. Roberto may have talked about issues in treatment he does not want anyone to know, especially in the context of a letter sent to his workplace from Dr. Freeman.

Companion Ethical Standard(s)

Standard 9.01: Basis of Assessment

> . . . (b) . . . [P]sychologists provide opinions of the psychological characteristics of individuals only after they

> have conducted an examination of the individuals adequate to support their statements or conclusions.

Could Dr. Freeman claim that conducting psychotherapy sessions for 3 months with Roberto is a form of examination? If yes, then could Dr. Freeman also claim sufficient professional knowledge has been gained in these 3 months of treatment to render an opinion? If Dr. Freeman believes this to be true, then he would have met requirements set forth in Standard 9.01 (b).

Standard 3.05: Multiple Relationships

> (a) A multiple relationship occurs when a psychologist is in a professional role with a person and . . . (1) at the same time is in another role with the same person. . .
>
> A psychologist refrains from entering into a multiple relationship if the multiple relationship could reasonably be expected to impair the psychologist's objectivity, competence, or effectiveness in performing his or her functions as a psychologist, or otherwise risks exploitation or harm to the person with whom the professional relationship exists. Multiple relationships that would not reasonably be expected to cause impairment or risk exploitation or harm are not unethical.

A letter summarizing treatment may be sufficient for the employer. However, if Roberto's employer is specifically requesting a psychological evaluation addressing Roberto's anger and workplace safety, Dr. Freeman would be entering into a multiple relationship by engaging in the role of a treating psychologist and a forensic psychologist through writing a letter. Standard 3.05 (a) does not explicitly prohibit Dr. Freeman from entering into such a role. However, it does require that Dr. Freeman decide if his existing treatment relationship with Roberto could impair his objectivity in forming an opinion regarding whether or not Roberto is at risk of losing his temper in a way that jeopardizes workplace safety.

Standard 4.05: Disclosures

> (a) Psychologists may disclose confidential information with the appropriate consent of the . . . individual client/patient.

In order for Dr. Freeman to provide Roberto's employer with any information about Roberto, the client would need to give consent, as specified in Standard 4.05 (a). Roberto could decide not to provide his workplace with a letter from Dr. Freeman if Dr. Freeman's opinion is contrary to what Roberto wants his workplace to know.

Standard 4.04: Minimizing Intrusions on Privacy

> (a) Psychologists include in written and oral reports and consultations, only information germane to the purpose for which the communication is made.

Whatever Dr. Freeman writes, Standard 4.04 directs him to only have conveyed information that directly relates to Roberto's ability to regulate his temper.

Legal Issues

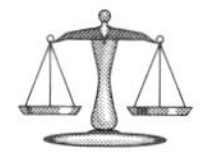

South Carolina

> *S.C. Code Ann. Regs.100-4 (2010).*
>
> C. Competence. . .
>
> (6) Sufficient professional information. A psychologist rendering a formal professional opinion about a person . . . shall not do so without direct and substantial professional contact with and a formal assessment of that person. . .
>
> J. Assessment procedures and reports. . .
>
> (3) Reservations concerning results. The psychologist shall include in his/her report of the results of an assessment procedure any deficiencies of the assessment norms for the individual assessed and any relevant reservations or qualifications which affect the validity, reliability, or other interpretations of results.

Texas

> *22 Tex. Admin. Code § 465.13 (2010). Personal Problems, Conflicts and Dual Relationships.*
>
> (b) Dual Relationships.
>
> (1) A licensee must refrain from entering into a dual relationship with a client . . . if such a relationship presents a risk that the dual relationship could impair the licensee's objectivity, prevent the licensee from providing competent psychological services, or . . . otherwise cause harm to the other party. . .
>
> (5) A licensee considering a professional relationship that would result in a dual . . . relationship shall take appropriate measures, such as obtaining professional consultation or assistance, to determine whether there

is a risk that the dual relationship could impair the licensee's objectivity or cause harm to the other party. If potential for impairment or harm exists, the licensee shall not provide services regardless of the wishes of the other party.

22 Tex. Admin. Code § 465.16 (2010). Evaluation, Assessment, Testing, and Reports.

(c) Limitations. . .

(5) Licensees provide opinions of the psychological characteristics of individuals only after they have conducted an examination of the individuals adequate to support their statements or conclusions. When such an examination is not practical, licensees document the efforts they made to obtain such an examination and clarify the probable impact of their limited information to the reliability and validity of their conclusions.

In both jurisdictions, Dr. Freeman violated the law by not engaging in a sufficient evaluation on behalf of his psychotherapy client. In addition, Texas would likely find that Dr. Freeman engaged in a multiple relationship if he conducted such an evaluation.

Cultural Considerations

Global Discussion

Singapore Psychological Society:
Code of Professional Ethics

Principle 9. Impersonal services.

Psychological services for the purposes of diagnosis, treatment, or personalised advice . . . are provided only in the context of a professional relationship. . .

1. The preparation of personnel reports and recommendations based on test data secured solely by mail is unethical. . . The reports must not make specific recommendations as to employment or placement of the subject which go beyond the psychologist's knowledge of the job requirements of the company.

Any report Dr. Freeman might issue about Roberto should only include information about the likelihood of Roberto's temper, rather than other information regarding his treatment for depression. Singapore's code states that Dr. Freeman "must not make specific recommendations as to employment." Therefore, Dr. Freeman may be in conflict with Singapore's code if he attempts to provide a letter about Roberto with recommendations regarding his job.

American Moral Values

1. What is Dr. Freeman expected to evaluate about Roberto? How would providing an evaluation of Roberto affect the therapeutic alliance in light of the preexisting treatment relationship? Has his previous treatment warranted a statement about how "safe" it is for Roberto to return to work?
2. How does depression relate to the incident that led to Roberto being put on leave? Could working in a racially hostile or aggravating workplace contribute to depression?
3. How does Dr. Freeman view Roberto's treatment at work? Should Roberto have submitted to serving on the Diversity Committee, and if so, on what basis? On what basis did Roberto have a reasonable claim not to be put on the committee?
4. Does Dr. Freeman believe Roberto reacted reasonably toward Ethel's accusation of being homophobic? Does Dr. Freeman weigh race and sexual orientation differently in terms of their importance for diversity? Or is there a problem with the way the committee was led to address these issues?
5. Does Dr. Freeman writing this letter indicate an acceptance of the company's view of the matter? Does it support the view of Roberto as the problem, as opposed to a larger problem for which the company was responsible?

Ethical Course of Action

Directive per APA Code

Standard 9.01(a) directs psychologists to render opinions based only on information and techniques sufficient to support their findings. It is questionable whether information obtained for one purpose, as in treatment, is appropriate to use for another purpose, such as rendering an expert opinion. Therefore, the technique upon which Dr. Freeman bases his opinion is suspect if only treatment information is used to render an opinion. To use an appropriate evaluation process, like a multiple measured approach used in a formal psychological evaluation, Dr. Freeman would need to conduct more than a review of his treatment notes. By engaging in a formal psychological evaluation after serving as a treating psychologist, Dr. Freeman would enter into a multiple relationship. To clearly meet the requirements of Standard 9.01 (a), it is best for Dr. Freeman to refer Roberto to another psychologist for the psychological evaluation.

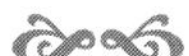

Dictates of One's Own Conscience

If you were Dr. Freeman, faced with such a request from a client, which of these would you do?

1. Consult with a colleague to determine whether the referral question and responding to the question as a treating psychologist would result in the appearance of a multiple relationship.
2. Talk to Roberto about the negative consequences of having his workplace know of the fact that he is in treatment that predates his temper outburst.
3. Tell Roberto your opinions about his temper if you thought he had temper control problems.
4. Write a treatment summary report for Roberto to take to work. In this treatment summary, note Roberto's previous problems, or lack of previous problems, with his temper.
5. Talk to Roberto about multiple relationship problems if you were to write a letter, and then refer him to another psychologist for assessment.

What if you were a female Dr. Antoinette, rather than Dr. Freeman, and you as a lesbian agree with Ethel that Roberto is discriminatory toward gays and lesbians? How might this affect your decision? Under such circumstance, would you

1. Not tell Roberto of your own opinion, and refer him to another psychologist for assessment?
2. Not tell Roberto of your own opinion about the content of the disagreement, but write a letter giving Roberto's history with controlling his temper?
3. Discuss with Roberto that you think Ethel is correct?
4. Combinations of the above-listed actions?
5. Or one that is not listed above?

If you were Dr. Freeman working in Singapore, you would need to tell Roberto that you could not write such a letter because your ethics code directs you not to "make specific recommendations as to employment" that "go beyond the psychologist's knowledge of the job requirements of the company."

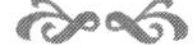

STANDARD 9.01: BASES FOR ASSESSMENTS

> . . . (b) Except as noted in 9.01c, psychologists provide opinions of the psychological characteristics of individuals only after they have conducted an examination of the individuals adequate to support their statements or conclusions. When, despite reasonable efforts, such an examination is not practical, psychologists document the efforts they made and the result of those efforts, clarify the probable impact of their limited information on the reliability and validity of their opinions, and appropriately limit the nature and extent of their conclusions or recommendations.

A CASE FOR STANDARD 9.01 (B): Too Much to Do, Not Enough Time to Do It

Dr. Wells provides psychological evaluations for colleagues in his practice. Lately his referrals have gone from 3 per month to 10. A full evaluation consists of a Minnesota Multiphasic Personality Inventory (MMPI), a Wechsler Adult Intelligence Scale (WAIS), a clinical interview, and a Beck Depression Inventory (BDI). Sheila, a referred client, needs an evaluation. Dr. Wells speaks with Sheila on the phone briefly, explains the assessment process and the fee, and schedules her assessment. However, when Sheila comes in, Dr. Wells realizes he has double-booked two assessments at once. He performs one assessment with another client, and assigns his assistant, Lee, a psychology intern, to conduct an assessment with Sheila. He instructs Lee to leave all raw data and notes from the interview on his desk. When Dr. Wells goes to write up Sheila's final report, he refers to the notes from the clinical interview and raw scores from the assessment tests. The scores for the BDI and WAIS are within normal range, but the computerized report on the MMPI reveal an elevation on the L and F-K scales. Dr. Wells speaks with Lee about Sheila's demeanor during the testing. He asks Lee whether she was open and frank with her answers, or if she appeared to present facts in a guarded light. Lee reports that Sheila was quiet and seemed tired toward the end of the 4-hour assessment period, and she complained about the length of the MMPI. Dr. Wells writes up his report of Sheila, noting her "reluctance to comply with parts of the exam" and that elevations on the MMPI scale are a possible indication of psychopathology she was trying to conceal during the exam. He signs and dates the report, and then bills for it under his own name.

Issues of Concern

Standard 9.01 (b) addresses situations in which the psychologist who is rendering an opinion does not personally conduct the interview or supervise the administration of any psychometric instrument. In this situation, the issue of concern includes whether relying on a report from a psychology assistant constitutes an examination of the individual, and whether or not writing the report without reference to Lee as the person who conducted the interview and administered the psychometric instruments violates this section of Standard 9.01 (b), which directs Dr. Wells to document such activities. Also of concern is whether sufficient note was taken of the limitations on reliability and validity; as well as whether billing for the report under the doctor's name only can be considered misleading.

APA Ethics Code

Companion General Principle

Principle B: Fidelity and Responsibility

> Psychologists uphold professional standards of conduct, clarify their professional roles and obligations.

Principle B suggests that Dr. Wells should compare his professional activities against those standards of the profession. Do the majority of psychologists in his geographic location use the services of a psychomatrician and bill for such services under their own license?

Principle C: Integrity

> Psychologists seek to promote accuracy, honesty, and truthfulness in the . . . practice of psychology. In these activities psychologists do not . . . engage in fraud . . . or intentional misrepresentation of fact. . .

Principle C directs psychologists to act with integrity in all areas of their professional activity. As such, hopefully Dr. Wells's report is accurate. However, in this case there may be reason to doubt whether the report is accurate because Dr. Wells's conclusion does not appear to match the information reported by Lee. At the same time, Dr. Wells, being more experienced, may have interpreted all relevant facts more accurately than his psychology assistant.

Companion Ethical Standard

Standard 2.05: Delegation of Work to Others

> Psychologists who delegate work to employees . . . take reasonable steps to . . . (2) authorize only those responsibilities that such persons can be expected to perform competently on the basis of their education, training, or experience, either independently or with the level of supervision being provided; and . . . (3) see that such persons perform these services competently.

Standard 2.05 would have Dr. Wells delegate Sheila's examination only to someone who is competent to perform the task. Unless otherwise indicated, it is usually safe to assume that a psychology assistant would be competent to conduct an interview and administer psychometric instruments independently. However, psychology assistants must also be adequately prepared to handle incidental situations competently. It is conceivable that Lee did not handle the circumstances of Sheila's fatigue adequately. Her fatigue during the testing may have adversely affected her test results. Should Lee have sought Dr. Wells's consultation at the time Sheila complained of fatigue? Should Dr. Wells have periodically checked in on Lee when he was evaluating Sheila?

Standard 9.07: Assessment by Unqualified Persons

> Psychologists do not promote the use of psychological assessment techniques by unqualified persons.

Standard 9.07 directs Dr. Wells not to use unqualified persons in his work except for training. The presumption is that Lee can use psychological assessment techniques in a competent manner. In the situation described, has Dr. Wells provided Lee with appropriate supervision to conduct the interview and administer the assessments?

Standard 9.10: Explaining Assessment Results

> Regardless of whether the scoring and interpretation are done by psychologists, by employees or assistants[,]. . . psychologists take reasonable steps to ensure that explanations of results are given to the individual.

Standard 9.10 directs Dr. Wells to personally conduct the interpretation session, even though he had not conducted any of the assessment sessions.

Standard 6.04: Fees and Financial Arrangements

> . . . (c) Psychologists do not misrepresent their fees.

Regardless of whether or not this is a third-party billing or private pay situation, it is a misrepresentation for Dr. Wells to bill for the full assessment under his name and at his rate of reimbursement. Given that the assessment was conducted by Lee and Dr. Wells, it would be more accurate for Dr. Wells to bill for the assessment with the assumption that services provided by Lee would be billed under a lesser rate than those performed by Dr. Wells.

Standard 1.04: Informal Resolution of Ethical Violations

> When psychologists believe that there may have been an ethical violation by another psychologist, they attempt to resolve the issue by bringing it to the attention of that individual.

If Lee was working as a psychology assistant/psychomatrician, he would not expect to see or review Dr. Wells's final report. However, as a psychology assistant it is reasonable to expect that Lee would be writing the report under Dr. Wells's supervision, or at a minimum be reading the report for educational purposes. If in reading the report, Lee disagreed with Dr. Wells's conclusions, or his billing practice, Standard 1.04 would direct Lee to bring the matter to Dr. Wells's attention.

Legal Issues 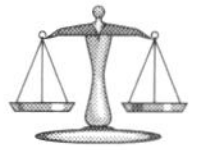

Washington

> *Wash. Admin. Code § 246-924-160 (2009). Continued Supervision of Persons. . .*
>
> (1) The law requires holders of a certificate of qualifications to perform psychological functions "under the periodic direct supervision of a psychologist licensed by the board." The board's interpretation of this statement is that a holder of a certificate of qualification, referred to as a "psychological assistant," is certified *in tandem* with a licensed psychologist and not in his or her own right. . .
>
> (3) Minimum supervision shall include discussion of the psychological assistant's work through regularly scheduled contacts with the supervisor at appropriate intervals. . . The supervisor shall be responsible for preparing evaluative reports of the psychological assistant's performance, which will be forwarded to the board on a periodic basis.
>
> (4) When a licensed psychologist assumes the responsibility of supervision, he or she shares the professional and ethical responsibility for the nature and quality of all of the psychological services the psychological assistant may provide. Failure to provide supervision as described in the agreement may result in appropriate action against the license of the supervisor. . .
>
> (6) In every case where psychological testing is done and a report is written based on that testing by a psychological assistant, the supervising licensed psychologist will countersign the report indicating his or her approval.
>
> *Wash. Admin. Code § 246-924-359 (2009). Client Welfare.*
>
> (1) Providing explanation of procedures. The psychologist shall upon request give a truthful, understandable, and reasonably complete account of the client's condition to the client or to those responsible for the care of the client.
>
> *Wash. Admin. Code § 246-924-364 (2009). Fees.*
>
> Disclosure of cost of services. The psychologist shall not mislead or withhold from the client, a prospective client, or third party payor, information about the cost of his/her professional services. . .
>
> (1) Reasonableness of fee. The psychologist shall not exploit the client or responsible payor by charging a fee that is excessive for the services performed.
>
> *Wash. Admin. Code § 246-924-366 (2009). Fraud, Misrepresentation, or Deception.*
>
> The psychologist shall not use fraud, misrepresentation, or deception . . . in providing psychological service . . . [or] in reporting the results of psychological evaluations or services.

Arkansas

> *Arkansas Psych. Board Rules and Reg. § 6 (2010) Supervision.*
>
> 6.2. C. The supervisor shall establish and maintain a level of supervisory contact consistent with professional standards, insuring the welfare of the public, and the ethical and legal protection of the supervision process.
>
> 6.2. C. 1 A minimum of 1 hour of face-to-face supervision per week for provisional licensure applicants who have not previously held a psychology license. . .

> 6.2. E. The Board requires the supervisor to be clearly aware of the professional skills, practices, ethics, and abilities of each person being supervised.
>
> 6.2. E. 1 Supervisors may only supervise those areas of practice indicated in their own Statement of Intent.
>
> 6.3. Requirements of Supervision...
>
> 6.3. B. 4 The Board recognizes that ... the variability of practice, level of professional skill, and personal/professional characteristics of the Psychological Examiner is such that individually tailored supervision is necessary... A.C.A. §17-97-102 requires supervision of Psychological Examiners for "overall personality appraisal or classification... " Supervisors are responsible for all these services provided by Psychological Examiners under their supervision, whatever the method of documentation of personality evaluations and treatment plans. Co-signature is one option for documenting this relationship and supervision.
>
> 6.3. B. 5 As required by law, when inquiry is made, users of the Psychological Examiner's services shall be informed when services provided are supervised.
>
> Section 16. Code of Ethics
>
> 16.1. The Arkansas Psychology Board adopts the Ethical Principles of Psychologists and Code of Conduct of the American Psychological Association as part of these Rules and Regulations. The principles shall constitute one standard by which appropriate professional practices are determined.

Dr. Wells violated the laws of both jurisdictions regarding supervision and fraud by failing to provide sufficient supervision for his assistant and charging for the evaluation under his name. The work done by Lee is not equivalent to the level of Dr. Wells's competency, and thus it is fraudulent to charge for work done by Lee at Dr. Wells's rate.

Cultural Considerations

Global Discussion

Code of Ethics for the Psychologist: Spain

> ***Article 48.*** Psychological Reports must be clear, precise, rigorous and intelligible to the addressee. They must state their range and limitations, the writer's degree of certainty of the various contents in the report, whether it is current or temporary in nature, the techniques used in its preparation, and always specifying the particulars of the professional issuing it.

Provided that Dr. Wells includes in his report information regarding Lee's role in performing the assessment with Sheila, and provided that the report is "clear, precise and rigorous" in its content, Dr. Wells would be in compliance with this portion of Spain's code. Spain's code is silent on whether it is a conflict for someone other than the assessing psychologist to write up the report, although Dr. Wells is obligated to express his "degree of certainty" regarding its contents. Among the "techniques used in preparation," it can be argued that Dr. Wells would state that Lee performed the assessment, and that he, Dr. Wells, did not interact with Sheila in person during that assessment. Provided that he does so, it would appear that Dr. Wells would be in compliance with Spain's code.

American Moral Values

1. Why does Dr. Wells believe Sheila's testing was billable as a service performed by him? Why does Dr. Wells accept Lee's report about Sheila's behavior? Is secondhand information good enough? Is there a particular quality to hiding symptoms that requires direct observation to assess?
2. Does Dr. Wells believe that tests like the MMPI can be delegated without distorting their results? Could Lee's judgment have been affected by how Sheila took her tests? Does Dr. Wells believe Lee can competently judge resistance to the test? Could Dr. Wells's experience and manner have put Sheila more at ease?
3. Does Dr. Wells believe that, given his schedule, it is better that Sheila be tested now rather than risk not getting tested by him or his psychology assistant at all? Does he believe his abilities, even through the interviewing of a psychology assistant, justify seeing her rather than referring her to someone else?
4. Is the reason for Sheila's referral a factor in Dr. Wells's decision to delegate the testing? If, instead of a simple assessment, she was referred to him as a possible suicide threat, would he have let Lee test her? Why is it acceptable for this case?
5. How much is Dr. Wells taking into account his status in the practice in seeing these referred clients? Is he afraid to turn down referrals from colleagues?

Ethical Course of Action

Directive per APA Code

Standard 9.01 (b) allows for circumstances in which the psychologist has not personally conducted the examination. In such situations, Standard 9.01 (b) directs Dr. Wells to have indicated in the report that the information is limited by the fact that he is basing his opinion on an interview and observation conducted by his psychology assistant. Provided he does include Lee's role in the assessment, Dr. Wells would be in compliance with Standard 9.01 (b). To be in compliance with Standard 6.04 (c), Lee's involvement with Sheila's assessment would also need to be reflected in the fees billed for the assessment.

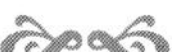

Dictates of One's Own Conscience

If you were Lee, after reviewing the report on Sheila written by Dr. Wells, which of these might you do?

1. Nothing beyond reading the report.
2. Discuss Dr. Wells's conclusions with him in order to learn more about how to write a report.
3. Point out to Dr. Wells that the report needed to contain the limitations and that the conclusions were based on Lee's observations, not Dr. Wells's own observations.
4. Ask Dr. Wells about the difference between what you thought and Dr. Wells's conclusions regarding Sheila, and possibly seek to have the report be adjusted if it has not already been released.
5. Wonder whether Dr. Wells was somehow biased against women who were getting evaluations, and thus arrived at a more negative conclusion than you did.
6. Combinations of the above-listed actions.
7. Or one that is not listed above.

If you were Dr. Wells practicing in Spain, you would make no changes in your behavior in the vignette, presuming that the report written was clear, precise, and rigorous.

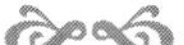

STANDARD 9.01: BASES FOR ASSESSMENTS

> . . . (c) When psychologists conduct a record review or provide consultation or supervision and an individual examination is not warranted or necessary for the opinion, psychologists explain this and the sources of information on which they based their conclusions and recommendations.

A CASE FOR STANDARD 9.01 (C): The Endless Court Case

Ellen contacts Dr. Webb for consultation on a previously conducted parent evaluation. Two years ago, Kyle, her ex-husband, hired Dr. Simpson to perform a parenting evaluation. Without consultation with Ellen, their children, or Ellen's treating psychiatrist, Dr. Simpson made the recommendation that Kyle should have custodial custody of their daughter. The judge considered the evaluation to be inadequate and did not admit the evaluation into the court proceedings. On the advice of her attorney, as protection against harm from this evaluation, Ellen has filed an ethics complaint against Dr. Simpson. The state examining board reviewed the case and decided not to investigate on grounds that no state standards for parenting evaluations exist, and therefore the state board cannot make any determination on this case.

Kyle has filed for another hearing to gain custody of the children. The previous judge has now retired, and a new judge is in charge. This new judge is admitting the evaluation from Dr. Simpson for consideration in the case. Ellen wants Dr. Webb to write an opinion regarding Dr. Simpson's parenting evaluation.

Issues of Concern

Standard 9.01 (c) speaks to a psychologist's assessment when such assessments do not include individual examination. The request made by Ellen for Dr. Webb to review the report is such a situation. Some of the issues for Dr. Webb to consider in this situation include the following: Is there any basis for the review, since the state board has already ruled on lack of standards to evaluate the adequacy of the evaluation technique? If Dr. Webb were to review the report and render an opinion on the technique used by Dr. Simpson, can he justify a review of Dr. Simpson's work?

Independent of Dr. Simpson's work, might Ellen be better served if Dr. Webb conducted a parenting evaluation that would potentially provide a more timely, accurate, or competent report from which the court could draw a more informed conclusion?

APA Ethics Code

Companion General Principle

Principle B: Fidelity and Responsibility

> Psychologists . . . are aware of their professional . . . responsibilities to society and to the specific communities in which they work. Psychologists uphold professional standards of conduct. . . They are concerned about the ethical compliance of their colleagues' scientific and professional conduct.

There are several ideas in Principle B relevant to this situation. The first idea entails Dr. Webb's responsibility to the community in which he works. One of those communities includes the community of psychologists. What effect might it have on Dr. Webb's relationship with other psychologists if he testifies against Dr. Simpson, another psychologist?

The second idea encompassed in Principle B suggests that Dr. Webb should be concerned about Dr. Simpson's conduct. In this case, if Dr. Webb, on review of the parenting evaluation, thought Dr. Simpson did not meet the professional standards of conduct, and Dr. Simpson demonstrated questionable competence, does Principle B guide Dr. Webb to show concern? In upholding professional standards of conduct, Dr. Webb would be guided by Principle B to act on whatever concerns he may have regarding Dr. Simpson's work.

Principle D: Justice

> Psychologists recognize that fairness and justice entitle all persons to access to and benefit from the contributions of psychology and to equal quality in the processes, procedures, and services being conducted by psychologists.

If Dr. Webb decides not to provide his professional opinion about the previous parenting evaluation on the same grounds as the state psychology board, might he be shying away from acting in the highest ideas of Principle D? The highest aspiration in Principle D would have Dr. Webb acting in such a manner that Ellen would have access to and benefit from the best kind of parenting evaluation that psychologists are able to perform.

Companion Ethical Standard(s)

Standard 1.04: Informal Resolution of Ethical Violations

> When psychologists believe that there may have been an ethical violation by another psychologist, they attempt to resolve the issue by bringing it to the attention of that individual.

Standard 2.01: Boundaries of Competence

> . . . (e) In those emerging areas in which generally recognized standards for preparatory training do not yet exist, psychologists nevertheless take reasonable steps to ensure the competence of their work and to protect clients . . . from harm.

The implementation for the relevant parts of Principle B is Standard 1.04. If Dr. Webb thought Dr. Simpson's parenting evaluation for Ellen violated Standard 2.01, Standard 1.04 directs Dr. Webb to contact Dr. Simpson in some way and call Dr. Simpson's attention to the ethical violation.

Regardless of whether Dr. Webb thought Dr. Simpson performed a competent parenting evaluation for Ellen, it is appropriate to consider whether Dr. Webb is competent himself to conduct a parenting evaluation, let alone critique someone else's. Does the ruling from the state psychology board regarding standards of parenting evaluations necessarily force Dr. Webb to base his argument on problems other than the competency of Dr. Simpson's parenting evaluation?

It could be argued that parenting evaluations for the jurisdiction in which Dr. Webb practices fall under an emerging area of practice. To be in compliance with Standard 2.01 (e), regardless of whether the state psychology board has established standards, Dr. Webb and Dr. Simpson should look to the profession for those emerging practices that increase competence in this area.

Standard 2.04: Bases for Scientific and Professional Judgments

> Psychologists' work is based upon established scientific and professional knowledge of the discipline.

Standard 2.04 would direct Dr. Webb to look toward the profession to determine the standards for parenting evaluations. If Dr. Webb were to undertake a review of Dr. Simpson's parenting evaluation for Ellen, Dr. Webb would need to ensure that he has enough information to substantiate his opinion on the grounds of scientific or professional knowledge.

Legal Issues 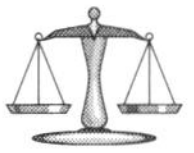

Florida

> *Florida Statute 61.122 (2010). Child custody evaluations; presumption of psychologist's good faith; prerequisite to parent's filing suit; award of fees, costs, reimbursement.*
>
> (1) A psychologist who has been appointed by the court to conduct a child custody evaluation in a judicial proceeding is presumed to be acting in good faith if the evaluation has been conducted pursuant to standards that a reasonable psychologist would have used as recommended by the American Psychological Association's guidelines for child custody evaluation in divorce proceedings.

Georgia

> *Ga. Comp. R. & Regs. 510-5-.08 (2010). Forensic Assessment.*
>
> (1) Psychologists' forensic assessment, recommendations, and reports are based on information and techniques . . . sufficient to provide appropriate substantiation for his/her findings.
>
> (2) Psychologists provide written or oral forensic reports or testimony of the psychological characteristics of an individual only after they have conducted an examination of the individual adequate to support his/her statements or conclusions. Provided, however, that when, despite reasonable efforts, such an examination is not feasible, psychologists clarify the impact of his/her limited information on the reliability and validity of his/her reports and testimony, and they appropriately limit the nature and extent of his/her conclusions or recommendations.
>
> (4) Whenever necessary, psychologists acknowledge the limits of his/her data or conclusions.

In Florida, Dr Webb would be expected to have reviewed Dr. Simpson's evaluation in a manner that did not conflict with the Guidelines for Child Custody Evaluations in Family Law Proceedings (see www.apa.org/practice/guidelines/child-custody.pdf). Dr. Webb would not be in violation of the law in Georgia as long as Dr. Webb's report delineated his methodology and focused upon whether Dr. Simpson's methodology was sufficient to evaluate Kyle's fitness as a parent. For Georgia, Dr. Simpson's evaluation depended upon only one measure: Kyle being interviewed and forming findings based upon one measure would violate the law.

Cultural Considerations

Global Discussion

The Professional Board for Psychology Health Professions of South Africa:
Ethical Code of Professional Conduct (April 2002)

> 1. Assessment within a professional context.
>
> 1. Psychologists shall provide opinions of the psychological characteristics of individuals only after they have conducted an examination of the individual that is professionally adequate to support their findings.

Dr. Simpson would be in violation of South Africa's code if his recommendation explicitly denied Ellen custody based upon only examining Kyle directly before issuing a report. However, South Africa's code is silent regarding correct protocol for a records review evaluation. If it can be assumed that assessment standards in South Africa hold true for a records review as well as an in-person assessment, then Dr. Webb would need to include information in the records review that discusses the limitations of the information he has used, as well as the impact of limited information on his findings in the report.

American Moral Values

1. What is Dr. Webb's role for Ellen? Should he conduct an examination of Ellen? Is he merely supposed to comment on Dr. Simpson's evaluations? What are the standards that he would cite in order to do that? Does he need to consider how the judge will consider his statement?
2. What would Dr. Webb's argument be? Is this argument the best way to help Ellen? Does Dr. Webb sympathize with her case, or only with the fact that she was unfairly harmed by an inadequate evaluation?
3. Does he let Dr. Simpson's evaluation stand? What is his sense of fairness and justice, and how will that impact his decision on what statement to write?
4. How does he consider the practice of psychologists writing evaluations in the first place? Will he improve the practice with his own statement? Does it risk damaging credibility, especially given the state board's statement that there are no standards for judging parental evaluations?

Ethical Course of Action

Directive per APA Code

Standard 9.01 (c) does not prohibit Dr. Webb from providing consultation to the courts based on a review of the report. It does direct Dr. Webb to stipulate the sources of information upon which he is judging Dr. Simpson's work. The state psychology board has already established that there are no state standards for parenting evaluations. Therefore, Dr. Webb would not be able to refer to his opinion based on state standards. Dr. Webb, then, would need to make his opinion based on professional standards of practice as stipulated in Standard 2.04 and the Guidelines for Child Custody Evaluations in Family Law Proceedings (see www.apa.org/practice/guidelines/child-custody.pdf).

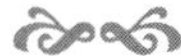

Dictates of One's Own Conscience

If you were Dr. Webb, faced with such a referral, which of these would you do?

1. Decline the referral based on any variety of reasons, which may include
    a. schedule already too full.
    b. no basis to render an opinion based on the state psychology board's opinion.
    c. not wanting to testify against a colleague.
2. Consult with Ellen and her attorney, stating that seeking to discredit Dr. Simpson's work is difficult to accomplish based on the state's stance on parenting evaluations.
3. Recommend that you perform an independent parenting evaluation for Ellen. This time you would include information from all relevant parties such as both parents, their interactions with their children, and various collateral people who know about the circumstances of the family.
4. Let the attorney know that you, as Dr. Webb, are well acquainted with Dr. Simpson, and know that he is typically predisposed to decide in favor of females in the interest of the child. How might this knowledge about Dr. Simpson affect Dr. Webb's decision regarding handling of the referral?
5. Combinations of the above-listed actions.
6. Or one that is not listed above.

If you were Dr. Webb practicing in South Africa, the above-listed options would still apply since the guideline for custody evaluation and psychological assessment is essentially the same as that listed in the APA Ethics Code.

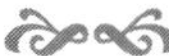

STANDARD 9.02: USE OF ASSESSMENTS

(a) Psychologists administer, adapt, score, interpret, or use assessment techniques, interviews, tests, or instruments in a manner and for purposes that are appropriate in light of the research on or evidence of the usefulness and proper application of the techniques.

A CASE FOR STANDARD 9.02 (A): Are There Any Valid Tests for Zachary?

Dr. Stevens's first job post graduation is in a community health center in a rural area of the West Coast. She is given a referral for Zachary, a 7-year-old Somali boy whose family migrated to the United States from a refugee camp in Kenya when Zachary was 5 years old. Zachary reports that he is often bored in school and does not like school at all. His teacher and the school principal report that Zachary appears to be very bright but does not tolerate frustration and is often aggressive at school. Dr. Stevens is aware of the limitations of standardized testing for refugee children for whom English is a second language and may compromise the validity of some types of testing for Zachary. She decides to administer the Draw-A-Person (DAP) test as a qualitative assessment tool to ascertain intellectual functioning as well as rule out other possible mental health diagnoses.

Issues of Concern

Standard 9.02 (a) directs Dr. Stevens to choose an assessment instrument that is appropriate for the question and situation. As part of an assessment for a 7-year-old child with behavioral problems at school, it is appropriate to ascertain intelligence level and to rule out other possible diagnoses such as attention deficit hyperactivity disorder (ADHD). Dr. Stevens knows the traditional assessment instruments used in the United

States are highly language dependent and are not appropriate or applicable to a child with Zachary's ethnic background and socioeconomic status. Is her choice of Draw-A-Person appropriate for use as a measure of intelligence in light of the research? Is it appropriate for use as a measure of ADHD in light of the research? Conversely, are there any valid assessment instruments to ascertain Zachary's level of intellectual functioning or to rule out ADHD, given his recent migration and limited English proficiency?

APA Ethics Code

Companion General Principle

Principle D: Justice

> Psychologists recognize that fairness and justice entitle all persons to access to and benefit from the contributions of psychology and to equal quality in the . . . services being conducted by psychologists.

Principle D: Justice guides Dr. Stevens to ensure that Zachary has access to a psychological evaluation and recommendations regarding intervention(s) for his school problems. To deny Zachary access on the grounds that traditional assessment measures used within the profession of psychology do not provide valid measures to assess him would be in violation of the aspiration behind Principle D.

Companion Ethical Standard(s)

Standard 2.01: Boundaries of Competence

> . . . (b) Where scientific or professional knowledge in the discipline of psychology establishes that an understanding of factors associated with age, gender[,] . . . ethnicity, culture, national origin[,] . . . disability, language, or socioeconomic status is essential for effective implementation of their services[,] . . . psychologists have or obtain the training, experience, consultation, or supervision necessary to ensure the competence of their services, or they make appropriate referrals.

To conduct a competent assessment of Zachary, Standard 2.01 (b) directs Dr. Stevens to consider factors that are associated with his age, his gender, his culture, his national origins, his ethnicity, and socioeconomic status as a refugee. If Dr. Stevens does not have knowledge or is not competent in understanding the relevance of these factors with regard to assessment, Standard 2.01 (b) directs Dr. Stevens to either obtain the training or refer Zachary to someone who is competent in these relevant areas.

Standard 2.02: Providing Services in Emergencies

> In emergencies, when psychologists provide services to individuals for whom other mental health services are not available and for which psychologists have not obtained the necessary training, psychologists may provide such services in order to ensure that services are not denied.

To ensure that services are not denied under certain circumstances, Standard 2.02 allows for psychologists who are not normally competent in an area to provide services. Does serving in a rural community constitute such a state of emergency in which psychologists would be permitted to provide services in which they are not normally competent or trained? Conversely, can it be argued that only a psychologist who is of Somali descent or an expert in Somali culture is competent to perform an assessment for Zachary?

Standard 2.04: Bases for Scientific and Professional Judgments

> Psychologists' work is based upon established scientific and professional knowledge of the discipline.

Does current research on validity of using Draw-A-Person versus other well-established intelligence tests support the use of this assessment to derive an intelligence quotient? Might Dr. Stevens find other tests of intelligence that are not language dependent and include nonverbal measures to be a more valid assessment to use with Zachary?

Legal Issues 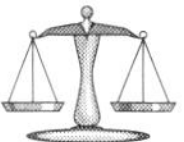

Colorado

> *Colo. Rev. Stat. Ann. § 12-43-222 (West, 2010). Prohibited Activities—Related Provisions.*
>
> (1) A person licensed . . . under . . . this article is in violation of this article if such person . . .
>
> (h) Has performed services outside of such person's area of training, experience, or competence . . .
>
> (m) Has failed to obtain a consultation or perform a referral when such failure is not consistent with generally accepted standards of care . . .

(t) Has engaged in any of the following activities and practices. . .

(III) Ordering or performing, without clinical justification, any service . . . that is contrary to the generally accepted standards of such person's practice.

Delaware

24 Dela. Code § 3514 (2010). Grounds for Refusal, Revocation or Suspension of Licenses and Registrations.

(a) A practitioner licensed . . . under this chapter shall be subject to disciplinary actions set forth in § 3516 of this title, if, after a hearing, the Board finds that the psychologist or psychological assistant . . .

(5) Has not conducted the practitioner's professional activities in conformity with the American Psychological Association's Ethical Principles of Psychologists and Code of Conduct (hereinafter referred to as the Ethics Code); and in conformity with the rules and regulations adopted by the Board to implement the Ethics Code.

Dr. Stevens has violated the law of both jurisdictions by not obtaining consultation in order for her to raise her level of competency. The selection of one measure, and reliance upon only one measure in light of the multicultural aspects of the case, and Dr. Stevens's limited experience would weigh heavily as factors for consideration in Delaware.

Cultural Considerations

Global Discussion

The Professional Board for Psychology Health Professions of South Africa:
Ethical Code of Professional Conduct (April 2002)

5.5. Cultural diversity.

5.5.1. Psychologists who . . . use assessment methods shall be familiar with the reliability, validation, and related standardization or outcome studies of, and proper applications and uses of, the methods they use.

i. Psychologists shall recognize limits to the certainty with which diagnoses, findings, or predictions can be made about individuals, especially where linguistic, cultural and socio-economic variances exist.

Dr. Stevens may be in violation of this portion of the code if the DAP assessment is found to be an improper application of an assessment method, even if she is using it in good faith and with the best of intentions to adequately assess and ascertain appropriate interventions for Zachary.

American Moral Values

1. Has Dr. Stevens chosen the best possible tests for establishing Zachary's intelligence level and explaining his frustration (e.g., detecting ADHD)? Does a Draw-A-Person test capture the forms of intelligence that Zachary displays? Can Dr. Stevens provide any evidence of intelligence beyond formal testing? How has he shown intelligence in his academic work?
2. Does Zachary deserve a chance to receive appropriate services even if the available tests cannot compensate for language differences and the experience of migration? Though this is a rural area, is there anyone who could help Dr. Stevens take into account Zachary's life in a refugee camp and the challenges of adjusting to a new country?
3. If this area has limited resources for accommodating Zachary's background, should Dr. Stevens take it upon herself to diagnose Zachary and provide services to him? Will he fail to thrive in the school system otherwise? Is there anyone else in the community who could do better?
4. What does Dr. Stevens believe is the most important issue to tackle with Zachary? Does she value reducing aggression over lessening his frustration? Does she believe that encouraging his intelligence is the main goal for making his life better?
5. What relationship should Dr. Stevens establish with Zachary's family? What are their views about school and Zachary's needs? Do they believe he needs to adjust to school and "fit in" instead of being pulled out for services? Do they believe a diagnosis like ADHD could be stigmatizing?

Ethical Course of Action

Directive per APA Code

It can be argued that, per Standard 2.02, the rural setting allows for Dr. Stevens to provide services to Zachary without violating the ethical standards of competency. Standard 9.02 (a) directs Dr. Stevens to choose an assessment instrument that is valid for the referral question. In the case of Zachary, Standard 2.01 (b) would direct Dr. Stevens to find assessment instruments that would be valid for his age (7 years old), gender (male), race (African), ethnicity (Somali), and socioeconomic status (recent refugee). Arguably, such a task is daunting, and it does not appear the selection of Draw-A-Person meets the directives of Standard 2.04. As directed by Standard 2.01 (e), Dr. Stevens would be well advised to consult other psychologists who may be more knowledgeable in using nonverbal instruments for measures of intelligence or doing assessments for ADHD, or who may be better trained in providing services for either refugees or individuals from Somalia.

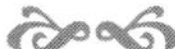

Dictates of One's Own Conscience

If you were Dr. Stevens, faced with a school referral for Zachary, which of these might you do?

1. Not conduct the assessment, but recommend treatment for Zachary's aggressive behavior.
2. Conduct the assessment using projective test instruments to assess emotional adjustment and not assess intelligence level.
3. Proceed with DAP, reasoning that given the fact that there are not valid tests of intelligence for Zachary, something is better than nothing.
4. Use academic and social classroom observations as a better indicator of innate intelligence as opposed to using any standardized measurement of intelligence.
5. Combinations of the above-listed actions.
6. Or one that is not listed above.

If you were Dr. Stevens practicing in South Africa and faced with a school referral for Zachary, you would look up all validity studies for nonverbal measures of intelligence before proceeding with further assessment.

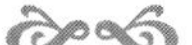

STANDARD 9.02: USE OF ASSESSMENTS

> . . . (b) Psychologists use assessment instruments whose validity and reliability have been established for use with members of the population tested. When such validity or reliability has not been established, psychologists describe the strengths and limitations of test results and interpretation.

A CASE FOR STANDARD 9.02 (B): The First Daughter

Mr. Bradley hired Dr. Tucker for a custody evaluation to obtain full custody of his children. The family consists of Mr. Bradley, the father; Mrs. Marjorie, the mother; a 7-year-old daughter; and a 5-year-old son. Dr. Tucker, a white female psychologist, has conducted many custody evaluations and has established a set of standard procedures including individual interviews with parents, Minnesota Multiphasic Personality Inventory–2 (MMPI-2) testing, and joint observation of each parent and his or her children on separate occasions. During this process, Dr. Tucker noted that Mrs. Marjorie took an excessive amount of time to complete the preliminary paperwork in the waiting room. She was also compulsive in completing the MMPI-2 as evidenced by her repeated questioning of the office support staff about the meaning of the test questions. The MMPI-2 revealed high scores on the scale for depression and on the Male/Female scale, an indication that she may be overly dependent/submissive and suffer from depression. Questioning the possible reasons for Mrs. Marjorie's struggles with the MMPI-2, Dr. Tucker administered a Wechsler Adult Intelligence Scale–Revised (WAIS-R), which revealed a full-scale score of 85, an indication that Mrs. Marjorie's intellectual functioning was in the low-average range. In the report, Dr. Tucker noted that Mr. Bradley was a warm and responsive parent, and that his MMPI-2 was normal. On the other hand, Dr. Tucker noted that Mrs. Marjorie was someone of low-average intelligence who suffers from depression. She also indicated that Mrs. Marjorie appeared distant and cold, as evidenced by her refusal to refer to her children by their names, referring to them instead as "first daughter" and "first son." In the social history section of the report, Dr. Tucker did note that Mr. Bradley is a white American male and that Mrs. Marjorie is Korean. The couple met and married while Mr. Bradley was stationed in Korea on military duty. Based on the evaluation results, Dr. Tucker recommended Mr. Bradley should be named as the custodial parent with Mrs. Marjorie having every other weekend visitation. Sometime after Dr. Tucker had released the parenting evaluation, an attorney for Mrs. Marjorie contacted her and requested her presence at a deposition.

Issues of Concern

Standard 9.02 (b) directs Dr. Tucker to have used assessment instruments that are valid and reliable.

The MMPI is a well-established standard assessment instrument used in assessing for psychopathology. It is reasoned that the MMPI profile for Mr. Bradley is most likely valid, as he falls within the normative population for MMPI-2. The same instrument does not include a Korean immigrant population as part of the normative sample. This is also true for the WAIS-R in that Mr. Bradley falls within the normative population sample for both assessment inventories, but Mrs. Marjorie does not. On the other hand, the use of MMPI-2 is a relatively standard evaluation protocol for psychological evaluations. What circumstances would justify Dr. Tucker's deviating from customary assessment protocol? Is Mrs. Marjorie's Korean ancestry a valid justification of such deviation? Does Dr. Tucker's interpretation of the test results take into consideration the different nationalities of Mr. Bradley and Mrs. Marjorie? Was Dr. Tucker competent to proceed with the evaluation without consultation since she did not obtain a cultural consultation and had no prior training or experience with Korean immigrants?

APA Ethics Code

Companion General Principle

Principle D: Justice

> Psychologists recognize that fairness and justice entitle all persons to access to and benefit from the contributions of psychology and to equal quality in the processes, procedures, and services being conducted by psychologists. Psychologists exercise reasonable judgment and take precautions to ensure that . . . the boundaries of their competence, and the limitations of their expertise do not lead to . . . unjust practices.

Principle D argues for equality in services rendered by psychologists. Dr. Tucker's procedure for parenting evaluation appears to give equal treatment since she has both parents use the same psychometric instrument and undergo the same interviews. Dr. Tucker might have favored Mrs. Marjorie by giving her extra attention with the administration of the WAIS-R.

Principle D further suggests psychologists guard against bias and limitations of their expertise in such a manner that those limitations do not result in unjust practice. Dr. Tucker, having conducted many parent evaluations, appears to be practicing within her area of competence. She allows for equal treatment in the assessment procedure to guard against bias. She went beyond her normal procedure in the decision to use the WAIS-R as a precautionary step to ensure that the limits of her procedures did not unduly bias the results against Mrs. Marjorie. In light of this situation, it appears Dr. Tucker has attempted to meet some of the aspirational guidelines set by Principle D.

Principle E: Respect for People's Rights and Dignity

> Psychologists are aware of and respect cultural, individual, and role differences, including those based on age, gender[,] . . . race, ethnicity, culture, national origin[,] . . . language . . . [and] consider these factors when working with members of such groups. Psychologists try to eliminate the effect on their work of biases based on those factors, and they do not knowingly participate in or condone activities of others based upon such prejudices.

Although Dr. Tucker's assessment procedure did meet the aspiration enumerated in Principle D, that of justice, it appears that she was less than exemplary in carrying out the principles articulated in Principle E. It is questionable as to whether Dr. Tucker was aware of or considered the limitations of the assessment instruments she used in terms of culture and language, and her own limitations in terms of knowledge about Korean culture.

Companion Ethical Standard(s)

Standard 2.01: Boundaries of Competence

> . . . (b) Where scientific or professional knowledge in the discipline of psychology establishes that an understanding of factors associated with age, gender[,] . . . race, ethnicity, culture, national origin[,] . . . language . . . is essential for effective implementation of their services[,] . . . psychologists have or obtain the training, experience, consultation, or supervision necessary to ensure the competence of their services.

Standard 2.01 (b) operationalizes the concept of respecting differences as articulated in Principle E. While Dr. Tucker seemed to demonstrate competency with regard to conducting parent evaluations, it is less clear whether her competence includes providing services to immigrants of Korean ancestry. Did the conclusions drawn by Dr. Tucker evidence an understanding of the cultural and linguistic differences? Was Dr. Tucker aware of the possibility that she may be predisposed to view Mr. Bradley more favorably given their shared cultural background? If there is a question regarding competence for any specific population, Standard 2.01 (b) directs Dr. Tucker to have obtained support through further training, extra consultation, or supervision.

Standard 9.02: Use of Assessments

> . . . (c) Psychologists use assessment methods that are appropriate to an individual's language preference and competence, unless the use of an alternative language is relevant to the assessment issues.

Per Standard 9.02 (c), Dr. Tucker needed to have considered the language competence of Mr. Bradley and Mrs. Marjorie. Mr. Bradley, who was raised in the United States, does not appear to have had difficulties with the use of the English language during the assessment. Regardless of Mrs. Marjorie's language competence, Standard 9.02 (c) directs Dr. Tucker to have considered the possibility that the questions Mrs. Marjorie's asked about the items on the MMPI may have been due to difficulty with understanding the language or the colloquialisms embedded in the stated questions. Given Mrs. Marjorie's background as an adult immigrant from Korea, Standard 9.02 (c) directs Dr. Tucker to have checked for the level of language competence with regard to her ability to complete the assessments.

Standard 9.06: Interpreting Assessment Results

> When interpreting assessment results[,] . . . psychologists take into account the purpose of the assessment as well as the various test factors, test-taking abilities, and other characteristics of the person being assessed, such as situational, personal, linguistic, and cultural differences, that might affect psychologists' judgments or reduce the accuracy of their interpretations. They indicate any significant limitations of their interpretations.

Even if Mrs. Marjorie's command of the English language justified administration of the assessments in English, Standard 9.06 directs Dr. Tucker to have evaluated whether the use of the MMPI and the WAIS-R with a Korean immigrant is within the scope of the tests' normative population. In addition, Standard 9.02 (c) directs Dr. Tucker to consider what, if any, are the limitations with regard to the interpretation of the results. Factors such as the linguistic and cultural differences as specifically named in Standard 9.06 would have affected the interpretation of the test results as well as the clinical observations.

Legal Issues 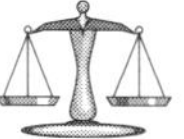

California

Cal. Fam. Code § 3110.5 (West 2004).

> (b) (1) On or before January 1, 2002, the Judicial Council shall formulate a statewide rule of court. . .
>
> (B) The rule shall require all evaluators to utilize comparable interview, assessment, and testing procedures for all parties that are consistent with generally accepted clinical, forensic, scientific, diagnostic, or medical standards.

Cal. Rules of Court, Rule 5.220 (West 2010). Court-Ordered Child Custody Evaluations.

> (h) Ethics
>
> In performing an evaluation, the child custody evaluator must:
>
> (1) Maintain objectivity, provide and gather balanced information for both parties, and control for bias. . .
>
> (6) Operate within the limits of the evaluator's training and experience and disclose any limitations or bias that would affect the evaluator's ability to conduct the evaluation. . .
>
> (11) Be sensitive to the socioeconomic status, gender, race, ethnicity, cultural values, religion, family structures, and developmental characteristics of the parties.

Hawaii

Haw. Code R. § 16-98-34 (2010). Unethical Practice of Psychology.

> (e) The psychologist shall respect the integrity and protect the welfare of the person or group with whom the psychologist is working. . .
>
> (6) The psychologist who requires the taking of psychological tests for . . . classification . . . purposes shall protect the examinees by insuring that the tests and test results are used in a professional manner.

Dr. Tucker is expected to indicate within the report Mrs. Marjorie's background as an adult immigrant from Korea and whether Dr. Tucker developed sufficient competence to interpret the results of the evaluation for such a person. For instance, Dr. Tucker could have obtained and mentioned the fact that cultural consultation occurred during the case. Since Dr. Tucker did not include limitations about the use of the evaluation measures with someone of Mrs. Marjorie's background, Dr. Tucker essentially broke the laws and failed to protect the welfare of Mrs. Marjorie by using comparable instruments, thus engaging in Eurocentric insensitivity (American Psychological Association [APA], 2002, Guideline #4: "[B]e aware of the limitations of assessment practices" [p. 48]).

Cultural Considerations

Global Discussion

The Professional Board for Psychology Health Professions Council of South Africa: Ethical Code of Conduct (April 2002)

> 5.5. Cultural diversity
>
> 5.5.1. Psychologists who . . . use assessment methods shall be familiar with the reliability, validation, and related standardization or outcome studies of, and proper applications and uses of, the methods they use.
>
> 1. Psychologists shall recognize limits to the certainty with which . . . predictions can be made about individuals, especially where linguistic, cultural and socio-economic variances exist.
>
> 2. Psychologists shall make every effort to identify situations in which particular assessment methods or norms may not be applicable or may require adjustment in administration, scoring and interpretation because of factors such as . . . culture[,] . . . ethnic and social origin, gender, language.

As directed by South Africa's code, Dr. Tucker is to make every effort to determine whether a Korean immigrant with less than fluent English being administered an MMPI is a situation where standard assessment methods are either not applicable or require adjustments. Not understanding the language the MMPI was given in could explain Mrs. Marjorie's repeated questioning of office staff, rather than the assumption that this makes her neurotic. Dr. Tucker's use of an assessment tool that is highly culture-bound and normed on those other than Korean immigrant women is evidence for Dr. Tucker's violation of the 5.5.1 section of the South African code. Once the MMPI is used, Dr. Tucker would need to explain its limitations, its likely lack of validity, and how cultural factors may account for much of the negative evidence against Mrs. Marjorie as a parent.

American Moral Values

1. Was Dr. Tucker's evaluation unfair to Mrs. Marjorie? Did Dr. Tucker take into account any linguistic or cultural factors that may have affected the MMPI results, or did she only mention Mrs. Marjorie's national origin and that she met her husband there?
2. As English is Mrs. Marjorie's second language, could this fact have hindered her ability to understand test questions? Did Dr. Tucker know that family titles (e.g., "first daughter") rather than proper names are common as forms of address in Korean culture? Was being "compulsive" more like a determination to understand questions that could affect a divorce judgment?
3. What does Dr. Tucker make of the MMPI finding that Mrs. Marjorie is depressed? Does Dr. Tucker believe that cultural isolation or alienation could affect scores for depression? How would an admission of depression affect the overall evaluation?
4. Does Dr. Tucker understand the cultural dimensions of referring to children by their family designation (e.g., "first son")? Does Dr. Tucker account adequately for how differing conceptions of family and privacy might affect Mrs. Marjorie's responses? How should Dr. Tucker broach these issues in her statement?
5. How will Dr. Tucker's representation of Mrs. Marjorie relate to her practice and her work with Asian American and Asian immigrant clients? Does she feel a special responsibility to fight against possible forms of discrimination?

Ethical Course of Action

Directive per APA Code

Following Principle D: Justice, Dr. Tucker's method for conducting the evaluation treated both Mr. Bradley and Mrs. Marjorie equally. In addition, Dr. Tucker aspired to meet Principle E by administering the WAIS-R to Mrs. Marjorie in recognition of the differences in the backgrounds between Mr. Bradley and Mrs. Marjorie. Standard 9.02 (b) does not prohibit the use of the MMPI-2 or the WAIS-R in cross-cultural situations such as this one. However, Standard 9.02 (b) directs Dr. Tucker to have described the limitations of the test results. Moreover, Standard 9.06 directs Dr. Tucker to acknowledge the limitations of the instruments themselves. Except for a possible violation of Standard 9.02 (c), in that Dr. Tucker did not check into Mrs. Marjorie's language preference, it appears Dr. Tucker is in compliance with the ethical standards pertaining to assessment.

Independent of the procedures and assessment instruments selected, the relevant question for this vignette is whether Dr. Tucker was practicing within the boundaries of her competency as identified in Standard 2.01 (b). If, at the deposition, the attorney cites Standard 2.06 (b), Dr. Tucker would then need to show evidence that she indeed had sufficient education, training, or experience demonstrating her competence in working with a member of the immigrant Korean population. Based on her stated interpretation of the assessment results, Dr. Tucker would have a difficult time defending her competence in working with Koreans who have immigrated to the United States.

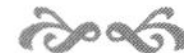

Dictates of One's Own Conscience

If you were Dr. Tucker, post receipt of the attorney's request but previous to appearing for the deposition, which of these would you do before the deposition?

1. Review your notes on the case to make sure that you remember all the relevant facts.
2. Reflect upon APA Multicultural Guideline #5: *"Psychologists strive to apply culturally appropriate skills in clinical and other applied psychological practices"(APA, 2003, p. 43) in which you are urged to consider that* "Eurocentric models may not be effective in working with other populations as well, and indeed, may do harm by mislabeling or misdiagnosing problems and treatments" (p. 45).
3. Consult with another psychologist to help you prepare for the deposition.
4. Ask a psychologist who is an expert in the area of Korean immigrants or Asian Americans to review your assessment.
5. Consult with a psychologist with a specialty in immigrants regarding possible questions about divorce practices in Korea that might surface at a deposition.
6. Combinations of the above-listed actions.
7. Or one that is not listed above.

If you were Dr. Tucker practicing in South Africa, you would not have administered the MMPI or the WAIS to Mrs. Marjorie.

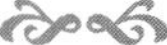

STANDARD 9.02: USE OF ASSESSMENTS

> . . . (c) Psychologists use assessment methods that are appropriate to an individual's language preference and competence, unless the use of an alternative language is relevant to the assessment issues.

A CASE FOR STANDARD 9.02 (C): Disabled or ESL?

The state disability office refers Monica for a routine annual disability examination. Monica is a 22-year-old immigrant from Mexico who came to the United States when she was 7 years old. At age 17, while walking home from high school, Monica was abducted, physically abused, sexually assaulted, and then left on the side of the road. Monica was diagnosed with post-traumatic stress disorder (PTSD) and major depressive disorder (MDD) secondary to the assault. She has lived at home with her mother since the assault because of an inability to leave the house without an escort, which has prevented her from engaging in gainful employment.

Monica arrives at Dr. Porter's office accompanied by Ray, her boyfriend. Monica is meticulously groomed and fashionably dressed. A Mental Status Exam reveals a euthymic mood with full range of affect, excellent sleep, no use of psychotropic medications, no report of acute emotional distress, a stable relationship with her boyfriend, enjoyment from hanging out and shopping with her friends, intermittent recollections of the assault, and no report of any significant problems in her life except discomfort in leaving the house by herself. A battery of standardized testing included the Millon Clinical Multiaxial Inventory–III (MCMI-III), the Minnesota Multiphasic Personality Inventory–2 (MMPI-2), the Beck Depression Inventory–II (BDI-II), and the Impact of Events Scale–Revised (IES-R), all of which revealed subclinical levels of psychiatric symptoms. With regard to work, Monica cites trouble concentrating and language as potential barriers, as well as uncertainty about her career path. Monica is concerned that if she loses her disability status, this will adversely affect her family because this is their only source of income.

Issues of Concern

Standard 9.02 (c) addresses the use of language in assessment. Presumably, Standard 9.02 (c) refers to the language used for the clinical interview as well as the tests themselves. Monica has been living in the United States for more than half of her life, was educated in the U.S. school system, and has used English throughout her educational career. Based on this, one might reasonably assume she has sufficient mastery of the English language and is able to participate in the clinical interview without using Spanish. However, are the selected assessments, all of which are written and administered in English, appropriate for the individual? In addition to English proficiency, are the tests normed for Mexican immigrants? If Monica is concerned about language proficiency on the job, is there sufficient reason to consider conducting the interview and the tests in Spanish, her native language? Or are PTSD and language problems a ruse to not go to work?

APA Ethics Code

Companion General Principle

Principle E: Respect for People's Rights and Dignity

> Psychologists are aware of and respect cultural, individual, and role differences, including those based on age, gender[,] . . . race, ethnicity, culture, national origin[,] . . . language, and socioeconomic status and consider these factors when working with members of such groups.

Principle E directs Dr. Porter's attention to considering whether he should take into account Monica's age, gender, ethnicity, national origin, language, and socioeconomic status in his work with her. Taking these factors into account would affect decisions regarding selection of a test battery and interpretation of the test results.

Principle D: Justice

> Psychologists exercise reasonable judgment and take precautions to ensure that their potential biases, the boundaries of their competence, and the limitations of their expertise do not lead to or condone unjust practices.

Principle D: Justice suggests that Dr. Porter consider his level of competency for working with the Mexican American population.

Companion Ethical Standard

Standard 3.07: Third-Party Requests for Services

> When psychologists agree to provide services to a person . . . at the request of a third party, psychologists attempt to clarify at the outset of the service the nature of the relationship with all individuals or organizations involved. This clarification includes the role of the psychologist[,] . . . an identification of who is the client, the probable uses of the services provided or the information obtained, and the fact that there may be limits to confidentiality.

The state disability service has requested an assessment for Monica. The professional role Dr. Porter holds depends on his contractual relationship with the state's disability services office. If Dr. Porter is an employee of the state, or if he holds a contract with the state to be paid directly for the evaluation, then Dr. Porter's client is not Monica, but the state. It is doubtful whether Monica holds the privilege of privacy and confidentiality with regard to anything she does with Dr. Porter, unless Monica has privately retained him. Standard 3.07 directs Dr. Porter to make attempts to clarify these stipulations. It is also up to Dr. Porter to define what constitutes "attempts" for clarification, and to make these clarifications in such a manner as to assure that Monica understands the role and limitations of the relationship.

Standard 9.03: Informed Consent in Assessments

> . . . (b) Psychologists inform persons . . . for whom testing is mandated by . . . governmental regulations about the nature and purpose of the proposed assessment services, using language that is reasonably understandable to the person being assessed.
>
> (c) Psychologists using the services of an interpreter obtain informed consent from the client/patient to use that interpreter.

Standard 9.03 augments Standard 3.07. Standard 3.07 (b) directs Dr. Porter to use the language that is reasonably expected to be understood, meaning that Monica is to understand that Dr. Porter's job is to recommend whether she receive disability benefits and services from the state.

Standard 9.03 (c) directs Dr. Porter to obtain consent from Monica should he decide to use an interpreter for any part of his work with her. Given that Monica reported some difficulty with the English language, it would be prudent for Dr. Porter to make sure she is aware of the option to receive the services of an interpreter. If Monica decided she would like an interpreter, then Dr. Porter would need to include in his report a description of any limitations that resulted from the use of an interpreter in the testing process.

Standard 2.01: Boundaries of Competence

> (b) Where . . . professional knowledge in the discipline of psychology establishes that an understanding of factors associated with age, gender[,] . . . race, ethnicity, culture, national origin[,] . . . language, or socioeconomic status is essential for effective implementation of their services[,] . . . psychologists have or obtain the training, experience, consultation, or supervision necessary to ensure the competence of their services, or they make appropriate referrals.

Standard 2.01 (b) is the operationalization of Principle E: Respect for People's Rights and Dignity. Standard 2.01 (b) sets the standard for the case with Monica. Dr. Porter is to be competent based on training, experience, consultation, or supervision to provide services to a client who is a young adult (22-year-old) female, whose native language is Spanish, whose socioeconomic status is at the poverty level, and whose national origin is Mexican. If Dr. Porter is not already competent to deliver services for the relevant population, then Standard 2.01 (b) directs him to secure consultation or supervision. The essential question for this assessment is whether, given the level of acculturation one expects for Monica, factors related to language fluency are relevant.

Standard 9.02: Use of Assessments

> . . . (b) Psychologists use assessment instruments whose validity and reliability have been established for use with members of the population tested. When such validity or reliability has not been established, psychologists describe the strengths and limitations of test results and interpretation.

Standard 9.02 (b) directs Dr. Porter to choose instruments that take into account Monica's status as a Mexican immigrant. It is unclear whether Dr. Porter determined if there are Spanish versions for some of the instruments or whether Mexican Americans were a part of the normative population for the instruments chosen. Regardless of the appropriateness of the instruments for Monica, Standard 9.02 directs Dr. Porter to include a description about any and all limitations of the instruments and the validity of his interpretations based on those instruments.

Legal Issues

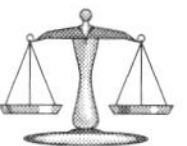

Indiana

868 Ind. Admin. Code 1.1-11-4.1 (2010). Relationships Within Professional Practice.

> (m) Where differences of:
>
> (1) age;
>
> (2) gender;
>
> (3) race;
>
> (4) ethnicity;
>
> (5) national origin[;] . . .
>
> (9) language; or
>
> (10) socioeconomic status . . .
>
> significantly affect a psychologist's work concerning particular individuals . . . the psychologist shall obtain the training, experience, consultation, or supervision necessary to ensure the competence of the psychologist's services concerning such individuals. . . If the psychologist cannot obtain the training, experience, consultation, or supervision necessary to ensure the competence of the psychologist's services, the psychologist shall decline to offer services and shall make appropriate referrals.

868 Ind. Admin. Code 1.1-11-5 (2010). Psychology Practice.

> (b) A psychologist's assessments, recommendations, reports, and psychological diagnostic or evaluative statements must be based on information and techniques (including personal interviews of the individual when appropriate) sufficient to appropriately substantiate the findings.

Kansas

Kan. Admin. Regs. § 102-1-10a (2010). Unprofessional Conduct.

> (f) ignoring client welfare, which shall include the following acts. . .
>
> (11) continuing to use . . . tests . . . not warranted by the client's . . . condition. . .
>
> (j) improperly using assessment procedures, which shall include the following acts:
>
> (1) Basing assessment, intervention, or recommendations on test results and instruments that are inappropriate to the current purpose or to the patient characteristics;

(2) . . . failing to make adjustments in administration or interpretation because of relevant factors, including gender, age, race, and other pertinent factors;

(3) failing to indicate significant limitations to the accuracy of the assessment findings . . .

(5) . . . submitting psychological . . . reports . . . on the basis of information and techniques that are insufficient to substantiate those findings. . .

(o) Engaging in improprieties with respect to forensic practice, which shall include the following acts:

(1) When conducting a forensic examination, failing to inform the examinee of the purpose of the examination and the difference between a forensic examination and a therapeutic relationship . . .

(3) failing to conduct forensic examinations in conformance with established scientific and professional standards.

To be in compliance with the law, Dr. Porter's evaluation report should take into account Monica's multicultural background and address whether the measures used were appropriate in light of their validity and reliability findings for someone with Monica's background.

Cultural Considerations

Global Discussion

The Professional Board for Psychology
Health Professions Council of South Africa:
Ethical Code of Conduct (April 2002)

1. Psychologists' assessments, recommendations, reports, and psychological diagnostic or evaluative statements shall be based on information and techniques sufficient to provide appropriate substantiation for their findings.

1. Informed consent in assessments.

5.3.2. Psychologists shall inform persons . . . for whom testing is mandated by law about the nature and purpose of the proposed assessment services, using language that is reasonably understandable to the person being assessed.

5.8. Interpreting assessment results.

When psychologists interpret assessment results[,] . . . psychologists shall take into account the various test factors and characteristics of the person being assessed, such as situational, personal, linguistic, and cultural differences that might affect psychologists' judgements or reduce the accuracy of their interpretations. They shall indicate any significant reservations they have about the accuracy or limitations of their interpretations.

Arguably, as Monica had been living in the United States for 15 years and she did not bring an interpreter with her to the assessment, her English proficiency is sufficient enough to understand Dr. Porter's questions. However, South Africa's code is silent on acculturation of immigrants, and how their experience and language acquisition may differ from other populations.

Next, Dr. Porter must account for the "personal, situational, linguistic and cultural" differences in his interpretation of the assessment results and in his final report. If Monica's inability to work seems to stem from her language proficiency, rather than her assault, then can an immigrant be assumed to be acculturated sufficiently enough that tests designed for English-speaking Americans are valid?

American Moral Values

1. How does Dr. Porter see his duty for this referral? Does he see Monica first and foremost as his patient, or does he see himself as a contracted employee of the state? How does his role inform his attitude toward Monica's fear about losing disability? What does he owe to the state, and what does he owe to Monica?

2. Are Dr. Porter's tests fair to Monica on a cultural and linguistic basis? Does Dr. Porter believe himself to have sufficient training for clients facing issues of gender, race, ethnicity, and language, in addition to the trauma Monica underwent? Does he believe her English is good enough to report her mood and experiences accurately and clearly? Do her test results give Dr. Porter enough reason not to consult another psychologist before making an evaluation?

3. How does Dr. Porter view language outside of the issue of testing in Monica's case? Does he believe hard work and determination will allow an individual to overcome language barriers? Or does he believe that Monica's job search is unfairly impeded by a work environment hostile to non-English or beginning English speakers?

4. How strong of a personal response does Dr. Porter have to Monica's abduction and assault? Does he believe she deserves more leeway from the state after having survived what was done to her? Does he believe that, indications from testing aside, this trauma will still take a toll on her overall well-being going forward? How much weight does he give to her inability to leave the house alone?

Ethical Course of Action

Directive per APA Code

Standard 9.02 (c) directs Dr. Porter to assess Monica's language competence before proceeding to conduct a psychological evaluation in English. Monica was educated in the U.S. school system for Grades K–12 and used English throughout her educational career. There is no reason to believe that she does not have sufficient mastery of English to participate in the clinical interview in English. Thus use of English does not violate the directives of Standard 9.02 (c). However, language proficiency is not equivalent to cultural competence. To be in compliance with the directives of Standard 9.02 (b), Dr. Porter needs to ascertain the validity of the English version of the MCMI-III, MMPI-2, BDI-II, and IES-R for Mexican Americans. In addition, he should address the cultural limitations of these instruments in his assessment report.

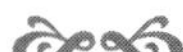

Dictates of One's Own Conscience

If you were Dr. Porter, how might you proceed?

1. Decide that the normal protocol is culture dependent and, regardless of language proficiency, is not valid for Monica.
2. Decide that the instruments selected are adequate for use with Monica, given her age at migration, and proceed with your normal protocol.
3. Decide that the linguistic problems, though relevant, are not severe enough to alter normal protocol and address them thus in the interpretation section of the report: Regardless of immigrant status, you do not see any reason that the test results are not valid, and you conclude that Monica no longer suffers from PTSD.
4. Regardless of the test results,
    a. you consider the combination of Monica's immigrant status and her residual subclinical PTSD symptoms to impact her daily functioning and conclude that she still suffers from PTSD.
    b. you take into consideration that she is subclinical for PTSD only because her family and boyfriend have sheltered her. You conclude that further treatment is needed to transition her to full independent functioning.
5. In consideration of the test results, you think enabling Monica to stay at home does her a disservice in the long term and conclude that the assessment does not support evidence of disability from PTSD.
6. In consideration of her socioeconomic status, the family's dependence on the disability income, and evidence of subclinical symptoms, you conclude there is sufficient reason to continue disability based on mental illness.
7. You are of Hispanic descent and are competent both linguistically and culturally to interpret the test results, which you do as follows:
    a. You think that people like Monica give Hispanics and Mexicans a bad name. You conclude there is no evidence to support continued diagnosis of PTSD.
    b. You think that Monica is acting culturally congruently, given the history of the assault, and conclude that Monica needs further time to recover from the trauma of the assault.
8. Combinations of the above-listed actions.
9. Or one that is not listed above.

If you were Dr. Porter practicing in South Africa, the above-listed options would still apply since the guidelines for selection and interpretation of assessment instruments are not substantially different from those listed by the APA Ethics Code.

STANDARD 9.03: INFORMED CONSENT IN ASSESSMENTS

(a) Psychologists obtain informed consent for assessments, evaluations, or diagnostic services, as described in Standard 3.10: Informed Consent, except when **(1) testing is mandated by law or governmental regulations;** (2) informed consent is implied because testing is conducted as a routine educational, institutional, or organizational activity (e.g., when participants voluntarily agree to assessment when applying for a job); or (3) one purpose of the testing is to evaluate decisional capacity. Informed consent includes an explanation of the nature and purpose of the assessment, fees, involvement of third parties, and limits of confidentiality and sufficient opportunity for the client/patient to ask questions and receive answers.

A CASE FOR STANDARD 9.03 (A) (1): Grounded

Frederick, a 31-year-old married Caucasian male, is a Navy pilot with 10 years of active duty service. Recently, Frederick was sent to Dr. Hunter by his flight surgeon for certification as psychologically fit to resume full flight status following a restriction to a 1-year provisional status. Frederick's restriction from flight is based on his diagnosis of post-traumatic stress disorder after a plane crash incident 4 years ago. He is now concerned that unless he is restored to full flight status, not only is his military career over, but the PTSD diagnosis also will prevent him from finding civilian employment as a pilot. Regulations specify a psychological evaluation as the only means to alter a diagnosis and change flight status. Military aviation policy stipulates non-flight status if a psychological evaluation finds any condition that may potentially place either Frederick or others at risk.

Frederick says he is free from all psychological symptoms and offers his stellar performance during the most recent Iraq deployment as evidence of his restored mental health. Scores on the Impact of Events Scale (IES), PTSD Checklist, and Beck Depression Inventory–II (BDI-II) corroborate this self-report. However when questioned further about his last deployment in Iraq, he appeared to be obviously distressed as he recounts several incidents involving his witnessing of horrific injuries of dead military personnel. Frederick's level of distress signifies residual PTSD. Fredrick admits to mild levels of PTSD symptoms after returning from Iraq a year ago, but not to a severity of the level that would impair his ability to function in the military. He does not think his postwar difficulties have any bearing on his capacity to fly.

Issues of Concern

Standard 9.03 (a) specifies that psychologists are to obtain informed consent before engaging in any psychological assessment services. Since the U.S. military is considered part of the government, and this assessment is being conducted under the criteria established by military regulations, then Standard 9.03 (a) (1) applies. This means Dr. Hunter is not required to obtain informed consent. Regardless of consent, does Dr. Hunter still have to explain to Frederick the purpose of the assessment, any fees, or the limits of confidentiality? Further, would she need to allow Frederick the opportunity to ask her questions about anything she does? Does this apply even if Dr. Hunter is not part of the military, or does the exception to informed consent only apply if Dr. Hunter has entered into an employment or contractual relationship with the military?

APA Ethics Code

Companion General Principle

Principle A: Beneficence and Nonmaleficence

> Psychologists strive to benefit those with whom they work and take care to do no harm. In their professional actions, psychologists seek to safeguard the welfare and rights of those with whom they interact professionally and other affected persons.

Guided by Principle A, Dr. Hunter would consider a course of action that benefits all parties concerned. While Frederick is free to focus on his concern with his potential to work and earn a living, Principle A suggests that Dr. Hunter is guided to focus on both Fredrick and those affected persons involved in this situation, which would include others in his military unit who may be harmed should Frederick not remain mentally stable throughout his active duty.

Principle B: Fidelity and Responsibility.

> They [psychologists] are aware of their professional and scientific responsibilities to society and to the specific communities in which they work. Psychologists uphold professional standards of conduct . . . [and] clarify their professional roles and obligations.

Principle B guides Dr. Hunter to consider her responsibility not only to Frederick, but also to the community of people who are affected by Dr. Hunter's work. In this situation, the community is not a vague group of people but very specifically those who will be going into combat situations with Frederick and whose lives will depend on Frederick's mental status and subsequent stability. Principle B points Dr. Hunter's attention to the fact that her work will affect the lives of both Frederick and those who are in his military unit.

Companion Ethical Standard(s)

Standard 3.07: Third-Party Requests for Services

> When psychologists agree to provide services to a person . . . at the request of a third party, psychologists attempt to

clarify at the outset of the service the nature of the relationship with all individuals . . . involved. This clarification includes the role of the psychologist . . . an identification of who is the client, the probable uses of the . . . information obtained, and the fact that there may be limits to confidentiality.

The military in the person of Frederick's commanding officer has requested an evaluation. This situation meets those specified in Standard 3.07. Standard 3.07 directs Dr. Hunter to clarify from the outset of her encounters with Frederick that she is providing a service to the commanding officer, which means her client is the military. Standard 3.07 also directs Dr. Hunter to inform Frederick that the limits of confidentiality are subject to military regulation. Thus, Dr. Hunter needs to be well aware of Fredrick's privacy rights in this evaluation situation and to inform him of such.

Standard 3.04: Avoiding Harm

Psychologists take reasonable steps to avoid harming their clients/patients . . . [and] organizational clients . . . and to minimize harm where it is foreseeable and unavoidable.

Standard 3.04 is the operationalization of Principle A: Beneficence and Nonmaleficence. Frederick is reporting to Dr. Hunter that a diagnosis of PTSD will harm him by negatively impacting his ability to continue in the military or find a job in a related civilian field. Standard 3.04 directs Dr. Hunter to be concerned about Frederick as well as the safety of other military personnel who will be serving with Frederick. Therefore, Dr. Hunter needs to be concerned about how to avoid or at least minimize harm to the military community as well as Frederick.

Legal Issues 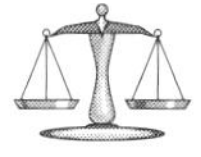

Kentucky

201 Ky. Admin. Regs. 26:145 (2010). Code of Conduct.

Section 2. Client Requirements.

(1) Identification of a client. A client shall be a person who receives:

(a) An evaluation, assessment, or psychological testing. . .

(2) A corporate entity or other organization shall be considered the client if the professional contract is to provide a psychological service of benefit to the corporate entity or organization. . .

(4) Services involving more than one (1) interested party. If more than one (1) party has an appropriate interest in the professional services rendered by the credential holder to a client or clients, the credential holder shall clarify to all parties prior to rendering the services the dimensions of confidentiality and professional responsibility that shall pertain in the rendering of services.

Michigan

Mich. Admin. Code r. 338.2515 (2010). Prohibited Conduct.

Rule 15. Prohibited conduct includes, but is not limited to, the following acts or omissions by any individual covered by these rules. . .

(c) Taking on a professional role when personal, scientific, professional, legal, financial, or other relationships could impair the exercise of professional discretion or make the interests of a patient, supervisee, or student secondary to those of the licensee.

In both jurisdictions, Dr. Hunter should engage in a thorough disclosure about the fact that the Navy is the client for the purposes of the evaluation, and that anything that is said or revealed in the evaluation is likely to be disclosed to the client. If Dr. Hunter does not engage in such a disclosure process, she would violate the law in Kentucky. It is unlikely that Dr. Hunter would be in violation of the law in Michigan, unless Frederick obtained evidence that Dr. Hunter's evaluative judgment was tainted by the financial relationship with the client, the Navy.

Cultural Considerations

Global Discussion

Code of Ethics for the Psychologist: Spain.

Article 42. When such assessment or intervention has been requested by other persons such as judges, educational professionals, parents, employers or anyone other than the person to be assessed, the latter . . . have the right to be informed about the assessment or intervention and the addressee of the resulting Psychological Report. The subject of a Psychological Report has the right to know its content, providing that this will not pose a grave danger to the subject or the Psychologist, even when the report has been requested by others.

Article 43. Psychological Reports prepared at the request of institutions or organisations in general, apart from

> the provisions of the preceding article, are subject to the same general duties and rights for confidentiality defined above. Both the Psychologist and the institution requesting are obliged not to divulge the report outside the strict range for which it was conceived.
>
> When enumerations or lists of assessed individuals, in which the diagnosis and assessments data must appear, are requested from the Psychologist by other agencies, for planning purposes, obtaining resources or for any other ends, these should be made omitting the subject's name and identification data, whenever those are not strictly necessary.

If Dr. Hunter and Frederick were in Spain, Dr. Hunter would be obligated to inform Frederick about the purpose of the assessment, and her report results (42); keep their results confidential outside the purpose of giving the results to the military (43); and omit Frederick's information and identifying data where it is not strictly necessary (43). Provided that harm will not come to Dr. Hunter or Frederick by doing so, Dr. Hunter may also release the report's findings to Frederick, if requested to do so (42).

American Moral Values

1. How does Dr. Hunter draw the line between her responsibility to Frederick and her responsibility to the military? How will she judge Frederick's pleas to fly while considering those who could be harmed by a poor flight performance?
2. How do Dr. Hunter's views about the military in general affect her willingness to lend weight to Frederick's self-report? How does she frame his desire to fly again—mostly as a concern for his career or as a sense of duty toward one's country? Does she believe the military has not paid enough attention to conditions like PTSD, including whether soldiers' self-reports have credibility? Or does she believe the military is too rule-bound and inflexible about "non-flight status" to consider that Frederick could manage his PTSD symptoms and fly?
3. Does Dr. Hunter fear for Frederick's quality of life if he does not fly? Given that a PTSD diagnosis might threaten his chance at a civilian pilot job, how will Frederick cope with the loss of his flying career? Is there a way for Dr. Hunter's evaluation to address that issue with his superiors?
4. How could Frederick's recurring symptoms of PTSD affect his flying and performance? How reckless would Dr. Hunter take herself to be if she were not extremely cautious in her diagnosis? If she believes that many other pilots are struggling with the condition but not reporting it, is Dr. Hunter more inclined to tout Frederick's self-report as good enough support to let him fly again?

Ethical Course of Action

Directive per APA Code

Through 9.03(a) (1), the APA Ethics Code supports the military policy in that, regardless of Dr. Hunter's findings, Frederick does not have an option pertaining to the release of the psychological evaluation. Standard 3.07 requires Dr. Hunter to have informed Frederick of the fact at the onset of services that her client is the military, not Frederick. As assigned by her client, Dr. Hunter's role as examiner is to ascertain the risk to safety Frederick poses to the other members of his military unit and himself. While Dr. Hunter's level of responsibility for informed consent is limited, it is clinically prudent for Dr. Hunter to provide Frederick with basic information about the nature and purpose of the assessment, as well as ascertaining if Frederick understands the military policies regarding full flight status.

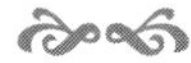

Dictates of One's Own Conscience

If you were Dr. Hunter, faced with this situation, within the parameters set by the APA Ethics Code and guided by your own moral stance, which of these might you do?

1. Not render an opinion, but recommend that Frederick receive further treatment and be reevaluated in 6 months.
2. Recommend Frederick reenlist for another term of duty; engage in another assessment regarding his PTSD before he is discharged into civilian life.
3. Render a finding of PTSD, in remission, with recommendation that he not be assigned to combat duties.
4. Render a finding of PTSD.
5. If you were in civilian private practice and Frederick retained the privilege of confidentiality,
    a. render diagnosis of PTSD and recommend permanent disability.
    b. render diagnosis of PTSD in remission and recommend avoidance of similar situations of the original trauma.

   c. render opinion that PTSD is no longer relevant since Frederick does not exhibit symptoms in civilian life.
6. Combinations of the above-listed actions.
7. Or one that is not listed above.

If you were Dr. Hunter, practicing in Spain, would you inform Frederick from the outset that although he has the right to see the final report, and the final report will not be seen outside of official purposes, that your client is the military, not Frederick, and you will likely release pertinent information to them?

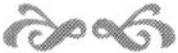

STANDARD 9.03: INFORMED CONSENT IN ASSESSMENTS

> (a) Psychologists obtain informed consent for assessments, evaluations, or diagnostic services, as described in Standard 3.10, Informed Consent, except when (1) testing is mandated by law or governmental regulations; **(2) informed consent is implied because testing is conducted as a routine educational, institutional, or organizational activity (e.g., when participants voluntarily agree to assessment when applying for a job)**; or (3) one purpose of the testing is to evaluate decisional capacity. Informed consent includes an explanation of the nature and purpose of the assessment, fees, involvement of third parties, and limits of confidentiality and sufficient opportunity for the client/patient to ask questions and receive answers.

A CASE FOR STANDARD 9.03 (A) (2): Job Skills

National Railways requires all employees to retake their preemployment assessments. The National Railways Company used to send preemployment packets to prospective applicants, but the company now has a proctored administration of preemployment assessments. National Railways has requested that all currently employed personnel update their personnel files with the current preemployment assessment packet, including current assessment results.

Edwin has worked at National Railways for the last 23 years. He has risen through the ranks to the status of an engineer. He is now 2 years away from retirement. After several weeks of procrastinating by Edwin, he is told by the company that he either takes the exam now or risks immediate dismissal. To the company's surprise, Edwin fails the proctored preemployment assessment.

Dr. Hicks, the psychologist in charge of overseeing the updating of personnel files, has routinely been referred any current employees who have problems with the preemployment exams. Edwin admits to Dr. Hicks he cannot really read and had someone else complete all of his preemployment paperwork in his initial interview 23 years ago. He asks Dr. Hicks to consider his outstanding work record of the past 23 years, and ignore his inability to read as he has been able to function well in his job duties. He also stated that, since taking the preemployment examination, he has had a psychological evaluation and was diagnosed with a reading disability. Edwin asks Dr. Hicks whether the company could exempt him from the preemployment tests in light of the fact that he has an excellent work record and that he has a diagnosis of a reading disability.

Issues of Concern

The conditions for Edwin's assessment meet the exception in the need for psychologists to obtain informed consent as stated in Standard 9.03 (a) (2). While Dr. Hicks does not need to obtain Edwin's consent to be tested because it is implied by Edwin's employment agreement, should she still inform Edwin of the purpose and nature of the assessment?

There are two different issues of concern for Dr. Hicks to consider. One has to do with the American Disabilities Act (ADA) and the other involves fraud. What responsibility does Dr. Hicks have for an after-the-fact ADA compliance? Also, how shall Dr. Hicks handle Edwin's fraudulent act 23 years ago? In the strictest view of this situation, the breach of trust was made by Edwin when he knowingly engaged in fraudulent activity 23 years ago by having someone else take his exam for him. Edwin continued the falsehood throughout his 23 years of employment by never revealing his inability to read. Presuming Edwin has been an honest person in all other respects of his job, is it really of benefit to the railroad company to terminate Edwin's employment?

APA Ethics Code

Companion General Principle

Principle E: Respect for People's Rights and Dignity

> Psychologists are aware of and respect . . . individual . . . and role differences, including those based on age . . . [and] language[,] . . . and consider these factors when working

> with members of such groups. Psychologists try to eliminate the effect on their work of biases based on those factors, and they do not knowingly participate in or condone activities of others based upon such prejudices.

Aspiring to the highest aspirations of Principle E, Dr. Hicks would need to consider the valid application of a standardized battery of tests for one individual who has a stated disability. Simultaneously, how does respect for individual differences justify overlooking Edwin's past dishonest conduct and his current honest disclosure?

Companion Ethical Standard(s)

Standard 3.11: Psychological Services Delivered to or Through Organizations

> (a) Psychologists delivering services to or through organizations provide information beforehand to clients . . . [including] (1) the nature and objectives of the services[,] . . . (3) which of the individuals are clients[,] . . . (4) the relationship the psychologist will have with each person and the organization[,] . . . (5) the probable uses of services provided and information obtained[,] . . . (6) who will have access to the information, and . . . (7) limits of confidentiality. As soon as feasible, they provide information about the results and conclusions of such services to appropriate persons.

As an employee of the company who has oversight of one aspect of their personnel policy, Dr. Hicks's work is essentially done at the request of her employer, National Railways. In terms of Standard 3.11, Dr. Hicks's client is the National Railways Company, not Edwin. Per Standard 3.11 (a), Dr. Hicks is directed to inform Edwin of her role as an agent of the railway company and the limits of confidentiality thereof.

Standard 2.01: Boundaries of Competence

> . . . (b) Where . . . professional knowledge in the discipline of psychology establishes that an understanding of factors associated with age, gender . . . [, and] disability . . . is essential for effective implementation of their services[,] . . . psychologists have or obtain the training, experience, consultation, or supervision necessary to ensure the competence of their services, or they make appropriate referrals.

Even though Dr. Hicks was not the psychologist who administered the assessments, she is in a position to interpret the test results and give recommendations to the company regarding Edwin. Standard 2.01 (b) brings into question Dr. Hicks's competency to interpret the test results and to give recommendations. The relevant areas of specialty required by this case are those concerning age (Edwin being close to retirement), gender (a male), class (someone who has worked all of his life at a semi-skilled job), and disability (reading).

Standard 3.01: Unfair Discrimination

> In their work-related activities, psychologists do not engage in unfair discrimination based on age, gender . . . disability . . . or any basis proscribed by law.

The original preemployment testing did not allow for accommodations. Though there was no reason to think accommodations were needed, now that Edwin has been diagnosed with a reading disability, do the original conditions of the testing unfairly discriminate against someone with a disability? Also, now that Dr. Hicks knows Edwin has a reading disability, should different methods of assessment be considered in order not to unfairly discriminate against Edwin? Even if an alternative assessment were given or accommodations were made, is it unethical to overlook Edwin's fraudulent acts just because he is disabled?

Legal Issues 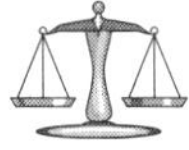

Minnesota

> *Minn. R. 7200.4600 (2010). Competence.*
>
> Subpart 1. Limits on practice.
>
> A psychologist shall limit practice to the areas of competence in which proficiency has been gained through education and training or experience.
>
> Subp. 4. Referrals.
>
> A psychologist shall recognize that there are other professional, technical, and administrative resources available to clients and make referrals to those resources when it is in the best interests of clients to be provided with alternative or complementary services.
>
> *Minn. R. 7200.5000 (2010). Assessments, Tests, Reports.*
>
> Subp. 1b. Administration and interpretation of tests.
>
> A psychologist must be qualified to administer and interpret tests employed and must be prepared to explain to the client the purposes, applications, scoring, and interpretation of those tests.

Missouri

Mo. Code Regs. Ann. tit. 20, § 2235-5.030 (2010). Ethical Rules of Conduct.

(3) Competence.

(A) Limits on Practice. The psychologist shall limit practice . . . to the areas in which competence has been gained through professional education, training derived through an organized training program and supervised professional experience. If important aspects of the client's problems fall outside the boundaries of competency, then the psychologist shall assist his/her client in obtaining additional professional consultation. . .

(12) Assessment Procedures.

(A) Competent Use of Assessment Techniques.

The psychologist shall use, administer and interpret psychological assessment techniques competently and maintain current knowledge about research developments and revisions concerning the techniques that are used.

Dr. Hicks would be held to the standard of being competent to interpret the test results of someone who is suffering from a significant learning disability. Unless Dr. Hicks met that competency or obtained sufficient consultation to engage in competent practice for someone with Edwin's issues, Dr. Hicks would violate the law in both jurisdictions.

Cultural Considerations

Global Discussion

Canadian Code of Ethics for Psychologists

Principle III: Integrity in relationships.

Straightforwardness/openness.

III.14. Be clear and straightforward about all information needed to establish informed consent. . .

III.15. Provide suitable information about the results of assessments, evaluations . . . [, and] findings to the persons involved, if appropriate and if asked. This information would be communicated in understandable language.

Dr. Hicks has not violated this portion of the Canadian code. Edwin's consent for assessment was assumed to be given since the exam is part of maintaining employment. Canada's code is silent on whether or not Dr. Hicks ought to administer the assessment to Edwin orally, as he is unable to use written English. What is difficult about Dr. Hicks's position is that Edwin is obviously able to function within his job role, having maintained employment for so long, as well as having been promoted. Dr. Hicks is obligated, according to Canada's code, to make the results of the assessment available to persons deemed "appropriate" and if asked (15).

American Moral Values

1. What does Dr. Hicks see as the most morally troubling part of Edwin's case? Is it that he lied about his preemployment 23 years ago, or that he did not become literate since then? Or is it that he now may be fired 2 years before retiring, even after having shown his competency at the job? What does her role as the company's in-house psychologist suggest should be her chief priority? Does that conform to what she would do as a psychologist *per se*?
2. How does Dr. Hicks view the preemployment assessment tests? Does the company need to update its files and obtain a consistent body of test results for its employees? Is this mainly a bureaucratic exercise for the sake of uniformity and organization, or is it meant to weed out undesirable employees who slipped through the cracks, as it were? How does Dr. Hicks see her work in this context? Is her report on Edwin's results a case of the company being rightfully informed of a longtime employee's condition, or does she also believe the company has been wronged by Edwin's deception? How will this affect her action?
3. How does Dr. Hicks weigh the relevance of Edwin's reading disability? Does this mitigate Edwin's responsibility for his literacy? Or is this a problem that Edwin should have had diagnosed well before failing the preemployment exams? What validity does the preemployment exam have for those who have this kind of disability? Should the company offer an alternative exam to better judge the work of those with learning disabilities?
4. What does Dr. Hicks think about the nature of work and loyalty to the company? Does 23 years of labor deserve too much respect to fire Edwin, or does she believe Edwin may have undeservedly held a job for too long already? Did Edwin's performance prove itself, or could a person who honestly took the preemployment tests have performed better for the company?
5. Does Dr. Hicks believe the shame of illiteracy, and the lengths to which those who are illiterate will go to hide it, outweigh the dishonesty of having someone else take a test? Does she view honesty as too important to be outweighed by consequences?

Ethical Course of Action

Directive per APA Code

Standard 9.03 (a) (2) allows for situations such as Edwin's. Dr. Hicks, a psychologist who is employed by the company Edwin works for, may engage in an employment assessment without Edwin's consent. It is doubtful that Dr. Hicks would find herself in this situation with Edwin if informed consent was required for assessment. The consequences of such exception brought Dr. Hicks face-to-face with an after-the-fact ADA compliance problem. Unless Dr. Hicks is competent to provide services to individuals with a disability, per Standard 2.01 (b), Edwin should be referred to another psychologist for assessment with someone who knows how to work with individuals with reading disabilities.

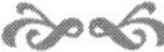

Dictates of One's Own Conscience

If you were Dr. Hicks, faced with this situation, which of these would you do?

1. Recommend that Edwin be terminated for fraud because disability does not justify lying.
2. Recommend that Edwin be disciplined in some manner for the fraudulent act 23 years ago, but not be terminated from employment.
3. Retest Edwin under conditions that meet the accommodation recommendations for his reading disability. What if Dr. Hicks has a learning disability? How might this affect her decision?
4. Combinations of the above-listed actions.
5. Or one that is not listed above.

If you were Dr. Hicks, faced with this situation in Canada, you would complete the assessment on Edwin and make the results known to appropriate persons, likely the employer and Edwin himself.

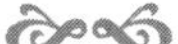

STANDARD 9.03: INFORMED CONSENT IN ASSESSMENTS

(a) Psychologists obtain informed consent for assessments, evaluations, or diagnostic services, as described in Standard 3.10, Informed Consent, except when (1) testing is mandated by law or governmental regulations; (2) informed consent is implied because testing is conducted as a routine educational, institutional, or organizational activity (e.g., when participants voluntarily agree to assessment when applying for a job); or **(3) one purpose of the testing is to evaluate decisional capacity.** Informed consent includes an explanation of the nature and purpose of the assessment, fees, involvement of third parties, and limits of confidentiality and sufficient opportunity for the client/patient to ask questions and receive answers.

A CASE FOR STANDARD 9.03 (A) (3): Exceptional Circumstances

Anita is a 22-year-old female police officer facing prosecution on charges of assault with a deadly weapon. Anita's attorney has referred her to Dr. Crawford for an assessment to determine if Anita is competent to stand trial and to determine whether decisional capacity was diminished at the time of the incident. Dr. Crawford was provided with Anita's arrest record.

During the interview, Anita told Dr. Crawford she has a history of sexual abuse. She was sexually molested as a child and in high school. Since employment with the state, she has been forced to work with a higher-ranking man who has been sexually harassing her. She explained that he talks to her in a demeaning manner, uses sexually explicit language, and has exposed himself to her. On the day in question, he had cornered her and tried, for the first time, to fondle her. She pulled out her gun and said she would pull the trigger if he did not stop the sexual harassment.

Issues of Concern

The situation with Anita may be an exception to Standard 3.10: Informed Consent. Standard 9.03 (a) (3) allows Dr. Crawford to conduct this assessment regardless of whether Anita wants to participate. Anita has not gone to trial yet. No sitting magistrate has ordered or requested such an evaluation. It appears that Anita's decisional capacity is not compromised at the time Dr. Crawford is doing the interview and that Anita is participating willingly. Even if Dr. Crawford finds that Anita's capacity was diminished at the time of the assault, should Standard 9.03 (a) (3) still apply? Should Dr. Crawford comply with Standard 3.10 regardless of whether Standard 9.03 (a) (3) allows for assessment without consent?

APA Ethics Code

Companion General Principle

Principle B: Fidelity and Responsibility

> They [psychologists] are aware of their professional and scientific responsibilities to society and to the specific communities in which they work. Psychologists uphold professional standards of conduct . . . [and] clarify their professional roles and obligations.

Principle B guides Dr. Crawford's attention not only to the client but to the profession and the society. Principle B makes a distinction between psychologists considering the welfare of the client only and simultaneously considering the welfare of the client and the implicit contract the profession of psychology holds with society. In this case, Principle B suggests Dr. Crawford will focus on Anita, the general public Anita will encounter in her line of work, and on upholding the standards of service for the profession.

Companion Ethical Standard(s)

Standard 3.10: Informed Consent

> (a) When psychologists . . . provide assessment[,] . . . they obtain the informed consent of the individual. . .
>
> (b) For persons who are legally incapable of giving informed consent, psychologists nevertheless (1) provide an appropriate explanation, (2) seek the individual's assent, (3) consider such persons' preferences and best interests, and (4) obtain appropriate permission from a legally authorized person.

Standard 3.10 (a) directs psychologists to obtain consent from clients before proceeding with an assessment of any kind. Standard 3.10 (b) requires psychologist to obtain assent, regardless of whether consent is necessary or is given.

Standard 9.03: Informed Consent in Assessments

> . . . (b) Psychologists inform persons . . . for whom testing is mandated by . . . governmental regulations about the nature and purpose of the proposed assessment services.

Standard 9.03 (b) modifies Standard 9.03 (a) slightly. Standard 9.03 (b) directs Dr. Crawford to act in the same manner as she would with anyone who is seeking an assessment up to the point of asking for consent. This means that Dr. Crawford is obligated to tell Anita all information required under Standard 3.10 (b).

Standard 3.04: Avoiding Harm

> Psychologists take reasonable steps to avoid harming their clients/patients, and to minimize harm where it is foreseeable and unavoidable.

Standard 3.04 is a narrower interpretation of Principle B. Standard 3.04 specifies that Dr. Crawford's responsibility is only to Anita, whereas Principle B guides Dr. Crawford to consider the implicit agreement psychologists have with society. To some extent, the combination of Principle B and Standard 3.04 directs Dr. Crawford's attention toward a balance between doing what is best for Anita and still protecting the general public interacting with Anita.

Standard 3.07: Third-Party Requests for Services

> When psychologists agree to provide services to a person . . . at the request of a third party, psychologists attempt to clarify at the outset of the service the nature of the relationship with all individuals . . . involved. This clarification includes the role of the psychologist (e.g., . . . expert witness), an identification of who is the client, the probable uses of . . . the information obtained, and the fact that there may be limits to confidentiality.

Dr. Crawford is doing this assessment at the request of Anita's attorney. Presumably, Anita is participating in this assessment on the advice of her attorney. As directed by Standard 3.07, Dr. Crawford needs to explain her role as a forensic psychologist and let Anita know of the high probability that information from Anita will be viewed both by the defense and the prosecuting attorney.

Legal Issues 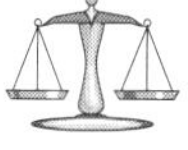

Montana

> *Mont. Admin. R. 24.189.2305 (2009). Professional Responsibility.*
>
> (2) In regard to respect for others, a licensee:
>
> (a) shall not exploit persons over whom they have . . . evaluative . . . authority such as . . . clients;

(b) who . . . administers, scores, interprets or uses assessment techniques shall be familiar with the reliability, validation and related standardization or outcome studies of, and proper applications and uses of, the techniques they use; and . . .

(iv) shall ensure . . . that an explanation of the results is provided using language that is reasonably understandable to the person assessed. . .

(7) In regard to forensic activities, a licensee:

(a) shall not render a formal professional opinion about the psychological and emotional characteristics of an individual without direct and substantial professional contact with or a formal assessment of that person.

New Jersey

N.J. Admin. Code § 13:42-10.5 (2010). Maintaining Competence in Testing Situations.

(g) A licensee shall administer . . . all testing material . . . consistent with accepted standards of practice.

In Montana, Dr. Crawford is expected to provide a full disclosure about the assessment and the likely uses of the assessment, which would include the distinct likelihood that details of the assessment would be released to the court and prosecution. New Jersey law is silent about the need for disclosure, although it might be argued that the accepted standards of practice would necessitate disclosures in light of the APA standards.

Cultural Considerations

Global Discussion

Code of Ethics: Netherlands

Principle III: Integrity.

III.2.3 Information and consent.

III.2.3.3 Equal information to the external principal and to the client.

If an external principal has contracted his services, the psychologist should ensure, prior to initiation of the professional relationship, that both the external principal and the client . . . have been issued the same information concerning the purpose and procedure of the professional relationship, as well as the intended work method. The psychologist only enters into such a contract if all parties involved agree upon purpose and procedure. . .

III.2.3.4 Content of the information.

The information should preferably be issued in writing and, where applicable, shall include:

* the purpose of the professional relationship and the context within which it will take place; the role of the client and psychologist herein;

* the procedure that is to be followed, the activities in which the client will be directly or indirectly engaged[;] . . .

* the methods of . . . evaluation . . . that may be applied, and their expected outcome and limitations;

* the kind of data concerning the client which will be collected and the way in which they will be stored;

* the way in which reports . . . will be drafted and to whom they will be issued;

* the stipulations in the Code of Ethics concerning access and copy, revision and blocking issuance of report;

* the institutions, if any, that have an interest in the professional relationship;

* the possible side effects of the professional activity;

* the psychologist's obligation to adhere to the Code of Ethics and client's right of complaint;

*any alteration of the above shall be discussed with the client.

If this situation occurred in the Netherlands, Dr. Crawford must adhere to the following steps: She must ensure that Anita, her attorney, and the prosecution have a clear and equal understanding of the purpose and methods of Dr. Crawford's role. Further, all involved parties, including Anita, must be in agreement before Dr. Crawford begins working with Anita.

American Moral Values

1. What kind of consent ought Dr. Crawford obtain from Anita? What should Anita understand about Dr. Crawford's role? What kind of information would undermine Dr. Crawford's ability to determine "decisional capacity"?

2. Would telling Anita that her decisional capacity is at issue cloud the results? Is Anita a threat to deceive based on what would help her legally? How much information would give Anita a maximum amount of consent without detracting from an objective assessment of her decisional capacity?

3. Does Dr. Crawford believe there is a principled stand against sexual harassment to be taken here? Would Anita being found incompetent excuse her superior

from having evidence presented against him? Or is it more important that Anita not be jailed for making an accusation of sexual assault?

4. Does Dr. Crawford believe that Anita's previous abuse, including at the hands of her supervisor, helped to drive her to react with a firearm? If these circumstances justify her action, do they also suggest she was not in control of her actions? Does Dr. Crawford believe this was a reasonable, justifiable act of self-defense, even though it was triggered by previous trauma?

Ethical Course of Action

Directive per APA Code

It appears that Anita's attorney may be exploring the possibility of claiming diminished capacity at the time of the incident between Anita and her superior. Diminished capacity is a form of decisional capacity. Therefore, Standard 9.03 (a) (3) could apply. Standard 9.03 (a) (3) allows Dr. Crawford to conduct this assessment regardless of whether Anita wants to participate.

Standards 3.10 (b) and 9.03 (b) require that Dr. Crawford give Anita information about the evaluation and obtain assent, not consent. Standard 3.07 requires that Dr. Crawford explain her role as the forensic psychologist, the assessment process, and how the information will most likely be used.

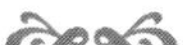

Dictates of One's Own Conscience

At this point of the intake session, if you were Dr. Crawford, which of these would you do?

1. Reassure Anita that you would do your best to help her, and proceed with the assessment.
2. Review with Anita what the process of the assessment will involve.
3. Discuss with Anita's attorney, with Anita in the room, the referral question and the probable use of the assessment results.
4. Obtain consent, regardless of whether the APA Ethics Code allows for exceptions to Standard 3.10.
5. Make sure Anita knows that the report will also go to the opposing attorney before proceeding with the assessment.
6. Combinations of the above-listed actions.
7. Or one that is not listed above.

If you were Dr. Crawford practicing in the Netherlands, you would not proceed until Anita, her attorney, a representative of the state, and most likely the opposing attorney have all signed consent to treatment.

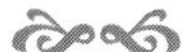

STANDARD 9.03: INFORMED CONSENT IN ASSESSMENTS

. . . (b) Psychologists inform persons with questionable capacity to consent or for whom testing is mandated by law or governmental regulations about the nature and purpose of the proposed assessment services, using language that is reasonably understandable to the person being assessed.

A CASE FOR STANDARD 9.03 (B): But I Need to Go Back

Esther, a 26-year-old single Caucasian female, is an Army mechanic with 8 years of active duty service. Her commanding officer referred her to Dr. Boyd for a psychological evaluation to determine if she is fit for active duty. Her last deployment was to Afghanistan where Esther was among a group of soldiers hit by a roadside ambush. The ambush involved active combat and resulted in horrific injuries and death. Since the ambush, there has been a noticeable drop in her performance. Dr. Boyd tells Esther that the purpose of the assessment is to ascertain her ability to safely resume active duty without endangering others. Esther says to Dr. Boyd, "I know you have to do this, but please be understanding because if you say I am not fit, then they will not want me anymore, and then I can't get a job when I get out either."

Issues of Concern

Esther is undergoing this psychological assessment at the behest of her commander. The order from a military commander constitutes a mandate by government regulation and meets the conditions for Standard 9.03 (b). Dr. Boyd does not need Esther's consent to conduct this assessment. Nonetheless, Dr. Boyd tells Esther about what he will be doing in the assessment and why she is being assessed. Has Dr. Boyd used language that is understood by Esther? Can one presume that she has understood Dr. Boyd's account of the nature and purpose of the proposed assessment process based on her response to Dr. Boyd?

APA Ethics Code

Companion General Principle

Principle B: Fidelity and Responsibility

> Psychologists establish relationships of trust with those with whom they work.

A part of establishing a relationship of trust with one's client is to explain the process and procedures to the extent that neither the process of assessment nor the use of the resulting information is a surprise.

Companion Ethical Standard(s)

Standard 3.07: Third-Party Requests for Services

> When psychologists agree to provide services to a person . . . at the request of a third party, psychologists attempt to clarify at the outset of the service the nature of the relationship. . . This clarification includes the role of the psychologist (e.g., . . . diagnostician . . .), an identification of who is the client, the probable uses of the . . . information obtained, and the fact that there may be limits to confidentiality.

Esther appears to know that she holds no privilege of confidentiality in this situation, and that the information will be used to determine her continued status in the military.

Standard 3.04: Avoiding Harm

> Psychologists take reasonable steps to avoid harming their clients/patients[,] . . . organizational clients, and . . . to minimize harm where it is foreseeable and unavoidable.

Dr. Boyd's responsibility to do no harm extends to both Esther and the state as a whole. The recommendations Dr. Boyd makes have significant implications for the welfare of those coworkers who work alongside Esther.

Legal Issues 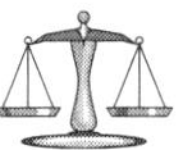

New Mexico

> *N.M. Code R. § 16.22.2.10 (2010). Patient Welfare.*
>
> A. Informed consent for therapy and evaluation.
>
> (1) The psychologist shall appropriately document and obtain appropriate informed consent for . . . evaluation. Informed consent means that the person:
>
> (a) has the capacity to consent;
>
> (b) has been informed of significant information concerning the therapy or evaluation in language that is understandable; and
>
> (c) has freely and without undue influence expressed consent. . .
>
> (3) In addition, the psychologist shall:
>
> (a) inform those persons who are legally incapable of giving informed consent about the proposed interventions or evaluations in a manner commensurate with the persons' psychological capacities;
>
> (b) seek or obtain their assent to those interventions or evaluations; and
>
> (c) consider such persons' preferences and best interests.
>
> B. Limits of confidentiality in forensic . . . evaluations.
>
> (1) The psychologist shall explain the limits of confidentiality to parties at the outset, before the evaluation begins, and the explanation should be documented. The psychologist shall also clarify how the information will be used and which parties or entities will have access to the evaluation. The procedures of the evaluation and their purpose should be described to the parties. . .
>
> J. Avoiding harm. Psychologists take reasonable steps to avoid harming . . . others with whom they work, and minimize harm where it is foreseeable and unavoidable.

New York

> *N.Y. Comp. Codes R. & Regs. tit. 8, § 29.1 (2010). General Provisions.*
>
> B. Unprofessional conduct . . . shall include . . .
>
> 1. willful or grossly negligent failure to comply with substantial provisions of Federal, State or local laws, rules or regulations governing the practice of the profession . . .
>
> 8. revealing of personally identifiable facts, data or information obtained in a professional capacity without the

> prior consent of the patient or client, except as authorized or required by law . . .
>
> 11. performing professional services which have not been duly authorized by the patient or client or his or her legal representative.

In both jurisdictions, Dr. Boyd is to obtain informed consent from Esther before the evaluation. In New Mexico, Dr. Boyd must additionally inform Esther about the likely use of data from the assessment. Dr. Boyd could disregard the additional explanation if the details about why the assessment included how the information would likely be used and who would have access to the evaluation data. New York's law is silent as to what details would entail adequate informed consent.

Cultural Considerations

Global Discussion

Canadian Code of Ethics for Psychologists

> Principle I: Respect for the dignity of persons.
>
> *Freedom of consent.*
>
> I.27. Take all reasonable steps to ensure that consent is not given under conditions of coercion [or] undue pressure.

In Canada, Dr. Boyd has the challenging task of determining if Esther's consent to his evaluation has been freely given, or whether Ester is under undue pressure since to refuse the evaluation would end Esther's career. Further, Dr. Boyd would be obligated to inform Esther that results of the evaluation for PTSD will be reported to Esther's superiors and will be documented. If she does not have PTSD, but submits to the evaluation only to ensure her employment, that can be considered undue pressure under Canada's code. However, if she actually does have PTSD, it is possible that her decision-making capacity has been temporarily impaired, and she would thus be more susceptible to giving consent to an assessment than she would otherwise.

American Moral Values

1. Has Dr. Boyd explained to Esther in understandable language what his assessment is meant to accomplish? Does Esther's worry about her job and future indicate that she understands the assessment? Does Dr. Boyd need to reassure her that his assessment need not result in the consequences she fears?
2. How much is Dr. Boyd responsible for Esther's worries about the results? Could her stress and anxiety distort her test results? Does he need to reassure her in order to make an accurate assessment of whether she has PTSD or not? Does he need to explain to her that he is testing for PTSD, not just "fitness" for a job in general? Does he need to explain that PTSD need not be permanent? Does he need to explain how bad it would be if Esther had PTSD and tried to resume her usual duties in the field?
3. What is Dr. Boyd's responsibility to the military? Are they his client? Could caring for Esther's state of mind come at the expense of helping the military remove a dangerously incapable mechanic? How important is competence on the battlefield? How many more people could be in danger if someone with PTSD is put back on duty?

Ethical Course of Action

Directive per APA Code

Dr. Boyd does not need consent for assessment from Esther to conduct this assessment as established in Standard 9.03 (b). Regardless of whether consent is required, Standard 9.03 (b) directs Dr. Boyd to tell Esther about the nature and purpose of the assessment. Evidenced from Esther's response, it appears that Esther understands that the assessment is requested by a third party (Standard 3.07), and the likely use of Dr. Boyd's assessment. It appears that Dr. Boyd did tell Esther about the purpose of the assessment in language she understood. Therefore, it appears Dr. Boyd has met conditions and is in compliance with Standard 9.03 (b).

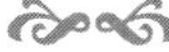

Dictates of One's Own Conscience

If you were Dr. Boyd, on the receiving end of such a plea, which action would you take?

1. Obtain an IQ to ascertain whether Esther has the cognitive ability to truly understand the nature of the assessment.
2. Explain that you cannot be flexible when other people's lives depend on your opinion.
3. Further explore Esther's understanding of the nature and purpose of the assessment to ascertain the probability that Esther is motivated to appear normal.

4. Combinations of the above-listed actions.
5. Or one that is not listed above.

If you were Dr. Boyd practicing in Canada, on the receiving end of such a plea, you would seriously consider not conducting the assessment since the circumstances for the assessment are coercive, and Esther is experiencing undue pressure to influence the outcome of the assessment.

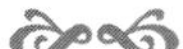

STANDARD 9.03: INFORMED CONSENT IN ASSESSMENTS

> . . . (c) Psychologists using the services of an interpreter obtain informed consent from the client/patient to use that interpreter, ensure that confidentiality of test results and test security are maintained, and include in their recommendations, reports, and diagnostic or evaluative statements, including forensic testimony, discussion of any limitations on the data obtained.

A CASE FOR STANDARD 9.03 (C): Misinterpretation

Dr. Mason is conducting a psychological evaluation on Eddie to determine his eligibility for special education. The student files indicate that Eddie is a 7-year-old bilingual Tagalog-speaking boy with an American father and a Filipino mother. The family recently moved back to the United States from the father's last assigned military base in Japan. Dr. Mason quickly discovers that Eddie speaks so little English that she cannot proceed with the assessment without the assistance of an interpreter. Luckily, Dr. Mason remembers that the school nurse is Filipino and speaks Tagalog. With the aid of the school nurse, Dr. Mason proceeds to administer the Wechsler Intelligence Scale for Children–IV (WISC-IV). Eddie's scores indicate a Full Scale IQ (FSIQ) of 80, which indicates lo-normal intelligence. His mother objects to the findings on the grounds that she knows the school nurse through the community and does not consider her to be a competent speaker of Tagalog.

Issues of Concern

Standard 9.03 (c) specifies conditions necessary for the use of an interpreter. Ethical issues raised by this situation are whether Dr. Mason needed the informed consent of the family for the use of the interpreter. As specified in Standard 9.03 (c), Dr. Mason did not need informed consent to conduct the assessment, as exempted by Standard 9.03 (a) (2). In addition, because testing was for special education services and considered a routine educational activity, it is also exempt from consent as specified by Standard 9.03 (a) (2). Clinical issues raised by this situation are whether the school nurse is competent to act as an interpreter; whether Dr. Mason is competent to conduct an assessment for a child for whom English is a second language (ESL); and finally, whether the WISC-IV is normed for Filipino and/or ESL children.

APA Ethics Code

Companion General Principle

Principle E: Respect for People's Rights and Dignity

> Psychologists . . . are aware of and respect cultural . . . differences, including those based on age, gender[,] . . . race, ethnicity, culture . . . [, and] language . . . and consider these factors when working with members of such groups.

Principle E guides Dr. Mason to consider the factors listed. In this case, the relevant factors include age (child of 7 years), ethnicity (biracial military), culture (both Filipino and American), and language (non-proficient English speaker). Might she be competent to provide service to this child? Competency in this specific instance would not only include knowing how to use an interpreter, but also selecting the age- and language-appropriate testing instruments, and understanding the limitations to interpretation of the test results.

Companion Ethical Standard(s)

Standard 9.03: Informed Consent in Assessments

> (a) Psychologists obtain informed consent for assessments, evaluations, or diagnostic services . . . except when . . . (2) informed consent is implied because testing is conducted as a routine educational . . . activity.

The question of relevance for this situation is whether conducting an assessment to determine eligibility or need for special education is considered a routine educational activity. When every child is administered some standardized test, then such assessment would be considered routine. However, only certain children are selected for special education. If routine, then Dr. Mason does not need consent from the client for the assessment. If it is routine and client consent is not needed, then certainly Dr. Mason would not need to obtain client consent for use of an interpreter as specified in Standard 9.03 (c).

Standard 3.10: Informed Consent

> . . . (b) For persons who are legally incapable of giving informed consent, psychologists nevertheless (1) provide an appropriate explanation, (2) seek the individual's assent, (3) consider such persons' preferences and best interests, and (4) obtain appropriate permission from a legally authorized person.

If Dr. Mason needed consent to assess Eddie, then Standard 3.10 directs Dr. Mason to have acquired consent from Eddie's parents. If Dr. Mason had obtained consent prior to testing, would it have been a reasonable expectation for either Dr. Mason or Eddie's parent(s) to raise the question of the need for an interpreter prior to the actual testing session?

Standard 2.05: Delegation of Work to Others

> Psychologists who . . . use the services of others, such as interpreters, take reasonable steps to (1) avoid delegating such work to persons who have a multiple relationship with those being served that would likely lead to . . . loss of objectivity; (2) authorize only those responsibilities that such persons can be expected to perform competently on the basis of their education, training, or experience . . . and (3) see that such persons perform these services competently.

A companion to Standard 9.03 (c), Standard 2.05 placed certain requirements on Dr. Mason when she used an interpreter. Standard 2.05 (1) directs Dr. Mason to have ascertained whether the school nurse knows Eddie's family and the nature of any relationship between them. Standard 2.05 (b) also directs Dr. Mason to have ascertained the school nurse's competence to function as an interpreter. In addition, Standard 2.05 (c) would include instructing the school nurse about the need to keep work information confidential and refrain from the sharing of this information with any personal contacts she may have in the Filipino community.

Standard 9.02: Use of Assessments

> . . . (b) Psychologists use assessment instruments whose validity and reliability have been established for use with members of the population tested. When such validity or reliability has not been established, psychologists describe the strengths and limitations of test results and interpretation.

Dr. Mason realized the limitation of her ability to conduct an assessment for Eddie, but it was only once she had started the assessment process. Upon realizing Eddie's language preference, Standard 9.02 (b) directs Dr. Mason to then consider the appropriateness of the instrument she had chosen. Could the use of a less language-dependent assessment of intelligence have been more appropriate for a child with limited English proficiency?

Standard 2.01: Boundaries of Competence

> . . . (b) Where scientific or professional knowledge in the discipline of psychology establishes that an understanding of factors associated with . . . language . . . is essential for effective implementation of their services[,] . . . psychologists have or obtain the training, experience, consultation, or supervision necessary to ensure the competence of their services, or they make appropriate referrals.

Standard 2.01 (b) directs Dr. Mason to assess whether she is competent to conduct a special education assessment for Eddie. Since Dr. Mason is employed as a psychologist in a school, she is presumed to be competent to conduct assessment for any educational service. Thus, the relevant question is whether she is competent to select and interpret test results for immigrant children with limited English proficiency. If Dr. Mason deemed herself not to be competent in this area, Standard 2.01 (b) directs her to seek additional consultation or supervision.

Legal Issues 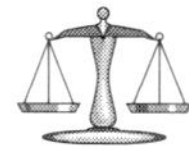

Ohio

> *Ohio Admin. Code 4732:17 (2010). Rules of Professional Conduct.*
>
> (B) Negligence:
>
> A psychologist . . . shall be considered negligent if his/her behaviors[,] . . . in the judgment of the board, clearly fall below the standards for acceptable practice of psychology. . .
>
> (C) Welfare of the client. . .
>
> (3) Informed client. A psychologist . . . shall give a truthful, understandable, and reasonably complete account of

a client's condition to . . . those responsible for the care of the client. The psychologist . . . shall keep the client fully informed as to the purpose and nature of any evaluation . . . and of the client's right to freedom of choice regarding services provided.

(5) Informed choice. A psychologist or school psychologist shall accord each client informed choice . . . [and] confidentiality. . .

(F) Testing and test interpretation:

(1) Assessment procedures:

(a) A psychologist . . . shall treat the results or interpretations of assessment regarding an individual as confidential information.

Pennsylvania

49 Pa. Code § 41.61 (2010). Code of Ethics.

Principle 8. Utilization of assessment.

(a) . . . Psychologists guard against misuse of assessment results.

In both jurisdictions, Dr. Mason will likely have broken the law by involving the nurse as an interpreter without the consent of Eddie's mother. Secondarily, misuse of the assessment results could occur from the nurse talking about Eddie's performance.

Cultural Considerations

Global Discussion

The Professional Board for Psychology
Health Professions Council of South Africa.
Ethical Code of Professional Conduct (April 2002)

5. Assessment activities.

5.1. Informed consent in assessments.

5.2.1. Psychologists shall refrain from the misuse of assessment techniques . . . and take reasonable steps to prevent others from misusing the information these methods provide. . .

5.3.3. Psychologists using the services of an interpreter obtain informed consent from the client/patient to use the interpreter. . . Psychologists always remain cognizant of the limits to data obtained via the use of an interpreter and frame their conclusions and recommendations accordingly.

5.5. Cultural diversity.

5.5.1. Psychologists who . . . use assessment methods shall be familiar with the reliability, validation, and related standardisation or outcome studies of, and proper applications and uses of, the methods they use.

5.5.2. Psychologists shall recognise limits to the certainty with which diagnoses . . . [and] findings . . . can be made about individuals, especially where linguistic, cultural and socio-economic variances exist. Psychologists shall make every effort to identify situations in which particular assessment methods or norms may not be applicable or may require adjustment in administration, scoring and interpretation because of factors such as age . . . culture, disability[,] . . . ethnic and social origin.

According to 5.2.1, Dr. Mason is not to misuse assessment techniques. Even with adequate translation, several parts of the WISC-IV are Eurocentric, and thus Dr. Mason's findings, particularly the FSIQ, are flawed (5.5.1, 5.5.3). Dr. Mason's use of an unqualified paraprofessional is also problematic. Ability to speak a language does not ensure competency to translate. The matter of informed consent (5.3.3) is also a concern: By definition, Dr. Mason needs consent from Eddie's parent or legal guardian, regardless of the language in which the tests are given. It also does not appear that Dr. Mason made an attempt to ensure that Eddie's test results would remain confidential, as per 5.3.3, or that the testing procedure itself would remain private. Finally, Dr. Mason's report would need to qualify her findings, diagnoses, and recommendations by stating clearly that they are likely invalid.

American Moral Values

1. Did Dr. Mason need to obtain consent from Eddie's mother for the translator who was available? Was Dr. Mason justified in getting someone whom she knew to translate? Does she know the nurse to be fluent in Tagalog?
2. How accurate does Dr. Mason believe the WISC-IV is when administered through a translator or interpreter? Should the interpreter be certified for this type of job? Did Dr. Mason believe it would be too difficult to obtain someone trained in time for Eddie's assessment?
3. How does Dr. Mason regard the mother's response to the test? Was the mother just searching for a reason to negate the results, or is she a fair judge of the nurse's Tagalog?
4. How does Eddie's mother know the nurse in the community? Is there a personal reason that the two

might be in conflict? Is the mother embarrassed about the results, and does she fear the results will become known in the community? Or is the mother risking communal disapproval by her objection, suggesting that she honestly believes the nurse is not competent to translate for her son?

5. What are Dr. Mason's views about Eddie's abilities and the need for special education? Is she more apt to accept the results if they mean better special education services for Eddie? Would she prefer to err on the side of his receiving too many services rather than not enough? Has she considered what the mother might think of special education, including its possible stigmatizing effect on her son?

Ethical Course of Action

Directive per APA Code

Standard 3.10 requires Dr. Mason to have obtained consent from the parent(s) for the assessment. In addition, Standard 9.03 (c) requires that Dr. Mason obtain consent from Eddie's parents for the use of the school nurse as an interpreter. Even if Eddie's parents had given consent, Dr. Mason, as directed by Standard 2.05, needed to have determined that the school nurse was qualified to function as an interpreter for psychological assessment. Beyond the logistics of appropriately setting the stage for the assessments, Dr. Mason needed to have made sure that the instrument selected was appropriate for the individual as directed in Standard 9.02 (b), and that she was competent, as required in Standard 2.01(b), to interpret the results of the test.

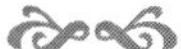

Dictates of One's Own Conscience

If you were Dr. Mason and were not specifically trained to conduct assessment on the special population of ethnic minority children, based on the mother's objections, which of these would you do?

1. Express sympathy for the mother's objections, and keep the test and report without further alterations.
2. Review the testing with a consultant to determine the appropriateness of the whole process.
3. Meet with the mother to decide if there was anyone in the community she would approve of for use as an interpreter.
4. Add an addendum to the testing report stating the limitation of the report based on the possible problems with the interpreter.
5. Given the mother's objection, retest Eddie with a different interpreter and a different assessment instrument.
6. Reinterpret the test result in light of the mother's objections.
7. Combinations of the above-listed actions.
8. Or one that is not listed above.

If you were Dr. Mason practicing in South Africa and faced with Eddie's mother's objections, you should meet with the mother to get consent for assessment, then redo the assessment with an agreed-upon interpreter using another psychometric instrument. In addition, you would qualify any findings and diagnoses in your report with a disclosure about the differences between Eddie and yourself culturally, socially, and linguistically.

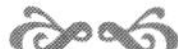

STANDARD 9.04: RELEASE OF TEST DATA

(a) The term test data refers to raw and scaled scores, client/patient responses to test questions or stimuli, and psychologists' notes and recordings concerning client/patient statements and behavior during an examination. Those portions of test materials that include client/patient responses are included in the definition of test data. Pursuant to a client/patient release, psychologists provide test data to the client/patient or other persons identified in the release. Psychologists may refrain from releasing test data to protect a client/patient or others from substantial harm or misuse or misrepresentation of the data or the test, recognizing that in many instances release of confidential information under these circumstances is regulated by law.

A CASE FOR STANDARD 9.04 (A): Limits on Help

Dr. Morales receives a referral from the school counselor to provide a special education evaluation for Troy to determine if he is experiencing emotional impairment. Troy is a 15-year-old Caucasian male who has been having some difficulties with social interactions in school.

Dr. Morales administers the Minnesota Multiphasic Personality Inventory–2 (MMPI-2) and the Behavior Assessment System for Children–2 (BASC-2), the Wechsler Intelligence Scale for Children–IV (WISC-IV), and the Wide Range Achievement Test–4 (WRAT-4), and the Connors Parent and Teachers Rating Scale (CPTRS). Results from the MMPI-2 indicate Major Depression. BASC-2 indicates evidence of some psychotic features such as hearing voices and having strange and unusual experiences. Symptomology for both diagnoses, depression and psychosis, was supported by the CPTRS. Dr. Morales submitted an assessment report diagnosing Troy with Major Depression and a Rule Out for Major Depression with Psychotic Features. He releases the report to the school counselor who is the referral source, to Troy, and to Troy's parents.

The school system's case review committee requests that Dr. Morales send all test data, including the raw scores as well as the specific responses to all items. Dr. Morales thinks the raw scores may argue for the existence of a psychotic disorder. He does not think there is sufficient support for psychotic disorder but fears a focus on the endorsement of psychotic symptoms may follow Troy, possibly adversely impacting his interactions with the school system in the future.

Issues of Concern

Standard 9.04 (a) allows for release of raw data with the specific request for release. Standard 9.04 also allows for psychologists to use their discretion in not releasing raw test data if there is the need to protect the client or if they fear the misuse of the raw data. Dr. Morales is faced with a request for the release of raw test data. Should Dr. Morales release the raw test data as requested? Can Dr. Morales consider that releasing the raw test data is authorized by Troy and his parents based on their permission to release the assessment report to the school? Are there substantiated reasons for Dr. Morales to withhold raw test data even if Troy and his parents have provided consent for the release?

APA Ethics Code

Companion General Principle

Principle A: Beneficence and Nonmaleficence

> Psychologists strive to benefit those with whom they work and take care to do no harm. In their professional actions, psychologists seek to safeguard the welfare and rights of those with whom they interact professionally. . . When conflicts occur among psychologists' obligations or concerns, they attempt to resolve these conflicts in a responsible fashion that avoids or minimizes harm.

Principle A: Beneficence and Nonmaleficence is one of the highest principles for psychologists. Dr. Morales is aware of the possible harm that could come to Troy should specific information from the raw test data be available to school personnel as well as possible others in the future who are untrained in the interpretation of psychological instruments and assessment inventories. Principle A guides Dr. Morales to guard against the misuse of information collected in the course of providing psychological services.

Companion Ethical Standard

Standard 3.04: Avoiding Harm

> Psychologists take reasonable steps to avoid harming their clients . . . and to minimize harm where it is foreseeable and unavoidable.

Standard 3.04 is the operationalization of Principle A: Beneficence and Nonmaleficence. Dr. Morales is concerned with the possibility that providing the raw data to the school review committee could cause harm to Troy because of misinterpretation of the data. As directed by Standard 3.04, Dr. Morales needs to take reasonable steps to avoid harm. Should Dr. Morales deny release of raw data to the school system, regardless of whether such release is authorized by Troy and his parents?

Standard 3.09: Cooperation With Other Professionals

> When indicated and professionally appropriate, psychologists cooperate with other professionals in order to serve their clients/patients effectively and appropriately.

At the outset, Dr. Morales's responsibility is to provide information to Troy and his legal guardians. Secondarily, Dr. Morales is to provide information to the school at the request and with the permission of Troy and his parents. Dr. Morales's responsibility to the school is limited by the consent of his client, and as specified in Standard 9.04 (a), is to be guided by his own sense of protection of his client. Only after these two considerations are met should Dr. Morales cooperate with the school system.

Legal Issues 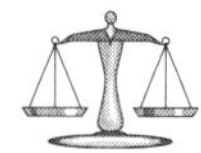

South Carolina

S.C. Code Ann. Regs.100-4 (2010). Code of Ethics.

J. Assessment procedures and reports.

(1) Confidential information. A psychologist shall treat an assessment result or interpretation regarding an individual as confidential information.

(2) Communication of results. The psychologist should accompany, subject to professional judgment[,] . . . communication of results of assessment procedures . . . to other agents of the client by adequate . . . explanations.

Texas

22 Tex. Admin. Code § 465.22 (2010). Psychological Records, Test Data and Test Protocols.

(b) Maintenance and Control of Records and Test Data. . .

(3) Licensees shall make all reasonable efforts to protect against the misuse of any record or test data.

(c) Access to Records and Test Data. . .

(4) Test data are not part of a patient's or client's record. Test data are not subject to subpoena. Test data shall be made available only:

(A) to another qualified mental health professional and only upon receipt of written release from the patient or client, or

(B) pursuant to a court order.

In both jurisdictions, Dr. Morales does not violate the laws by not releasing the raw data. Although the Texas law is more explicit, South Carolina's law also permits Dr. Morales to use his professional judgment about what data to provide from the evaluation to the school.

Cultural Considerations

Global Discussion

Singapore Psychological Society: Code of Professional Ethics

Principle 14. Test interpretation.

Test scores, like test materials, are released only to persons who are qualified to interpret and use them properly.

1. Materials for reporting test scores . . . are closely supervised by qualified psychologists. . .

2. Test results or other assessment data used for evaluation or classification are communicated . . . in such a manner as to guard against misinterpretation or misuse. In the actual case, an interpretation of the test result rather than the score is communicated.

Dr. Morales must be qualified (Principle 14) to use and interpret these assessments, carefully (1) safeguard the reporting of Troy's scores to his parents and to those necessary employees of Troy's school, and (2) ensure that these results are communicated in such a way that they will not be misused. Dr. Morales must communicate an interpretation of what the test scores mean, rather than the scores themselves. Therefore, if Dr. Morales was practicing in Singapore, he would cite the ethics code and decline the request from the school system case review committee.

American Moral Values

1. What are Dr. Morales's views about how the educational system handles diagnoses of psychosis? What does he fear could happen to Troy if the diagnosis "follows" him? Does that outweigh any risks of not telling the school about psychotic tendencies indicated by the raw data?
2. What role does Dr. Morales's assessment play in the rest of Troy's life? Is there a difference in how Troy's diagnosis will function in larger society? Should he inform Troy's parents of the tendencies the tests picked up? Is Dr. Morales at all responsible for Troy receiving adequate and appropriate treatment for what the tests indicated?
3. Does Dr. Morales believe the school system is competent enough to interpret raw data? Could giving over the data strengthen the school's presumption to do so in other students' cases? Is Dr. Morales responsible for helping to defend psychologists from being pressured in the future?
4. Is there a value in transparency when it comes to data and diagnosis? Is Dr. Morales threatened by a possible challenge to his status as a trained, socially legitimized interpreter of this data? Could sharing the data help to build trust between the school system and Dr. Morales, as well as show his confidence in his own analysis? Could Dr. Morales and the school develop a more constructive, collaborative relationship in deciding what Troy needs?

Ethical Course of Action

Directive per APA Code

Since Dr. Morales is not an employee of the school and the test data therefore does not belong to the school system, Standard 9.04 (a) allows Dr. Morales to release the raw data only after he receives a release from Troy or Troy's parents. Even with such a release, Standard 9.04 (a) also provides Dr. Morales room to consider the possible harm that may result with regard to Troy should the raw test data be released. Given Dr. Morales's concerns, he is within the ethical dictates to refuse to release the raw test data as requested by the school system.

Dictates of One's Own Conscience

What would you do if you were Dr. Morales?

1. Offer to meet with the school review committee to respond to their concerns instead of sending raw test data?
2. Offer to release the raw test data only to the school psychologist?
3. Release the test data after consulting with Troy and his parents?
4. Explain to Troy and his parents the possible use of the test data and the possible harm from the presence of raw test data in his permanent school files, and then request that Troy resend his authorization to release raw test data?

What if, in addition to your already stated concerns, Troy's mother is Native American, and Troy was raised predominately in her culture? Would you

1. Have additional concerns for possible misinterpretation of the raw test data?
2. Incorporate a culturally congruent explanation of the endorsed psychotic responses in your test report and release the raw test data as evidence of cultural congruence, not as evidence of psychosis?
3. Enact combinations of the above-listed actions?
4. Or respond in a way that is not listed above?

If you were Dr. Morales practicing in Singapore, you would send the relevant section of the Singapore Ethics Code, noting that you could not send the actual raw data.

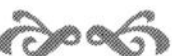

STANDARD 9.04: RELEASE OF TEST DATA

> . . . (b) In the absence of a client/patient release, psychologists provide test data only as required by law or court order.

A CASE FOR STANDARD 9.04 (B): A Tale of Two Brothers

Corey, an 11-year-old Caucasian male, has been referred to the school psychologist, Dr. Kennedy. Corey has been disruptive in class, seems unable to sit still, and is often angry. With Corey's verbal agreement, Dr. Kennedy administers the Behavior Assessment System for Children–2 (BASC-2), the Wechsler Intelligence Scale for Children–IV (WISC-IV), the House-Tree-Person, and the Kinetic Family Drawing. The images that emerge from both the House-Tree-Person and Kinetic Family Drawing are troubling. Upon further questioning, Corey reveals to Dr. Kennedy that he is currently experiencing physical abuse at home from his older brother. His father works the evening shift, and his mother left home some time ago. He is in his older brother's care after school until his father gets home, which is usually sometime around 11:00 p.m. Corey has experienced many episodes of being hit, kicked, and punched. Upon request, Corey shows Dr. Kennedy faded bruises and scrapes on his arm and torso. Corey says he doesn't want Dr. Kennedy to tell his father what is happening, as this will only make his older brother angrier and upset his father.

Issues of Concern

In most states, psychologists are mandated reporters of child abuse. The results from the projective tests are part of the evidence supporting the need for the reporting of child abuse to the state protective services. Dr. Kennedy has explicit prohibition from her minor client not to reveal any information. Would Dr. Kennedy be required by the laws in her state to ignore Corey's request for confidentiality and release test data as well as report to the state authorities?

APA Ethics Code

Companion General Principle

Principle A: Beneficence and Nonmaleficence

> In their professional actions, psychologists seek to safeguard the welfare and rights of those with whom they interact professionally.

Psychologists aspire to protect and safeguard the welfare of their clients. On behalf of those who are vulnerable and unable to protect themselves, such as a child, Principle A seeks to have psychologists hold their safety and welfare uppermost in mind as they do their work. In this case with Corey, for Dr. Kennedy to uphold the highest ideal of Principle A, she would act in such a way as to seek Corey's safety.

Principle E: Respect for People's Rights and Dignity

> Psychologists are aware that special safeguards may be necessary to protect the rights and welfare of persons or communities whose vulnerabilities impair autonomous decision making.

Children, due to the nature of their dependency, are a vulnerable population whose ability for autonomous decision making is impaired. Principle E points Dr. Kennedy to taking special safeguards to protect Corey's welfare. Part of the special safeguard may be breaking confidentiality in order to address physical abuse of a child.

Companion Ethical Standard

Standard 4.05: Disclosures

> . . . (b) Psychologists disclose confidential information without the consent of the individual only as mandated by law, or where permitted by law for a valid purpose such as to . . . (3) protect the client . . . from harm.

Physical abuse of a child is a clear case of harm. Standard 4.05 allows for Dr. Kennedy to break confidentiality without Corey's permission. In addition, certain states mandate Dr. Kennedy to report the abuse, regardless of Corey's wishes.

Standard 4.02: Discussing the Limits of Confidentiality

> (a) Psychologists discuss with persons (including, to the extent feasible, persons who are legally incapable of giving informed consent and their legal representatives) . . . (1) the relevant limits of confidentiality . . .
>
> (b) . . . and thereafter as new circumstances may warrant.

Standard 4.02 (a) directs Dr. Kennedy to have discussed with Corey and/or his father, at the onset of the assessment, the conditions under which their confidentiality will not be honored. It should come as no great surprise to Corey's father that Dr. Kennedy would break confidentiality once Corey revealed the evidence of physical abuse in the home. Standard 4.02 (b) reminds psychologists to have these conversations regarding limits of confidentiality repeatedly as each new situation arises. Thus, Dr. Kennedy needs to have another conversation with Corey and his father regarding the previous discussion of the limits of confidentiality and to discuss the current ramifications of breaking confidentiality through a report of child abuse.

Legal Issues 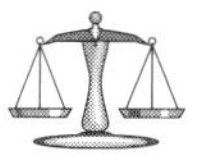

Florida

Fla. Admin. Code Ann. r. 64B19-19.002 (2010). Definitions.

> A "client" . . . is that individual who, by virtue of private consultation with the psychologist, has reason to expect that the individual's communication with the psychologist during that private consultation will remain confidential, regardless of who pays for the services of the psychologist.

Fla. Admin. Code Ann. r. 64B19-19.006 (2010). Confidentiality

> (1) One of the primary obligations of psychologists is to respect the confidentiality of information entrusted to them by service users. Psychologists may disclose that information only with the written consent of the service user. The only exceptions to this general rule occur in those situations when nondisclosure on the part of the psychologist would violate the law.

Florida Statute 39.201 (2010). Mandatory reports of child abuse, abandonment, or neglect; mandatory reports of death; central abuse hotline . . .

> (1) (a) Any person who knows, or has reasonable cause to suspect, that a child is abused . . . or neglected by a parent . . . shall report such knowledge . . . to the department.

Hawaii

> *Haw. Code R. § 16-98-34 (2010). Unethical Practice of Psychology.*
>
> (d) Safeguarding information about an individual that has been obtained by the psychologist in the course of . . . investigation is a primary obligation of the psychologist. Such information shall not be communicated to others unless certain important conditions are met:
>
> (1) Information received in confidence may be revealed only . . . where there is a clear and imminent danger to an individual . . . and then only to appropriate . . . public authorities.
>
> *Haw. Rev. Stat. § 350-1.1 (2010). Reports.*
>
> (a) Notwithstanding any other state law concerning confidentiality to the contrary, the following persons who, in their professional . . . capacity, have reason to believe that child abuse or neglect has occurred . . . shall immediately report the matter orally to the department or to the police department:
>
> (1) Any licensed . . . professional of . . . any health- related occupation who . . . treats, or provides . . . services, including but not limited to . . . psychologists.

Dr. Kennedy is a mandatory reporter in both Florida and Hawaii. If she failed to make a report, she would violate the laws of those jurisdictions. The circumstances of Corey's disclosure are irrelevant in light of the mandatory reporting duties.

Cultural Considerations

Global Discussion

The Professional Board for Psychology Health Professions Council of South Africa: Ethical Code of Professional Conduct (April 2002)

> 5. Assessment Activities
>
> 1. Release of test data.
>
> Test data refer to the test protocols, record forms, scores and notes regarding an individual's responses to test item data in any media. Psychologists may release test data to other psychologists or other qualified professionals based on a client release. Psychologists shall refrain from releasing test data to persons who are not qualified to use such information except (1) as required by law or a court order, (2) by a client release to an authorised person such as an attorney or employer, or (3) to the client as appropriate. Psychologists may refrain from releasing test data to protect a client from harm.

If Dr. Kennedy was treating Corey in South Africa, she would have a difficult path to navigate between protecting 11-year-old Corey from possibly greater harm by releasing the results of the assessments to his father, and agreeing to keep Corey's confidentiality and risking further abuse. At issue here is whether or not Dr. Kennedy has permission to release the assessment results to someone other than the client. If it is part of South Africa's law to report all known or suspected abuse of a minor child to authorities, as it is in many other countries, then Dr. Kennedy may release that information. However, Corey's father may not be considered an "authorized" person under South Africa's code, and again, potential harm to Corey may come from Dr. Kennedy's release of test data without permission.

American Moral Values

1. How does Dr. Kennedy view Corey's request for privacy as a way to avoid further abuse? How much of Corey's statement is a reasonable attempt at self-protection, and how much of it is a fearful by-product of the abuse itself? How can Dr. Kennedy convey her respect for Corey's request while acting responsibly to help prevent further abuse? What kind of trust and support will Dr. Kennedy need to maintain in order to work with Corey, his family, and his school going forward?
2. How do Dr. Kennedy's views and experiences relating to physical abuse inform her assessment of Corey's situation? On what conditions would it be worth getting Corey out of his current situation? Is physical abuse too detrimental to risk "toughing it out" or finding new arrangements with his father? What is her gut reaction to his wounds? Does Dr. Kennedy take being beaten by an older sibling as "normal" enough to seek a solution without releasing the data?
3. What are Dr. Kennedy's views about Corey's father? How much does she sympathize with his predicament as a working single parent? Would Corey's case present differently if it were Corey's mother who was the parent? How does Dr. Kennedy assess Corey's worry about his father's stress? Does that indicate a fear of the father being abusive? Is the father's work situation understandable enough to see him as part of a solution (different child care arrangements)?
4. How would an intervention from Child Protective Services (CPS) affect Corey's family relationships,

both short and long term? Does Dr. Kennedy believe that Corey's abuse is mitigated by the structure and support he gets from his family? Or does his current situation lend him no significant stability, negating any general value of "family"?

5. Should Dr. Kennedy tell Corey what the law has instructed her to do with cases of abuse? Would that help reassure him that her report was not his fault? Does Corey, as an 11-year-old, need to be told along with his father in order not to be overwhelmed? Would it be right to use the threat of reporting to pressure the father to change Corey's situation?

Ethical Course of Action

Directive per APA Code

Standard 9.04 (b) gives two conditions under which test data may be released. One condition is when a client has given a signed release of information. The second condition is when law or court order requires such release. If Dr. Kennedy was practicing in Virginia, then she would be permitted under Standard 9.04 (b) to release Corey's projective drawings, the stories with the drawings, and any other information gathered in the course of conditions related to the assessment to state protective services.

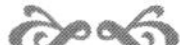

Dictates of One's Own Conscience

If you were Dr. Kennedy, which action would you take?

1. Immediately make a report to the state Child Protective Services.
2. Remind Corey that you have to tell someone he is being physically abused to try to stop the abuse.
3. Attempt to contact Corey's father immediately to let him know of the allegations of abuse before contacting any state protective services.
4. Inform Corey's father that you are reporting Corey's allegations to Child Protective Services, and that you are also concerned that Corey is being neglected due to the father's work schedule. Suggest that Corey's father be present in the room when you make the report to CPS.
5. Request a family meeting with Corey and his father to disclose the abuse allegations, and suggest to Corey's father that he manage this situation with his other son on his own, suggest a specific timeline, and state that you will follow up on any future abuse incidents by reporting them to Child Protective Services.
6. Combinations of the above-listed actions.
7. Or one that is not listed above.

If you were practicing in South Africa, you would likely not release the assessment results to Corey's father if you thought doing so would place Corey in harm's way. However, you would also consider that by not releasing the results of the drawings to the appropriate persons, harm is also coming to Corey.

STANDARD 9.05: TEST CONSTRUCTION

Psychologists who develop tests and other assessment techniques use appropriate psychometric procedures and current scientific or professional knowledge for test design, standardization, validation, reduction or elimination of bias, and recommendations for use.

A CASE FOR STANDARD 9.05: Stereotype, Self-Fulfilling Prophecy, or Reality

The clinic at the Modern School of Psychology provides career counseling, psychological assessments for adults, and learning disability testing for school-age children. These services are available to the public and facilitate training for graduate students taking assessment classes. Development of assessment techniques does not stop at the actual instrument, but includes the whole process of assessment such as paperwork, consent forms, where testing is conducted, and so on. The clinic's standard procedure for assessment thus is part of the development of assessment techniques. The Modern School of Psychology's clinic requires that the receptionist give clients a demographic questionnaire to complete. The student evaluators are then to review the demographic information for accuracy in their first interview. On the demographic sheet are the U.S. Census questions pertaining to age, sex, and race.

Issues of Concern

The development of a test is a long and arduous process. For this reason, the vast majority of psychologists will not engage in the development of an instrument. However, for every psychologist who ever administers a test or conducts a psychological assessment, psychologists participate in developing of assessment procedures. Standard 9.05 directs psychologists to use procedures that are based on current relevant scientific or professional knowledge. Standard 9.05 applies to the simple gathering of demographic information. What considerations do all psychologists who conduct psychological assessments need to be aware of per Standard 9.05?

APA Ethics Code

Companion General Principle

Principle B: Fidelity and Responsibility

> Psychologists . . . are aware of their professional and scientific responsibilities to society and to the specific communities in which they work.

Principle B guides psychologists to be aware of their responsibilities. What these specific responsibilities are at any given time may be nebulous and up for debate. One responsibility that most states espouse through their continuing education requirement is for psychologists to keep abreast of the scientific knowledge related to their areas of competency. In this respect, to approach the aspiration of knowing the scientific basis of one's work as guided by Principle B requires the clinical faculty of the school to have thought through the available evidence for adopting their intake procedures.

Companion Ethical Standard

Standard 2.04: Bases for Scientific and Professional Judgments

> Psychologists' work is based upon established scientific and professional knowledge of the discipline.

Standard 2.04 interprets part of Principle B and obligates psychologists to not only be aware, but also to apply scientific knowledge to all aspects of their work. An example of such an application in the situation with assessment procedures is the research about stereotypes and their impact on performance (Huang, 2004; Steele, 1997; Walton & Spencer, 2009). What changes to the standard intake procedures might the clinic adopt in order to apply the findings on stereotypes and their impact on the performance?

Standard 3.01: Unfair Discrimination

> In their work-related activities, psychologists do not engage in unfair discrimination based on age, gender, gender identity, race, ethnicity, culture, national origin, religion, sexual orientation, disability, socioeconomic status, or any basis proscribed by law.

Including questions pertaining to age, sex, and race in a similar manner to the U.S. Census demographic questions may be common practice. If psychologists are to enact the directives of Standard 3.01 and Principle E: Respect for People's Right and Dignity, then psychologists need to be aware of the most recent research on discrimination and eliminate stereotyping questions at intake.

Legal Issues 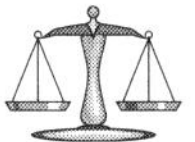

Virginia

> *18 Va. Admin. Code § 125-20-150 (2010). Standards of Practice.*
>
> B. Persons licensed by the board shall . . .
>
> 6. Avoid harming patients . . . for whom they provide professional services and minimize harm when it is foreseeable and unavoidable . . .
>
> 12. Construct, maintain, administer, interpret and report testing and diagnostic services in a manner and for purposes which are appropriate.

Washington

> *Wash. Admin. Code § 246-924-359 (2009). Client Welfare.*
>
> (3) Stereotyping. In their work-related activities, psychologists do not engage in unfair discrimination based on age, gender, race, ethnicity, national origin, religion, sexual orientation, disability, socioeconomic status, or any basis proscribed by law.
>
> *Wash. Admin. Code § 246-924-365 (2009). Assessment Procedures.*
>
> (2) Limitations regarding assessment results. When reporting of the results of an assessment procedure,

the psychologist shall include any relevant reservations, qualifications, or limitations which affect the validity, reliability, or other interpretation of results.

In both jurisdictions, the licensing board would likely find that the laws were broken. The intake procedure of the school clinic is not in compliance with nondiscrimination laws of both states based on evidence of bias being created through use of race categories immediately before the assessment.

Cultural Considerations

Global Discussion

The Professional Board for Psychology Health Professions Council of South Africa: Ethical Code of Conduct (April 2002)

> 5. Assessment activities.
>
> Psychologists have responsibility for . . . assessment, including . . . tests . . . [and] instruments. . . Psychologists have a particular responsibility to ensure cultural . . . competence in the provision of these services.
>
> 5.4. Test development.
>
> Psychologists who develop . . . tests and other assessment methods shall use scientific procedures and current professional knowledge for test design, standardisation, validation, reduction or elimination of bias, and recommendations for use.

Using census questions related to race prior to any sort of performance-based assessment is arguably in violation of both scientific procedures and elimination of bias. The Modern School would also be in violation of South Africa's code if they allowed the demographic information (race, etc.) to influence the sorts of assessments given.

American Moral Values

1. What is the value of demographic information for exploring the significance of a test? Is the accurate collection of that information best ensured through a questionnaire filled out before the test? If recent research suggests that filling out demographic information affects the test that follows, is there another way to collect such information? Would asking for that information after the test be just as effective?

2. What is the best way to avoid the negative cuing effect of demographic information requests? Again, would procuring that information after the test avoid that effect? Or would it create another mystique about such tests that might carry over to future tests?

3. How should graduate students and professionals think about this issue for their assessments? Is current research authoritative enough as a reason for not collecting demographic information beforehand? Will there be resistance to this move, and those who dismiss its attempt at bias elimination as instead a "special" measure for minorities who have absorbed negative biases about themselves? Are dominant groups positively cued by demographic requests, implying that bias could be lessened in both directions by avoiding such requests before testing?

4. What other types of cuing need to be addressed to improve future testing? What are the power dynamics at work between test subjects and administrators that might skew subjects' abilities to perform?

Ethical Course of Action

Directive per APA Code

Standard 9.05 requires those who develop assessment techniques to use current scientific knowledge for elimination of bias. Procedures followed in all aspects of conducting a psychological assessment fall under the dictates of Standard 9.05, including the simple gathering of demographic information. In order to be in compliance with Standard 9.05, the clinic procedures need to be in line with current scientific knowledge regarding the effect of stereotyping on test performance.

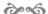

Dictates of One's Own Conscience

If you were the clinic director and became aware of the effect of stereotyping on test performance, which action would you take?

1. Do nothing because demographic information has to be gathered in some way, and stereotyping is so prevalent that it is almost impossible to avoid.

2. Mail the demographic information questions to the client prior to intake and request that he or she bring the questionnaire to the first session. In this way, separate the time between the mention of stereotype factors and the assessment.

3. Do not require the students to review demographic information with the client prior to assessment procedures.
4. Have every assessment report contain a statement regarding the limits of test interpretation based on stereotype triggers.
5. Administer the demographic information sheet at the end of the assessment process instead of the beginning.
6. Combinations of the above-listed actions.
7. Or one that is not listed above.

If the clinic was located in South Africa, the above-listed options would still apply since the guidelines for nondiscrimination as well as test construction are not substantially different from those listed by the APA Ethics Code.

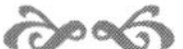

STANDARD 9.06: INTERPRETING ASSESSMENT RESULTS

> When interpreting assessment results, including automated interpretations, psychologists take into account the purpose of the assessment as well as the various test factors, test-taking abilities, and other characteristics of the person being assessed, such as situational, personal, linguistic, and cultural differences, that might affect psychologists' judgments or reduce the accuracy of their interpretations. They indicate any significant limitations of their interpretations.

A CASE FOR STANDARD 9.06: Perseverating Bats

Regina has been assigned to administer a practice test for her Rorschach class. Subjects are recruited through the school clinic, and volunteers receive feedback on their results. Regina administers the Rorschach to Dan, who is an artist. On the second Rorschach percept, Dan says, "It's a bat." On the third image, Dan repeats, "It's a bat. In fact, I think it's the same bat I just saw." On the fourth image, Dan, becoming agitated, exclaims, "It's that same bat again! Is it going to follow me throughout this whole thing?" Then on one more subsequent card, Dan shakes his head in dismay, and with evident sorrow on his face, says, "The bat has been killed. Killed by some idiot on the road who didn't look where they were going. Why do people do that? Now I guess that bat won't follow me anymore. Why did you do this to me? Why did you make that bat follow me, only to end up like this?"

Later that week, Regina bumps into Dan in front of the elevator in their apartment building. To both of their surprise, Dan and Regina live in the same apartment complex. Regina tells her supervisor, Dr. Dixon, of Dan's responses on the Rorschach and also informs her that Dan lives in the same apartment building that she does. Dr. Dixon looks troubled while Regina asks, "What do we tell him?"

Issues of Concern

Learning the administration and interpretation of a complex test like the Rorschach is difficult at best. Arguably, the best training for students is to immediately and directly apply classroom-based material. In the case of practicing assessments with actual human subjects, this can often lead to surprises. Standard 9.06 requires that in the interpretation of Dan's performance on the Rorschach, the assessor needs to take into account the purpose and relevant characteristics of Dan as a subject. What factors need to be taken into account for Dan? Given that this is a learning exercise for Regina, is it appropriate to even give Dan any feedback?

APA Ethics Code

Companion General Principle

Principle C: Integrity

> Psychologists seek to promote accuracy, honesty, and truthfulness in the . . . practice of psychology.

Principle C guides Dr. Dixon to be accurate in her supervision of Regina regarding Dan. It also guides Regina to be accurate in her interpretation of Dan's test results as well as any feedback she might give to Dan. Given that this is a training situation where Regina is not conducting a full assessment and does not have other necessary and relevant information to make an accurate interpretation of the Rorschach, is there anything accurate in what she might say to Dan?

Companion Ethical Standards

Standard 10.01: Informed Consent to Therapy

> . . . (c) When the therapist is a trainee and the legal responsibility for the services provided resides with the

> supervisor, the client . . . is informed that the evaluator is in training and is being supervised and is given the name of the supervisor.

Whatever the situation with Dan and Regina is, Dr. Dixon holds the legal responsibility as the supervisor. Standard 10.01 dictates that Regina tell Dan about the existence and role of Dr. Dixon.

Standard 9.07: Assessment by Unqualified Persons

> Psychologists do not promote the use of psychological assessment techniques by unqualified persons, except when such use is conducted for training purposes with appropriate supervision.

By definition, as a student and as a supervisee, Regina is unqualified to perform independently. Standard 9.07 allows for Regina to function professionally under supervision where she is not competent to perform any of the activities. Standard 9.07 also requires that Regina be under Dr. Dixon's supervision to interact with Dan.

Standard 9.10: Explaining Assessment Results

> Regardless of whether the scoring and interpretation are done by . . . assistants[,] . . . psychologists take reasonable steps to ensure that explanations of results are given to the individual.

Standard 9.10 directs Dr. Dixon to ensure that Dan is given an explanation of his Rorschach results. Is it appropriate for Regina to give Dan interpretation, given that (1) this is a training situation, (2) Rorschach was given in isolation of other tests, and (3) there is the existence of a multiple relationship between Dan and Regina?

Standard 3.05: Multiple Relationships

> . . . (b) If a psychologist finds that . . . a potentially harmful multiple relationship has arisen, the psychologist takes reasonable steps to resolve it with due regard for the best interests of the affected person and maximal compliance with the Ethics Code.

Dan and Regina's relationship as neighbors in the same apartment building was unknown to either of them at the time of testing. The situation qualifies as a multiple relationship as defined in standard 3.05 (b). Standard 3.05 (b) directs Regina to resolve the situation with maximum compliance with the ethics code. Standard 3.05 does not prohibit the existence of a multiple relationship, and the fact that Regina and Dan live in the same apartment building does not necessarily obligate Regina to withdraw from the case.

Legal Issues 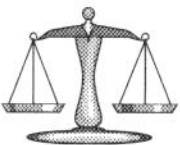

California

> *Cal. Admin. Rules § 1387.1 (2010). Qualifications and Responsibilities of Primary Supervisors.*
>
> (f) Primary supervisors shall be responsible for monitoring the welfare of the trainee's clients.
>
> (g) Primary supervisors shall ensure that each client or patient is informed, prior to the rendering of services by the trainee
>
> (1) that the trainee is unlicensed and is functioning under the direction and supervision of the supervisor.

Florida

> *Fla. Admin. Code Ann. Sect. 64b19-18.004. Use of Test Instruments.*
>
> (2) A psychologist who uses test instruments in the psychologist's practice of psychology:
>
> (a) Must consider whether research supports the underlying presumptions which govern the interpretive statements which would be made by the test instrument as a result of its completion by any service user . . .
>
> (c) Must integrate and reconcile the interpretive statements made by the test instrument based on group norms, with the psychologist's independent professional knowledge, evaluation and assessment of the individual who takes the test. . .
>
> (4) In performing the functions listed at subsection (2) of this rule, the psychologist must meet with the test subject face-to-face in a clinical setting unless the psychologist has delegated the work to a . . . psychological trainee . . . in a doctoral psychology program approved by the American Psychological Association.

In California, the supervisor must monitor the welfare of the client, and the client must be informed of Dr. Dixon's involvement. In Florida, the law calls for an integration and reconciliation of test data in the course of an assessment. A few statements about "bats" on a Rorschach are insufficient data to suggest any conclusion. To meet the requirements set out in the Florida code, Dr. Dixon must encourage further testing and other assessment procedures to occur before any results are conveyed about the evaluation. In addition, in light of Regina finding out that Dan lives in her building, Dr. Dixon would be wise to reassign the case for further evaluation by another student to avoid any appearance of multiple relationships.

Cultural Considerations

Global Discussion

Singapore Psychological Society:
Code of Professional Ethics

> Principle 7. Client welfare.
>
> The psychologist respects the integrity and protects the welfare of the person . . . with whom work is undertaken. . .
>
> 1. The psychologist who asks that an individual reveal personal information in the course of . . . testing . . . does so only after making certain that the responsible person is fully aware of the purposes of the . . . testing . . . and of the ways in which the information may be used.
>
> 5. The psychologist who requires others to take psychological tests for didactic . . . purposes protects the examinees by ensuring that the test results are used appropriately.

If Regina was performing this practice assessment in Singapore, it would be incumbent upon Regina (and Dr. Dixon as the supervising psychologist) to ensure that Dan fully understands that the purpose of the Rorschach is for Regina to practice giving and interpreting the assessment. In this particular case, neither Dan nor Regina fully knew the possible results of such an exercise. What use of this information is now considered appropriate? What might be the possible harm to Dan in learning that his Rorschach results are unexpectedly negative? Within the context of Dan's being an artist, is it completely accurate to interpret his results in a similar manner as those of non-artists? Regina and Dr. Dixon agreed to give direct feedback to Dan before Regina knew that Dan was her neighbor. It may be an appropriate use of the test results to discard all of the assessment materials after Regina is done with the practice administration and scoring.

American Moral Values

1. What results are owed to Dan as a volunteer subject? Have Dr. Dixon and Regina committed to giving him a full interpretation of the results by one or both of them? Is it important for him to receive some feedback as acknowledgment of the terms of his participation? Or is it more important for him to know Regina's limitations as an interpreter and to be prevented from being given misleading results? If the latter, do they owe him an apology if he was not clear on those limitations and conditions?
2. How do Dr. Dixon and Regina anticipate Dan will react to their various responses? How do the results of his Rorschach test itself shape their expectations? Could he be paranoid that they were withholding important information from him? Will he feel exploited as a test subject, having gone through an apparently distressing test experience while not receiving the kind of feedback that could help him understand the ordeal?
3. Does Dan need treatment for the kind of symptoms he showed during the Rorschach? Does not revealing the results due to insufficient expertise risk his not getting that treatment?
4. How does Regina's living in Dan's building feature as a question of multiple relationships? Should this be cited as a reason for Regina not giving Dan results? Will this be a scrupulous way to preserve professionalism, or is this a way to get Regina out of an uncomfortable social situation? Could it be a way to protect Regina from a negative reaction by Dan? If the results had been positive, should the issue of multiple relationships come into play?
5. How does the cultural significance of the Rorschach test inform Dr. Dixon and Regina's take on Dan's status? Should Dan have understood this test as more of a personal experience with a famous exercise, one that depends on one's own way to make meaning out of a pattern? Is the Rorschach in this context more like narrating what one sees in the clouds than, say, talking about one's mother to a psychotherapist (to use another cultural cliché)? How much responsibility do psychologists bear for using a test that elicits the kind of reaction Dan showed? Is this a psychic risk that could have been made known ahead of time?
6. How do Dr. Dixon and Regina's ideas about artists affect their view of Dan's situation? Does a subject being an artist lead one to take such results more seriously or less seriously in terms of treatment?
7. What kind of training is Dr. Dixon providing Regina in this episode? Does Dr. Dixon owe Regina a chance to score the results as part of her training? Or does Regina need to understand when more expertise is needed before moving forward with one's assessment? Does Dr. Dixon need to address the program itself, which puts students like Regina in a difficult situation when faced with disturbing results?

Ethical Course of Action

Directive per APA Code

Standard 10.01 directs that Dan be informed of Regina's status as a student under supervision. In addition, Standard 9.07 requires Regina, as a student under supervision, to adhere to Dr. Dixon's directives. Regina has acted appropriately in asking Dr. Dixon what she should say to Dan. Standard 3.05 does not require Regina to alter her current relationship with Dan since living in the same apartment building is a very distant relationship.

Standard 9.06 directs psychologists to take into account the purpose of the assessment. In this case, the purpose of the assessment is entirely for Regina's training benefit. The subject is not drawn from a clinical population; there is no referral question to be answered; and therefore there is no clinical need for interpretation.

Standard 9.06 also directs psychologists to consider other characteristics of the person being tested in making interpretations of any test results. Factors that place significant limitation on the accuracy of any interpretation include the absence of necessary background material to appropriately interpret the test responses and uncertainty regarding how the extent of Dan's artistic training may influence his responses to the percepts. In addition, given the presence of a multiple relationship, it may be prudent not to make an interpretation.

To aspire to the full intent of Principle C, the class might consider avoiding unwise or unclear commitments. In this situation, it would be prudent for the students not to promise that practice tests will be accompanied by test interpretation or feedback sessions with subjects.

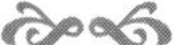

Dictates of One's Own Conscience

If you were Dr. Dixon, which of these would you do?

1. Direct Regina to score the responses before determining what to say to Dan.
2. Direct Regina to score the responses, recontact Dan for more background information and a standardized clinical interview, and then attempt an interpretation.
3. Consult with a colleague regarding the normative range of responses for artists.
4. Direct Regina to research artist responses to the Rorschach test.

If you were Regina, which action would you take?

1. Score the response to pass the class.
2. Tell your supervisor that an interpretation has to be given to Dan because you told him that you would let him know of the results.
3. Argue that you do not want to do any interpretation because you fear Dan's subsequent relationship with you in the apartment building if he does not like the interpretation.
4. Tell Dan that the results indicate he has unusual thought processes but that such unusual thoughts may be a reflection of his artistic training.
5. Combinations of the above-listed actions.
6. Or one that is not listed above.

If you were Dr. Dixon teaching in Singapore, you would direct yourself to "ensure that the test result are used appropriately" by directing Regina to remind Dan that (1) Regina is a student, (2) the administration of the test is not always accurate, and (3) Regina is not able to give Dan interpretation of his Rorschach.

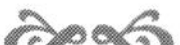

STANDARD 9.07: ASSESSMENT BY UNQUALIFIED PERSONS

Psychologists do not promote the use of psychological assessment techniques by unqualified persons, except when such use is conducted for training purposes with appropriate supervision.

A CASE FOR STANDARD 9.07: Conflicting Opinion

Dr. Ramos is a licensed psychologist working for the school system. Amber is entering first grade. She has had a difficult year in kindergarten. Amber's parents have asked Dr. Ramos for a psychological evaluation to help Amber obtain special support services as she enters into the first grade. In reviewing Amber's school records provided by Amber's mother, Dr. Ramos found that her primary teacher and her special education teacher at the beginning of kindergarten completed a Gillian Asperger's Disorder Scale (GADS). The special education teacher gave Amber a provisional diagnosis of autism based on the GADS. Dr. Ramos completed a full battery of tests. The full battery included the completion of the Krug Asperger's Disorder Index (KADI) by both the parents and teacher, and an Autism Diagnostic Observation Schedule (ADOS). Dr. Ramos's report does not confirm a diagnosis of autism or Asperger's. Amber's parents file a complaint with the school board, charging that Amber has unfairly lost her special support services based on Dr. Ramos's assessment.

Issues of Concern

Standard 9.07 directs Dr. Ramos not to promote the use of assessment techniques by unqualified persons. The GADS is a simple paper-and-pencil questionnaire that can be completed by anyone who has consistent contact with the child. Amber's mother would argue that it was appropriate for Amber's teachers and for the previous assessor to have used the instruments. Indeed, she is making the argument that Dr. Ramos's assessment is not accurate. On what grounds would Dr. Ramos defend her findings? What argument would she use to demonstrate that the previous GADS results were invalid?

APA Ethics Code

Companion General Principle

Principle B: Fidelity and Responsibility

> Psychologists . . . cooperate with other professionals and institutions to the extent needed to serve the best interests of those with whom they work. They are concerned about the ethical compliance of their colleagues' scientific and professional conduct.

Principle B guides Dr. Ramos to consider the professional community in which she works. Aspiring to the ideals of fidelity and responsibility, Dr. Ramos would seek to consult with both Amber's primary and special education teachers. Amber's teachers have their own code of ethics governing their work as education professionals. Should a teacher's code of conduct prohibit his or her use of instruments like the GADS, a psychological assessment tool, to help the students perform in school? Does Principle B steer Dr. Ramos toward action in this particular case?

Companion Ethical Standard

Standard 3.09: Cooperation With Other Professionals

> When indicated and professionally appropriate, psychologists cooperate with other professionals in order to serve their clients/patients effectively and appropriately.

Standard 3.09 reminds Dr. Ramos as a professional that her work does not occur in a vacuum. When it is in the best interest of the client, Standard 3.09 directs psychologists to cooperate with other professionals. To best serve Amber, it is essential for Dr. Ramos to work with Amber's parents and teacher(s) to, at a minimum, obtain information. For Amber to be best served within a school system, it is essential for Dr. Ramos to work collaboratively with all parts of the school system.

Standard 9.01: Bases for Assessments

> (a) Psychologists base the opinions contained in their . . . reports . . . on information and techniques sufficient to substantiate their findings.

With regard to Standard 9.01, Dr. Ramos is obligated to choose the battery of assessment instruments that is sufficient to substantiate her reported results. Presumably, if Dr. Ramos utilized another instrument to assess for symptoms of autism/Asperger syndrome, she must provide sound scientific reasoning for choosing to do so.

Standard 9.10: Explaining Assessment Results

> Psychologists take reasonable steps to ensure that explanations of results are given to the individual or designated representative

Standard 9.10 requires Dr. Ramos to provide an explanation of her results to Amber's parents. Standard 9.10 does not require that Dr. Ramos's explanation be in agreement with the opinion of Amber's parents.

Legal Issues 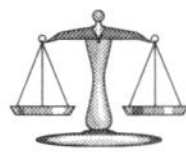

Hawaii

> *Haw. Code R. § 16-98-34 (2010). Unethical Practice of Psychology.*
>
> (k) Test scores, like test materials, may be released only to persons who are qualified to interpret and use them properly:

(1) Materials for reporting test scores to parents, or which are designed for self-appraisal purposes in schools . . . shall be closely supervised by qualified psychologists. . .

(2) Test results . . . shall be communicated to . . . relatives . . . in such a manner as to guard against misinterpretation or misuse. . .

(3) When test results rather than the score are communicated directly to parents and students, they shall be accompanied by adequate interpretive aids or advice.

Indiana

868 Ind. Admin. Code 1.1-11-5 (2010). Psychology Practice.

Sec. 5. . . (b) A psychologist's . . . report . . . must be based on information and techniques . . . sufficient to appropriately substantiate the findings.

868 Ind. Admin. Code 1.1-11-6 (2010). Psychological Testing.

Sec. 6. . . (c) Except as otherwise provided by law, psychological testing may be administered and interpreted only by a licensed psychologist who is endorsed as a health service provider in psychology, or by a person under the direct supervision of a health service provider in psychology, provided that such supervision is in compliance with this article.

In both jurisdictions, Dr. Ramos has not broken any of the laws. As long as she produces an evaluation report that is based upon multiple-measure corroboration, she would satisfy the laws, even though other employees within her school system appeared to have acted beyond the scope of their training. Dr. Ramos was not charged with the supervision of those employees so is only responsible for her work product. In Hawaii, she is further obligated by the law to meet with the parents and provide direct explanations of the results of the evaluation.

Cultural Considerations

Global Discussion

Code of Ethics for the Psychologist: Spain.

Article 19. The use of any kind of strictly psychological material . . . must be reserved exclusively for psychologists, and they in turn must refrain from providing it to non-competent persons. Psychologists must manage psychological documentation, or when appropriate, guarantee its safekeeping.

According to the Spanish code, teachers may not use psychological tests or give psychological diagnoses. Dr. Ramos did not violate the code by allowing an unqualified person to diagnose or use the assessment. Although Spain's code is silent on the method or the means, it seems that Dr. Ramos is charged with safeguarding psychological documentation and assessments so that they are not used by untrained non-psychologists. Therefore, Dr. Ramos may need to have a conversation about this ethical breach with the special education teacher's supervisor, or the school administrator, to attempt to ensure that any future misuse does not occur, and the current misuse is corrected within the record.

American Moral Values

1. How does Dr. Ramos relate her assessment to that of the special education teacher? Does she need to overrule the judgment of an unqualified practitioner? Would it set a harmful precedent not to contest an untrained teacher administering "provisional" tests for conditions like autism and Asperger's? Does the prior "provisional" test have any validity?
2. Even if she regards her testing as complete, should Dr. Ramos try to collaborate with Amber's family and the school system? Should she agree, as a gesture of goodwill, to consult with another psychologist to corroborate her findings? Is there any additional data that could be provided by Amber, her family, and her teachers that could fill out and nuance Dr. Ramos's results? Does the special education teacher have any expertise that Dr. Ramos thinks would be relevant for determining Amber's need for special services? Or does a collaborative effort act as a concession, encouraging challenges like the one Amber's mother has leveled against Dr. Ramos?
3. What are Dr. Ramos's views of this school system and the educational system in general? Does she want to stand with the school system against a family seeking services? Does she believe students by and large receive the services they need, or do more students, with or without formal diagnoses, deserve more assistance in order for them to function well in school? What degree of diagnostic inaccuracy or vagueness is justified in order for a student to receive the right services? Does Amber's case merit such diagnostic "slack"?
4. Does Dr. Ramos believe the school board challenge will harm her career? Should she stand up on principle for her practice and established modes of testing, or

does she risk too much damage to her reputation and that of other psychologists in the school district? How will her actions affect future conflicts over testing in the district?

5. What are Dr. Ramos's views about how society treats autism and Asperger's? Does she believe the conditions are being denied or categorized differently (e.g., "socially awkward"), or does she think it more likely that parents and teachers are too quick to reach for those labels? Is there a social stigma that Dr. Ramos believes would attach to Amber if she were incorrectly diagnosed as being on the spectrum?

Ethical Course of Action

Directive per APA Code

Dr. Ramos, as specified by Standard 2.01, is presumably competent to perform the assessment. Having earned her credentials to work as a psychologist, she is by training more qualified to administer psychological assessments than the special education or kindergarten teachers. It is unclear as to who exactly gave Amber the diagnosis of Asperger's. However, unless it was a psychologist duly certified and competent to perform child assessments, Dr. Ramos is obligated per Standard 9.07 not to support the previous work by untrained persons. Refusing to endorse the previous diagnosis without a fully independent assessment, as was done by Dr. Ramos, is a way of not promoting the use of psychological assessment techniques by unqualified persons.

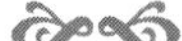

Dictates of One's Own Conscience

If you were Dr. Ramos, faced with complaint from a disgruntled mother, which would you do?

1. Recommend that she solicit another assessment from a psychologist who is independent of the school.
2. Meet with Amber's mother again to explain the full assessment.
3. Meet with Amber's mother to explain why you used the KADI instead of the GADS if you suspect she questions the validity of the instrument.
4. Meet with the school special education team for consultation on your work.
5. Consult with another school psychologist to review your work.
6. Meet with the kindergarten and special education teachers to reaffirm the information upon which you based your results.
7. Combinations of the above-listed actions.
8. Or one that is not listed above.

If you were Dr. Ramos practicing in Spain, faced with a complaint from a disgruntled mother, you are obligated to explain that previous use of the psychological test material was inappropriate and produced unsubstantiated results.

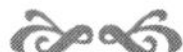

STANDARD 9.08: OBSOLETE TESTS AND OUTDATED TEST RESULTS

(a) Psychologists do not base their assessment or intervention decisions or recommendations on data or test results that are outdated for the current purpose.

A CASE FOR STANDARD 9.08 (A): One Assessment Fits All

Dr. Reyes completed a full neuropsychological assessment of Mr. Don, a Native American, 9 months ago. This assessment was performed after Mr. Don suffered a head injury during an earthquake. Evaluation with the Halstead-Reitan Neuropsychological Test Battery and parts of the Luria-Nebraska battery indicated that Mr. Don had sustained some cognitive impairment. Subsequent testing indicated overall improvement, but with intermittent problems in some areas of functioning. Mr. Don works as an air traffic controller. Recently, he complained that he is very worried he might make an error at work that may result in the death or injury of others. He stated that he has already made some errors, and he had reported them to his supervisor, who did not seem terribly concerned. Mr. Don also currently meets criteria for clinical depression, although the symptoms are mild at this time.

Issues of Concern

Standard 9.08 (a) addresses itself to the use of prior test data in formulating new decisions regarding diagnosis. Relevant questions for Dr. Reyes to consider may include the following: Is Don asking for a work competency statement from Dr. Reyes? Does the directive of 9.08 require Dr. Reyes to conduct another full battery of tests? Should a neuropsychological assessment performed 9 months ago be considered outdated? If the previous assessment contained recommendations for work accommodations, could Dr. Reyes refer to or use the previous recommendations? Regardless of what Mr. Don requests, should Dr. Reyes recommend a medical leave based on imminent danger?

APA Ethics Code

Companion General Principle

Principle B: Fidelity and Responsibility

> Psychologists . . . are aware of their professional . . . responsibilities to society. . . Psychologists uphold professional standards of conduct, clarify their professional roles and obligations, accept appropriate responsibility for their behavior, and seek to manage conflicts of interest that could lead to exploitation or harm.

Principle B calls Dr. Reyes's attention to the notion that she has a responsibility to her client, as well as to society. In this situation, Dr. Reyes should be aware of her responsibility to protect the lives of travelers from any potential error Mr. Don may make due to the condition of his mental health. The concern for public safety should be balanced with Dr. Reyes's awareness of Mr. Don's personal need to be engaged in gainful wage work.

Companion Ethical Standard

Standard 4.05: Disclosures

> (a) Psychologists may disclose confidential information with the appropriate consent of the . . . individual client. . .
>
> (b) Psychologists disclose confidential information without the consent of the individual only as mandated by law, or where permitted by law for a valid purpose such as to . . . (3) protect the client/patient, or others . . . from harm . . . in which instance disclosure is limited to the minimum that is necessary to achieve the purpose.

Standard 4.05 enables Dr. Reyes to discharge her responsibility to society by allowing her to disclose confidential information obtained through the course of her work. Dr. Reyes could collaborate with Mr. Don's supervisor if Mr. Don gives consent, which is the condition for Standard 4.05 (a). If Mr. Don is hesitant to have his workplace know about his evaluation, Dr. Reyes could still contact his workplace, but only if she believed it was necessary in order to protect people from harm, as specified in Standard 4.05 (b).

Standard 9.06: Interpreting Assessment Results

> When interpreting assessment results . . . psychologists take into account the purpose of the assessment as well as the various test factors, test-taking abilities, and other characteristics of the person being assessed, such as situational, personal[,] . . . and cultural differences, that might affect psychologists' judgments or reduce the accuracy of their interpretations. They indicate any significant limitations of their interpretations.

Whether in a new assessment or using a previous assessment, Standard 9.06 directs Dr. Reyes to take into account the purpose and individual circumstances when making interpretations. Looking at the previous evaluation for head injury, it appears that Dr. Reyes did not focus on any of Mr. Don's personal or cultural factors. Regarding the current question of concentration level, do Mr. Don's personal and cultural differences have any relevance? When addressing the question of whether or not Mr. Don possesses the ability to concentrate at work, does it make any difference whether Mr. Don is of Native American ancestry?

Legal Issues 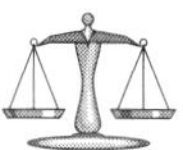

Kansas

> *Kan. Admin. Regs. § 102-1-10a (2010). Unprofessional conduct.*
>
> (j) improperly using assessment procedures, which shall include the following acts:
>
> (1) Basing assessment, intervention, or recommendations on test results and instruments that are inappropriate to the current purpose or to the patient characteristics;
>
> (2) failing to identify situations in which particular assessment techniques or norms may not be applicable or failing to make adjustments in administration or interpretation because of relevant factors, including . . . race . . .
>
> (3) failing to indicate significant limitations to the accuracy of the assessment findings . . .

> (5) endorsing, filing, or submitting psychological assessments, recommendations, reports, or diagnostic statements on the basis of information and techniques that are insufficient to substantiate those findings.

Kentucky

> *201 Ky. Admin. Regs. 26:145 (2010). Code of Conduct.*
>
> Section 5. Client Welfare.
>
> (3) Stereotyping. The credential holder shall not impose on the client a stereotype of behavior, values, or roles related to . . . race . . . which would interfere with the objective provision of psychological services to the client.

Dr. Reyes would be in violation of Kansas code if the previous assessment results were used to determine Mr. Don's current functioning. At times, an individual's race category may be irrelevant to the question at hand, as is the case for Mr. Don. If Dr. Reyes allowed Mr. Don's status as a Native American somehow to influence her deliberations, then Dr. Reyes also would be in violation of Kentucky code.

Cultural Considerations

Global Discussion

The New Zealand Psychological Society Code of Ethics

> 9. Psychological assessment.
>
> Psychologists guard against any misuse or bias in selection, administration, scoring and interpretation of assessment instruments or procedures. They are prepared to justify, in terms of current scientific literature, their use and interpretation of any assessment instrument or procedure. They avoid using instruments which are obsolete or of dubious scientific status.

Although both the Luria-Nebraska and the Halstead-Reitan are appropriate to assess cognitive functioning and levels of possible neurological impairment, neither is currently used to assess or diagnose depression. If Dr. Reyes uses the results from this assessment, along with Mr. Don's self-report of errors at work, she risks violating this portion of New Zealand's code. Although these test instruments may be valid, the results from the first exam, given 9 months ago, might arguably be considered obsolete.

American Moral Values

1. How does Dr. Reyes view the limits of an assessment? Should she adhere to the relevance of Halstead-Reitan and Luria-Nebraska to cognitive impairment, given that they are not tests for depression? Or are there some kinds of information that are too important not to mention, even if they are incidental to the formal tests administered?
2. Should Dr. Reyes perform another assessment, both to be up to date and to include tests more suited to measuring depression or anxiety? Will this satisfy demands for accuracy while addressing the possible problems Mr. Don is facing?
3. Do the tests for cognitive impairment adequately account for differences of culture? If not, could Dr. Reyes be more inclined to include information not measured by those tests to compensate for that bias? What is Dr. Reyes's particular experience with Native American clients or culture, and to what degree should she reconsider Mr. Don's testing in light of it?
4. What role does Mr. Don's occupation play in Dr. Reyes's judgment? Is an air traffic controller subject to more urgent statements about possible mental health problems? What is the culture of air traffic controllers when it comes to these issues? Should Dr. Reyes consider whether the supervisor will dismiss her assessment without formal test measures?

Ethical Course of Action

Directive per APA Code

Nine months is an extended period of time in terms of any cognitive changes post head injury. There could be any number of possible reasons for Mr. Don's poor concentration, including depression, drug and alcohol abuse, anxiety or caffeine overdose, and so forth. The question of poor concentration is very different from the question of possible neurological impairment. For Dr. Reyes to follow the directives of Standard 9.08, she needs to develop her current opinion based on more than the previous test data.

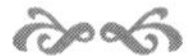

Dictates of One's Own Conscience

What if you were Dr. Reyes and had grown up around several Native American reservations. Based on life experience, you know that many Native Americans struggle with alcoholism. Which of these would you do?

1. Know that for this situation, Mr. Don's culture is of no relevance, and proceed in your usual and customary treatment regime.
2. Contact the employer to inquire about Mr. Don's work performance.
3. Write a medical leave of absence letter for Mr. Don to take to his workplace.
4. Conduct a second battery of assessments to determine the possible reasons and extent of Mr. Don's concentration problems.
5. Discuss with Mr. Don your mandated duty to warn if you are practicing in such a state.
6. Discuss with Mr. Don his alcohol use and its effects on cognitive functioning.
7. Know that almost all American Indians suffer from alcoholism, regardless of whether Mr. Don is currently using, and refer Mr. Don to Alcoholics Anonymous and inpatient alcohol treatment.
8. Combinations of the above-listed actions.
9. Or one not listed above.

If you were Dr. Reyes practicing in New Zealand, ideally, you would administer a test appropriate for depression, or issue a report with details about the cognitive impairment with data to justify the current conclusions, regardless of whether the depression information was included.

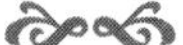

STANDARD 9.08: OBSOLETE TESTS AND OUTDATED TEST RESULTS

> . . . (b) Psychologists do not base such decisions or recommendations on tests and measures that are obsolete and not useful for the current purpose.

A CASE FOR STANDARD 9.08 (B): Culturally (In)Competent

Dr. Burns teaches the multicultural counseling course in the Modern School of Psychology. With an eye on publishing, Dr. Burns uses the Multicultural Awareness Knowledge Skills Scale (MAKSS) as a pre and post measure of multicultural competency. He has MAKSS scores from the last 5 years.

Dr. Gordon, the new chair of the department, questions Dr. Burns's competency to teach the multicultural course. Dr. Gordon cites recently published articles questioning the validity of the MAKSS and the low student ratings as evidence of his questionable teaching ability. Dr. Burns argues that he needs to continue to use the MAKSS in order to maintain instrument consistency for comparison studies.

Issues of Concern

There are two primary issues in this vignette. Both concern the use of this instrument by Dr. Burns and by Dr. Gordon. The purposes for which Dr. Burns is using the MAKSS are to measure student progress, acquisition of classroom knowledge, and possibly accumulation of data for research on teaching methodology. Discovering that one's assessment tool may be biased, obsolete, or inadequate can be troubling for psychologists, particularly if multicultural competence is an area without many assessments tools. What might be the outcome to Dr. Burns's study if he decides to switch to a different assessment tool based on Dr. Gordon's remarks? Which study would be likely seen as more flawed—one in which an outdated tool is used correctly for the pre- and posttest consistency that is the scientific gold standard, or one in which two different tools are used, thereby reducing overall comparability? If Dr. Burns's intention with his study is to attempt to bolster the credibility of this particular tool, or to perhaps begin an investigation into the development of a sounder scientific tool, then his use of this assessment could be justified.

One of the purposes for use of the MAKSS is to measure Dr. Burns's effectiveness as a teacher of multicultural competency. Is the MAKSS designed to measure acquisition of knowledge or teaching ability? Can an instrument designed to measure multicultural competency be used to measure knowledge acquisition? Moreover, is knowledge acquisition a good measure of teaching effectiveness?

The other measure used by Dr. Burns is student ratings. The student ratings in many University settings are typically measures of student satisfaction with the course. Dr. Gordon's attempt to discredit Dr. Burns by pointing to low scores on student evaluations does not take into account the many reasons, both personal and professional, that could cause such evaluations. Is Dr. Gordon's use of student ratings contrary to Standard 3.08 (b)?

APA Ethics Code

Companion General Principle

Principle B: Fidelity and Responsibility

> Psychologists . . . are concerned about the ethical compliance of their colleagues' scientific and professional conduct.

Principle B would support Dr. Gordon's suggestion to Dr. Burns about the current research on the MAKSS. Linking the use of a measure of knowledge acquisition with the student ratings may not, at face value, be motivated by the ideals of Principle B.

Principle C: Integrity

> Psychologists seek to promote accuracy, honesty, and truthfulness in the science . . . [and] teaching . . . of psychology.

Dr. Burns's responsibility as a teaching psychologist is to provide students with a curriculum that accurately reflects the most current research and practices. As the department chair, it is Dr. Gordon's responsibility to ensure that faculty members educate students about the most current research and practices. If indeed Dr. Burns is using an obsolete or invalid measure in his teaching and the reason for continued use of MAKSS is for his own personal research interest, would he be ignoring the intent of Principle C? On the other hand, if all of the developed instruments for multicultural competence have the same problem as the MAKSS, is Dr. Gordon's critique irrelevant?

Companion Ethical Standard

Standard 7.03: Accuracy in Teaching

> . . . (b) When engaged in teaching or training, psychologists present psychological information accurately.

As directed by Standard 7.03 (b), Dr. Burns needs to provide his students with the most accurate information. This includes considerations as to whether or not the inclusion of the MAKSS is warranted based on the most current research. Such consideration is in line with Standard 2.04: Bases for Scientific and Professional Judgment, which obliges Dr. Burns to base his work on the established scientific and professional knowledge of the discipline.

Regardless of the validity of the instrument, Dr. Burns's use of any outcome measure supports the goal of Standard 7.03 (b).

Standard 7.04: Student Disclosure of Personal Information

> Psychologists do not require students . . . to disclose personal information in course- . . . related activities, either orally or in writing, regarding . . . relationships with . . . peers . . . except if (1) the program . . . has clearly identified this requirement in its admissions and program materials or (2) the information is necessary to evaluate or obtain assistance for students whose personal problems could reasonably be judged to be preventing them from performing their training- or professionally related activities in a competent manner or posing a threat to the students or others.

Standard 7.04 directs Dr. Burns not to use the MAKSS to obtain personal information about relationships with peers unless one of two standards is met. The vignette does not indicate whether the admissions or program materials specified in advance that data would be collected from students to determine the increase in their multicultural awareness. It appears that Dr. Gordon should have raised one more criticism of Dr. Burns's pedagogy.

Standard 9.02: Use of Assessments

> (a) Psychologists . . . use . . . instruments . . . for purposes that are appropriate in light of the research on or evidence of the usefulness and proper application of the techniques.

Standard 9.02 (a) directs Dr. Burns to use instruments that are appropriate for the intended purpose. It appears that Dr. Burns is using the MAKSS for two purposes. One is to measure multicultural competency, and the other is probably for research purposes given that he noted he has accumulated data across a 5-year period. At the heart of Dr. Gordon's criticism is whether Dr. Burns has violated Standard 9.02 (a). Hopefully, the intent of Dr. Gordon's comments is to assure that Dr. Burns is in compliance with Standard 2.03: Maintaining Competence.

Standard 1.04: Informal Resolution of Ethical Violations

> When psychologists believe that there may have been an ethical violation by another psychologist, they attempt to resolve the issue by bringing it to the attention of that individual.

As directed by Standard 1.04, Dr. Gordon has brought his concern to Dr. Burns's attention.

Legal Issues 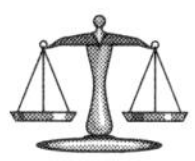

Maryland

Md. Code Regs. 10.36.05.04 (2010). Competence.

A. Professional Competence. A psychologist shall . . .

(4) Use . . . assessment techniques only when the psychologist knows that the circumstances are appropriate for applications of those . . . techniques, supported by reliability, validation, standardization, and outcome studies.

Md. Code Regs. 10.36.05.06 (2010). Psychological Assessment.

A. A psychologist shall . . .

(2) Administer psychological tests in keeping with accepted standards of practice and avoid use of obsolete measurement techniques;

(3) Use appropriate or specialized assessment instruments when working with individuals from special populations[;] . . .

(5) Select scoring and interpretive programs and services on the basis of evidence of the validity of the programs and procedures.

Michigan

Mich. Admin. Code r. 338.2515 (2010). Prohibited Conduct.

Rule 15. Prohibited conduct includes, but is not limited to, the following acts or omissions by any individual covered by these rules[:] . . .

(c) Taking on a professional role when personal, scientific, professional, legal, financial, or other relationships could impair the exercise of professional discretion or make the interests of a patient, supervisee, or student secondary to those of the licensee.

In both jurisdictions, Dr. Burns may be in violation of the laws for using an obsolete measure. Maryland's law clearly expects that Dr. Burns continue to develop his competence, and the use of an obsolete measure that may also be unreliable demonstrates that he has failed to maintain a reasonable level of competence. In Michigan, the evidence would have to show that the use of the measure served Dr. Burns's role in a manner that impaired the interests of his students. In light of APA Standard 7.04, the licensing board may view Dr. Burns as violating student privacy interests.

Cultural Considerations

Global Discussion

The New Zealand Psychological Society Code of Ethics

9. Psychological assessment. . .

9.2 Psychologists guard against any misuse or bias in selection, administration, scoring and interpretation of assessment instruments or procedures. They are prepared to justify, in terms of current scientific literature, their use and interpretation of any assessment instrument or procedure. They avoid using instruments which are obsolete or of dubious scientific status.

In order to comply with New Zealand's code, Dr. Burns would need to justify his choice of this particular assessment tool for his pre and post measures. Dr. Burns will need to carefully weigh his own scientific judgment in continuing to use this tool and the consistency of his pre- and posttest study design in light of Dr. Gordon's characterization that the instrument is obsolete.

Likewise, Dr. Gordon would need to justify his interpretation of the student satisfaction ratings and Dr. Burns's use of the MAKSS as valid measures of Dr. Burns's teaching skills.

American Moral Values

1. Why does Dr. Burns value the consistency of the MAKSS in the face of recent criticism? Does Dr. Burns find the value in an imperfect test to outweigh the risks of not having a standardized test at all? How should Dr. Burns weigh the value of his previous research? How valuable are comparison studies when the instrument itself may not be a reliable measure? How much of Dr. Burns's resistance stems from his reluctance to abandon years' worth of publishable research?
2. How does Dr. Gordon come to evaluate Dr. Burns on the basis of his using MAKSS and receiving low evaluations? What kind of evaluations do multicultural courses usually get? How do students generally react to a course (especially one that is required) that confronts difficult issues of culture and pluralism?
3. Given the lack of alternative tests for the MAKSS, can Dr. Gordon reasonably expect Dr. Burns to have already abandoned the research he had conducted with that test? How much consideration is Dr. Burns's career owed in terms of his position on MAKSS? Does

Dr. Gordon believe in measures for multicultural competency? If so, should there be alternative tests presented? Lacking such alternatives, should Dr. Burns hold off on any testing rather than base his evaluations on a faulty test?

Ethical Course of Action

Directive per APA Code

Standard 9.08 (b) directs psychologists to consider whether the test is either obsolete or not useful for its intended purpose. The published literature on the topic of MAKSS is inconclusive (Boysen & Vogel, 2008; Diaz-Lazaro & Cohen, 2001). Thus, both Dr. Burns and Dr. Gordon are correct in their positions regarding the instrument, per Standard 9.08 (b), 9.02 (a): Use of Assessment, and Standard 7.03 (b): Accuracy in Teaching. Dr. Burns is in keeping with Standard 9.02 (a) in the purpose for which the instrument is being used. Depending on the construction and procedures of the university's use of student ratings of the courses, Dr. Gordon may or may not be in compliance with 9.08 (b).

As directed by Standard 1.04, Drs. Gordon and Burns should attempt mutual resolution of the disagreement.

Dictates of One's Own Conscience

If you were Dr. Burns, would you:

1. Forward the published literature to Dr. Gordon to support your argument for use of the instrument?
2. Cite the published literature on the drawbacks and difficulties of using student ratings as a valid measure of student learning?
3. Meet with Dr. Gordon to:
   a. ascertain the source of his information regarding the MAKSS, and whether the studies calling into question the validity and reliability of the measure provide compelling evidence about the MAKSS?
   b. determine if there are other concerns about your teaching, and if the results of the MAKSS could in anyway identify specific students rather than the aggregate changes of the attitudes of the class?
   c. Determine if there are wider concerns about your job performance?
4. Meet with the dean to argue racial discrimination by the new chair, citing that if the instrument was a measure of anti-Semitism, Dr. Gordon would not be questioning its validity.

If you were Dr. Gordon, which action would you take?

1. Meet with Dr. Burns in person to discuss your concerns.
2. Ask Dr. Burns to present his research findings at a university symposium so you can become more knowledgeable about his use of the MAKSS.
3. Acknowledge the difficulty of teaching multicultural courses, and consider as faculty how to improve the curricula throughout the program in line with the APA's multicultural guidelines.
4. Discuss how best to measure Dr. Burns's teaching abilities in light of the low student ratings, and whether such low ratings suggest that the students are feeling individually singled out in contravention of APA Standard 7.04.
5. Combinations of the above-listed actions.
6. Or one that is not listed above.

If you were either Dr. Burns or Dr. Gordon teaching in New Zealand, you would produce a review of the literature to justify the use each of you is making of the MAKSS and the student ratings.

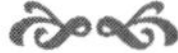

STANDARD 9.09: TEST SCORING AND INTERPRETATION SERVICES

(a) Psychologists who offer assessment or scoring services to other professionals accurately describe the purpose, norms, validity, reliability, and applications of the procedures and any special qualifications applicable to their use.

A CASE FOR STANDARD 9.09 (A): (Un)Professional Consultation

Dr. Shaw conducts assessments in her private practice. Ms. Leslie, a clinical social worker, routinely requests Dr. Shaw to provide an MMPI-2 for all of Ms. Leslie's clients. For these assessments, Dr. Shaw usually receives a summary of client background from Ms. Leslie. Dr. Shaw administers the MMPI-2 and provides Ms. Leslie with a short interpretation paragraph and a copy of the computer-generated interpretation.

Leroy, a new client, has come to Dr. Shaw with symptoms of depression after a very difficult divorce. Leroy reports he ruminates about parts of the child custody evaluation, which hurts his relationship with his children and his parenting skills. Leroy shows Dr. Shaw a copy of the child custody evaluation. Dr. Shaw recognizes an MMPI-2 interpretation paragraph she wrote for Ms. Leslie with a copy of the computer-generated interpretation attached.

Issues of Concern

Assessments are an important service provided by psychologists. It is within a psychologist's scope of practice to administer psychological tests and provide interpretation for these tests. Ms. Leslie's request for such services for use in her clinical practice certainly seems appropriate. In addition, Dr. Shaw's administration and interpretation of the MMPI–2 is within the scope of practice designated for a psychologist's work. The issues of note are whether the interpretation paragraph is inclusive of all elements specified in Standard 9.09 (a), whether it is appropriate to release the actual computer-generated interpretation printout, and whether Dr. Shaw has sufficient information regarding the client to generate an interpretation. Arguably, Dr. Shaw cannot control the use of information contained within a psychological report once it leaves her office. However, is there anything Dr. Shaw could do to minimize the inappropriate use of a psychological assessment? Once such misuse is known, is there anything Dr. Shaw should/could do about the seemingly inappropriate use of a psychological assessment?

APA Ethics Code

Companion General Principle

Principle B: Fidelity and Responsibility

> Psychologists . . . cooperate with other professionals . . . to the extent needed to serve the best interests of those with whom they work.

Guided by Principle B, Dr. Shaw's collaboration with Ms. Leslie would be based on the best interest of clients. Ms. Leslie may be able to provide better service if she had Dr. Shaw's MMPI–2 interpretation for her client(s). Can Dr. Shaw be assured that her interpretation of the MMPI–2 used in isolation actually serves the best interest of Ms. Leslie's clients? As seen with Leroy, the use of Dr. Shaw's MMPI–2 interpretation turned out to be of disservice to Ms. Leslie's client. How far does Dr. Shaw's responsibility extend in terms of guarding against inappropriate use of the psychologist's work?

Standard Principle A:
Beneficence and Nonmaleficence

> When conflicts occur among psychologists' obligations or concerns, they attempt to resolve these conflicts in a responsible fashion that avoids or minimizes harm.

Certainly most psychologists would be troubled by the inappropriate use of an assessment instrument and the subsequent interpretation. Aspiring to the principle of nonmaleficence, how might Dr. Shaw conduct herself in relation to Ms. Leslie's use of the psychological assessment in Leroy's parenting evaluation and in response to any future referrals from Ms. Leslie for MMPI–2?

Companion Ethical Standard

Standard 9.01 (b): Bases for Assessment

> Psychologists provide opinions of the psychological characteristics of individuals only after they have conducted an examination of the individuals adequate to support their statements or conclusions.

Would most psychologists consider the administration of an MMPI-2 and summary statements of the client background gathered by another mental health service professional to be adequate to meet Standard 9.01 (b)'s requirement for examination of the individual? Also, would it be sufficient to support an interpretation statement about a client?

Standard 9.06: Interpreting Assessment Results

> When interpreting assessment results, including automated interpretations, psychologists take into account the purpose of the assessment as well as the various test factors, test-taking abilities, and other characteristics of the person being assessed, such as situational, personal, linguistic, and cultural differences, that might affect psychologists' judgments or reduce the accuracy of their interpretations. They indicate any significant limitations of their interpretations.

Standard 9.06 pertains, in part, to the activities Dr. Shaw performs for Ms. Leslie's clients. Unless

Ms. Leslie's background summary contains either the client's presenting problem or a specific assessment question, it is doubtful Dr. Shaw is able to specify the purpose of the assessment besides a general wish to know how an individual performed on the MMPI-2. In addition, Dr. Shaw would need to address test factors listed in Standard 9.06 in order to be in compliance.

Standard 9.10: Explaining Assessment Results

> Psychologists take reasonable steps to ensure that explanations of results are given to the individual or designated representative unless the nature of the relationship precludes provision of an explanation of results . . . and this fact has been clearly explained to the person being assessed in advance.

Per Standard 9.10, as part of the assessment, Dr. Shaw should have provided an explanation about how the client should receive the results of the testing. It is conceivable that Dr. Shaw provides this explanation through the process of obtaining informed consent by specifying that results for each assessment client will be forwarded to Ms. Leslie. If Dr. Shaw had some arrangement in which the client and Dr. Shaw do not meet face-to-face, Leroy would have known it was Dr. Shaw who provided Ms. Leslie with the MMPI-2 information used in the parenting evaluation. Is a report sent to Ms. Leslie with an explanation to the client that results will be forward to Ms. Leslie sufficient to meet the directives of Standard 9.10?

Standard 3.05: Multiple Relationships

> (a) A multiple relationship occurs when a psychologist is in a professional role with a person and . . . (2) at the same time is in a relationship with a person closely associated with or related to the person with whom the psychologist has the professional relationship. . . A psychologist refrains from entering into a multiple relationship if the multiple relationship could reasonably be expected to impair the psychologist's objectivity . . . or effectiveness in performing his or her functions as a psychologist. . . Multiple relationships that would not reasonably be expected to cause impairment . . . are not unethical.

As described in Standard 3.05 (a) (2), Dr. Shaw is in a multiple relationship with Leroy. It is unclear whether Dr. Shaw enters into a multiple relationship with Ms. Leslie as described in Standard 3.05 (a) (3) if Dr. Shaw accepts another testing client from Ms. Leslie while Leroy is in treatment with Dr. Shaw. While Standard 3.05 does not categorically prohibit multiple relationships, it does give some parameters for consideration. Is there a reasonable expectation that knowing the history between Ms. Leslie and Leroy would impair Dr. Shaw's objectivity with Leroy? Would Leroy's knowledge of the source of the MMPI-2 information impair Dr. Shaw's effectiveness with him? How does knowledge of Ms. Leslie's use of the MMPI-2 report affect Dr. Shaw's relationship with Ms. Leslie?

Standard 1.01: Misuse of Psychologists' Work

> If psychologists learn of misuse or misrepresentation of their work, they take reasonable steps to correct or minimize the misuse or misrepresentation.

Regarding the basis upon which she conducted the MMPI-2 reports for Ms. Leslie, Dr. Shaw believed that the information would be used for general clinical understanding of the client. Dr. Shaw's report on Leroy's MMPI-2 results was not done with the knowledge that the purpose of the assessment was for parenting evaluations. Such use of the interpretation is a misuse of Dr. Shaw's work. Standard 1.01 directs Dr. Shaw to do something about this misuse.

Standard 1.04: Informal Resolution of Ethical Violations

> When psychologists believe that there may have been an ethical violation by another psychologist, they attempt to resolve the issue by bringing it to the attention of that individual, if an informal resolution appears appropriate and the intervention does not violate any confidentiality rights that may be involved.

Ideally, Dr. Shaw would contact Ms. Leslie directly and address any misunderstanding Ms. Leslie may hold about the appropriate use of the MMPI-2 testing and interpretation information provided by Dr. Shaw. Standard 1.04 permits this informal resolution only if Leroy agrees to a release of information about the fact that he is now in treatment with Dr. Shaw.

Legal Issues 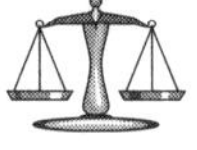

Minnesota

> *Minn. R. 7200.5000 (2010). Assessments, Tests, Reports.*
>
> Subp. 1a. Computerized testing services.
>
> A psychologist who uses computerized testing services is responsible for the legitimacy and accuracy of the test

interpretations. Computer-generated interpretations of tests must be used only in conjunction with professional judgment. A psychologist must indicate when a test interpretation is not based on direct contact with the client, that is, when it is a blind interpretation.

Subp. 3. Reports.

The provision of a written . . . report . . . is a psychological service. The report must include:

A. a description of all . . . procedures upon which the psychologist's conclusions are based;

B. any reservations or qualifications concerning the validity or reliability of the conclusions formulated and recommendations made[;] . . .

D. a statement as to whether the conclusions are based on direct contact between the psychologist and the client.

Missouri

Mo. Code Regs. Ann. tit. 20, § 2235-5.030 (2010). Ethical Rules of Conduct.

(12) Assessment Procedures.

(D) Reservations Concerning Results. The psychologist shall include in his/her report of the results of an assessment procedure any deficiencies of the assessment norms for the individual assessed and any relevant reservations or qualifications which affect the validity, reliability or other interpretation of results . . .

(F) Information for Professional Users. The psychologist offering an assessment procedure or automated interpretation service to other professionals shall accompany this offering with a manual or other printed material which fully describes the development of the assessment procedure[,] . . . the rationale, evidence of validity and reliability, and characteristics of the normative population. The psychologist shall explicitly state the purpose and application for which the procedure is recommended and identify special qualifications required to administer and interpret it properly.

In both jurisdictions, it appears that Dr. Shaw has broken the law by not informing Ms. Leslie in writing about the limitations of such a testing approach. In Minnesota, Dr. Shaw failed to note any reservations about drawing conclusions from the findings of an MMPI, absent multiple-measure corroboration. She failed to note that she had not met with the client directly but had provided a blind interpretation. In Missouri, she failed to note any reservations about providing a blind interpretation, and failed to provide the manual or other printed matter that fully describes the development, validity and reliability, and characteristics of the normative group for the MMPI, and its use in high-conflict family law cases.

Cultural Considerations

Global Discussion

The Professional Board for Psychology Health Professions Council of South Africa: Ethical Code of Professional Conduct (April 2002)

5.10. Test scoring and interpretation services.

1. Psychologists who offer assessment or scoring procedures to other professionals shall accurately describe the purpose, norms, validity, reliability, and applications of the procedures and any special qualifications applicable to their use. They shall explicitly state the language, cultural and any other limitations of the norms.

2. Psychologists shall select scoring and interpretation services (including automated services) on the basis of evidence of the validity and reliability of the programme and procedures as well as on other appropriate considerations.

3. Psychologists shall retain responsibility for the . . . use of assessment instruments, whether they administer, score and interpret such tests themselves or use automated or other services.

Regardless of whether Dr. Shaw sees Leroy in person to evaluate him or is scoring and interpreting his assessment for someone else, Dr. Shaw is still responsible for the use and safety of that information. Even though the social worker is the person charged with explaining the assessment results to Leroy, ultimately it is Dr. Shaw who bears responsibility for the quality, accuracy, and use of those assessment results. To fully comply with South Africa's code, Dr. Shaw should not have released testing results on Leroy to Ms. Leslie.

American Moral Values

1. Does Dr. Shaw support the use of the MMPI-2 she administered as a part of Leroy's child custody evaluation? How exactly does this test reflect on Leroy's parenting skills and relationship with his children? What limits does Dr. Shaw believe one can put on the MMPI-2's relevance?

2. Does Dr. Shaw believe Ms. Leslie used her evaluation correctly? Did she read Dr. Shaw's interpretation paragraph competently? Was there anything that Dr. Shaw could have made clearer in that paragraph? What issues does Dr. Shaw need to address with Ms. Leslie moving forward?
3. Does Leroy remember taking this test with Dr. Shaw? Is he possibly here out of a sense of revenge? If he does not remember, should Dr. Shaw tell Leroy that she administered the MMPI-2? Is it deceitful not to tell him?
4. If Leroy lacks an understanding of how the MMPI-2 was used or misused, would telling him she administered it unnecessarily drive him to reject treatment from Dr. Shaw? Would it lead him to mistrust psychologists in general?
5. If Dr. Shaw does not believe her test was used fairly, how does this affect her treatment of Leroy? Would her guilt or outrage be constructive, or at least not obstructive?

APA Ethics Code

Directive per APA Code

The service Dr. Shaw provides to Ms. Leslie's clients is allowable under Standard 9.09 (a). In addition, as directed by Standard 9.09 (a), Dr. Shaw is to describe the purpose of the testing, the norms, validity, reliability, applications of the MMPI-2, and qualifiers regarding proper use of the MMPI-2 interpretation. It is unclear what Dr. Shaw included in her interpretation statement that was sent to Ms. Leslie. Thus, it is not possible to determine if Dr. Shaw is in violation of Standard 9.09 (a). However, it is doubtful that Dr. Shaw had conducted a face-to-face examination of the individuals, as required by Standard 9.01 (b). A summary of a client's background provided by Ms. Leslie is not a substitute for a direct examination of the client and would be inadequate to support Dr. Shaw's interpretation of the MMPI-2. Therefore, Dr. Shaw appears to be in violation of Standard 9.01 (b). In addition, it appears Dr. Shaw is in violation of Standard 9.10 because it is evident Dr. Shaw never met Leroy, and thus she could not have given him the test results.

Dr. Shaw is now in a multiple relationship, as defined by Standard 3.05 (a) (2), with Leroy. Since she did not remember having provided an MMPI-2 interpretation of Leroy to Ms. Leslie, it is doubtful if her prior relationship would negatively impact their current treatment relationship. Therefore, continued treatment with Leroy would not be in violation of Standard 3.05 (a) (2).

While Dr. Shaw has no control over how Ms. Leslie uses her MMPI-2 interpretations, Standard 1.01 does direct Dr. Shaw to correct Ms. Leslie's unaltered use of the MMPI-2 interpretations and computer-generated results. The way to correct misuse of her MMPI-2 report, as required by Standard 1.04, is for Dr. Shaw to bring the problem to Ms. Leslie's attention.

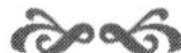

Dictates of One's Own Conscience

If you were Dr. Shaw, which action would you take?

1. Tell Leroy that you were the one who generated the MMPI-2 and interpretation for Leslie.
2. Explain to Leroy how the MMPI-2 works and how it fits into his parenting evaluation.
3. Offer to refer Leroy to another psychologist for a new parenting custody evaluation.
4. Conduct clinical interviews and MMPI-2 administration and interpretations for all future consultations for Ms. Leslie.
5. Ask Leroy for permission to cite his parent evaluation when you talk to Ms. Leslie about the inclusion of the MMPI-2 information in a parent evaluation.
6. Meet with Ms. Leslie and discuss your concerns over a business lunch.
7. Write Ms. Leslie a letter citing your concerns and ask her to stop using MMPI-2 interpretations with computer printouts in her parenting evaluations.
8. Combinations of the above-listed actions.
9. Or one that is not listed above.

If you were Dr. Shaw practicing in South Africa, you would know that psychologists retain responsibility for the use of assessment instruments, and thus would probably not have provided such service to Ms. Leslie.

STANDARD 9.09: TEST SCORING AND INTERPRETATION SERVICES

. . . (b) Psychologists select scoring and interpretation services (including automated services) on the basis of

> evidence of the validity of the program and procedures as well as on other appropriate considerations.

A CASE FOR STANDARD 9.09 (B): Why Can't I Use It?

Dr. Holmes conducted an evaluation of Francisco, a 10-year-old immigrant from Mexico. Dr. Holmes determined Francisco's intelligence quotient (IQ) to be functioning in the low-average range based on the Draw-A-Person Quantitative Scoring System (DAP-QSS). He had purchased the scoring materials overseas while doing his APA-accredited internship. He now scores and interprets the tests himself because the automated scoring software he was trained on is not available in the United States. This evaluation was used to request special education services for Francisco. The school psychologist, Dr. Rice, has questioned the validity of the IQ score, and based upon reliance on the DAP-QSS, has denied special education services. Dr. Holmes argues that he routinely uses the DAP-QSS as a measure of intelligence because it is not dependent on language proficiency.

Issues of Concern

Standard 9.09 (b) focuses on the selection of scoring software and services for an assessment. While overseas, Dr. Holmes was apparently trained in the scoring method of the DAP enough to derive an IQ quotient. Now he does his own scoring and interpretation. Dr. Rice is questioning the use of the DAP as a measure of intelligence. If Dr. Holmes was able to produce evidence for the validity of the scoring procedures, would he have satisfied the requirements of Standard 9.09 (b) and addressed Dr. Rice's concerns? Having satisfied the requirements of Standard 9.09 (b), would Dr. Rice be obligated to accept Francisco's low-average IQ score?

APA Ethics Code

Companion General Principle

Principle E: Respect for People's Rights and Dignity

> Psychologists are aware of and respect cultural . . . differences, including those based on age[,] . . . ethnicity[,] . . . national origin . . . [, and] language[,] . . . and consider these factors when working with members of such groups.

Dr. Holmes has complied with Principle E. He has taken into consideration Francisco's unique position based on his age, ethnicity, and language by selecting an appropriate test and scoring method. Is the present difficulty due to the lack of recognition of the cultural differences necessary to accurately assess Francisco on the school system's end? Or is the difficulty due to Dr. Holmes's selection of a particular test to assess intelligence that suggests he is incompetent?

Principle B: Fidelity and Responsibility

> Psychologists . . . cooperate with other professionals . . . to the extent needed to serve the best interests of those with whom they work.

Principle B would have both Dr. Holmes and Dr. Rice cooperate with each other in order to best serve Francisco's educational needs. It is doubtful that the best practice in cooperation could accurately describe the work relationship between Dr. Rice and Dr. Holmes.

Companion Ethical Standard(s)

Standard 3.09: Cooperation With Other Professionals

> When indicated and professionally appropriate, psychologists cooperate with other professionals in order to serve their clients/patients effectively and appropriately.

Standard 3.09 is the companion to Principle B: Fidelity and Responsibility. In this specific situation, it can be argued that the best practice with regard to cooperation is one of collaboration. To what extent should Dr. Holmes have consulted with Dr. Rice before the selection of the assessment instrument? To what extent should Dr. Rice have consulted with Dr. Holmes before the denial of services for Francisco? How might they proceed now to cooperate in the best interest of Francisco?

Standard 9.02: Use of Assessments

> . . . (c) Psychologists use assessment methods that are appropriate to an individual's language preference and competence, unless the use of an alternative language is relevant to the assessment issues.

Per Standard 9.02 (c), Dr. Holmes's selection method is appropriate given Francisco's limited English proficiency. However, the caveat in Standard 9.02 (c) stipulates use of an alternative language if relevant. Instead of arguing for a nonverbal IQ assessment instrument, might Dr. Holmes have used the Spanish-language version of a U.S.-accepted intelligence measure? Alternatively, would Dr. Rice's self-education regarding the uses of the DAP as a measure of IQ in other countries be relevant for the purpose of obtaining supportive educational services for Francisco?

Legal Issues 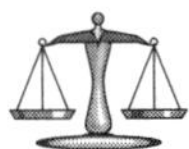

Nebraska

> *172 Neb. Admin. Code §§ 156-010 (2010). Regulations Defining Unprofessional Conduct by a Psychologist.*
>
> 010 ASSESSMENT AND TREATMENT TECHNIQUES. A psychologist shall make reasonable efforts to preclude misuse in the . . . utilization of psychological assessment techniques for use with clients. Unprofessional conduct includes but is not limited to:
>
> 010.01 Failure . . . to indicate any serious concerns or special circumstances that exist regarding validity or reliability because of the circumstances of the assessment or the inappropriateness of the norms for the person tested . . .
>
> 010.05 In presenting psychological information, failure to make reasonable efforts to present such information objectively, fully, and accurately.

Nevada

> *Nev. Admin. Code § 641.234 (2010). Assessment Procedures: Communication of Results to Patient; Limitations on Use.*
>
> 3. If a psychologist offers to other professionals an assessment procedure or automated interpretation service, he shall:
>
> (a) Provide a manual or other written material which fully describes the development of the procedure or service, the rationale therefor, evidence of the validity and reliability thereof, and characteristics of the group of persons which the procedure or service uses as a norm;
>
> (b) Explicitly state the purpose and application for which the procedure or service is recommended;
>
> (c) Identify special requirements which are necessary to administer and interpret the procedure or service properly.

In Nebraska, it is unlikely that Dr. Holmes could provide sufficient evidence about the validity of the DAP-QSS for arriving at his interpretation, thus violating the law, because he had not provided sufficient information about the measure and justification for its use. In Nevada, he broke the law by failing to provide the manual or other printed matter to Dr. Rice that fully describes the development, validity and reliability, and characteristics of the normative group for the DAP-QSS.

Cultural Considerations

Global Discussion

Canadian Code of Ethics for Psychologists

> Principle IV: Responsibility to society.
>
> IV.26. Exercise particular care when reporting the results of any work regarding vulnerable groups, ensuring that results are not likely to be misinterpreted or misused in the development of . . . practices (e.g., . . . reinforcing discrimination against any specific population).

Dr. Holmes must use particular care when reporting work with vulnerable groups (IV.26), for example, with an immigrant child, so as to ensure that such results (low intelligence among immigrants, for example, which may in fact be an issue of language proficiency) are not misinterpreted or misunderstood by larger systems, or that they do not reinforce already-existing stereotypes regarding lower intelligence among immigrants, particularly immigrants of color.

American Moral Values

1. What aspects of intelligence does Dr. Holmes believe the DAP adequately evaluates? Are these comprehensive enough to justify not using tests more dependent on language proficiency? Would it be possible to use language-based tests that are in Francisco's first language? Is there a way Dr. Holmes can present the specific virtues of the DAP-QSS to the school psychologist?
2. What does Dr. Holmes think about the school's motives for refusing services? Wouldn't a test more dependent on language proficiency produce an even lower score for Francisco if his proficiency with English was low? Does the school's position acknowledge Dr. Holmes's methodological reasoning?
3. Does Dr. Holmes view his interactions with the school in terms of Francisco or an ongoing relationship with

the school that will affect many subsequent clients? Are there measures he would take to get Francisco services that would subvert longer-term goals for changing how the school regards tests?

Ethical Course of Action

Directive per APA Code

Standard 9.09 (b) directs Dr. Holmes to select scoring and interpretation software and services that ensure the validity of the assessment results. Dr. Holmes has elected to do his own scoring and interpretation because he is unable to find a software program or scoring service in the United States that has satisfactory validity for the assessment he is using. Not only has he met the specifics of the directives in Standard 9.09 (b), but he has also demonstrated value for accuracy in terms of scoring and interpretation. Dr. Rice, however, is not concerned about the accuracy of Dr. Holmes's scoring or the validity of the interpretation. Dr. Rice is concerned about the appropriateness of the instrument selected, as stated in Standard 9.01 (a). Dr. Holmes's counterargument is based on Standard 9.02 (c). This standard directs Dr. Holmes to consider the use of an alternative language, if relevant. For assessment of Francisco, who speaks Spanish, Dr. Holmes could have used the Spanish-language version of an instrument that is much more widely accepted in the United States.

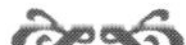

Dictates of One's Own Conscience

If you were Dr. Holmes faced with a request from Francisco's parents to help with the school system, which of these would you do?

1. Contact Dr. Rice to find out more specifics of the school system's denial of services to Francisco.
2. Contact Dr. Rice to find out why the IQ score was not accepted.
3. Write a supplemental report to Dr. Rice that provides reference for the validity and reliability of DAP-QSS for the assessment of intelligence, per Standard 9.02 (b).
4. Acknowledge that the DAP is not an accepted instrument for measuring IQ in the United States, and write a supplemental report to Dr. Rice describing the strengths and limitations of the instrument for IQ measurement, per Standard 9.02 (b).
5. Reassess Francisco using the Spanish version of the WISC.
6. Combinations of the above-listed actions.
7. Or one that is not listed above.

If you were Dr. Holmes practicing in Canada, reassess Francisco using the Spanish version of the WISC to double-check that the low IQ is still present. This is so as not to perpetuate or reinforce the stereotype that Mexicans, being mostly nonwhite, are of lower intelligence.

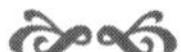

STANDARD 9.09: TEST SCORING AND INTERPRETATION SERVICES

> . . . (c) Psychologists retain responsibility for the appropriate application, interpretation, and use of assessment instruments, whether they score and interpret such tests themselves or use automated or other services.

A CASE FOR STANDARD 9.09 (C): I Did What the Test Said!

Dr. Robertson is a newly licensed psychologist. Prior to attending graduate school, he worked in the human resources department of a company and has some background and experience in organizational psychology. Dr. Robertson provides strategic organizational support based on a combined knowledge of clinical psychology and human resources. Some of his clients are seeking job enhancement or retraining skills in a tough economic environment. As part of his support services, Dr. Robertson conducts an assessment that uses the Myers-Briggs Type Indicator Test (MBTI). For scoring, he uses an Internet website that also gives automated interpretation. Dr. Robertson gives the printout from the website to the client without further analysis.

Ida is unhappy with her job. She is depressed and fears that in an economic downturn she will likely lose her job. Dr. Robertson administers the Myers-Briggs Type Indicator test. Based on the automated interpretation, Myers-Briggs indicates the likelihood that Ida would do best in a leadership-oriented position where she is encouraged to supervise and provide organization to others. Based on the type indicator, Ida is advised to be more assertive and ask for more money and/or an increase in responsibility during her next performance evaluation. After her annual review, Ida tells Dr. Robertson that not only did she not get the salary raise, but her supervisor informed her she was insubordinate and lucky to have a job, and he put her on a performance revision rather than a promotion track. Ida meekly says to Dr. Robertson, "I thought you knew this test really well. You told me what to say, and I said that. Now I could lose my job. Well, I sure can't pay you anymore if I don't have a job."

Issues of Concern

Standard 9.09 (c) places responsibility for the appropriate application of the assessment instrument on the psychologist. This means Dr. Robertson cannot hand off responsibility for the interpretation of the Myers-Briggs to a web-based scoring and interpretation program.

Regardless of scoring and interpretation software, Dr. Robertson is responsible for his choice to use the Myers-Briggs and the interpretation he gave to Ida. Could her probationary status have been avoided with more careful interpretation of the Myers-Briggs, and the integration of other data from his interactions with her? In light of the fact that Ida is depressed, unhappy with her work, and anxious about losing her job, might he have chosen different instruments to assess her job enhancement possibilities and how her depression affects her work?

APA Ethics Code

Companion General Principle

Principle A: Beneficence and Nonmaleficence

> Psychologists strive to benefit those with whom they work and take care to do no harm.

Principle A articulates the psychologist's primary value, which is to benefit others. Beyond all other considerations, Dr. Robertson's primary consideration is to provide services that would be of benefit. Failing that, psychologists are to, at a minimum, do no harm. It is unrealistic to think that psychologists are omnipotent and can foresee all the possible effects of their actions. Therefore, it may be unreasonable to place all of the responsibility for Ida's negative evaluation on Dr. Robertson. However, at a minimum, is it possible to link *some* of the harm to Dr. Robertson's actions?

Companion Ethical Standard(s)

Standard 2.01: Boundaries of Competence

> (a) Psychologists provide services . . . in areas only within the boundaries of their competence, based on their education, training, supervised experience, consultation, study, or professional experience.

It is clear that Dr. Robertson had experience through his previous work in human resources. His training in psychology may not necessarily have provided the educational expertise or supervision for career enhancement or organizational potential counseling. Could some of the harm that befell Ida have been related to Dr. Robertson practicing outside of his competence?

Standard 9.02: Use of Assessments

> (a) Psychologists administer, adapt, score, interpret, or use assessment . . . instruments in a manner and for purposes that are appropriate in light of the research on or evidence of the usefulness and proper application of the techniques.

Although the Myers-Briggs is a well-known and often-cited assessment of personality type, it is not a typical tool utilized by most clinical psychologists. It is more commonly used by human resources and other training professionals who are interested in personnel development, workplace morale, and improved management of human conflict. At issue here is the choice of the assessment tool, as well as Dr. Robertson's questionable decision to perform scoring with a website scoring system. Assuming Ida paid him for his services, is it within ethical guidelines for Dr. Robertson to collect money for an assessment tool he neither scored nor interpreted himself? How is what Dr. Robertson did any better than if Ida found the website herself, took the test, and used the information from it to make decisions about her professional potential? Does Dr. Robertson's position as a psychologist lend more seeming credibility to his use of this assessment tool than would otherwise be the case? Regardless of who scored the assessment, Dr. Robertson is still responsible for using these techniques in a manner that upholds Standard 9.02 and the principles of beneficence and nonmaleficence. He is in violation of Standard 9.02 both for his choice of this particular assessment tool and for not being clear that he was in fact charging her for a general computerized interpretation of her results, rather than applying the actual assessment skills as an organizational and clinical psychologist that he likely has.

Legal Issues 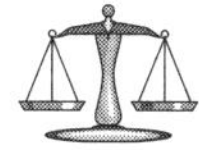

New Jersey

N.J. Admin. Code § 13:42-10.5 (2010). Maintaining Competence in Testing Situations.

(c) . . . Licensees shall present the results of assessments and their interpretations in such a way as to minimize the potential for misuse by others. . .

(e) Licensees who employ computerized narrative reports shall have the knowledge, skill and ability to interpret the scales of the instrument independently. Licensees shall not rely on the interpretations contained in a computerized narrative report as though the report were individually tailored specifically for that examinee. Statements in the narrative shall be evaluated in the context of the facts of the case and the licensee's own impressions of the test subject. Licensees shall be responsible for conclusions and recommendations based on computerized narrative reports and shall not be relieved of such responsibility by the use of a computerized narrative report. . .

(g) A licensee shall administer . . . all testing material . . . consistent with accepted standards of practice.

New Mexico

N.M. Code R. § 16.22.2.15 (2010). Assessment Procedures.

B. Use of assessment in general and with special populations. Psychologists who administer, score, interpret, or use assessment techniques shall be familiar with reliability, validity, standardization, comparative, and outcome studies of the techniques they use and with the proper application and use of those techniques.

(1) The psychologist shall recognize limits of the confidence with which . . . predictions can be made about individuals.

(2) The psychologist shall identify situations in which particular assessment techniques or norms may not be applicable or may require adjustment in administration or interpretation because of factors such as an individual's . . . disability . . . status.

C. Communication of results. The psychologist shall communicate results of the assessment to the client . . . in as clear and understandable a manner as reasonably possible and with respect for the client. . .

D. Reservations concerning results. The psychologist shall include in the assessment report the results of any limitations of the assessment procedures as may apply to the reliability or validity of the assessment techniques or the interpretation of results.

(1) Issues of individual differences, such as . . . disability[,]. . . should be carefully considered and addressed whenever relevant.

In both jurisdictions, Dr. Robertson has violated the laws. In New Jersey, he relied upon a computer-generated report and failed to meet reasonable standards of practice in conducting an assessment and providing the results of the evaluation to the client. In New Mexico, not only did he violate the law, but in addition, Dr. Robertson did not consider the individual differences of disability—in Ida's case, her depression, and how her depression may have affected the testing. In both jurisdictions, Dr. Robertson would be expected to conduct a much more thorough evaluation before making the type of recommendations that were made.

Cultural Considerations

Global Discussion

New Zealand Psychological Society Code of Ethics

Principle 9: Assessment

9.5 Psychologists do not normally release uninterpreted data from assessments to persons who are not specifically trained in the use and interpretation of the instruments concerned.

9.6 Psychologists are responsible for ensuring adequate supervision of assessment instruments of procedures administered, scored or interpreted by others under their direction unless such persons are themselves properly trained in their use.

Dr. Robertson would likely be in violation of New Zealand's code, although the code is silent with regard to automated assessment scoring services. If it can be assumed that Dr. Robertson used a computerized scoring tool that was valid (9.6), he would still be found in violation of 9.5, as he allowed data from a computerized assessment to be released and used by Ida without adding his own interpretation of the material.

American Moral Values

1. Why does Dr. Robertson offer job advice as part of his treatment? Does he see a conflict of interest between providing therapy and offering "organizational support"? Could he miss aspects of his patients' conditions by concentrating too much on job advice? Does he need to take a closer look at Ida's depression?
2. Why does Dr. Robertson rely on automated results for the Myers-Briggs? Is he shirking his duty as a medical authority by not interpreting the results of this test for his patients? How does he justify not providing such results? Does Dr. Robertson believe Myers-Briggs is a lightweight test, one that patients are free to take with a grain of salt? Do patients understand what he thinks of the test before he offers it to them?
3. Has Dr. Robertson researched how the website arrives at its results? Did he inform Ida that the website was reliable? Could she feel he is giving her case short shrift by referring her to a website evaluation?
4. What role did the Myers-Briggs results play in Dr. Robertson advising Ida to ask for a raise? Would he have advised her to do that regardless? Was such direct advice warranted by the results? Was it therapeutically appropriate? Could Ida have felt pressured to act as Dr. Robertson suggested?
5. Why did Dr. Robertson suggest that she might ask for a raise? Had he considered whether she deserved a raise? Was his use of the word "might" intended to imply she should make the final decision herself? Had he considered the details of her work environment, including what kind of a person her boss was? How did this advice relate to Ida's long-term career plans and goals? Was it helpful to have a therapist guide her to take "initiative," or should Dr. Robertson have let Ida initiate her own actions in this context?
6. Is Dr. Robertson responsible for Ida's current plight, given the consequences for her raise request? Does Dr. Robertson think Ida might be trying to pass off her own part in the raise request? Does he believe she is telling the truth about how she asked, the context, and so forth? Did he warn her of the possible negative consequences of asking for a raise? Was his advice an implicit promise that results would be positive? Or should she have realized that no one can predict how such things will turn out?
7. If Dr. Robertson does accept some degree of responsibility, what would be adequate compensation for Ida's situation? Is she owed free therapy? Does he need to settle to avoid a malpractice suit? Should he intervene with her boss, or would that further damage her prospects at work? Is an apology all that he can offer, given that the damage cannot be undone?
8. Should Ida still be Dr. Robertson's client? Can their relationship recover from this problem? How will Ida be able to trust his advice? Should Dr. Robertson refer her to another therapist?

Ethical Course of Action

Directive per APA Code

Per Standard 9.09 (c), Dr. Robertson needs to do more than just provide Ida with a computer-generated interpretation of the Myers-Briggs. Even if the web-based scoring program was accurate, Dr. Robertson still needed to select parts of the computerized interpretation that were specifically applicable to Ida. In addition, Dr. Robertson is still responsible for appropriately translating the test results as they apply to Ida and her specific life situation.

Though Ida did present with dissatisfaction of her job, the selection of the test instrument may have been less than useful in helping Ida in the context of her depression and anxiety, thus violating Standard 9.02. The poor decision in choosing a test instrument may reflect Dr. Robertson's limited competency in this area, and it places him in violation of Standard 2.01 (a).

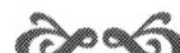

Dictates of One's Own Conscience

If you were Dr. Robertson faced with the course of events reported by Ida and her implied threat of treatment termination, which of these would you do?

1. Explore in more detail what transpired in the performance evaluation, with an eye to ways in which Ida may have sabotaged herself, regardless of the assessment results from the Myers-Briggs.
2. Explain that the information from the Myers-Briggs does not dictate a course of action, and speculate on why Ida might have surmised that she was told by you to assertively ask for a raise.
3. Explain that the Myers-Briggs may not have been sufficient in light of her depression and suggest further testing.

4. Proceed to problem solve on how to respond to her supervisor's feedback.
5. Combinations of the above-listed actions.
6. Or one that is not listed above.

If you were practicing in New Zealand, you would refrain in the future from using the Myers-Briggs, at least without adding your own interpretation and commentary to the computerized results before giving them to clients. Regarding Ida, you would likely offer to give another assessment, or redo the Myers-Briggs and add your own interpretation to the computerized results.

STANDARD 9.10: EXPLAINING ASSESSMENT RESULTS

> Regardless of whether the scoring and interpretation are done by psychologists, by employees or assistants, or by automated or other outside services, psychologists take reasonable steps to ensure that explanations of results are given to the individual or designated representative unless the nature of the relationship precludes provision of an explanation of results (such as in some organizational consulting, pre-employment or security screenings, and forensic evaluations), and this fact has been clearly explained to the person being assessed in advance.

A CASE FOR STANDARD 9.10: A Missing Step

The Modern School of Psychology provides psychological assessments to indigents applying for state welfare. The local welfare department provides a steady supply of assessment clients for the students. In trade, the Modern School of Psychology charges the state welfare department a nominal fee for a full-battery assessment. The clients are predominately homeless, and routinely do not return for their feedback session. These clients are showing up at the welfare office in desperate straits, and the department cannot give them support because it is waiting on the psychological evaluation. However, the evaluations are being held at the clinic awaiting client feedback sessions. The state welfare department has requested that test reports not be held for the feedback session. To facilitate the welfare department's request, the Modern School of Psychology has adopted a policy that reports are sent directly to the welfare office, and no feedback sessions are offered to welfare applicants themselves.

Issues of Concern

Standard 9.10 sets the general requirement that when psychologists conduct an assessment, test results are to be provided to the clients. The exception to this requirement is when the assessment is done within a context that precludes interpretation feedback. The examples given in Standard 9.10 include organizational consulting, preemployment or security screenings, and forensic evaluations. The nature of the relationship between these psychology students and welfare applicants does not preclude interpretation feedback. Indeed, scheduling feedback sessions had been part of the standard assessment procedure. The reality of the situation with a very transient population in urgent need of support not only resulted in an inability to actually give feedback interpretation, but it was also harming the clients by creating a barrier to their receiving public assistance support. Could the specific circumstances of the client's life meet the exception requirement set forth in Standard 9.10? Does the inconvenience of trying to coordinate a return visit justify not offering a client feedback session? Given the characteristics of the population, could the Modern School of Psychology alter its test protocol to facilitate a same-day feedback session?

APA Ethics Code

Companion General Principle

Principle D: Justice

> Psychologists recognize that fairness and justice entitle all persons to access to and benefit from the contributions of psychology and to equal quality in the processes, procedures, and services being conducted by psychologists.

One of the procedures in the assessment process is a feedback interpretation. Making an exception to this process based on generalized characteristics of a specific group of individuals, namely, those who are applying for public assistance, does not appear to satisfy the ideals of Principle D: Justice, which asks psychologists to attempt the giving of equal quality of care to all clients. How is altering an assessment process for one individual in order to address the specific needs of that individual different from establishing an agency policy that alters this procedure for a whole class of people? Does the school policy violate the spirit of Principle D?

Principle E: Respect for People's Rights and Dignity

> Psychologists are aware of and respect cultural, individual, and role differences, including those based on . . . socioeconomic status, and consider these factors when working with members of such groups. Psychologists try to eliminate the effect on their work of biases based on those factors, and they do not knowingly participate in or condone activities of others based upon such prejudices.

Aspiring to the ideals of Principle E, the School of Modern Psychology has indeed taken into consideration the socioeconomic status of the welfare assessment clients in its policies regarding assessments. Yet in the very act of respecting differences, the school may have established a practice that is prejudicial. In this situation, does there appear to be a conflict between Principles D and E?

Companion Ethical Standard(s)

Standard 3.07: Third-Party Requests for Services

> When psychologists agree to provide services to a person . . . at the request of a third party, psychologists attempt to clarify at the outset of the service the nature of the relationship with all individuals . . . involved. This clarification includes the role of the psychologist (e.g., . . . diagnostician . . .), an identification of who is the client, the probable uses of . . . information obtained, and the fact that there may be limits to confidentiality.

The students of the School of Modern Psychology are providing assessments for clients at the request of the welfare office. This situation meets the requirements and falls under Standard 3.07. In addition, as required by Standard 3.07, students need to clearly explain that they are doing the testing for the welfare office and that all information provided by the client will go to the welfare office.

Standard 1.03: Conflicts Between Ethics and Organizational Demands

> If the demands of an organization . . . for whom they are working are in conflict with this Ethics Code, psychologists clarify the nature of the conflict, make known their commitment to the Ethics Code, and take reasonable steps to resolve the conflict consistent with the General Principles and Ethical Standards of the Ethics Code.

It is conceivable that either a student would object to unequal treatment for welfare clients or that a client would want feedback and object to clinic policy. In such situations, the supervising psychologist of a student or the student him- or herself is required to voice his or her concerns and to take steps to resolve the differences so that he or she could comply with the APA Ethics Code.

Standard 3.01: Unfair Discrimination

> In their work-related activities, psychologists do not engage in unfair discrimination based on . . . socioeconomic status.

While it is commendable that the school's clinic has the intent of facilitating the most expedited process possible for clients to complete the welfare application and possibly receive much-needed assistance, such intentions do not necessarily justify a practice that may be discriminatory to clients in that it does not provide them with comparable quality of service. By adopting a policy that eliminates feedback interpretation sessions, the students who follow this policy and the creators of it may have engaged in unfair discrimination.

Legal Issues 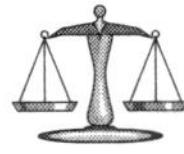

Montana

> *Mont. Admin. R. 24.189.2309 (2009). Professional Responsibility.*
>
> (2) In regard to respect for others, a licensee . . .
>
> (b) who . . . administers, scores, interprets or uses assessment techniques . . .
>
> (ii) shall attempt to identify situations in which particular . . . assessment techniques . . . may not be applicable . . . because of factors such as . . . disability . . . or socioeconomic status . . .
>
> (iv) shall ensure, unless the nature of the relationship is clearly explained to the person being assessed in advance and precludes provision of an explanation of results, that an explanation of the results is provided using language that is reasonably understandable to the person assessed or to another legally authorized person on behalf of the client.

Virginia

> *18 Va. Admin. Code § 125-20-150 (2010). Standards of Practice.*
>
> B. Persons licensed by the board shall . . .
>
> 6. Avoid harming patients . . . and minimize harm when it is foreseeable and unavoidable . . .
>
> 12. Construct, maintain, administer, interpret and report testing and diagnostic services in a manner and for purposes which are appropriate.

In both jurisdictions, the psychologist supervisor of the clinic has violated the laws. This occurred by providing the results of the evaluations to the welfare office without providing the results to the subjects. Such a process may harm those clients. In particular, the interpretations of the evaluation may be contested by the clients, and the disagreements could have affected the final results of the evaluation.

Cultural Considerations

Global Discussion

The Professional Board for Psychology
Health Professions Council of South Africa:
Ethical Code of Professional Conduct (April 2002)

> 5. Assessment activities.
>
> 5.9. Explaining assessment results.
>
> Unless the nature of the relationship is clearly explained to the person being assessed in advance and precludes provision of an explanation of results[,] . . . psychologists shall ensure that the explanation of the results . . . is reasonably understandable to the person assessed. . . [P]sychologists shall take reasonable steps to ensure that appropriate explanations of results are given.

Even with a prior agreement as part of informed consent to not have feedback sessions after these assessments are given, the Modern School would likely not be found in violation of South Africa's code. Standard 5.9 states that assessment results are to be given to all subjects in language easily understood. The code does not allow psychologists to dispense with feedback sessions due to the socioeconomic status of the person undergoing the assessment, no matter how helpful the intentions of the clinic or welfare office may be. However, South Africa's code states that if the preclusion of explanation of results is explained in advance, it is permitted. Psychologists, however, are still obligated to take "reasonable steps" to ensure appropriate explanations are given, which may be situationally contraindicated when the test population is unlikely to return for feedback.

American Moral Values

1. What is the value of a feedback session? What weight does that value have compared to homeless clients receiving speedier assistance at the welfare office? Does it have less weight given that homeless clients have usually not shown up for their feedback session? Or does it have more weight given what good those sessions could have done for such clients?
2. Could feedback sessions help homeless clients understand their condition better? How important could that understanding be for their pursuit of a better life? Could it change what type of assistance they seek, both from the welfare office and other agencies?
3. Even if the feedback session has been underappreciated, is it feasible to increase the numbers of clients returning for them? How much time and energy are needed to increase attendance, and is that worth the delays these clients would have in receiving welfare assistance?
4. Is the welfare office sufficiently aware of the value of feedback sessions? Is the New School being too complicit with the welfare office in terms of how clients are being treated? Are homeless clients being considered as individuals who can learn and benefit from knowing more about their mental health condition?
5. Is the school doing everything it can to facilitate clients getting their results? Would it be possible, for example, to have quicker turnaround times, so that students could administer tests, look at the results, and give feedback within a 6-hour block? How much coordination and labor would this require? Is this an investment the school can make, given its other priorities?

Ethical Course of Action

Directive per APA Code

Standard 9.10 requires that assessment procedures provide an explanation of results. It further requires these results to be given either to the individual or his or her designated representative. Maybe on a case-by-case basis, some clients may request that the welfare office serve as their designated representative for the purpose of feedback. However, for the clinic to adopt such a policy violates the requirement for feedback established in Standard 9.10. Exceptions do exist, and Standard 9.10 does provide for exceptions to the rule. But the circumstance of a high no-show rate for feedback sessions does not meet the provisions for the exception as stated in Standard 9.10. Therefore, regardless of the intent, the policy established by the school regarding no feedback sessions for welfare applicants violates the directives of Standard 9.10.

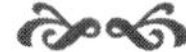

Dictates of One's Own Conscience

If you were the director of the clinic with administrative responsibility for review of policy, and you were reading this section of this book for ethics continuing education (CE) credits, which of these would you do?

1. Require students to inform the assessment clients of the policy regarding feedback sessions at the outset of treatment.
2. Alter the policy to allow students to give a feedback session if a client so requests.
3. Tell everyone concerned that you are in violation of Standard 9.10, and stop the service to welfare applicants completely.
4. Require that students and supervisors not take on welfare assessments for the purpose of training unless all steps in the assessment procedure could be done within 6 hours. You reason that if everyone could get such a quick turnaround time, then clients would not need to return to the clinic for a feedback session but would receive their feedback on the day of the testing.

If you were a supervisor of a student or a student faced with a client who wants to know the result of the tests, which action would you take?

1. Object to the policy of no feedback session, per Standard 1.03.
2. Let the clinic know that you think this policy is discriminatory based on the client's socioeconomic status.
3. After letting your objections be known, proceed with the feedback session.
4. Tell the client that you disagree with the policy but are not in a position to alter it.
5. Recommend that the client get the feedback from the welfare office.
6. Offer to mail the client a copy of your report.
7. Combinations of the above-listed actions.
8. Or one that is not listed above.

If you were a supervisor of a student or a student conducting these evaluations in South Africa and were faced with a client who wants to know the result of the tests, you would remind the client that, as previously discussed, the report has already been sent to the state welfare department. Further, regardless of who is in receipt of the report, you will hold an assessment feedback session with the client.

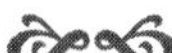

STANDARD 9.11: MAINTAINING TEST SECURITY

> The term test materials refers to manuals, instruments, protocols, and test questions or stimuli and does not include test data as defined in Standard 9.04: Release of Test Data. Psychologists make reasonable efforts to maintain the integrity and security of test materials and other assessment techniques consistent with law and contractual obligations, and in a manner that permits adherence to this Ethics Code.

A CASE FOR STANDARD 9.11: Incomplete Results

Alexander started having difficulties in school this year. Debbie, Alexander's mother, believes Alexander's problems are due to the unstructured nature of middle school. Debbie reports that Alexander has always had some problems, and she had worked very closely with his elementary school teacher to structure the classroom environment to help support Alexander. However, since beginning middle school, where Alexander has multiple classrooms with multiple teachers, Alexander has had numerous emerging academic and social problems. Debbie has requested special accommodations for Alexander.

Alexander was referred to Dr. Hunt by the pediatrician. Dr. Hunt has requested that Debbie provide him with Alexander's school records and reports from any previous psychological assessments. Debbie provides Dr. Hunt with school report cards, special education reports, and summaries of a previous psychological evaluation. Attached to the psychological evaluation are the raw scores and the original answer sheets.

At the end of the feedback session, Dr. Hunt gives Debbie and Alexander a copy of his report. Debbie asks, "Is that all there is? Where are all of the original answers? The other doctor gave us everything. Isn't that part of what I pay for?"

Issues of Concern

Standard 9.11 makes a distinction between test materials and test data. Depending on the instrument used, the actual answer protocols, which often contain data, may also contain raw test material. The client's responses to the test material recorded in the answer protocols are defined as raw test data. Providing a client with the completed protocols could conflict with Standard 9.11. Standard 9.04: Release of Test Data obligates Dr. Hunt to provide his client with the test data. Under what conditions should Dr. Hunt provide Debbie with Alexander's test data? If the answer protocol contained both the raw test data and some test material, should Dr. Hunt release the answer protocols? It would be reasonable for Debbie to expect Dr. Hunt to provide her with the answer protocols if she previously received these from an earlier assessment. Should Dr. Hunt be concerned about the previous assessment results if the answer protocols from the earlier assessment contain raw test data?

APA Ethics Code

Companion General Principle

Principle B: Fidelity and Responsibility

> Psychologists . . . are aware of their professional . . . responsibilities . . . to the specific communities in which they work. . . They are concerned about the ethical compliance of their colleagues' scientific and professional conduct.

The community within which Dr. Hunt works includes those psychologists who develop assessment instruments, those who will be using the instruments, and the future clients who will be administered the assessments. Principle B: Fidelity and Responsibility calls Dr. Hunt's attention to all of these individuals by calling for the protection of proprietary material and the prevention of contamination from practice effects. Principle B also suggests that Dr. Hunt would need to help the psychologist who conducted the previous assessment to uphold the values in Principle B.

Principle D: Justice

> Psychologists recognize that fairness and justice entitle all persons to access to and benefit from the contributions of psychology and to equal quality in the processes, procedures, and services being conducted by psychologists.

Principle D suggests that psychologists aspire to provide equal access in the provision of services to all clients. This includes ensuring that future clients have access to services. Dr. Hunt's decision to protect raw test material allows for future clients to be tested accurately.

Companion Ethical Standard(s)

Standard 9.04: Release of Test Data

> Pursuant to a client . . . release, psychologists provide test data to the client . . . or other persons identified in the release.

Standard 9.04 allows for Dr. Hunt to release test data to the client if he or she requests it. Thus, Dr. Hunt's providing Debbie with Alexander's test data is not unethical.

Standard 1.04: Informal Resolution of Ethical Violations

> When psychologists believe that there may have been an ethical violation by another psychologist, they attempt to resolve the issue by bringing it to the attention of that individual, if an informal resolution appears appropriate and the intervention does not violate any confidentiality rights that may be involved.

Standard 1.04 directs Dr. Hunt to bring the matter to the psychologist who conducted the previous assessment, if Dr. Hunt thinks he or she has committed an ethical violation.

Legal Issues 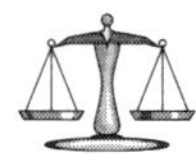

Ohio

Ohio Admin. Code 4732-17. Rules of Professional Conduct.

(F) Testing and test interpretation. . .

(2) Test security. . . Psychologists . . . make reasonable efforts to maintain the integrity and security of test materials and other assessment techniques consistent with law and contractual obligations. Access to such devices is limited to persons with professional interests who will safeguard their use.

Pennsylvania

Pa. Admin. Code 41.61. Code of Ethics.

Principle 8. Utilization of assessment.

(a) In the . . . utilization of psychological assessment techniques, psychologists observe relevant professional standards and make every effort to promote the welfare and best interests of the client. A person who has been examined has the right to receive, and the psychologist has the responsibility to provide, explanations of the nature, purpose, results and interpretations of assessment techniques in language the person can understand. Psychologists . . . avoid imparting unnecessary information which would compromise test security, but they provide requested information that explains the basis for decisions that may adversely affect the person examined or that person's dependents. . .

(f) . . . The psychologist makes every effort to avoid misuse of test reports.

In both jurisdictions, Dr. Hunt is complying with the laws by not providing raw test data to Debbie, Alexander's mother. Pennsylvania law suggests that Dr. Hunt should meet with Debbie and talk with her about the procedures used that assured the validity of the findings.

Cultural Considerations

Global Discussion

Singapore Psychological Society:
Code of Professional Ethics

Principle 13. Test security.

Psychological tests and other assessment devices, the value of which depends in part on the naiveté of the subject. . . Access to such devices is limited to persons with professional interests who will safeguard their use.

1. The psychologist is responsible for the control of psychological tests . . . when their value might be damaged by revealing to the general public their specific contents or underlying principles.

According to Singapore's code, Dr. Hunt cannot give raw scores to Debbie and Alexander, as doing so might reveal specific contents or underlying principles. Although he cannot control such actions by the previous psychologist, it is incumbent upon Dr. Hunt to uphold test security by limiting access to these psychological tests to only other psychologists who are also charged with safeguarding them. Revealing raw scores and other pieces of the tests to members of the general public is clearly in violation of Singapore's code and is not allowable, regardless of the actions of the previous psychologist.

American Moral Values

1. Does Dr. Hunt believe sharing raw scores threatens the security of a test? Did Alexander's previous psychologist make a mistake by sharing raw scores with Debbie? Does Dr. Hunt need to take action against this psychologist? How would such action affect Debbie and Alexander?
2. What does Dr. Hunt owe Debbie, given her understanding of what feedback constituted? When Dr. Hunt saw that raw scores were attached to the materials Debbie gave him, should he have addressed the issue of raw data with Debbie before moving forward? If so, does he owe Debbie an apology or partial refund for that oversight? Or is the confidentiality of scores not a question Dr. Hunt could have been expected to address ahead of time, given how unusual it is to share scores?
3. What considerations might have led Dr. Hunt to share data with Debbie? Is she trained enough to know how the tests work anyway? Is she knowledgeable enough to identify particular answers from Dr. Bernard that could complicate or distort overall evaluative tallies or classifications? How much power should parents have in that context? Is there a way to go over data without compromising the test or allowing Debbie to prepare Alexander for specific questions?
4. How will keeping raw scores confidential affect Dr. Hunt's work with Alexander? Will Dr. Hunt seem secretive or aloof? How can he maintain and rebuild trust with Debbie?

Ethical Course of Action

Directive per APA Code

Standard 9.11 prohibits the release of raw test material. Standard 9.04 allows for the release of raw test data with a proper request for such a release. Debbie, as a parent, is probably requesting test data, not test material. Dr. Hunt is obligated, per Standard 9.04, to provide the test data to Debbie. The situation becomes problematic if the answer sheets with the test data also contain test material, as defined in Standard 9.11. Under such circumstances, the prudent course of action is to maintain security of the test material by not releasing the answer protocol.

Secondarily, if the previously released answer protocol contained test material, Standard 1.04 and Principle D require that Dr. Hunt bring his concerns to the attention of the psychologist who conducted the previous assessment.

Dictates of One's Own Conscience

If you were Dr. Hunt, faced with such a request, which action would you take?

1. Give the answer sheet to Debbie after redacting all test material from the answer sheet.
2. Offer to extract the test data from the answer sheet, and then give Debbie only the test data in a different format.
3. Explain to Debbie that the previous psychologist violated regulations and should not have given her the answer sheet.
4. Engage in informal intervention with the psychologist who conducted the previous assessment.
5. Write a letter of complaint to the psychologist who conducted the previous assessment.
6. Combinations of the above-listed actions.
7. Or one that is not listed above.

If you were Dr. Hunt practicing in Singapore, faced with such a request, you would explain that access to such devices is limited to persons with professional interests. Therefore, based on professional standards of conduct, you cannot release test material except to another psychologist.

CHAPTER 10

Therapy

Ethical Standard 10

CHAPTER OUTLINE

- Standard 10.01: Informed Consent to Therapy
- Standard 10.02: Therapy Involving Couples or Families
- Standard 10.03: Group Therapy
- Standard 10.04: Providing Therapy to Those Served by Others
- Standard 10.05: Sexual Intimacies With Current Therapy Clients/Patients
- Standard 10.06: Sexual Intimacies With Relatives or Significant Others of Current Therapy Clients/Patients
- Standard 10.07: Therapy With Former Sexual Partners
- Standard 10.08: Sexual Intimacies With Former Therapy Clients/Patients
- Standard 10.09: Interruption of Therapy
- Standard 10.10: Terminating Therapy

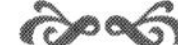

STANDARD 10.01: INFORMED CONSENT TO THERAPY

(a) When obtaining informed consent to therapy as required in Standard 3.10: Informed Consent, psychologists inform clients/patients as early as is feasible in the therapeutic relationship about the nature and anticipated course of therapy, fees, involvement of third parties, and limits of confidentiality and provide sufficient opportunity for the client/patient to ask questions and receive answers.

A CASE STANDARD 10.01 (A): The Betrayal

Lillian is an intern at a comprehensive treatment facility for those with cancer. One of her rotations is working on the crisis telephone line, which provides support to callers. Most callers contact the facility only once; crisis hotline policy is that no demographic information is requested unless the same person calls three times or more. At the third call from the same person, Lillian is to obtain demographic information and to review informed consent to treatment and discuss limits of confidentiality with the phone-in client. This informed consent is conducted in the presence of another crisis telephone hotline staff member, who will briefly verify with the client that he or she understands the consent form and agrees to it. Verbal consent is followed up with a hardcopy mailed to the caller for signature. Today, Lillian is speaking with Jimmy, who had called once before. Jimmy has been diagnosed with lung cancer. He opens the call with "I can't do this anymore. Nothing in my life is working. My mother is dying; my marriage is breaking up; I can't get a job; and I just don't see the point. I have to talk to someone about this, and right now you're the only one I trust. You can't tell anyone about this, right?"

Issues of Concern

The design of the telephone program and the policies regarding Lillian's tasks suggest that little difference exists between providing supportive counseling versus therapy. Further, it appears that the agency policy notes that the nature of the therapeutic relationship changes at the third telephone call. Standard 10.01 requires psychologists to obtain informed consent to therapy as early as is feasible in the therapeutic relationship. Does a psychologist not need to obtain consent if the service provided is supportive counseling? Or do psychologists need to obtain consent regardless of whether the service is deemed to be supportive counseling or therapy? Does waiting to obtain consent for treatment until the third contact meet the requirement of Standard 10.01, which calls for such consent to be obtained as early as feasible?

A second focus for Lillian with Jimmy is whether a duty to protect has been triggered. For the purposes of this vignette, it is assumed that Lillian and Jimmy reside in the same state. Depending on the state, a mandate to report Jimmy may exist if he is a danger to himself. Even if Jimmy is actively suicidal, does Lillian have sufficient demographic information to determine how to initiate an on-site intervention?

APA Ethics Code

Companion General Principle

Principle B: Fidelity and Responsibility

> Psychologists establish relationships of trust with those with whom they work. They are aware of their professional . . . responsibilities to society. . . Psychologists uphold professional standards of conduct, [and] clarify their professional roles and obligations.

Principle B calls psychologists' attention to the fact that they hold responsibilities to two different entities, the client and society. Lillian's responsibility to Jimmy is to establish a relationship of trust. Her responsibility to society is to uphold the law when it mandates Lillian to prevent Jimmy from harming himself.

Companion Ethical Standard(s)

Standard 4.01: Maintaining Confidentiality

> Psychologists have a primary obligation and take reasonable precautions to protect confidential information obtained through . . . any medium, recognizing that the extent and limits of confidentiality may be regulated by law.

Standard 4.01 directs Lillian to protect Jimmy's privacy by not revealing information he divulges. In fact, Jimmy explicitly inquires about his right to privacy. The caveat contained in Standard 4.01 is that Lillian is not required to keep Jimmy's information confidential if there is a law relevant to the type of information shared. Most states have regulations regarding client information related to harm to self. If Jimmy is calling from a state that mandates psychologists' reporting of a client's intent to harm him- or herself, then Lillian must answer Jimmy, "No, I have to tell someone you are going to hurt yourself."

Standard 1.02: Conflicts Between Ethics and Law, Regulations, or Other Governing Legal Authority

> If psychologists' ethical responsibilities conflict with law[,] . . . psychologists clarify the nature of the conflict, make known their commitment to the Ethics Code and take reasonable steps to resolve the conflict consistent with the General Principles and Ethical Standards of the Ethics Code.

Standard 1.02 gives Lillian the directive for resolving the dual responsibility articulated in Principle B. Lillian's ethical responsibility is to uphold the ethical code. In this case, Standard 4.01 allows Lillian to break confidentiality.

Standard 1.03: Conflicts Between Ethics and Organizational Demands

> If the demands of an organization . . . for whom they are working are in conflict with this Ethics Code, psychologists clarify the nature of the conflict, make known their commitment to the Ethics Code, and take reasonable

> steps to resolve the conflict consistent with the General Principles and Ethical Standards of the Ethics Code.

Standard 1.03 directs Lillian to discuss with the internship site and her supervisor the problems with waiting until the third session to inform callers of her status as an intern and the limits of confidentiality. After the discussion, Standard 1.03 directs Lillian to take reasonable steps to negotiate a resolution that allows her to act in accordance with the ethics code. What steps are considered reasonable for Lillian to take in order to satisfy the dictates of Standard 1.03?

Standard 4.02: Discussing the Limits of Confidentiality

> . . . (b) Unless it is not feasible or is contraindicated, the discussion of confidentiality occurs at the outset of the relationship and thereafter as new circumstances may warrant.

Standard 4.02 (b) requires Lillian to tell Jimmy at the very beginning of the relationship the limits to confidentiality. This means knowing the state law in which Lillian is practicing and letting Jimmy know whether psychologists are mandated to report harm to self. To be in compliance with Standard 4.02, Lillian needs to have reviewed the limits of confidentiality with Jimmy at the beginning of the first call. Also, the limits of confidentiality should be repeated when Jimmy hints that he is suicidal during the second call.

Standard 10.01: Informed Consent to Therapy

> . . . (c) When the therapist is a trainee and the legal responsibility for the treatment provided resides with the supervisor, the client/patient, as part of the informed consent procedure, is informed that the therapist is in training and is being supervised and is given the name of the supervisor.

In addition, Lillian is required by Standard 10.01 (c) to tell Jimmy that she is a trainee under supervision, and that her supervisor will be told about his situation.

Standard 4.05: Disclosures

> . . . (b) Psychologists disclose confidential information without the consent of the individual only as mandated by law, or where permitted by law for a valid purpose such as to . . . (3) protect the client/patient, psychologist, or others from harm.

Should Jimmy live in a state that mandates or permits a report about harm to self, then Standard 4.05 (b) (3) allows Lillian to break confidentiality regardless of whether Jimmy wants anyone else to know about his suicidal ideation.

Legal Issues 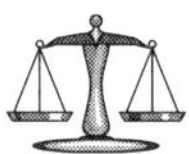

South Carolina

> *S.C. Code Ann. Regs.100-4 (2010). Code of Ethics.*
>
> G. Protecting confidentiality of clients. . .
>
> (2) Disclosure without informed written consent. The psychologist may disclose confidential information without the informed written consent of the psychologist when the psychologist judges that disclosure is necessary to protect against a clear and substantial risk of imminent serious harm being inflicted by the client on the client. . . In such case, the psychologist shall limit disclosure of the otherwise confidential information to only those persons and only that content which would be consistent with the standards of the profession in addressing such problems.

Texas

> *22 Tex. Admin. Code § 465.1 (2010). Definitions.*
>
> (4) "Informed Consent" means the written documented consent of the . . . client . . . only after the . . . client . . . has been made aware of the purpose and nature of the services to be provided, including but not limited to: the . . . right of access of . . . client . . . to the records of the services.

> *22 Tex. Admin. Code § 465.11 (2010). Informed Consent/ Describing Practices.*
>
> (b) Licensees provide appropriate information as needed during the course of the services about changes in the nature of the services to the patient . . . to ensure informed consent.

> *22 Tex. Admin. Code § 465.1 (2010). Definitions*
>
> (b) Licensees must inform their patients . . . about . . . foreseeable limitations on confidentiality created by existing and reasonably foreseeable circumstances prior to the commencement of services as part of the informed consent process described in Rule 465.11.
>
> (c) Licensees keep . . . clients informed of all changes in circumstances affecting confidentiality as they arise. . .
>
> (e) Licensees disclose confidential information without the consent of a . . . client only in compliance with applicable state and federal law. . .
>
> (g) Licensees may share information for consultation purposes without a consent only to the extent necessary

to achieve the purposes of the consultation. Licensees shall exclude information that could lead to the identification of the patient or client.

In South Carolina, psychologists may disclose confidential information if the client intends to commit a crime, or harm the self or another, and disclosure is necessary to prevent the harm from occurring (S.C. Code Ann. § 19-11-95(C) [2010]). The emergency admission procedures for South Carolina permit a psychologist who cannot gain access to a physician (who provides certification that a client requires involuntary treatment) to execute an affidavit for a probate court judge to issue an order of detention, and within the affidavit, the psychologist must indicate that the client is mentally ill, and because of this condition is likely to cause serious harm to the self or others, if not immediately hospitalized; it also should indicate why the usual examination procedures could not be followed at the local mental health center (S.C. Code Ann. § 44-17-430 [2010]).

In Texas, a qualified immunity exists for psychologists who act in good faith, and reasonably believe that disclosure of confidential information is necessary because a client may need involuntary treatment. Any peace officer may apprehend a person for emergency detention, at the nearest mental health facility, if a psychologist indicates that the client is mentally ill and poses a substantial risk of harm to self or others unless immediate restraint occurs (Tex. Health & Safety Code Ann. § 576.021 [Vernon 1998]). Mental illness means a disease or condition that either grossly impairs a person's behavior or substantially impairs the person's thought, perception of reality, emotional process, or judgment (Tex. Health & Safety Code Ann. §571.003 [Vernon 1998]). In both jurisdictions, Lillian would be expected to attempt to obtain informed consent for treatment, which would include disclosing to Jimmy the limits of her being able to protect his confidences. If he proceeded with treatment, Lillian would engage in an evaluation of Jimmy's suicidal ideation and launch a reasonable set of interventions in light of the evaluation's results (Benjamin, Kent, & Sirikantraporn, 2009).

Cultural Considerations

Global Discussion

Canadian Code of Ethics for Psychologists

Principle I: Responsible caring.

I.19. Obtain informed consent from all independent . . . persons for any psychological services provided to them except in circumstances of urgent need (e.g., disaster or other crisis). In urgent circumstances, psychologists would proceed with the assent of such persons, but fully informed consent would be obtained as soon as possible.

I.21. Establish and use signed consent forms that specify the dimensions of informed consent or that acknowledge that such dimensions have been explained and are understood, if such forms are required by law or if such forms are desired by the psychologist, the person(s) giving consent, or the organization for whom the psychologist works.

I.22. Accept and document oral consent, in situations in which signed consent forms are not acceptable culturally or in which there are other good reasons for not using them.

With regard to the issues surrounding informed consent, Canada's code makes clear that although it is most preferable that signed consent forms are explained and understood (I.21), in certain situations, the use and acceptance of oral consent forms are permissible (I.22), including in crisis situations (I.19), although it would be necessary to obtain informed consent as soon as the crisis has passed. Though Canada's code does not specify that consent is to occur on the first interaction, it does state that full consent must occur as soon as an emergency has passed. Arguably, waiting until the third telephone call puts Lillian at risk of being in violation of I.19.

American Moral Values

1. How does Lillian evaluate Jimmy's call and question about confidentiality? Is it necessary to breach policy and inform Jimmy now, during his second call, regarding consent and disclosures about the possible exceptions to confidentiality for suicide? Or should Lillian try to deflect the issue of consent and concentrate on talking Jimmy through his situation?
2. What does Lillian think is the most important consideration in trying to dissuade Jimmy from suicide? Is it building trust? Getting Jimmy to keep talking?
3. Will telling Jimmy about the consent and disclosure process build trust with Lillian or threaten it? How exactly should she word her information about consent and the disclosure process? Is there any justification for just mentioning "exceptions" to confidentiality without specifying suicide risk?
4. Would Lillian promise Jimmy not to tell anyone else about his condition if she thought it would save his

life? What would be the consequences of having to break that promise if it did not work?

5. Assuming Jimmy's condition improves, what will be the ongoing effect of Lillian's approach for how Jimmy thinks of counseling/psychologists? How could it affect those who know Jimmy or who learned about how Lillian handled the situation?
6. Should Lillian oppose the clinic's policy regarding the third visit? Or does the high number of non-returning callers make the policy a key for efficiency, which in turn aids in helping more people?

Ethical Course of Action

Directive per APA Code

Standard 10.01 (a) requires that Lillian obtain informed consent to therapy as early as possible. In the present situation, in accordance with organizational policy, the earliest time under the policy is at the beginning of the third call with the same person.

Standard 4.01 directs Lillian to protect Jimmy's privacy unless Lillian practices in a state that mandates Lillian to break confidentiality in order to protect Jimmy from harming himself. Standard 4.02 (b) directs Lillian to have told Jimmy the limits of confidentiality at the beginning of the first call.

Because organizational policy dictates that no consent to treatment or disclosures about the limits of confidentiality are reviewed until the third repeat call, Lillian has violated Standard 4.01. In addition, presumably, Lillian does not collect demographic information until she seeks the client's consent to treatment, and thus Lillian does not have the information to report Jimmy's suicidal ideation. If Lillian practiced in South Carolina or Texas, Lillian would not be in violation of state law if she did not disclose Jimmy's suicidal threats in light of the permissive nature of the duty to protect. However, in all jurisdictions, whether they have enacted a mandatory, permissive, or no duty to protect, prudent psychological practice would entail a thorough assessment of the suicidal threat and the implementation of a reasonable course of action to address the threat.

Standard 1.03 directs Lillian to negotiate with the agency to allow for discussion regarding the limits of confidentiality at the beginning of the first call, regardless of when informed consent to treatment is obtained.

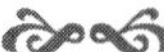

Dictates of One's Own Conscience

If you were Lillian and you have not discussed limits of confidentiality nor obtained informed consent to treatment with Jimmy, would you:

1. Consult with your supervisor on a second line?
2. Consult with any psychologist in the facility at the time?
3. Tell Jimmy you are not sure if you have to tell someone?
4. Tell Jimmy that you might have to tell someone, depending on what type of duty to protect the state has enacted (mandatory, permissive, or no duty at all)?
5. Ask Jimmy to name the location where he is physically located; then tell him if you have to report his suicidal ideation, and send out the first responder team identified by the state's law?
6. Talk with your supervisor about the need to review limits of confidentiality at the beginning of the first phone call?
7. Talk to the agency about the difference between obtaining informed consent to treatment and discussing the limits of confidentiality?
8. Combinations of the above-listed actions?
9. Or one that is not listed above?

If you were Lillian, and your internship was in Canada, would you

1. Attempt to get consent to treatment over the phone with Jimmy, and document this for the case file; attempt to do a suicide intervention with Jimmy?
2. Do not mention consent with Jimmy until you can ascertain the seriousness of his suicidality, instead attempting to get demographic information from Jimmy in order to help him?
3. Inform your supervisor that consent policy at your internship site is out of alignment with the code of ethics, and should be changed immediately?

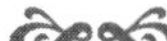

STANDARD 10.01: INFORMED CONSENT TO THERAPY

> ... (b) When obtaining informed consent for treatment for which generally recognized techniques and procedures have not been established, psychologists inform their clients/patients of the developing nature of the treatment, the potential risks involved, alternative treatments that may be available, and the voluntary nature of their participation.

A CASE FOR STANDARD 10.01 (B): The Therapeutic Touch

Robin was referred to Dr. Duncan for treatment of chronic back pain. The referring medical physician also reported that Robin has been diagnosed with dissociative identity disorder (DID). Dr. Duncan initially engaged in systematic relaxation and some biofeedback with Robin. This course of treatment brought on some measure of relief for Robin. After about eight months, Robin asked Dr. Duncan if there were any other types of therapy that could produce greater pain relief. Dr. Duncan told Robin that he has been learning a new technique called "healing touch." Although he reported that the therapy was very new and experimental, Dr. Duncan also mentioned that the preliminary outcomes of the approach were good. One complication of this therapy is the necessity for Dr. Duncan to physically touch Robin without the interference of any material between his hand and her skin over any and all parts of her body. Dr. Duncan disclosed that some patients have reported being sexually aroused by "healing touch," partly because patients who suffer from pain often are not used to being physically touched and because they experience such intense relief from their physical pain.

Issues of Concern

It appears that after 8 months of treatment, a therapeutic alliance has been established. The treatment has achieved a measure of success in addressing the presenting problem of chronic back pain which indicates reasons for Robin to have confidence in Dr. Duncan's competency. Robin is a bit impatient and maybe a bit desperate to achieve increased levels of pain relief.

In compliance with the requirements of Standard 10.01 (b), Dr. Duncan informed Robin of the experimental state of the new treatment, as well as the potential risks, and assured her that if she agrees to try the new technique, she can stop the "healing touch" approach at any time without consequence to their treatment relationship. Though it appears that Dr. Duncan has followed the directives of Standard 10.01 (b), most psychologists would be uncomfortable with the potentially sexual nature of the treatment. Is Dr. Duncan's prescription for "healing touch" in accord with those who practice touch therapy? Has Dr. Duncan violated the directives of the code of ethics?

APA Ethics Code

Companion General Principle

Principle D: Justice

> Psychologists recognize that fairness and justice entitle all persons to access to and benefit from the contributions of psychology and to equal quality in the processes, procedures, and services being conducted by psychologists.

As a profession, psychology has a body of knowledge and service that is provided for the treatment of those who are suffering. Dr. Duncan is applying the knowledge he has gained in the field of psychology when he provides treatment. Principle D suggests that psychologists apply such knowledge to all of their clients. If touch therapy is indeed based on contributions psychology as a profession has made to the alleviation of mental suffering, then, according to Principle D, Dr. Duncan should offer this treatment to all clients with similar symptoms who may benefit. If touch therapy is not based on established standards and accepted knowledge of the field, then Dr. Duncan should not be offering this treatment to any of his clients.

Principle A: Beneficence and Nonmaleficence.

> Because psychologists' . . . actions may affect the lives of others, they are alert to and guard against personal . . . factors that might lead to misuse of their influence.

Unless touch therapy as outlined by Dr. Duncan is within the established guidelines for treatment, Dr. Duncan may be using the treatment technique to disguise his personal interest in sex. This suspicion presumes Dr. Duncan is heterosexual and interested in a sexual encounter with Robin. If Dr. Duncan is heterosexual, then Dr. Duncan's behavior may be seen as sexual in nature and thus contrary to the value of Principle A: Beneficence and Nonmaleficence.

Principle B: Fidelity and Responsibility

> Psychologists uphold professional standards of conduct . . . and seek to manage conflicts of interest that could lead to exploitation or harm.

Principle B guides psychologists to be vigilant against exploitation and harm by examining the treatment of their clients in comparison to those established standards of the field. In the subspecialty of touch therapy, does Dr. Duncan's proposed procedure conform to the established guidelines? Is there established evidence for the effectiveness of touch therapy in treating chronic back pain?

Companion Ethical Standard(s)

Standard 2.04: Bases for Scientific and Professional Judgments

> . . . Psychologists' work is based upon established scientific and professional knowledge of the discipline.

Standard 2.04 dictates that Dr. Duncan be able to directly reference studies based on established methods that suggest touch therapy is helpful, and hopefully efficacious for the relief of back pain. However, to date there is controversial and limited scientific evidence about the safety or effectiveness of touch therapy (Lilienfield, Lynn, & Lohr, 2003; Singh & Ernst, 2008). To the best of professional knowledge to date, Dr. Duncan has violated Standard 2.04 by introducing the possibility of touch therapy as a viable treatment.

Standard 2.01: Boundaries of Competence

> . . . (e) In those emerging areas in which generally recognized standards for preparatory training do not yet exist, psychologists nevertheless take reasonable steps to ensure the competence of their work and to protect clients/patients . . . from harm.

Dr. Duncan argues that touch therapy is an experimental and emerging form of treatment. As such, he could argue that no established standards of competency or treatment protocols exist. Yet, even in such circumstances, Standard 2.01 requires that Dr. Duncan articulate steps he has taken to become competent in touch therapy and that his execution of touch therapy will not harm Robin. Otherwise, such a practice is outside the scope of his competency. Another example is the practice of moving the "qi" (life force energy) as described in Chinese medicine and often referred to in the United States as touch therapy. It does not involve the removal of clothing or actual physical contact between the healer and patient. In the current example, it is doubtful that Dr. Duncan is proposing to engage in the technique commonly referred to as touch therapy.

Standard 10.05: Sexual Intimacies With Current Therapy Clients/Patients

> Psychologists do not engage in sexual intimacies with current therapy clients/patients.

The protocol suggested by Dr. Duncan violates Standard 10.05 because he is requesting consent to make physical contact with Robin in ways that could be sexually arousing.

Standard 3.08: Exploitative Relationships

> Psychologists do not exploit persons over whom they have . . . authority such as clients/patients.

In the absence of established scientific knowledge within psychology of the efficacious use of physical touch for treatment, there is no known basis for Dr. Duncan to introduce his brand of touch therapy. In the presence of Standard 10.05, and in light of Dr. Duncan's own statement to Robin that the touch may sexually arouse her, the behavior appears exploitative and violates Standard 3.08.

Legal Issues 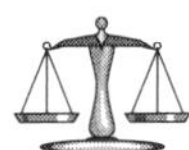

Vermont

> *26 Vt. Stat. § 3016 (2010). Unprofessional Conduct.*
>
> (4) Engaging in any sexual conduct with a client, or with the immediate family member of a client, with whom the licensee has had a professional relationship within the previous two years.

Virginia

> *18 Va. Admin. Code § 125-20-150 (2010). Standards of Practice.*
>
> B. Persons licensed by the board shall . . .
>
> 5. Avoid harming . . . clients . . . for whom they provide professional services. . . Not exploit or mislead people for whom they provide professional services. Be alert to and guard against misuse of influence . . .
>
> 8. Not engage in sexual intimacies with a . . . client . . . while providing professional services.

In both jurisdictions, Dr. Duncan's statement that the touch may be sexually arousing to his client would be viewed as a telling admission. He would break the law in both jurisdictions by engaging in "healing touch" treatment.

Cultural Considerations

Global Discussion

Hong Kong Psychological Society:
Professional Code of Practice

> 8. Any physical contact (e.g., hug or pat) made by the psychologist should be made as a gesture of support and only if the clients indicate that they feel comfortable with such contact. It should be withdrawn if the client indicates any degree of discomfort with it.
>
> 9. If physical contact goes beyond that described in (8) then:
>
> (a) it must be an agreed, integral part of therapy and
>
> (b) a third party must be present or in the immediate vicinity. Clients and psychologists must reach agreement on the identity of the third party.
>
> 10. Procedures involving nudity of the client ordinarily go beyond the bounds of established therapeutic practice.

Hong Kong's code is clear with regard to physical touch by a psychologist: If contact goes beyond a hug or a pat, it must be clinically indicated, agreed upon in advance, and must take place in the presence of a third party that both Robin and Dr. Duncan agree on. Finally, Hong Kong's code specifies that psychological interventions that involve removal of clothing by a client go beyond "established therapeutic practice," and that likely even in the presence of a third party would be difficult to justify within the bounds of established scientific knowledge. Therefore, even if a mutually acceptable third party joined them in the treatment room, as soon as Robin removes her clothes at the direct suggestion of Dr. Duncan, he is in violation of Hong Kong's code, and likely most other existing ethical codes of psychological societies.

American Moral Values

1. Does Dr. Duncan believe this therapy is the best way to treat Robin, or is he just providing Robin with information? Is the information he provides likely to convince Robin to receive treatment? What is Dr. Duncan's responsibility as far as managing expectations for a "new and experimental" method? Is Robin in a vulnerable state of mind as she looks for other methods of treatment, or is she just seeking information to improve her condition?
2. How would the "healing touch" treatment relate to the other aspects of Dr. Duncan's treatment of Robin? Is Dr. Duncan treating Robin's back pain alone, or does he have a larger view of her mental health that he imagines he could address? To what degree does Dr. Duncan need to consider Robin's DID before moving forward with the "healing touch" treatment? What relationship between DID and prior abuse should Dr. Duncan take into account? Will the use of skin-to-skin touch raise the risk of flashbacks or triggering for a client like Robin? Would it be more efficacious to have Robin engage the services of a licensed massage therapist, and schedule further psychotherapy sessions a few hours after the massage?
3. Is Dr. Duncan's training sufficient to begin this treatment? Will Robin be a "guinea pig" of sorts as he learns the practice? Should he refer her to someone adequately experienced? If he knows no such practitioner, should he bring up the method at all? Or should Robin be trusted to decide for herself whether to receive treatment from Dr. Duncan, knowing his qualifications?
4. How can Dr. Duncan be confident of Robin's full consent to "healing touch," especially given the type of physical contact it requires? Should she be asked to decide anything in his office, where his status might influence her decision making? How does her back pain and DID affect her decision-making abilities? Does Dr. Duncan believe there are special reasons to be careful when it comes to physical contact between therapist and client?
5. How does Dr. Duncan view the sexual arousal experienced by some "healing touch" patients? How would such arousal affect the client–therapist relationship? Does he have experience with this coming up in other forms of treatment? Should he be confident in his own ability as a practitioner to work through that issue with a client? Does Dr. Duncan's expertise in pain relief invest him with more legitimacy in Robin's eyes to touch a patient? Does Dr. Duncan need to take extra precaution not to exploit such authority or legitimacy?

Ethical Course of Action

Directive per APA Code

Dr. Duncan has followed procedure as specified in Standard 10.01 (b) for informed consent for experimental treatment. He does not violate the requirement for obtaining consent for treatment from Robin. However,

Dr. Duncan appears to use his authority and trust of patients for his self-interest, violating Principle A: Beneficence and Nonmaleficence, as well as Principle B: Fidelity and Responsibility. In that touch therapy is not a practice based on scientific and professional knowledge, Dr. Duncan would violate Standard 2.04. In that the movement of qi as described in Chinese Medicine does not involve removal of clothing, it is clear that Dr. Duncan is attempting to engage in another practice that suggests he lacks competence, and would violate Standard 2.01. The suggestion that Dr. Duncan may touch his client in such a way that would induce sexual arousal in Robin violates Standard 10.05. That Dr. Duncan could introduce this experimental treatment is based on his authority as a psychologist, and the violation of patient trust also would violate Standard 3.08.

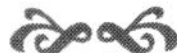

Dictates of One's Own Conscience

If you were a postdoctoral psychologist working part-time for Dr. Duncan running his biofeedback sessions with Robin, and Robin tells you she may not see you as much because she is going to try this new touch therapy with Dr. Duncan, which of these would you do?

1. Figure that Robin does not know what she is talking about.
2. Figure that Robin is working out her sexual problems with Dr. Duncan.
3. Ask Robin further questions as you set up the biofeedback equipment for her.
4. Become alarmed by Robin's story, and tell Dr. Duncan of Robin's fantasies.
5. Wonder about Dr. Duncan's motives and if Robin's story is accurate, be concerned about her sexual exploitation, and ask Dr. Duncan what is going on with Robin's treatment.
6. Ask Dr. Duncan whether he is proposing to engage in touch therapy with Robin.
7. Discuss Robin's claims with other psychologists for consultation.
8. Report Dr. Duncan to the licensing board for sexual misconduct.
9. Combinations of the above-listed actions.
10. Or one that is not listed above.

If you were this same postdoctoral psychologist working in Hong Kong, would you:

1. Immediately instruct Robin that any treatment that requires the removal of her clothing is not common practice for psychologists, and report Dr. Duncan to the licensing board?
2. Inform Robin that it is her right to have a third person present in the room during any proposed physical touch between her and Dr. Duncan?

STANDARD 10.01: INFORMED CONSENT TO THERAPY

> . . . (c) When the therapist is a trainee and the legal responsibility for the treatment provided resides with the supervisor, the client/patient, as part of the informed consent procedure, is informed that the therapist is in training and is being supervised and is given the name of the supervisor.

A CASE FOR STANDARD 10.01 (C): Volunteer Psychology Student

The Modern School of Psychology requires that all students in the doctoral psychology program participate in community practicum placements. Dawn, a first-year student, has chosen to do her practicum placement at the New City Suicide and Crisis Hotline. As a member of the unpaid staff working at the hotline, she is considered a volunteer. The New City Suicide and Crisis Hotline has a memorandum of understanding with the Modern School of Psychology that the Crisis Hotline will provide the experience and the same on-site supervision for all of their volunteers. The school also will provide consultation from licensed psychologists for all doctoral psychology students placed at the Crisis Hotline.

Dawn, like all hotline volunteers, has undergone the 1-month intensive training program. The hotline staff treats Dawn as a volunteer, even though Dawn is also a psychology practicum student. Her first week has gone well in that no major mishaps occurred. Dawn is now into her third week and has gotten to know Stanley, a repeat caller. This night, in the middle of a conversation without much consequence, Dawn casually mentions that she is a doctoral psychology student. Stanley reacts to this information with alarm and much offense, saying, "Have you been psyching me out and diagnosing me? Did you not tell me earlier so you could get me to tell you all my problems? Here I have been telling you everything, and you think I'm crazy!"

Issues of Concern

Dawn is interacting with Stanley as a lay volunteer for the crisis call-in center. Her status as a graduate psychology student is considered incidental. However, Dawn's reason for working at the crisis center is because of her training program in psychology. For Dawn, her status as a graduate psychology student is not incidental to her presence at the crisis call center. In addition, she is receiving supervision time with a licensed psychologist. Is Stanley's reaction understandable and foreseeable? Regardless of how the New City Suicide and Crisis Hotline considers Dawn, should Dawn have regarded her work at the crisis center as being under the auspices of her psychology program, and should she have told Stanley about herself and her supervisor?

Standard 10.01 (c) is relevant when the legal responsibility for the treatment provided resides with the supervisor. Dawn's work with Stanley is under the supervision of the volunteer on-site supervisor, not the psychologist who is supervising/consulting with her at her graduate program. Does Standard 10.01 (c) apply to the current situation?

APA Ethics Code

Companion General Principle

Introduction and Applicability

> Membership in the APA commits members and student affiliates to comply with the standards of the APA Ethics Code and to the rules and procedures used to enforce them.

All parts of the APA ethics code apply to Dawn as a graduate student regardless of whether her placement recognizes or treats her as a psychology graduate student. As such, these principles and standards apply to Dawn in her work at the crisis center.

Principle C: Integrity

> Psychologists seek to promote accuracy, honesty, and truthfulness in the . . . practice of psychology. In these activities psychologists do not . . . engage in . . . intentional misrepresentation of fact.

Principle C guides psychologists to ultimately build therapeutic alliance with their clients. Stanley's reaction to the information that Dawn is a doctoral psychology student indicates that he thinks Dawn has misrepresented herself and the facts about their relationship.

Companion Ethical Standard(s)

Standard 7.01: Design of Education and Training Programs

> Psychologists responsible for education and training programs take reasonable steps to ensure that the programs are designed to provide the . . . proper experiences, and to meet the requirements for licensure.

The experience provided to Dawn through her placement at the crisis center may be invaluable to her education. The arrangement between the New City Suicide and Crisis Hotline and the Modern School of Psychology appears to place the graduate student in a status that is more than a volunteer but less than a graduate psychology student. To be in compliance with Standard 7.01, might the graduate program have made other arrangements with the crisis center to better define Dawn's role and position?

Standard 3.10: Informed Consent

> (a) When psychologists . . . provide . . . therapy [and] counseling. . . they obtain the informed consent of the individual.

Regardless of whether the crisis center regards Dawn as a volunteer or not, Dawn is still obligated to follow Standard 3.10 (a). By neglecting to obtain informed consent, Dawn not only has violated Standard 3.10 (a), but ultimately she has failed Stanley.

Legal Issues 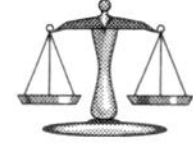

Washington

> *Wash. Admin. Code § 246-924-030 (2009). Guidelines for the Employment and/or Supervision of Auxiliary Staff.*
>
> (3) Responsibilities of the supervisor: The supervisor accepts full legal and professional responsibility for all services that may be rendered by the auxiliary staff. To this end, the supervisor shall have sufficient knowledge of all clients, including face-to-face contact when necessary, in order to plan and assure the delivery of effective services. The supervisor is responsible for assuring that appropriate supervision is available or present at all times. . .

(5) Conduct of services that may be provided by auxiliary staff: Procedures to be carried out by the auxiliary staff shall be planned in consultation with the supervisor. Clients of the auxiliary staff shall be informed as to his/her status and shall be given specific information as to his/her qualifications and functions. Clients shall be informed of the identity of the supervisor. They shall be informed that they might meet with the supervisor at their own request, the auxiliary staff person's or the supervisor's request.

California

Cal. Code Regs. tit. 16, § 1387.1 (West 2010). Qualifications and Responsibilities of the Primary Supervisors.

(f) Primary supervisors shall be responsible for monitoring the welfare of the trainee's clients.

(g) Primary supervisors shall ensure that each client or patient is informed, prior to the rendering of services by the trainee (1). that the trainee is unlicensed and is functioning under the direction and supervision of the supervisor; (2). that the primary supervisor shall have full access to the treatment records in order to perform supervision responsibilities.

In both jurisdictions, Dawn's primary supervision would be in violation of the laws and subject to licensing board sanctions. Not only was Stanley unaware that Dawn was being supervised, but he also was not informed of the identity of the supervisor, and that Dawn was acting under the direction of the supervisor.

Cultural Considerations

Global Discussion

Canadian Code of Ethics for Psychologists

Principle III: Integrity in relationships.

III.22. Make no attempt to conceal the status of a trainee and, if a trainee is providing direct client service, ensure that the client is informed of that fact.

Dawn has clearly violated this portion of the Canadian code, although responsibility lies mainly with her supervisor. Despite her status as a volunteer in the eyes of the hotline, Dawn is there under the auspices and license of a clinical psychologist as part of her doctoral training, and thus she and her supervisor are both in violation of this portion of Canada's code. Clearly, the client in this vignette would likely feel that Dawn's status has been concealed, and this would likely cause harm to the therapeutic relationship. In traditional clinical placement sites, an informed consent is likely to be done during the first visit, and little opportunity for misunderstanding exists. In situations where psychology students are placed in "nontraditional" sites, such as in the case of a site that uses both telephone and in-person sessions with potential clients, it behooves the student and supervising psychologist to take greater pains to clarify the nature of the relationship as early as possible.

American Moral Values

1. Was Dawn trained as a volunteer not to share personal information unless necessary? Does this training override the standard of informed consent for psychologists? Which role—volunteer or doctoral student—takes precedence in this context?
2. Would disclosing her status as a doctoral student in psychology from the beginning have been fairer to Stanley? Did he in any way expect to be talking to a psychologist? Would callers like him be reluctant to talk to such a person in any case? Or would it help build trust with the caller, displaying some sense of honesty? To what degree is Dawn responsible for the opinion of psychologists held by Stanley and callers like him?
3. Did the New School give Dawn adequate instruction about how to negotiate conflicting standards of conduct? If instructed to follow the training site's rules, how does Dawn decide whether or not to act according to the code's informed consent standard?
4. Does Dawn believe informed consent is more valuable to uphold as a practitioner than the clinic's rules? How would breaking the clinic's rules affect her work life there? Does she appear to be elevating herself above volunteer status by making such a decision?
5. Do psychologists have a special obligation to let a client know their occupation? In the context of this clinic, will clients need to be told they are talking to a trainee rather than a psychologist? What is Dawn's status as a psychologist-in-training when it comes to this setting?

Ethical Course of Action

Directive per APA Code

For Standard 10.01 (c) to apply, two conditions need to be met. One is that the therapist is a trainee. The other is that the legal responsibility for the treatment resides with the supervisor. The first condition is met in that Dawn is a therapist and is also a trainee. The second condition is not satisfied in that the supervisor/consultant at the graduate program does not hold legal responsibility for the work Dawn does at the crisis center. However, the on-site supervisor does hold legal responsibility. Standard 10.10 (c) would apply, and Dawn has violated this ethical standard by failing to tell Stanley that she is under supervision.

By virtue of Dawn's status as a graduate psychology student, all parts of the APA Ethics Code apply to her professional work. Regardless of whether Standard 10.01 (c) specifically applies to these circumstances, all other principles and standards apply. As such, Dawn and her supervisor/consultant also failed to uphold the intent of Principle C: Integrity, and were in violation of Standard 3.10 (a). In addition, the Modern School of Psychology might take a closer examination of their memorandum of understanding with the New City Suicide and Crisis Hotline within the context of Standard 7.01.

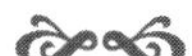

Dictates of One's Own Conscience

If you were Dawn, how would you respond:

1. To Stanley?
   a. Apologize to Stanley for the unintentional concealment of your graduate student status.
   b. Reassure Stanley that you do not think he is crazy.
   c. Reassure Stanley that you do not have any ulterior motive that involves deception.
   d. Let Stanley know that you are indeed a graduate psychology student, and though you do not think he is crazy, you have learned a great deal from him and would like to continue phone contact with him.
   e. Tell Stanley you would like to have the on-site supervisor join the call to explain the situation to him.
   f. Combinations of the above-listed actions.
   g. Or one that is not listed above.
2. To the on-site supervisor?
   a. Consult offline while on the phone with Stanley.
   b. Ask him or her to join in on the call to best guide you through this interaction with Stanley.
   c. Handle the call with Stanley and then debrief with him or her.
   d. Request that you be allowed to conduct informed consent to treatment with clients at the very beginning of the first call.
   e. Discuss the ramifications of your graduate student status for future callers.
   f. Combinations of the above-listed actions.
   g. Or one that is not listed above.
3. To the supervisor/consultant at the graduate program?
   a. Discuss how to handle informed consent to treatment with future callers.
   b. Request that he or she talk to the crisis center supervisor to gain mutual understanding of how you should handle future calls regarding informing the caller of your graduate student status.
   c. Ask why the program and the crisis center made the supervision/consultation arrangement.
   d. Combinations of the above-listed actions.
   e. Or one that is not listed above.

If you were Dawn and the crisis clinic was in Canada, would you inform your supervisor at the hotline that although you are considered a volunteer, your school and code of ethics require that each caller be told of your trainee status as a doctoral student in psychology?

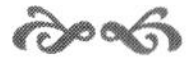

STANDARD 10.02: THERAPY INVOLVING COUPLES OR FAMILIES

(a) When psychologists agree to provide services to several persons who have a relationship (such as spouses, significant others, or parents and children), they take reasonable steps to clarify at the outset (1) which of the individuals are clients/patients and (2) the relationship the psychologist will have with each person. This clarification includes the psychologist's role and the probable uses of the services provided or the information obtained.

A CASE FOR STANDARD 10.02 (A): Male Bonding

Dr. Snyder is the treating psychologist for Bryan, a 15-year-old boy who has been diagnosed with oppositional behaviors and substance abuse problems. Dr. Snyder has recommended that treatment include family sessions interspersed with individual sessions with Bryan. Peggy, Bryan's mother, has sole custody; Tony, the father, lives one block away and has full visitation. This week in the family session, Bryan is very sullen, having been grounded after his father "snitched" on him to his mother for using marijuana. In an angry outburst in the family session, Bryan says to his father, "You are such a hypocrite!" Then Bryan turns to Dr. Snyder, saying, "I smoke with him all the time, and he is my best customer."

Issues of Concern

Dr. Snyder is providing treatment services that include several members of an estranged family. This situation is within the scope of Standard 10.02 (a). In accordance with Standard 10.02 (a), Dr. Snyder is to have identified which of the family members is the client, the nature of the relationship with members who are not identified as the client, and how confidential information will be used. Dr. Snyder may consider himself fortunate to have the drug relationship between son and father revealed in everyone's presence. It is fortunate because Dr. Snyder does not have to address individual confidentiality of information obtained from each family member within the context of family therapy. What he does have to address is confidentiality in the context of a possible mandated report of child abuse.

In most states, psychologists are mandated reporters of child abuse. This situation may not be so difficult clinically if Dr. Snyder has followed the dictates of Standard 10.02 (a) and clearly informed and negotiated his role in relation to each individual in the room and informed the family of the probable use and limitations of confidential information. If this has been done, Dr. Snyder's job is to determine whether a child abuse situation has arisen. If the reverse were the case in which Tony gave Bryan illegal drugs, then child abuse is clear. Has Tony abused his teenage son by purchasing illegal drugs from him?

APA Ethics Code

Companion General Principle

Principle E: Respect for People's Rights and Dignity

> Psychologists respect the dignity and worth of all people, and the rights of individuals to privacy, confidentiality, and self-determination. Psychologists are aware that special safeguards may be necessary to protect the rights and welfare of persons or communities whose vulnerabilities impair autonomous decision making.

Principle E calls Dr. Snyder's attention to the topic of privacy. In general, Dr. Snyder should respect each person's right to confidentiality as well as the right of the family as a whole to confidentiality. In addition, when a member of the treatment group involves a child, in this case, Bryan, Dr. Snyder takes care to protect his welfare. Welfare may be broadly defined in terms of Dr. Snyder's responsibility to safeguard Bryan from his father's abuse.

Companion Ethical Standard(s)

Standard 4.01: Maintaining Confidentiality

> Psychologists have a primary obligation . . . to protect confidential information . . . recognizing that the extent and limits of confidentiality may be regulated by law.

Depending on the state in which Dr. Snyder is practicing, the law may regulate information related to child abuse. If so, Dr. Snyder does not violate Standard 4.01 by contacting authorities regarding information obtained within the treatment session.

Standard 10.01: Informed Consent to Therapy

> (a) When obtaining informed consent to therapy . . . psychologists inform clients/patients as early as is feasible in the therapeutic relationship about the . . . limits of confidentiality.

Standard 10.01 (a) directs Dr. Snyder to have had a conversation about mandated reporting of child abuse at the outset of treatment.

Standard 4.02: Discussing the Limits of Confidentiality

> . . . (b) Unless it is not feasible or is contraindicated, the discussion of confidentiality occurs . . . thereafter as new circumstances may warrant.

Standard 4.02 (b) requires Dr. Snyder to remind this family of the mandate for him to report child abuse at this point in treatment.

Legal Issues 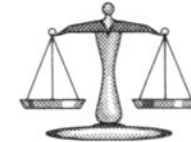

Florida

> *Fla. Admin. Code Ann. r. 64B19-19.002 (2010). Definitions.*
>
> A "client" . . . is that individual who, by virtue of private consultation with the psychologist, has reason to expect that the individual's communication with the psychologist

during that private consultation will remain confidential, regardless of who pays for the services of the psychologist.

Fla. Admin. Code Ann. r. 64B19-19.006 (2010). Confidentiality.

(1) One of the primary obligations of psychologists is to respect the confidentiality of information entrusted to them by service users. Psychologists may disclose that information only with the written consent of the service user. The only exceptions to this general rule occur in those situations when nondisclosure on the part of the psychologist would violate the law.

Florida Statute 39.201 (2010). Mandatory Reports of Child Abuse, Abandonment, or Neglect; Mandatory Reports of Death; Central Abuse Hotline.

(1) (a) Any person who knows, or has reasonable cause to suspect, that a child is abused, abandoned, or neglected by a parent . . . shall report such knowledge or suspicion to the department.

Hawaii

Haw. Code R. § 16-98-34 (2010). Unethical Practice of Psychology.

(d) Safeguarding information about an individual that has been obtained by the psychologist in the course of . . . investigation is a primary obligation of the psychologist. Such information shall not be communicated to others unless certain important conditions are met:

(1) Information received in confidence may be revealed only after careful deliberation and where there is a clear and imminent danger to an individual . . . and then only to appropriate professional workers or public authorities.

Haw. Rev. Stat. §350-1.1 (2010). Reports.

(a) Notwithstanding any other state law concerning confidentiality to the contrary, the following persons who, in their professional or official capacity, have reason to believe that child abuse or neglect has occurred . . . shall immediately report the matter orally to the department or to the police department:

(1) Any licensed . . . professional of . . . any health-related occupation who . . . treats, or provides . . . services, including but not limited to . . . psychologists.

In both jurisdictions, Dr. Snyder is a mandatory reporter. If he failed to make a report, he would violate the laws of those jurisdictions. The circumstances of Bryan's disclosure are irrelevant in light of the mandatory reporting duties. Dr. Snyder must file the report because of the admission. At least one of the parents or Child Protective Services will be likely to file an ethics complaint with the licensing board if he fails to make the report.

Cultural Considerations

Global Discussion

Canadian Code of Ethics for Psychologists

Principle I: Responsible caring.

Confidentiality.

I.44. Clarify what measures will be taken to protect confidentiality, and what responsibilities family . . . members have for the protection of each other's confidentiality, when engaged in services to . . . families.

If Dr. Snyder were seeing this family in Canada, what he would be called upon to do is help this family clarify with each other and himself what protections of each other's confidentiality would be agreed upon and maintained. Dr. Snyder would also clarify his role in maintaining the family's confidentiality, and would facilitate the co-creation of that responsibility with the entire family, regardless of whether he was seeing one or all of them. Hopefully, if Dr. Snyder is in compliance with the Canadian code, he would have had such a conversation early on in his therapy with the family that would have involved himself, both parents, and Bryan. Then, at Bryan's introduction of new information about one parent, Dr. Snyder would be well-served to remind Bryan, and both parents, of whatever confidentiality agreement they had all come to.

American Moral Values

1. Does Dr. Snyder give priority to Bryan's treatment or the family's treatment? Has Dr. Snyder made clear to his parents that Bryan is an individual client in a way they are not?
2. Does Bryan's statement obligate Dr. Snyder to report Tony's behavior? Does it make a difference whether it was made in an individual or family session? How can Dr. Snyder verify that Bryan's claim is true? What kind of verification would be useful and constructive? Is Tony's status as a client overridden by Bryan's status, especially given Bryan's age?

3. How will reporting Tony affect future treatment of the family? Does Dr. Snyder feel that he would have to rebuild trust with the parents? How will this affect family sessions with Bryan?

4. How do Dr. Snyder's beliefs about family support and cohesion affect his decision? Does he believe Bryan needs a stronger relationship with Tony to become better? Do they both need to obtain treatment for abuse before moving forward?

5. How does Bryan's selling drugs affect Dr. Snyder's view of his problems, both with substance abuse and oppositional behavior?

6. Is Dr. Snyder obligated to report Tony for child abuse, given that Bryan has reported smoking with Tony? Is smoking with Bryan any better than if Tony were giving Bryan the drugs himself? Or is Bryan fully capable and responsible for his own smoking of marijuana? What if the shared drug the father and son were using was alcohol? Oxycontin? What difference would this make to Dr. Snyder's actions?

7. How does the cultural and legal framing of marijuana use, for better or for worse, play a role in this situation? (Marijuana is illegal for all people to possess and use, while alcohol is not illegal for adults.)

8. Has Dr. Snyder used marijuana in the past himself? Has he found it to be mostly harmless? Can he draw upon that experience to judge the seriousness of this charge?

Ethical Course of Action

Directive per APA Code

Standard 10.02 (a) requires that Dr. Snyder identify the client, the nature of the relationship with members who are not identified as the client, and how confidential information will be used. It seems that Dr. Snyder has identified Bryan as the client, and that his role with Bryan's mother and father is to help them improve their parenting relationship with Bryan. If Dr. Snyder followed the directives of Standards 10.01 (a), 4.01, and 4.02, he would have discussed the limits of confidentiality already. At this juncture in treatment, Dr. Snyder is required to follow the directive of Standard 4.02 and hold another conversation about the limits of confidentiality, and break confidentiality to report that child abuse or neglect may be occurring.

It is not within the purview of the standards to direct clinical judgment. Whether Dr. Snyder reports this situation as child abuse, or decides that no child abuse has occurred, is guided by sources other than the APA Ethics Code. Dr. Snyder can exercise his clinical judgment about how to make the mandatory report so that the therapeutic alliance is not ruptured, and both of the parents are not surprised by the mandatory report.

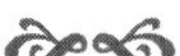

Dictates of One's Own Conscience

If you were Dr. Snyder sitting in the room with Bryan angrily blurting out the information about (1) Bryan selling illegal drugs, and (2) his father having supported his son's illegal behavior by purchasing the illegal drugs from him, which action would you take?

1. Remind Bryan and Tony that you are a mandatory reporter of child abuse and neglect, and plan out how you can convey the admission to Child Protective Services within the session so that the report is made and the therapeutic alliance is protected.
2. Ask Bryan and Tony if Peggy knew of this arrangement.
3. Ask Tony if Bryan's accusation was true.
4. Ask the parents to individually respond to Bryan's accusation.
5. Consider that Bryan is the perpetrator, so no child abuse situation is in evidence; and respond with a focus on inappropriate parenting.
6. Consider that Tony's supporting of Bryan's illegal behavior is a form of child abuse, and decide to contact local child protective authorities.
7. Combinations of the above-listed actions.
8. Or one that is not listed above.

If this situation were occurring in Canada, would you

1. Remind the family of whatever agreement regarding confidentiality you had previously come to at the start of family therapy?
2. Remind the family that if in fact you believe harm of a minor child was or is occurring, you may need to break confidentiality?

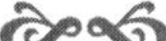

STANDARD 10.02: THERAPY INVOLVING COUPLES OR FAMILIES

> . . . (b) If it becomes apparent that psychologists may be called on to perform potentially conflicting roles (such as family therapist and then witness for one party in divorce proceedings), psychologists take reasonable steps to clarify and modify, or withdraw from, roles appropriately.

A CASE FOR STANDARD 10.02 (B): Incest

Crystal is a 10-year-old who lives with her mother in California during the school year and with her father in Arizona during summer breaks. Crystal started treatment with Dr. Gladys in California after a summer spent in Arizona with her father. Rita, Crystal's mother, complained bitterly about not liking the length of time Crystal is out of contact during the summer. Then Rita reports to Dr. Gladys that she is sure that Crystal has been sexually abused by her father during the summer visit. Privately, without Rita present, Dr. Gladys asks Crystal about her mother's concerns, and Crystal says, "I had a really fun visit with my Dad. I know that my mom thinks he is a weirdo or something, but Mom is uptight and Dad is just more huggier than my mom."

Issues of Concern

It appears that Dr. Gladys is providing treatment to Crystal. It is unclear as to the status of the parental relationship; therefore, the legal status of either the father or mother in the matter of authority to enter Crystal into treatment with Dr. Gladys is also unclear. Is it Dr. Gladys's responsibility to ascertain whether treatment is legally permissible? Or does Dr. Gladys rely on the authority of the custodial parent to provide the permission for Crystal to enter into treatment?

With Rita's concerns and allegations against the father, the probability of eventual court involvement is extremely high. Knowing the directive of Standard 10.02 (b), how should Dr. Gladys clarify her role? What stance and steps should she take now or before a court summons, to set parameters so that Dr. Gladys, Crystal, and Rita can decide whether the relationship needs to be modified or whether treatment should even continue? One possible modification is the establishment of a treatment relationship with the father in Arizona and the mother and daughter, in light of the emerging conflict between the parents.

APA Ethics Code

Companion General Principles

Principle B: Fidelity and Responsibility

> Psychologists . . . clarify their professional roles and obligations.

In cases where a dependent person, such as a child, is involved, there usually are other concerned parties also directly involved, such as the child's parents. Principle B calls Dr. Gladys's attention to and suggests the need for clarification of her professional role. For this case, Dr. Gladys might consider clarifying her role and relationship to Crystal, Rita, and the father in Arizona.

Principle E: Respect for People's Rights and Dignity

> Psychologists are aware that special safeguards may be necessary to protect the rights and welfare of persons . . . whose vulnerabilities impair autonomous decision making.

Aspiring to Principle E, Dr. Gladys is to take special safeguards to protect Crystal's rights and welfare. What privacy rights does Crystal, a 10-year-old child, have? How would it affect Crystal's greater welfare for Dr. Gladys to be pulled into what may be the start of a custody conflict?

Companion Ethical Standard(s)

Standard 3.10: Informed Consent

> (a) When psychologists . . . provide . . . therapy . . . they obtain the informed consent of the individual or individuals. . .
>
> (b) For persons who are legally incapable of giving informed consent, psychologists nevertheless (1) provide an appropriate explanation[,] . . . (2) seek the individual's assent[,] . . . (3) consider such persons' preferences and best interests, and . . . (4) obtain appropriate permission from a legally authorized person.

Standard 3.10 (a) requires that Dr. Gladys obtain informed consent for treatment. In the case of a child, as in Crystal, Standard 3.10 (b) requires that Dr. Gladys obtain consent from Crystal herself as well as from a legally authorized person. In a case where parents are separated, Dr. Gladys is required to determine who holds legal authorization to consent for Crystal to enter into treatment. It is unclear whether Dr. Gladys clarified the legal relationship with either the mother or the father. If Dr. Gladys missed the step of obtaining consent from the appropriate person(s), then she is in violation of Standards 3.10 (a) and 3.10 (b). If Dr. Gladys has determined the legal status of custody, how might that information influence her current dilemma?

Standard 10.02: Therapy Involving Couples or Families

> (a) When psychologists agree to provide services to several persons who have a relationship (such as . . . parents and children), they take reasonable steps to clarify at the outset . . . (1) which of the individuals are clients/ patients and . . . (2) the relationship the psychologist will have with each person. This clarification includes the psychologist's role and the probable uses of the services provided or the information obtained.

Part of the procedure to accomplish Standard 3.10 (a) includes the dictates of Standard 10.02 (a). Based on the description of Dr. Gladys's interactions with Crystal, it appears that Crystal is the identified client. Dr. Gladys, from the outset, is required to communicate the fact that Crystal is the client; as a result, Dr. Gladys must identify Crystal as the client, describe the extent to which information from Crystal will be treated as individually confidential, and establish how Dr. Gladys will relate to each parent.

Standard 4.01: Maintaining Confidentiality

> Psychologists have a primary obligation and take reasonable precautions to protect confidential information . . . recognizing that the extent and limits of confidentiality may be regulated by law.

Regardless of the agreement established under Standard 10.02 (a), Standard 4.01 allows Dr. Gladys to break confidentiality should state law mandate psychologists to report possible child abuse.

Standard 10.01: Informed Consent to Therapy

> (a) When obtaining informed consent to therapy[,] . . . psychologists inform clients . . . as early as is feasible in the therapeutic relationship about the . . . involvement of third parties, and limits of confidentiality.

If Dr. Gladys had followed the directive of Standard 10.01 (a), before treatment began, Dr. Gladys would have discussed the limits of confidentiality, which would include whether Dr. Gladys is required by law to report suspected child abuse. Rita and Crystal would already know Dr. Gladys might be mandated to break confidentiality and report child abuse. Has such knowledge motivated Rita to make the accusation? Does the accusation and Rita's belief that Dr. Gladys must report her concerns to the authorities set the stage for Rita to pursue legal action and attempt to prohibit contact between the father and Crystal? If Rita pursues legal action, then Dr. Gladys surely will be called to testify.

Standard 3.05: Multiple Relationships

> (a) A multiple relationship occurs when a psychologist is in a professional role with a person and . . . (2) at the same time is in a relationship with a person closely associated with or related to the person with whom the psychologist has the professional relationship, or (3) promises to enter into another relationship in the future with the person or a person closely associated with or related to the person.

A psychologist refrains from entering into a multiple relationship if it could reasonably be expected to impair the psychologist's objectivity, competence, or effectiveness in performing his or her functions as a psychologist, or otherwise risks exploitation or harm to the person with whom the professional relationship exists. Multiple relationships that would not reasonably be expected to cause impairment or risk exploitation or harm are not unethical.

If Rita engages in legal action, unless a stipulation exists that precludes all involvement in the possible future discovery and litigation about her client (i.e., the parents have agreed to and signed the stipulation before any pending litigation was threatened), Dr. Gladys may find herself in a multiple relationship. She would be the treating psychologist, yet Rita's lawyer may call upon Dr. Gladys to render an opinion about custody or contact and access to her client, a multiple relationship per Standard 3.05 (a) (2). At that point in the treatment, unless Dr. Gladys stays in a "fact" rather than an "expert" witness role, she would appear to have engaged in a multiple relationship.

Standard 3.05 does not specifically prohibit entering into a multiple relationship. However, will Dr. Gladys's objectivity be influenced by the high probability of having to report a possible child abuse situation or testifying in a custody hearing as a fact witness?

Legal Issues 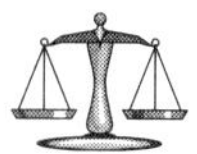

Indiana

Ind. Code Ann. § 16-39-2-3. Confidentiality.

Sec. 3. A patient's mental health record is confidential and shall be disclosed only with the consent of the patient.

Ind. Code Ann. § 25-33-1-17. Privileged Communications; Exceptions.

Sec. 17. A psychologist licensed under this article may not disclose any information acquired from persons with whom the psychologist has dealt in a professional capacity, except under the following circumstances . . .

(5) If the psychologist has the expressed consent of the client or . . . express consent of the client's legal representative.

(6) Circumstances under which privileged communication is abrogated under the laws of Indiana.

Ind. Code Ann. § 31-34-1-3 (LexisNexis Supp. 2010). Victim of Sex Offense; Living in Household With Victim of Sex Offense.

Sec. 3. (a) A child is a child in need of services if, before the child becomes eighteen (18) years of age:

(1) the child is the victim of a sex offense under [the law].

Ind. Code Ann. § 35-42-4-3 (LexisNexis Supp. 2010). Child Molesting.

Sec. 3. (a) A person who, with a child under fourteen (14) years of age, performs . . . sexual conduct commits child molesting, a Class B felony. However, the offense is a Class A felony if:

(1) it is committed by a person at least twenty-one (21) years of age;

(b) A person who, with a child under fourteen (14) years of age, performs . . . any fondling or touching, of . . . the child . . . with intent to arouse or to satisfy the sexual desires of either the child or the older person, commits child molesting, a Class C felony.

Kansas

Kan. Admin. Regs. § 102-1-10a (2010). Unprofessional Conduct.

(e) failing to obtain informed consent, which shall include the following acts:

(1) Failing to obtain and document . . . informed consent from the client or legally authorized representative for clinical psychological services before the provision of any of these services . . .

(g) failing to protect confidentiality, which shall include the following acts:

(1) Failing to inform each client . . . [of] the limits of client confidentiality, the purposes for which the information may be obtained, and the manner in which it may be used.

Kan. Stat. Ann. § 74-5323 (2010). Privileged Communication.

(a) The confidential relations and communications between a licensed psychologist and the psychologist's client are placed on the same basis as provided by law for those between an attorney and the attorney's client. Except as provided in subsection (b), nothing in this act shall be construed to require such privileged communications to be disclosed.

(b) Nothing in this section or in this act shall be construed to prohibit any licensed psychologist from testifying in court hearings concerning matters of . . . child abuse. There is no privilege under this section for information which is required to be reported to a public official.

Kan. Stat. Ann. § 21-3501 (2010): Definitions.

The following definitions apply in this article . . .

Kan. Stat. Ann. § 21-3502 (2010) (a). Rape is. . .

(2) sexual intercourse with a child who is under 14 years of age.

In both jurisdictions, Dr. Gladys must obtain informed consent. In light of Rita's complaint that included information about her daughter spending the entire summer visiting her father, it is quite likely that both parents have health care decision-making authority for their 10-year-old child. If indeed both parents hold health care decision authority, then Dr. Gladys would be obligated legally to obtain consent for treatment from both parents.

Cultural Considerations

Global Discussion

Association for Greek Psychologists

7. The psychologist is not allowed to testify in court as a witness for the defense or prosecution of his client.

If this situation were to unfold in Greece and become a litigious one or part of a divorce proceeding, Dr. Gladys could not participate. It is unclear whether Dr. Gladys is mandated to report possible sexual abuse in Greece, as is legally obligated in the United States and most other countries.

American Moral Values

1. How does Rita's charge affect Dr. Gladys's treatment of Crystal? Is it advisable to ask Crystal about her mother's concerns if Crystal did not initiate discussion on that subject? Is it advisable to ask about her relationship with her father if such inquiry could affect possible future investigations? How does this exchange affect Crystal's relationship with Dr. Gladys? Will she consider Dr. Gladys a representative of her mother's concerns? An arbiter of her parents' views?

2. How can Dr. Gladys clarify her role as Crystal's therapist to Rita? What kind of relationship does Dr. Gladys think will be most constructive? Should she be concerned that Rita will be less forthcoming if she does not feel Dr. Gladys takes her concerns seriously enough? How can Dr. Gladys convey that she takes sexual abuse claims very seriously and also strongly supports appropriate father–daughter physical affection?

3. Does Rita expect Dr. Gladys to report back regarding what Crystal said about her summer visit? How does Dr. Gladys preserve client–therapist privacy? Does Crystal understand the nature of that privacy? Does Dr. Gladys need to reestablish some ground rules so that Crystal does not wonder what comments will be known by which parent?

4. How does Dr. Gladys view the role of Crystal's father in this treatment? Has he contacted Dr. Gladys at all? To what degree does he need to be informed of Dr. Gladys's role and its limits?

Ethical Course of Action

Directive per APA Code

If Dr. Gladys had followed the directives of Standards 3.10 (a) and 3.10 (b), she would know the legal status of the father. She would either already have contact with the father if he has any legal custody of Crystal, or know that she does not need to concern herself with him because he does not have legal custody.

If Dr. Gladys had followed the directive of Standard 10.02, father, mother, Crystal, and Dr. Gladys would already know how such accusations would be handled among the four of them. And after due diligence, all would know that Dr. Gladys will make a clinical judgment as to whether the accusation of sexual abuse warrants breaking confidentiality with a report to Child Protective Services.

At this point in treatment, it is or should be apparent to Dr. Gladys that she may be called upon to function in roles in addition to that of a treating psychologist. At a minimum, she is called upon to step into the role of a possible mandated reporter if reasonable suspicion of sexual abuse exists. She also may be called upon to fulfill the role of treating psychologist and fact witness for probable custody litigation, while at least one of the lawyers attempts to blur these boundaries by asking questions that only an expert witness could answer. She must avoid entering into a multiple relationship per Standard 3.05. Standard 10.02 (b) requires that Dr. Gladys take reasonable steps to clarify her role and also, should it be necessary, to either modify her role or withdraw from her role as treating psychologist.

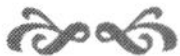

Dictates of One's Own Conscience

If you were Dr. Gladys, having complied with the directives of Standard 3.10 and stated the limit of confidentiality in regards to child abuse, what reasonable steps would you take as directed by Standard 10.02 (b) to clarify future roles?

1. Tell Rita that, based on Crystal's report, there does not appear to be sufficient grounds for you to make a report of child abuse?

2. Tell Rita that, in order to determine the best course of treatment for Crystal, you would need to make contact with Crystal's father?

3. Tell Rita and Crystal that you are a mandated reporter and that you will be making a report against the father?

4. Tell Crystal that the situation seems to be a bit messy between the mother and father, and ask how their conflict affected her in the past?

5. Seek to modify the relationship to include a stipulation that precludes either Rita or the father from seeking to involve you in any future discovery or

court actions so that you can maintain your therapeutic alliance with Crystal?

6. Combinations of the above-listed actions?
7. Or one that is not listed above?

If you were Dr. Gladys, and this situation occurred in Greece, would you directly remind all family members, including Crystal, that regardless of the situation, you cannot testify in court for or against your client, Crystal?

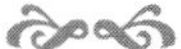

STANDARD 10.03: GROUP THERAPY

> When psychologists provide services to several persons in a group setting, they describe at the outset the roles and responsibilities of all parties and the limits of confidentiality.

A CASE FOR STANDARD 10.03: The High School Sweetheart

Dr. Cunningham practices in a small town in the Rocky Mountains. He has noticed that, during the last few years, his caseload has been populated by males who are all struggling with problems regarding intimacy. To facilitate a more universal experience, Dr. Cunningham decides to set up an ongoing men's support group. Because of the small-town setting of the group, they have all agreed to strict confidentiality in regards to membership and to contents of the group sessions. In the last year, this ongoing men's group has been quite successful in helping the men achieve greater levels of intimacy in their private lives. After 8 months of individual therapy with Nathan, assisting him in dealing with his intense feelings of jealousy, Dr. Cunningham decides that Nathan may benefit from hearing what other men have to say about this type of insecurity. Dr. Cunningham makes sure that Nathan does not have a first-degree relative in the group. Nathan walks into the group, only to be confronted by Dale. Dale is another member of the group, and Nathan's wife's former high school sweetheart.

Issues of Concern

When conducting group therapy, Standard 10.03 directs Dr. Cunningham to specify not only the role and responsibility of the therapist, but also the group members to each other. Within the clarification of roles must be a discussion and explication of privacy and confidentiality expectations between group members. The role and the limits of confidentiality for the therapist are detailed in the APA Ethics Code, but the role and limits of confidentiality among group members are not. Given the discovery of Nathan and Dale's past relationship, how might Dr. Cunningham guide the discussion regarding roles, responsibilities, and confidentiality among group members?

Does Nathan and Dale's past relationship fundamentally alter Dr. Cunningham's role? Does it impose a situation of multiple relationships? If so, would this multiple relationship be expected to affect Dr. Cunningham's competence to provide group therapy?

APA Ethics Code

Companion General Principle

Principle E: Respect for People's Rights and Dignity

> Psychologists respect the . . . rights of individuals to privacy, confidentiality, and self-determination.

Dr. Cunningham has established therapeutic alliances with both Nathan and Dale. A consequence of the therapeutic alliance is an increased degree of influence over Nathan and Dale. Depending on what Dr. Cunningham does, he could violate Principle E by failing to guard against using his influence to decrease the degrees of freedom for either Nathan or Dale to independently determine whether to stay in the group.

Companion Ethical Standard(s)

Standard 3.05: Multiple Relationships

> (a) A multiple relationship occurs when a psychologist is in a professional role with a person and . . . (2) at the same time is in a relationship with a person closely associated with or related to the person with whom the psychologist has the professional relationship . . .
>
> A psychologist refrains from entering into a multiple relationship if the multiple relationship could reasonably be expected to impair the psychologist's objectivity, competence, or effectiveness in performing his or her functions as a psychologist, or otherwise risks exploitation or harm to the person with whom the professional relationship exists.

> Multiple relationships that would not reasonably be expected to cause impairment or risk exploitation or harm are not unethical.
>
> . . . (b) If a psychologist finds that, due to unforeseen factors, a potentially harmful multiple relationship has arisen, the psychologist takes reasonable steps to resolve it with due regard for the best interests of the affected person and maximal compliance with the Ethics Code.

Dr. Cunningham appears to have entered into a multiple relationship with Nathan and Dale, as defined by Standard 3.05 (a) (2). It is doubtful that Dr. Cunningham could have discovered the past connection between the two group members. Due to unforeseen circumstances, Dr. Cunningham finds himself in this multiple relationship. As directed by Standard 3.05 (b), Dr. Cunningham must take reasonable steps to resolve the situation in the best interests of both Nathan and Dale.

Legal Issues 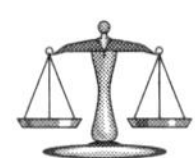

Kentucky

> *201 Ky. Admin. Regs. 26:145 (2010). Code of conduct.*
>
> Section 4. Impaired Objectivity and Dual Relationships. . .
>
> (2) Prohibited dual relationships.
>
> (a) The credential holder shall not . . . continue a professional relationship with a client if the objectivity or competency of the credential holder is impaired because of the credential holder's present . . . relationship with the client or a relevant person associated with or related to the client. . .
>
> Section 5. Client Welfare.
>
> (1) Providing explanation of procedures. The credential holder shall give a truthful, understandable, and appropriate account of the client's condition to the client. . . The credential holder shall keep the client fully informed as to the purpose and nature of . . . treatment . . . and of the client's right to freedom of choice regarding services provided. . .
>
> Section 7. Protecting the Confidentiality of Clients. . .
>
> (5) Multiple clients. If service is rendered to more than one (1) client during a joint session, the credential holder shall at the beginning of the professional relationship clarify to all parties the manner in which confidentiality shall be handled.

Maryland

> *Md. Code Regs. 10.36.05.04 (2010). Competence.*
>
> **B. Impaired Competence. . .**
>
> (2) A psychologist may not:
>
> (a) Undertake or continue a professional relationship with a client when the competence or objectivity of the psychologist is or could reasonably be expected to be impaired due to . . .
>
> (ii) The psychologist's present . . . relationship with the client or a person associated with or related to the client.
>
> *Md. Code Regs. 10.36.05.07 (2010). Client Welfare.*
>
> A. F. Termination of Services. A psychologist shall:
>
> (1) Make or recommend referral to another professional . . . if the referral is clearly in the best interest of the client; and
>
> (2) Unless precluded by the actions of the client, terminate the professional relationship in an appropriate manner, notify the client in writing of this termination, and assist the client in obtaining services from another professional, if:
>
> (b) A multiple relationship develops or is discovered after the professional relationship has been initiated.

In both jurisdictions, Dr. Cunningham must clarify the multiple relationships that unexpectedly emerged when Nathan or Dale disclosed that Nathan's wife was Dale's old girlfriend. The validity of a complaint about violating the law in either jurisdiction would be determined by an examination of the processing regarding the multiple relationship by Dr. Cunningham, its possible impact upon Nathan and Dale and other group members, and the exploration of alternatives to proceeding with the group treatment of Nathan and Dale.

Cultural Considerations

Global Discussion

Code of Ethics for the Psychologist: Spain

> ***Article 25.*** On accepting an intervention on individuals . . . [or] groups . . . psychologists must provide adequate information about the essential features of the relationship established, the problems being faced, the proposed objectives and the method used.

According to this portion of the Spanish code, what Dr. Cunningham would need to do to comply with this article is to "provide adequate information" about the group therapy relationship, the sorts of difficulties the group might face, what the hoped-for outcomes are, and what method he is using to facilitate the group. Spain's code is silent with regard to discussing the limits of confidentiality in a group versus an individual setting, although it is possible this could be part of what is implied with "problems being faced."

American Moral Values

1. Can Nathan be expected to work in a group with Dale in it? Could it be therapeutically constructive? Even if it were a useful challenge for Nathan in terms of his treatment, is it fair to ask Nathan to continue? How can Dr. Cunningham be sure that Nathan is making this decision on his own and not from social pressure? Should Dr. Cunningham make sure Nathan understands he is not obligated to join?
2. Does Dr. Cunningham view this situation as unavoidable given the connections among people in a small town? Is he more likely to encourage Nathan to try the group than if they were in a large city? Is this fair to Nathan, or is it an appropriate way to address a challenge of small-town life?
3. What will be the consequences of waiting for Nathan to find other men to talk to? Can Dr. Cunningham start another group? Is there another psychologist who has a men's group? How would this case be different if it were a women's group? Are there beliefs about therapy or psychology that Dr. Cunningham has to account for in managing the group? How will this affect his approach with Nathan?
4. If Nathan decides not to join the group, what will be the effect on the group itself? Will Dale assume it was because of him that Nathan couldn't join? What if that "fact" becomes a piece of gossip in the town? Will Dale trust Nathan to remain confidential about Dale being in the group?

Ethical Course of Action

Directive per APA Code

Standard 10.03 directs Dr. Cunningham to clarify roles, responsibilities, and limits of confidentiality among group members. Dr. Cunningham was careful to prevent multiple relationships in the group by assuring that no first-degree relatives are members of the group at the same time. Unforeseen by him, as defined in Standard 3.05 (a) and 3.05 (b), a multiple relationship has arisen. Guided by Principle E to assure group members' rights to self-determination, Standard 10.03 directs Dr. Cunningham to now describe each person's role, his responsibility to other group members, and the agreed-upon confidentiality rules among group members.

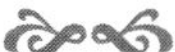

Dictates of One's Own Conscience

If you were Dr. Cunningham, in which of these ways might you describe the roles, responsibilities, and limits of confidentiality in the presence of this multiple relationship?

1. Ask Nathan if he wishes to stay for just this one group session.
2. Ask Nathan if he wishes to leave before the group even starts.
3. Ask Dale whether he wishes for Nathan to leave the group.
4. Ask the group as a whole whether they think Nathan should stay, and explore with Dale his connection to Nathan and whether one of them should leave.
5. Invite Dale to discuss his relationship with Nathan's wife before Nathan decides whether to join or leave the group.
6. Specify that group members are there to work on their own problems, and the presence of a past conflict that is still relevant today is a good chance to work on resolution of the problem.
7. Specify that group members are responsible for the well-being of each other and that everyone has to consent for Nathan to stay in the group.
8. Remind everyone that what happens in the group stays in the group, and that Nathan and Dale are not to mention the identity of members outside of group, to anyone, even a spouse.
9. Work on developing another men's group, or possibly splitting this one in two.
10. Combinations of the above-listed actions.
11. Or one that is not listed above.

If you were Dr. Cunningham running this group in Spain, you would inform the group that such occurrences, especially in small towns, are some of the problems the group might reasonably be expected to encounter, and ask if members want to continue working through their issues with each other as before.

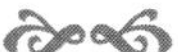

STANDARD 10.04: PROVIDING THERAPY TO THOSE SERVED BY OTHERS

In deciding whether to offer or provide services to those already receiving mental health services elsewhere, psychologists carefully consider the treatment issues and the potential client's/patient's welfare. Psychologists discuss these issues with the client/patient or another legally authorized person on behalf of the client/patient in order to minimize the risk of confusion and conflict, consult with the other service providers when appropriate, and proceed with caution and sensitivity to the therapeutic issues.

A CASE FOR STANDARD 10.04: The Magic Pill

Jeffrey, a 17 year old, is in treatment with Dr. Lane. Dr. Lane refers Jeffrey to Dr. Thelma, a new psychiatrist in town who specializes in working with children, to consider whether a trial of medication should be started with Jeffrey for symptoms of bipolar disorder. Jeffrey reports that Dr. Ruiz has placed him on some medications that are helping tremendously. Jeffrey's mother reports that Jeffrey no longer has temper outbursts. Jeffrey also reports that Dr. Ruiz thinks treatment with Dr. Lane is not necessary since "I can take care of everything with the medications."

Issues of Concern

Jeffrey now has two doctors providing him treatment for the same problem. Standard 10.04 suggests that Dr. Lane should proceed with caution with due consideration for Jeffrey's welfare when confusion and conflict arises with another treatment professional. Indeed, the confusion has already arisen with the conflicting recommendation for Jeffrey's treatment regime. Before responding, should Dr. Lane clarify whether he thinks the recommendation for medication only without psychotherapy for Jeffrey is warranted? What does he think of Dr. Ruiz's stance regarding psychotherapy? What type of relationship does he want to have with Dr. Ruiz?

APA Ethics Code

Companion General Principle(s)

Principle E: Respect for People's Rights and Dignity

> Psychologists respect the dignity and worth of all people, and the rights of individuals to privacy, confidentiality, and self-determination.

Principle E establishes the right of self-determination as a value for psychologists. This means Dr. Lane is to grant Jeffrey the right to choose the type of treatment he wishes, be it medication only or medication with psychotherapy.

Principle B: Fidelity and Responsibility

> Psychologists consult with, refer to, or cooperate with other professionals and institutions to the extent needed to serve the best interests of those with whom they work.

Principle B recognizes that psychologists work within a community of health care providers. Within this community, Dr. Lane collaborates by consulting with, referring to, or otherwise cooperating with other treatment providers for the benefit of their mutual clients. Dr. Lane has already exhibited collaboration by referring Jeffrey to consult with Dr. Ruiz. It may be desirable for Dr. Lane now to conduct further consultation with Dr. Ruiz.

Companion Ethical Standard(s)

Standard 3.09: Cooperation With Other Professionals

> When indicated and professionally appropriate, psychologists cooperate with other professionals in order to serve their clients/patients effectively and appropriately.

Standard 3.09 advises Dr. Lane to cooperate with Dr. Ruiz, when indicated and appropriate. Does the current situation indicate it is appropriate for Dr. Lane to cooperate with Dr. Ruiz? One way to cooperate with Dr. Ruiz is to transfer Jeffrey completely to Dr. Ruiz's care. Might it be appropriate to confirm Jeffrey's report of Dr. Ruiz's recommendation with Dr. Ruiz herself? Might a joint coordinated treatment regime better serve Jeffrey in the long run?

Standard 2.04: Bases for Scientific and Professional Judgments

> Psychologists' work is based upon established scientific and professional knowledge of the discipline.

The value of basing treatment recommendations on established knowledge of the discipline is prevention of unnecessary or harmful procedures. Are either Dr. Lane's or Dr. Ruiz's treatment recommendations based on current knowledge of effective interventions for Jeffrey? Diagnosis of bipolar disorder for children is still somewhat controversial, so should Dr. Lane inquire about the controversial aspects of such a diagnosis with Dr. Ruiz (Ghaemi & Martin, 2007; Olfman, 2007; Stringaris et al., 2010)?

Standard 10.10: Terminating Therapy

> (a) Psychologists terminate therapy when it becomes reasonably clear that the client/patient no longer needs the service, is not likely to benefit, or is being harmed by continued service.

Jeffrey and his mother have raised the question of termination of services with Dr. Lane. Per Standard 10.10 (a), Dr. Lane is to end treatment if continuing treatment will harm Jeffrey. Will harm occur to Jeffrey from working with both Dr. Lane and Dr. Ruiz, especially when their individual treatment recommendations are different?

Legal Issues

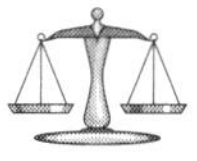

Michigan

> *Mich. Admin. Code r. 338.2515 (2010). Prohibited Conduct.*
>
> Rule 15. Prohibited conduct includes, but is not limited to, the following acts or omissions by any individual covered by these rules[:] . . .
>
> (c) Taking on a professional role when personal, scientific, professional, legal, financial, or other relationships could impair the exercise of professional discretion or make the interests of a patient, supervisee, or student secondary to those of the licensee.

Minnesota

> *Minn. R. 7200.4810 (2010). Impaired Objectivity, Effectiveness.*
>
> Subpart 1. Psychological services prohibited.
>
> A psychologist must not provide psychological services to a client . . . when the psychologist's objectivity or effectiveness is impaired.
>
> Subp. 2. Elements of impaired objectivity, effectiveness.
>
> A psychologist's objectivity or effectiveness is impaired whenever: . . .
>
> B. the psychologist misuses the relationship with a client due to a relationship with another individual or entity.

> *Minn. R. 7200.4900 (2010). Client Welfare.*
>
> Subp. 4. Preferences and options for treatment.
>
> A psychologist shall disclose to the client preferences of the psychologist for choice of treatment . . . and shall present other options for the consideration or choice of the client.
>
> Subp. 5. Conflict between psychologist and client.
>
> A psychologist who becomes aware of a divergence of interests, values, attitudes, or biases between a client and the psychologist sufficient to impair their professional relationship shall so inform the client. Either the client or the psychologist may terminate the relationship. . .
>
> Subp. 9. Coordinating services with other professionals.
>
> A psychologist shall ask a client whether the client has . . . a professional relationship with another mental health professional. If it is determined that the client had or has a professional relationship with another mental health professional, the psychologist shall, to the extent possible and consistent with the wishes and best interests of the client, coordinate services for that client with the other mental health professional.

Both Minnesota and Michigan direct Dr. Lane to put the interests of Jeffrey first when working out the coordination of services. In Minnesota, if Dr. Lane disagrees with Jeffrey's wish to receive medication treatment only, Dr. Lane is obligated to state the difference of opinion. If Jeffrey wanted to terminate treatment with Dr. Lane, Dr. Lane is to coordinate services for Jeffrey. If Dr. Lane impeded his client's relationship with Dr. Ruiz, he would violate the law in both jurisdictions through failing to support his client's interests. It could appear as if Dr. Lane were attempting to assert his own financial interests first.

Cultural Considerations

Global Discussion

Hong Kong Psychological Society:
Professional Code of Practice

> 3.4. Members do not normally offer professional services to an individual already receiving psychological assistance from another professional except by agreement amongst all parties concerned.
>
> *Other Disciplines*
>
> 3.5. Members shall ensure that they are aware of the knowledge and skills of professionals of related disciplines (e.g., law and medicine) and that, when appropriate, clients are referred for advice.
>
> 3.6. Members shall respect the professional standards of other disciplines, and great care shall be taken to develop and strengthen harmonious inter-disciplinary relations.

If Drs. Ruiz and Lane were treating Jeffrey in Hong Kong, several issues would be in play. First, can a psychiatrist who confines her treatment plan for bipolar disorder to prescribing psychotropic drugs be seen as giving "psychological assistance"? If so, then Dr. Lane would likely need to have a conversation with Jeffrey about only being treated by one person at a time. If, however, as a medical doctor, Dr. Ruiz is a member of a "related discipline," then Dr. Lane's obligation to her as a professional would be to respect her standards of practice, and attempt to develop and strengthen relationships between himself and Dr. Ruiz. Hong Kong's code, however, is silent on how specifically to proceed should a member of a related but different discipline attempt to tell one's client to end treatment or only accept treatment from that other provider. In other words, Dr. Lane is bound first to refer clients to allied professionals, which he did. Next, Dr. Lane is obligated to discuss with his client potential concerns and issues arising from having two treatment providers, which he presumably did, as Jeffrey agreed to the referral. Finally, Dr. Lane is called upon to take "great care" in developing and strengthening his relationship with Dr. Ruiz, which may be somewhat challenging, given their two different treatment approaches. Could Dr. Lane advise Jeffrey to stop seeing Dr. Ruiz, even though the medications are helping significantly? Should Dr. Lane refer Jeffrey to a psychiatrist who is more open to psychological scopes of practice, including talk therapy?

American Moral Values

1. How has Dr. Ruiz assessed Jeffrey's therapeutic needs? Has she determined that the only problems Jeffrey faces are those the drugs have seemed to treat? How can she make the claim to "take care of everything"? What is the obligation of Dr. Lane to challenge this view?
2. Has Dr. Ruiz seen Jeffrey's records? Have Jeffrey and his mother signed releases for Dr. Lane and Dr. Ruiz to exchange information?
3. How does Dr. Lane pursue Jeffrey's best interests? Is his therapy complementary to Dr. Ruiz's? How can Dr. Lane persuade Jeffrey and his mother that he is looking out for Jeffrey, not just his own business? Will criticizing Dr. Ruiz force Jeffrey to choose between them?
4. Does Dr. Lane believe that another doctor could provide medication as ably as Dr. Ruiz? Would Dr. Lane suggest switching to a doctor who will work better with him, while prescribing the same medications?
5. Is Dr. Ruiz's comment part of a larger debate between practitioners about medication versus talk therapy? Are Dr. Lane and Dr. Ruiz susceptible to fighting a professional battle through Jeffrey?

Ethical Course of Action

Directive per APA Code

Standard 10.04 gives procedural directions for situations where a psychologist is providing treatment services to a client who is also receiving mental health services elsewhere. Mental health services encompass work by individuals in many other allied professions, one of which is psychiatry. The procedural steps as stated in Standard 10.04 are as follows: (1) Carefully consider treatment issues, (2) consider potential damage to client's welfare, (3) discuss treatment issues with the client, (4) discuss problems with receiving treatment from two different mental health professionals so as to minimize risk of confusion and conflict, and (5) consult with the other service provider when appropriate. After completing steps 1 through 5, proceed with caution.

Dr. Lane considered the treatment issue of how best to rule out or treat bipolar disorder in a teenager and decided to refer for a medication consultation, thus accomplishing the first step required by Standard 10.04. The referral was in keeping with providing the best treatment possible to Jeffrey, thus complying with the second step of Standard 10.04 as well as Standard 2.04. Presumably, Dr. Lane discussed the reasons for his referral with Dr. Ruiz and the confusion that could arise from having potentially two different recommendations. If so, he has satisfied the third and fourth steps of the Standard 10.04 process.

What a mental health professional says to a client and what a client understands about what is said can be different. Following the directive of Standard 10.04 as well as Standard 3.09, Dr. Lane now needs to consult with Dr. Ruiz. Only after consultation with Dr. Ruiz, Jeffrey, and Jeffrey's mother should Dr. Lane proceed. Should he decide the ensuing confusion from two different treatment providers is harmful to Jeffrey, Dr. Lane should move to end treatment as directed by Standard 10.10 (a). Should Jeffrey and his mother decide to transfer treatment to Dr. Ruiz, regardless of Dr. Lane's opinions and recommendations, Dr. Lane is to respect Jeffrey's right to make such a decision, per Principle E.

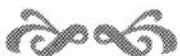

Dictates of One's Own Conscience

If you were Dr. Lane, hearing such a report from your teenage client, which of these would you think and do?

1. Wonder if Jeffrey understood Dr. Ruiz correctly.
2. Think Dr. Ruiz competitive and threatened by the profession of psychology.
3. Agree with Dr. Ruiz and move to terminate Jeffrey.
4. Refer Jeffrey to another psychiatrist.
5. Discuss with Jeffrey and his mother the pros and cons of medication only versus medication and psychotherapy.
6. Discuss with Jeffrey and his mother whether they have found psychotherapy to be helpful.
7. Offer to refer Jeffrey to another psychologist if he and his mother have found treatment with you to be unhelpful.
8. Request a consultation note from Dr. Ruiz regarding your patient Jeffrey.
9. Contact Dr. Ruiz for a conversation regarding Jeffrey after obtaining a signed release.
10. Combinations of the above-listed actions.
11. Or one that is not listed above.

If you were Dr. Lane treating Jeffrey in Hong Kong, would you:

1. Attempt to foster a more harmonious relationship with Dr. Ruiz by calling her, introducing yourself, and consulting with her about your mutual client?
2. Attempt to ascèrtain from Dr. Ruiz what her perspectives are on the efficacy of psychotherapy versus medications, and attempt to build a stronger relationship with her based on your mutual status as allied professionals?
3. Decide that referring Jeffrey to Dr. Ruiz was not appropriate, and inform Jeffrey that you will refer him to a psychiatrist who is more favorable toward psychotherapy?

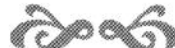

STANDARD 10.05: SEXUAL INTIMACIES WITH CURRENT THERAPY CLIENTS/PATIENTS

Psychologists do not engage in sexual intimacies with current therapy clients/patients.

A CASE FOR STANDARD 10.05: Hearsay

Dr. Harper has joined a group of mental health service providers who share an office suite. The others in the office consist of a psychiatrist, a clinical social worker, and two other psychologists. Dr. Harper has a cordial relationship with everyone. The relationship with Edna, a clinical social worker, has been slightly strained since a previous conversation in which Dr. Harper decided to talk to Edna about her inappropriate use of psychometricians for parenting evaluations.

Tiffany has been a client of Dr. Harper's for approximately a year. Tiffany's diagnosis is borderline personality disorder. During one session, she begins to describe a particular sex act in great detail, complete with sexually explicit noises of arousal. Dr. Harper decides not to interrupt her, having learned from previous sessions that interrupting Tiffany in the middle of one of her stories is generally counterproductive. Instead, it is their usual therapeutic pattern to examine the meaning of Tiffany's stories after she is done relaying the details of the situation. At the end of the session, as Dr. Harper is walking Tiffany down the hallway to the waiting room, Dr. Harper notices Edna's office door standing open and Edna looking at Dr. Harper with both curiosity and suspicion. About a month later, Dr. Harper receives notification from the state licensing board that a complaint has been made alleging improper sexual conduct with a client.

Issues of Concern

Standard 10.05 is very simple and direct: Do not have sex with your current clients. Given that treatment is conducted behind closed doors, how would anyone know that Dr. Harper is or is not having sex with Tiffany? Presuming that it was the concern about Tiffany that generated the complaint, was it reasonable for Edna who overheard the vocalizations that indicated sexual arousal to conclude that Dr. Harper was engaged in sexual contact with his client?

APA Ethics Code

Companion General Principle

Principle B: Fidelity and Responsibility

> Psychologists . . . are concerned about the ethical compliance of their colleagues' scientific and professional conduct.

Principle B guides Dr. Harper to be concerned about the practices of his office mates. Although Edna is not a psychologist, she is a colleague and within the arena of Principle B. Dr. Harper's conversation with Edna was, hopefully, motivated by the value of fidelity to the profession of mental health services. Likewise, might Edna's concern be similarly motivated?

Companion Ethical Standard(s)

Standard 3.02: Sexual Harassment

> Psychologists do not engage in sexual harassment. Sexual harassment is sexual solicitation, physical advances, or verbal or nonverbal conduct that is sexual in nature, that occurs in connection with the psychologist's activities or roles as a psychologist, and that either (1) is unwelcome, is offensive, or creates a hostile workplace or educational environment, and the psychologist knows or is told this or (2) is sufficiently severe or intense to be abusive to a reasonable person in the context. Sexual harassment can consist of a single intense or severe act or of multiple persistent or pervasive acts.

As defined in Standard 3.02 it appears that Dr. Harper's behavior with Tiffany does not meet the definition of sexual harassment. Does allowing a client to graphically report a sexual encounter hold any therapeutic value? Might Tiffany's behavior in Dr. Harper's office be experienced as sexual harassment by Dr. Harper?

Standard 1.04: Informal Resolution of Ethical Violations

> When psychologists believe that there may have been an ethical violation by another psychologist, they attempt to resolve the issue by bringing it to the attention of that individual, if an informal resolution appears appropriate and the intervention does not violate any confidentiality rights that may be involved.

Keeping with the spirit of Standard 1.04, even though Edna is not a psychologist, Dr. Harper took the initiative to address a concern informally with Edna. Could Edna have handled this situation in a way that was more protective of Tiffany? For example, might Edna have knocked and/or entered Dr. Harper's office when she thought he was having sex with a client? Might such an act have been more protective of Tiffany?

Standard 1.05: Reporting Ethical Violations

> If an apparent ethical violation has substantially harmed . . . and is not appropriate for informal resolution under Standard 1.04[,] . . . psychologists take further action appropriate to the situation. Such action might include referral . . . to state licensing boards. . . This standard does not apply when an intervention would violate confidentiality.

If it was Edna who made the ethics complaint against Dr. Harper, might it be prudent for Edna to have informally discussed her concerns with Dr. Harper? Or is it reasonable to expect someone who would engage in sex with one's client to categorically deny any such accusations, and therefore, it may not be appropriate to intervene informally with psychologists who engage in sex with their clients?

Standard 1.06: Cooperating With Ethics Committees

> Psychologists cooperate in ethics investigations . . . and resulting requirements by the APA or any affiliated state psychological association to which they belong. In doing so, they address any confidentiality issues. Failure to cooperate is itself an ethics violation.

Regardless of whether or not Edna could have engaged in informal resolution, now that Dr. Harper is notified of a complaint, he is obligated to respond.

Legal Issues

Montana

Mont. Admin. R. 24.189.2305 (2009). Practice of Psychology.

(1) In regard to conduct in the integrity of the profession, a licensee: . . .

(c) shall not participate in activities in which it appears likely that the psychologist's skills or data will be misused by others, unless corrective mechanisms are available.

Mont. Admin. R. 24.189.2314 (2009). Relationships.

(2) In regard to sexual relationships, a licensee: . . .

(b) shall not engage in sexual intimacies with current clients.

Nebraska

172 Neb. Admin. Code §§ 156-008 (2010). Sexual Misconduct.

A psychologist shall in no circumstances engage in sexual acts with clients. . . Specifically with regard to the clients, such unprofessional conduct includes but is not limited to: . . .

008.04 Engaging in any sexual act with a client.

Montana's and Nebraska's Administrative Codes mirror APA Ethics Code Standard 10.05. All disallow any sexual contact between Dr. Harper and Tiffany. The more relevant question may concern how the state licensing boards might proceed with their investigations of the complaint. More likely than not, the licensing boards would look to the record of the case to determine whether Dr. Harper's objectivity had been compromised and his involvement in the case violated the law. If the record showed that the interests of Tiffany were not served and Dr. Harper was encouraging the prurient conduct of Tiffany, the licensing boards in both jurisdictions would likely find that he acted unethically.

Cultural Considerations

Global Discussion

Canadian Code of Ethics for Psychologists

Principle II: Responsible caring.

II.27. Be acutely aware of the power relationship in therapy and, therefore, not encourage or engage in sexual intimacy with therapy clients.

Principle III: Integrity in relationships.

Avoidance of conflict of interest

III.31. Not exploit any relationship established as a psychologist to further personal . . . interests at the expense of the best interests of their clients. . . This includes, but is not limited to: . . . taking advantage of trust or dependency to encourage or engage in sexual intimacies.

The Professional Board for Psychology
Health Professions Council of South Africa:
Ethical Code of Professional Conduct (April 2002)

6.5. Sexual Intimacies With Current Therapy Clients.

Psychologists shall not engage in sexual intimacies of any nature (whether verbal, physical or both) with current therapy clients.

Canada's code is clear with regard to sexual contact between client and psychologist: It is prohibited due to an acute imbalance of power, risk of exploitation, and harm to the best interests of the client. The code is not explicit, however, regarding what constitutes "sexual intimacy." At issue here is the concern about Dr. Harper's possible exploitation of Tiffany: By allowing her to reenact sex acts in his office, is he acting in her best clinical interests, or is he "taking advantage of trust . . . to encourage . . . sexual intimacies"? Could he effectively do therapy with Tiffany without allowing such extensive sexual content to be voiced in his office? Ultimately, it is Dr. Harper's responsibility to provide a safe boundary and limit interactions with clients that could in any way be harmful or not in their best interests, which he has likely failed to do in this situation.

By contrast, South Africa's code is much less subjective and nebulous than the Canadian one on this point: Sexual intimacy, whether physical or verbal, is forbidden between Dr. Harper and Tiffany; thus, Dr. Harper, by allowing Tiffany to describe a sex act in his office, is in violation of South Africa's code.

American Moral Values

1. Does Dr. Harper assume this complaint comes from Edna overhearing Tiffany making suggestive sounds in his office? Should he wait to hear more details about the complaint before acting on that assumption?

2. What does Dr. Harper believe a professional colleague should do when he or she suspects sexual misconduct

on the part of another colleague? Assuming this is Edna complaining about Dr. Harper and Tiffany, what does Dr. Harper think Edna should have done if she was suspicious? Did she owe it to him to talk to him in person about her concerns?

3. Did Dr. Harper make a mistake by not talking directly to Edna as soon as he saw her reaction? Does that violate Tiffany's confidentiality, or would it be just a professional discussion of a case?
4. Does Dr. Harper highly value the privacy of his office? Does he need to apologize to Edna for the noise, or does he believe on principle that what goes on in his office is his professional decision? Did he resent Edna's look at him, especially if she was assuming he was acting inappropriately with Tiffany?
5. Does Dr. Harper need to address his previous criticism of Edna? Was there a lack of respect that Edna felt that, assuming she filed the complaint, led her to lash out against what she perceived was his lack of professionalism?

Ethical Course of Action

Directive per APA Code

Standard 10.05 is very clear. The question is whether allowing Tiffany to make a sexually graphic report is a form of sex that implicates Dr. Harper. As defined in Standard 3.02, what happened in treatment with Tiffany is not considered sexual harassment. Arguably, however, listening to Tiffany repeatedly describe sexually graphic material was probably not good clinical judgment in the confines of an office in which sounds are overheard between offices.

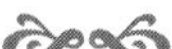

Dictates of One's Own Conscience

If you were Dr. Harper, faced with Tiffany's preoccupation with making a sexually graphic report, which action would you take?

1. Do nothing different from what Dr. Harper has done in this vignette.
2. Invite someone into the room as a witness until Tiffany finishes her story.
3. Interrupt Tiffany's story and ask her to convey her sexually graphic report more quietly.
4. Ask Tiffany about her motives for making such a sexually graphic report to you.
5. Suggest that henceforth you will audiotape Tiffany's sessions and obtain consultation from a peer to make sure you provide the very best treatment for her.

If you were Dr. Harper, faced with your own sexual attraction toward Tiffany and witnessing her preoccupation with making a sexually graphic report, would you:

1. Do nothing different from Dr. Harper in this vignette?
2. Ask that the sessions be audiotaped so that you could obtain consultation about how to best treat Tiffany while also reflecting upon your countertransference?
3. Talk to Edna as soon as Tiffany leaves the office, for a debriefing session?
4. Refer Tiffany to another colleague?

If you were Dr. Harper, after receipt of the complaint, which of these would you do?

1. Talk to Edna to ask if she was the person who made the complaint.
2. Regardless of whether it was Edna or not, ask to talk to Edna about Tiffany and the recent situation.
3. Contact your malpractice insurance company.
4. Contact an independent attorney.
5. Cooperate with the ethics committee.
6. Combinations of the above-listed actions.
7. Or one that is not listed above.

If you were Dr. Harper, practicing in Canada, would you

1. Recognize that although it is an issue of clinical judgment, allowing Tiffany to graphically relate sexual material to you repeatedly may be exploitative of her, and address it as a therapeutic issue with Tiffany?
2. Speak to Edna after the session to inquire as to what she overheard, and what her thoughts about what she overheard might be?

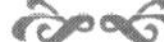

STANDARD 10.06: SEXUAL INTIMACIES WITH RELATIVES OR SIGNIFICANT OTHERS OF CURRENT THERAPY CLIENTS/PATIENTS

> Psychologists do not engage in sexual intimacies with individuals they know to be close relatives, guardians, or significant others of current clients/patients. Psychologists do not terminate therapy to circumvent this standard.

A CASE FOR STANDARD 10.06: The Seduction

Carmen fills the therapy hour with a litany of complaints about her husband, Manuel. Dr. Fox has been listening to Carmen's complaints for about 3 months and has assessed them as petty and Carmen's expectations to be unreasonable. One day, Carmen shows up to the session with her husband, Manuel, in tow. Carmen then requests a couples session. Carmen's implicit request for the couples session is for Dr. Fox to tell Manuel what is wrong with him. Dr. Fox is already predisposed to view Manuel in a more favorable stance, and unsurprisingly finds herself experiencing more positive regard for Manuel than for her client Carmen. At the end of the session, both Carmen and Manuel think it is a good idea for Manuel to come in for individual sessions with Dr. Fox to "give more background about the marriage." In these sessions, Manuel talks about his problems with his wife, and also asks questions about Dr. Fox's relationship with her husband. During the next few therapy sessions, Dr. Fox and Manuel find themselves discussing their own marital problems. They mutually agree that "it may be more productive to aim for peace in marriage instead of dialogue and understanding." After a month of individual sessions with Manuel, Carmen tells Dr. Fox that she has done miracles, that Manuel is a changed husband, and that she is now very happy. With much appreciation, Carmen says they do not intend to return for any further sessions.

Six months later, Dr. Fox runs into Manuel at a film festival. Manuel reports that he and Carmen are now separated. Dr. Fox is now also separated from her husband. They decide to have a late-night dinner after the movie. At the end of the evening, Manuel and Dr. Fox make plans for another date.

Issues of Concern

Acting congruently with Standard 10.06, Dr. Fox is not to engage in sexual intimacies with Manuel while Carmen is in treatment with Dr. Fox. Dr. Fox also did not terminate with Carmen in order to pursue a romantic relationship with Manuel. Carmen terminated treatment after her presenting complaint was resolved. The scenario as described does not indicate any violation of Standard 10.06.

Could it be argued that Dr. Fox allowed therapy to terminate with the hopes of having a romantic relationship with Manuel? Based on her two individual sessions with Manuel, did Dr. Fox know Carmen and Manuel's marital problems were not adequately addressed, but allowed Carmen to end the sessions? Did she hope that such a move would lead to a separation and divorce? Did Manuel terminate sessions with fantasies of having intimate relations with Dr. Fox? Might Manuel's seeming solicitation of Carmen be a guilty reaction to the attraction he and Dr. Fox felt for each other? Regardless of whether Dr. Fox and Manuel ever met each other again, might it be argued that the attraction Dr. Fox felt toward Manuel played some part in his separation, and thus harmed Carmen and resulted in a violation of Standard 10.06?

APA Ethics Code

Companion General Principle

Principle B: Fidelity and Responsibility

> Psychologists . . . seek to manage conflicts of interest that could lead to exploitation or harm.

In the absence of knowing or meeting Manuel, Dr. Fox's assessment of Carmen and opinion of Manuel were clinical judgments. A conflict of interest arose once Dr. Fox met Manuel and had an inkling of attraction toward him. Although it may not be unusual to have positive regard for a client, Principle B suggests that if such positive regard evolves toward attraction, then Dr. Fox would seek ways to manage such conflicts so as to prevent harm to either Carmen or Manuel.

Companion Ethical Standard(s)

Standard 10.02: Therapy Involving Couples or Families

> (a) When psychologists agree to provide services to several persons who have a relationship (such as

> spouses . . .), they take reasonable steps to clarify at the outset (1) which of the individuals are clients/patients and (2) the relationship the psychologist will have with each person.

At the point where Carmen arrived at therapy with her husband in tow, Standard 10.02 required Dr. Fox to have clarified her role in the relationship with Carmen and Manuel. Since the treatment topic was to find out more about the marriage, it appears that Dr. Fox considered Carmen to be the client, and the meetings with Manuel were collateral to Carmen's treatment. Could it be argued that regardless of how Dr. Fox considered Manuel's sessions, once he walked into her treatment room, he was a client?

Standard 3.05: Multiple Relationships

> (a) A multiple relationship occurs when a psychologist is in a professional role with a person and . . .
>
> (2) at the same time is in a relationship with a person closely associated with or related to the person with whom the psychologist has the professional relationship, or . . .
>
> (3) promises to enter into another relationship in the future with the person or a person closely associated with or related to the person. A psychologist refrains from entering into a multiple relationship if the multiple relationship could reasonably be expected to impair the psychologist's objectivity, competence, or effectiveness in performing his or her functions as a psychologist, or otherwise risks exploitation or harm to the person with whom the professional relationship exists.

It is the nature of couples and family therapy that the therapist is in multiple relationship with the couple/family members, as defined by Standard 3.05 (a) (2). While Carmen was in treatment with Dr. Fox, the multiple relationship with Manuel was not expected to impair Dr. Fox's competence in treatment of Carmen and lead to a violation of Standard 3.05.

Once Dr. Fox and Manuel met again, their relationship met the definition of multiple relationship of Standard 3.05 (a) (3). Since Carmen is no longer in treatment, her relationship with Manuel would not be expected to impair Dr. Fox's objectivity, competence, or effectiveness in doing her job. However, it could be argued that Dr. Fox's relationship with Manuel could and most probably would harm Carmen, regardless of whether she is in treatment with Dr. Fox or not.

Standard 10.08: Sexual Intimacies With Former Therapy Clients/Patients

> (a) Psychologists do not engage in sexual intimacies with former clients/patients for at least two years after cessation or termination of therapy.

For Dr. Fox to argue that Manuel remained a collateral contact and not a client may be self-protective. Dr. Fox held several treatment sessions with Manuel in her office, which means she engaged in a professional relationship with Manuel. Bumping into someone at a movie is serendipity, but making plans for a future date is engaging in sexual intimacies. While such a thing is not prohibited by Standard 10.08 (a), it requires a waiting time of 2 years between termination of treatment and beginning of sexual intimacies. Dr. Fox is in violation of Standard 10.08 (a).

Legal Issues 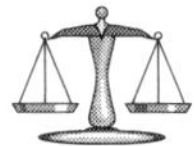

Nevada

> *Nev. Admin. Code § 641.229 (2010). Impairment of Licensee; Limitation on Contact With Current or Former Patient.*
>
> 3. If a psychologist has rendered professional services to a person, the psychologist shall not:
>
> (a) Engage in any verbal or physical behavior with the person which is sexually seductive . . .
>
> (c) Enter into a . . . potentially exploitive relationship with the person, for at least 2 years after the termination of the professional relationship, or for an indefinite time if the person is clearly vulnerable to exploitive influence by the psychologist because of an emotional or cognitive disorder.

New Jersey

> *N.J. Admin. Code § 13:42-10.9 (2010). Sexual Misconduct.*
>
> (a) As used in this section, the following terms have the following meanings unless the context indicates otherwise:
>
> "Client" means any person who is the recipient of a professional psychological service rendered by a licensee. . .
>
> (b) A licensee shall not engage in sexual contact with a current client, [or] a former client to whom psychological services were rendered within the immediately preceding 24 months. . .
>
> (j) It shall not be a defense to any action under this section that:

1. The client solicited or consented to sexual contact with the licensee; or

2. The licensee was in love with or had affection for the client.

Dr. Fox violated the law in Nevada. She provided professional services to Manuel, and she engaged in sexually seductive behavior. In New Jersey, Dr. Fox provided a service to Manuel, and thus he is considered a client. As long as Dr. Fox does not engage in sexual contact for 24 months after the termination of her service to the couple, she would not be viewed as having broken the law in New Jersey. However, such a position would be hard to sustain in light of their beginning a dating relationship, the likely ire of Carmen that could fuel a complaint, and an absence of some sort of record that would establish no sexual contact occurred.

Cultural Considerations

Global Discussion

Lithuanian Psychological Association

d) he/she shall avoid informing clients about his/her private life, except the cases when this represents a definite purpose advantageous to client;

e) he/she shall not abuse client's confidence and/or possible dependence to satisfy his/her personal interests or to benefit from it;

f) if it turns out that Psychologist's relations cannot retain their professional character, he/she shall direct client to another competent professional.

g) Psychologist shall not enter into professional interaction or use psychological techniques if his/her own emotional factors may hinder professional or ethical interactions with clients. Psychologist shall not enter into professional interaction if:

- he/she is closely related to client by kin;
- he/she strongly dislikes client or is strongly attracted to client;
- unsettled emotional conflicts of Psychologist may exercise influence upon client.

Lithuania's code is clear in this case: Dr. Fox has violated the intent and letter of the code. First, by disclosing information about herself and her marriage (d) for reasons other than therapeutic effect or benefit; next, by benefiting her own personal interests by using confidential information from Manuel, who, as a client, was in a position of less power than she (e); then, by recognizing that she was both averse to Carmen and highly favorable to Manuel, but choosing not to refer one or both clients to another psychologist (f); and finally, by allowing her own emotions and attractions to Manuel to conflict with her ethical obligation as a psychologist in charge of working with a couple (g), Dr. Fox has certainly strayed from both the letter and intent of Lithuania's code.

American Moral Values

1. How does Dr. Fox evaluate her work with Carmen and Manuel? Was it a good idea to do individual sessions with Manuel? Was it appropriate to discuss her marriage with Manuel? Why did she conclude with the idea that "peace" was better than "understanding" in marriage? Did she actually believe that would be a sustainable view for Carmen and Manuel's marriage, or her own?
2. How did Dr. Fox's feelings about Carmen affect her view of Manuel? Did her sympathies for Manuel lead to her sharing details of her own marriage? Did she serve Carmen's best interest as her client at every point?
3. Does Dr. Fox believe she did whatever she could to help Carmen and Manuel's marriage? Did she think that Carmen's grasp of the situation was realistic or correct? Did she advise Carmen to think through carefully whether or not ending therapy was correct? If Dr. Fox does not conclude she did quality work with this couple, how will this affect her subsequent work as a psychologist?
4. How will a relationship with Manuel be viewed by both ex-spouses? Will Dr. Fox be seen as an unscrupulous practitioner? Will it sow more conflict between the former couples? Will it lead to a complaint against Dr. Fox?

Ethical Course of Action

Directive per APA Code

If Dr. Fox mistakenly considers her relationship with Manuel as collateral in nature, and does not define Manuel as a client, then Dr. Fox could reason that she has not violated Standard 10.06. Moreover, if Dr. Fox considers that her attitude toward Carmen and her attraction to Manuel have not compromised her objectivity, then Dr. Fox could reason that she is not in violation of Standard 3.05. It is quite likely that Carmen would feel betrayed by Dr. Fox once Carmen discovered Manuel is involved in a romantic relationship with her former marriage counselor. The harm done to Carmen would have been due to Dr. Fox's violation of Standards 3.05 and 10.08 (a) and the intent of Principle B.

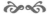

Dictates of One's Own Conscience

If you were Carmen and you discover that Manuel is dating Dr. Fox, which of these would you do?

1. Reason that it is one more example of how Manuel is inconsiderate, and proceed with a divorce.
2. Ask Manuel whether his feelings for Dr. Fox started when they were in therapy.
3. Write a letter to Dr. Fox telling her how you feel about her dating Manuel, especially when you and Manuel are not even divorced.
4. File a complaint against Dr. Fox for unethical practice.
5. Combinations of the above-listed actions.
6. Or one that is not listed above.

If you were Dr. Fox practicing in Lithuania, would you

1. Refer both Carmen and Manuel, once you ascertained that you were averse to Carmen and attracted to Manuel?
2. Avoided this situation by following Lithuania's code and not reveal any personal information about yourself to Manuel, as it is not clinically relevant or prudent?
3. Refer Manuel to a different therapist, disclosing your attraction to him?
4. Refer Manuel to a different therapist, disclosing only a conflict of interest in continuing therapy with him?

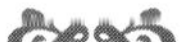

STANDARD 10.07: THERAPY WITH FORMER SEXUAL PARTNERS

> Psychologists do not accept as therapy clients/patients persons with whom they have engaged in sexual intimacies.

A CASE FOR STANDARD 10.07: We'll Always Have Rome

Dr. Armstrong, a resident training for his degree in family practice medicine, met Dr. Carpenter, a clinical psychologist, at an international convention in Rome. The conference theme was collaborative treatment of care providers for terminally ill patients. Drs. Armstrong and Carpenter discovered that they were both scheduled to return to the United States a day after the convention ends. They decided to spend the day together exploring Rome. The day was filled with exciting adventures and ended with a kiss—and exchanges of contact information with a parting line of "Call me if you ever visit my town."

Two years later, Dr. Carpenter receives a call from Dr. Armstrong. Dr. Armstrong has now moved across the country to the same town as Dr. Carpenter. Dr. Armstrong moved because his residency has ended and his wife got a very good job offer. Dr. Armstrong is having some problems adjusting to his wife's success and his feelings of isolation in a new town. Dr. Armstrong asks if Dr. Carpenter would accept him for individual psychotherapy to help with these life adjustments.

Issues of Concern

Standard 10.07 prohibits treating one's former sexual partner(s). The relevant ethical question is whether spending one day together that ends with a parting kiss meets the condition of having engaged in sexual intimacies. The clinical question is whether one is able to be objective with a person for whom one has had any sexual or romantic feelings, regardless of how brief or long-lived. Even if Dr. Carpenter does not now have any romantic interest in Dr. Armstrong, or vice versa, would it violate Standard 10.07 for her to accept him into treatment?

APA Ethics Code

Companion General Principle

Principle B: Fidelity and Responsibility

> Psychologists uphold professional standards of conduct, clarify their professional roles and obligations, accept appropriate responsibility for their behavior, and seek to manage conflicts of interest that could lead to exploitation or harm.

Principle B would have Dr. Carpenter examine her personal feelings toward Dr. Armstrong. Part of the examination needs to include an appraisal of her personal interest in Dr. Armstrong. Is she wishing for further relations with him in any capacity? Is she low on her client count and needs the extra income of a potentially full-paying client, and thus might reason that the relationship was so fleeting and so long ago that it is of no consequence now?

Companion Ethical Standard(s)

Standard 3.05: Multiple Relationships

> (a) A multiple relationship occurs when a psychologist is in a professional role with a person and (1) at the same time is in another role with the same person... A psychologist refrains from entering into a multiple relationship if the multiple relationship could reasonably be expected to impair the psychologist's objectivity ... in performing his or her functions as a psychologist... Multiple relationships that would not reasonably be expected to cause impairment or risk exploitation or harm are not unethical.

Dr. Carpenter was in a romantic relationship with Dr. Armstrong, albeit briefly. That brief romantic encounter established a connection between the two of them that still exists. Dr. Carpenter is now asked to enter into a professional relationship with Dr. Armstrong. If Dr. Carpenter consents to accept Dr. Armstrong into treatment, the condition for multiple relationship will have been met per Standard 3.05 (a) (1). Would having had a brief romantic encounter impair Dr. Carpenter's objectivity?

Standard 3.06: Conflict of Interest

> Psychologists refrain from taking on a professional role when personal ... relationships could reasonably be expected to (1) impair their objectivity, competence, or effectiveness in performing their functions as psychologists.

Standard 3.06 makes the same demand of Dr. Carpenter as Principle B in terms of self-examination. Then, based on the results of such self-examination, Standard 3.06 requires Dr. Carpenter not to accept Dr. Armstrong into treatment if there is any hint of conflict of interest on her part.

Legal Issues 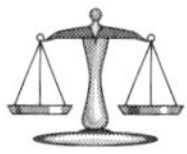

New Mexico

> *N.M. Code R. § 16.22.2.9 (2010). Impaired Objectivity and Dual Relationships.*
>
> B. Prohibited dual relationships.
>
> (1) The psychologist shall not undertake or continue a professional relationship with a client or patient when the objectivity or competency of the psychologist is compromised because of the psychologist's ... previous ... social, sexual, [or] emotional ... relationship with the client.

New York

> *N.Y. Comp. Codes R. & Regs. tit. 8, § 29.1 (2010). General Provisions.*
>
> b. Unprofessional conduct in the practice of any profession licensed ... shall include: ...
>
> 5. conduct in the practice of a profession which evidences moral unfitness to practice the profession.

In both jurisdictions, Dr. Carpenter's prior social relationship with Dr. Armstrong would result in her violating the laws that preclude multiple relationships. The laws of New Mexico clearly preclude Dr. Carpenter establishing a treatment relationship with a colleague with whom she had an earlier romantic relationship. New York's law raises the question about whether such boundary confusion would be evidence of moral unfitness. In light of the APA 10.07 standard, Dr. Carpenter's entering a treatment relationship with Dr. Armstrong would be considered an act of moral unfitness.

Cultural Considerations

Global Discussion

Lithuanian Psychological Association

> (g) Psychologist shall not enter into professional interaction or use psychological techniques if his/her own emotional factors may hinder professional or ethical interactions with clients. Psychologist shall not enter into professional interaction if:
>
> - he/she strongly dislikes client or is strongly attracted to client;
> - unsettled emotional conflicts of Psychologist may exercise influence upon client.

As in the previous vignette, Lithuania's code specifies that if a psychologist has unresolved emotional conflicts within themselves, these may exercise influence over that therapeutic relationship, and it is ill-advised for Dr. Carpenter to accept Dr. Armstrong as a client if she is still attracted to him.

American Moral Values

1. How does Dr. Carpenter classify her previous relationship to Dr. Armstrong? Was it a collegial relationship that had a fleeting romantic element, or was it mostly personal given the time they spent

together? Was the exchange of information and invitation to "look each other up" meant personally or professionally?

2. Does their sharing the day together present an obstacle for therapy? Did it cross a line of romantic intention that would be hard to undo as Dr. Armstrong's therapist? Or it is too long ago to refuse Dr. Armstrong treatment for his pain and suffering?
3. Is Dr. Armstrong calling on Dr. Carpenter because she is the only psychologist he knows in town? Does Dr. Carpenter believe he is desperate? Does he respect her as a professional, or is he reaching out based more on his personal connection to her?
4. How does Dr. Armstrong's marital status affect Dr. Carpenter's framing of her decision? Was Dr. Armstrong married when he and Dr. Carpenter met? If not, does the fact that Dr. Armstrong is having trouble in his marriage make their personal history more problematic or less problematic?
5. Does Dr. Carpenter have a special proficiency in issues like handling spousal success? Could she maintain a more professional stance if she had a therapeutic interest in his case? If Dr. Armstrong's problems are ones she feels she is the best in town at handling, is their previous contact enough to outweigh the help she could offer?
6. Should Dr. Carpenter recommend marriage counseling, given Dr. Armstrong's issues?

Ethical Course of Action

Directive per APA Code

Standard 10.07 is direct in its prohibition against accepting former romantic partners into treatment. Several questions need to be answered in the affirmative for Dr. Carpenter to violate Standard 10.07 if Armstrong entered into treatment with her. Examining the length of the encounter or the extent of sexual involvement may not answer the question of whether there were any sexual intimacies between Drs. Carpenter and Armstrong. Standard 3.05 (a) poses the criterion of whether their previous encounter would impair her clinical judgment, regardless of the previous relationship's brevity or her current feelings toward Dr. Armstrong. Given the nature of their previous relationship, even if Dr. Carpenter is now not interested in a romantic relationship with Dr. Armstrong, it is difficult to imagine that their previous encounter would not influence her clinical judgment of Dr. Armstrong.

Dictates of One's Own Conscience

If you were Dr. Carpenter, happily married for a year but in need of practice income, would you:

1. Determine the status of Dr. Armstrong's feelings toward you now?
2. Discuss the situation with your husband before making a decision?
3. Assess the probability of future encounters with Dr. Armstrong in other professional settings?
4. Protect yourself from complications, regardless of how much you might need the money now, and refuse to accept Armstrong as a client?
5. Combinations of the above-listed possible courses of action?
6. Or one that is not listed above?

If you were Dr. Carpenter practicing in Lithuania, would you explain to Dr. Armstrong that your previous romantic relationship makes it impossible for him to be your client, and offer him several referrals to colleagues?

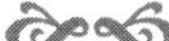

STANDARD 10.08: SEXUAL INTIMACIES WITH FORMER THERAPY CLIENTS/PATIENTS

> (a) Psychologists do not engage in sexual intimacies with former clients/patients for at least two years after cessation or termination of therapy.

A CASE FOR STANDARD 10.08 (A): A Relationship Dance

Dr. Weaver attends a "Gay Salsa" class every Thursday night. She goes for exercise rather than the romantic connections that happen in the class. However, on this day Dr. Weaver finds herself attracted to Wendy. They exchange contact information and Dr. Weaver hopes Wendy will call, which she does. However, Wendy's call is for treatment, not for a date. Wendy requests treatment for her generalized anxiety. Dr. Weaver reasons that the meeting and attraction to Wendy were very fleeting, and Dr. Weaver does need to build up her practice so as to increase her income; Dr. Weaver therefore sets an appointment with Wendy.

Halfway into the session, Dr. Weaver realizes that her attraction to Wendy is not mild, that it is interfering with her objectivity, and that ethically Dr. Weaver should not engage in therapy with Wendy. Dr. Weaver stops the session and tells Wendy that she is too attracted to her as a possible romantic partner to be her treating psychologist. Dr Weaver then refunds Wendy's co-pay, does not charge for the session, and ends the therapeutic relationship. The next day, Dr. Weaver gets another call from Wendy; this time it is for dinner and a movie.

Issues of Concern

Standard 10.08 (a) prohibits sexual intimacies with former clients for 2 years after termination of treatment. The relevant question for this situation is whether half of an unsuccessful session of therapy renders Wendy a therapy client.

It is difficult to determine the intensity of one's attraction from a fleeting encounter at a dance class. Based on this reasoning, Dr. Weaver accepted Wendy into treatment. Of related concern that was not considered by Dr. Weaver is the high probability of multiple relationships should both Dr. Weaver and Wendy continue to attend the Thursday Night Gay Salsa.

Now that treatment has ended and Wendy has called for a date, of relevant concern is whether Wendy was unduly influenced by that treatment encounter to consider Dr. Weaver as a romantic partner, or whether that brief therapeutic encounter gave Dr. Weaver sufficient information about Wendy to render any future equal-status relationship impossible.

APA Ethics Code

Companion General Principle

Principle A: Beneficence and Nonmaleficence

> Because psychologists' . . . actions may affect the lives of others, they are alert to and guard against personal . . . factors that might lead to misuse of their influence.

Principle A calls Dr. Weaver's attention to the fact that whatever she does will have some type of effect on Wendy. In choosing her actions, Principle A suggests Dr. Weaver will be alert to potential harm to Wendy generated by her personal situation. It seems two personal items have already affected Wendy—one being Dr. Weaver's need for clientele and the other being Dr. Weaver's attraction to Wendy.

Companion Ethical Standard(s)

Standard 3.05: Multiple Relationships

> . . . (b) If a psychologist finds that, due to unforeseen factors, a potentially harmful multiple relationship has arisen, the psychologist takes reasonable steps to resolve it with due regard for the best interests of the affected person and maximal compliance with the Ethics Code.

Unforeseen by Dr. Weaver was the intensity of her attraction to Wendy. But once that awareness had arisen, Standard 3.05 (b) requires that Dr. Weaver take steps to resolve the multiple relationship in favor of Wendy's interests.

Standard 3.08: Exploitative Relationships

> Psychologists do not exploit persons over whom they have . . . authority such as clients.

Dr. Weaver has made an effort to mitigate her personal conflict of interest with Wendy by choosing not to engage in treatment. Could her admission of attraction to Wendy be so seductive that it virtually invited the second phone call for a date? If so, then Dr. Weaver could be said to have used her authority as a treating psychologist to exploit the situation for a date with Wendy.

Standard 10.08: Sexual Intimacies With Former Therapy Clients/Patients

> Psychologists who engage in such activity after the two years following cessation . . . of therapy . . . bear the burden of demonstrating that there has been no exploitation, in light of all relevant factors, including . . .
>
> (1) the amount of time that has passed since therapy terminated . . . (2) the nature, duration, and intensity of the therapy . . . (3) the circumstances of termination . . . (4) the client's/patient's personal history . . . (5) the client's/patient's current mental status . . . (6) the likelihood of adverse impact on the client/patient . . . and (7) any statements or actions made by the therapist during the course of therapy suggesting or inviting the possibility of a post-termination sexual or romantic relationship with the client/patient.

If Dr. Weaver's brief session with Wendy is considered a therapeutic encounter, then Standard 10.08 (b) would apply to deciding whether she accepts Wendy's invitation for a date.

Legal Issues 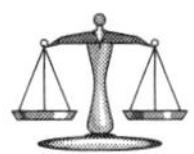

Ohio

> *Ohio Admin. Code 4732:17-01 (2010).*
>
> (C) Welfare of the client:
>
> (13) Unforeseen multiple relationships. If a psychologist . . . determines that, due to unforeseen factors, a prohibited multiple relationship has developed[,] . . . she shall take reasonable steps to resolve it with due regard for the welfare of the person(s) with whom there . . . was a professional psychological role. . .
>
> (E) Multiple relationships. A multiple relationship exists when a psychologist . . . is in another relationship with the same person. . .
>
> (2) Prohibited multiple relationships. The board prescribes that certain multiple relationships are expressly prohibited due to inherent risks of exploitation, impaired judgment by clients[,] . . . and/or impaired judgment, competence or objectivity of the psychologist. . .
>
> (c) A psychologist or school psychologist shall not:
>
> (i) Engage in sexual intercourse or other sexual intimacies; or, verbal or nonverbal conduct that is sexual in nature with any person with whom there has been a professional psychological role at any time within the previous twenty-four months. . .
>
> (e) The prohibitions established in paragraphs (E)(2)(b) and (E)(2)(c) of this rule extend indefinitely beyond twenty-four months after termination of the professional role if the person, secondary to emotional, mental, or cognitive impairment, remains vulnerable to exploitative influence.

Pennsylvania

> *49 Pa. Code § 41.61 (2010). Code of Ethics.*
>
> Principle 6. Welfare of the consumer.
>
> (b) Psychologists are continually cognizant of their own needs and their inherently powerful position vis a vis clients . . . in order to avoid exploiting their trust and dependency. Psychologists make every effort to avoid dual relationships with clients or relationships which might impair their professional judgment or increase the risk of exploitation. . . Sexual intimacies with clients are unethical.

In both jurisdictions, Dr. Weaver would be in violation of the laws if after ending her clinical relationship with Wendy, however brief, she then allowed the relationship to change to a dating relationship. Wendy sought Dr. Weaver out in the role of a psychologist, and Dr. Weaver wisely ended the relationship because of her emerging countertransference. Dr. Weaver could not then enter into a romantic relationship that is precluded by the laws.

Cultural Considerations

Global Discussion

Canadian Code of Ethics for Psychologists

> Principle II: Responsible caring.
>
> II.27. Be acutely aware of the power relationship in therapy and, therefore, not encourage or engage in sexual intimacy with therapy clients, neither during therapy, nor for that period of time following therapy during which the power relationship reasonably could be expected to influence the client's personal decision making.

If Dr. Weaver and Wendy live in Canada, the responsibility falls on Dr. Weaver to refrain from having an intimate relationship with Wendy for as long as there remains an imbalance in the power dynamics of their relationship. Although their therapeutic relationship lasted for only half of one session, nonetheless it may be assumed that during that session, Wendy fully believed and acted upon her understanding of Dr. Weaver as her psychologist, not her friend or potential partner. When a client puts him- or herself in the therapeutic role and begins working with a psychologist, even for one session, it can be argued that a power differential between the client and psychologist exists. Where Canada's code on this point differs from many is that it does not specify a minimum amount of time that a psychologist must wait before initiating intimacy with a former client. Canada's code, rather, holds the psychologist accountable to the power dynamics of the therapeutic relationship itself, and primarily to the protection of the client. It is possible that the power differential may cease to be influential rather quickly in Dr. Weaver and Wendy's situation, and therefore Dr. Weaver could ethically accept Wendy's invitation after discussion of this issue. It is also possible in other situations that even after the oft-prescribed

"2-year waiting period," such a power differential remains that no intimate relationship between the client and his or her former therapist is possible without risking harm to the client.

American Moral Values

1. How does Dr. Weaver sort out the personal and professional lines with Wendy before deciding what to do next? Her first contact with Wendy was personal. Even though she considered it "fleeting," was it enough of a personal connection to rule out therapy?

2. Even though Wendy now seems interested in Dr. Weaver, how does she believe Dr. Weaver acted? Does she believe that Dr. Weaver accepted her request for treatment at least partially out of romantic interest? Were Dr. Weaver's actions above-board from Wendy's perspective? Could Dr. Weaver's actions negatively affect Wendy's opinion of therapy and psychologists?

3. How does Dr. Weaver interpret the sequence of Wendy's actions? Why would Wendy ask her out after initially asking her for treatment? Why did she prefer a professional relationship first? Should Dr. Weaver consider possible issues around therapy, authority, and power that Wendy is working through before entering into a romantic relationship?

4. Knowing that Wendy has generalized anxiety, to what degree should Dr. Weaver help Wendy find other means of treatment? Can she refer her to other professionals and resources? What if these referrals (perhaps to a rival) somehow conflict with Dr. Weaver's desire to be with Wendy? Will she sacrifice the quality of her advice in order to maintain a connection to Wendy? Does that violate her professional duty?

Ethical Course of Action

Directive per APA Code

Psychologists obtain referrals from a variety of sources. Some of those sources may be chance encounters at dance classes. Once Dr. Weaver makes the decision to accept Wendy as a client, she should not engage in any interactions that may lead to sexual intimacies (Principle A and Standard 3.05). Once Wendy engages in treatment with Dr. Weaver, no matter how brief, she is a client. Standard 10.08 (a) prohibits Dr. Weaver from sexual intimacies with Wendy for 2 years post termination. For Dr. Weaver to accept Wendy's invitation for dinner and a movie would violate the directive of Standard 3.08. If Dr. Weaver and Wendy meet up again in 2 years, Dr. Weaver would need to meet all the requirements of Standard 10.08 (b) to engage ethically in any type of romantic relationship with Wendy.

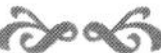

Dictates of One's Own Conscience

If you were Dr. Weaver, unencumbered and able to freely enter into a romantic relationship, what would you do in response to Wendy's invitation for dinner and a movie?

1. Reason that the therapeutic encounter was sufficiently brief to constitute a very casual relationship; decline the invitation to dinner, but say that you will see her at Thursday Gay Salsa dance class?

2. Reason that the attraction is sufficiently strong that you cannot risk further contact; decline the invitation to dinner and look for another dance group?

3. Explain to Wendy the nature and reason for the ethics code, and invite her to call you in 2 years should she wish to explore a further relationship?

4. Combinations of the above-listed actions?

5. Or one that is not listed above?

If you were Dr. Weaver, practicing in Canada, would you:

1. Decline the date with Wendy, citing your therapeutic relationship of one session and your strong feelings for Wendy?

2. Decline the date with Wendy, citing the likely power imbalance between you because of your previous therapeutic relationship?

3. Tell Wendy that when that imbalance has been resolved to your mutual satisfaction, you would be free to date her?

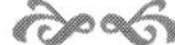

STANDARD 10.08 (B): SEXUAL INTIMACIES WITH FORMER THERAPY CLIENTS/PATIENTS

. . . (b) Psychologists do not engage in sexual intimacies with former clients/patients even after a two-year interval except in the most unusual circumstances. Psychologists who engage in such activity after the two years following cessation or termination of therapy and of having no sexual contact with the former client/patient bear the burden of demonstrating that there has been no exploitation, in light of all relevant factors, including (1) the amount of time that has passed since therapy terminated; (2) the nature, duration, and intensity of the therapy; (3) the circumstances of termination; (4) the client's/patient's personal history; (5) the client's/patient's current mental status; (6) the likelihood of adverse impact on the client/patient; and (7) any statements or actions made by the therapist during the course of therapy suggesting or inviting the possibility of a post-termination sexual or romantic relationship with the client/patient.

A CASE FOR STANDARD 10.08 (B): Kissing Cousins

Dr. Greene is treating 16-year-old Victoria, who, after experiencing sexual assault, ran away from home. The home situation is very difficult, so 3 months into treatment, Dr. Greene facilitates a foster care placement for Victoria. Victoria moves in with Kim, who is Victoria's mother's cousin. Victoria and Kim engage in family sessions once a month to address any relationship difficulties. During the course of treatment, Dr. Greene and Kim are clearly mutually attracted but neither acts on this attraction. After a year and a half of treatment, Victoria successfully enters college. During the school holidays, Victoria returns to her mother's home, and she sees Dr. Greene for occasional therapy sessions during that first year of school.

Three years after her last treatment session with Dr. Greene, and with much gratitude, Victoria invites Dr. Greene to her college graduation party. Dr. Greene meets up with Kim at the graduation party. They remember their mutual attraction for each other and begin dating.

Issues of Concern

Standard 10.08 (b) allows for relationships, including ones of sexual intimacy, with former clients under some circumstances. The allowable circumstances suggest the relationship could resume as a romance 2 years post termination of the therapy relationship. This case is 3 years post termination, no previous sexual contact had occurred, Dr. Greene and Kim never acted on their attraction, Dr. Greene's treatment relationship to Kim was distant, and no circumstances arose that suggested exploitation.

However, is it possible that once Dr. Greene is in a relationship with Kim, he could use his prior knowledge and authority to exploit family situations for Kim's benefit? The exploration of factors enumerated in Standard 10.08 (b) can be focused on two different people, on Kim and on Victoria. Should Standard 10.08 (b) apply only to Victoria since she was the identified client? Or should Standard 10.08 (b) apply also to Kim since at one point she could be considered as in some way a client of Dr. Greene? Or should Dr. Greene never have accepted Victoria's invitation to the graduation party, thus circumventing any of the ensuing complications?

APA Ethics Code

Companion General Principles

Principle A: Beneficence and Nonmaleficence

> Because psychologists' . . . actions may affect the lives of others, they are alert to and guard against personal . . . factors that might lead to misuse of their influence.

Principle A suggests that Dr. Greene think through the consequences of his actions, such as the potential of undue influence within Victoria's extended family because of his private knowledge yielded from years of therapy with various members of the family.

Principle B: Fidelity and Responsibility

> Psychologists . . . seek to manage conflicts of interest that could lead to exploitation or harm.

Principle B guides Dr. Greene to manage his very personal wish to pursue an intimate relationship with Kim and the professional directive to avoid situations where there is high potential for exploitation of Victoria's family.

Companion Ethical Standard(s)

Standard 10.08: Sexual Intimacies With Former Therapy Clients/Patients

> (a) Psychologists do not engage in sexual intimacies with former clients/patients for at least two years after cessation or termination of therapy.

It has been 3 years since Dr. Greene provided treatment to Victoria and 4 years since Kim has been in treatment as a collateral contact. Thus, 10.08 (a) does not apply.

Standard 3.05: Multiple Relationships

> (a) A multiple relationship occurs when a psychologist is in a professional role with a person and . . .
>
> (2) at the same time is in a relationship with a person closely associated with or related to the person with whom the psychologist has the professional relationship. . . A psychologist refrains from entering into a multiple relationship if the multiple relationship . . . risks exploitation or harm to the person with whom the professional relationship exists. Multiple relationships that would not reasonably be expected to cause impairment or risk exploitation or harm are not unethical.

After such a long treatment relationship, Victoria will probably always consider Dr. Greene to be her treating psychologist with the possibility of reengaging in treatment as life circumstances dictate. As Dr. Greene pursues a romantic relationship with Kim, he enters into multiple relationships with Kim as defined in Standard 3.05 (a) (2). The criteria for allowable multiple relationships are that the presence of the relationship does not cause impairment or risk exploitation or harm. By entering into a romantic relationship with his client after conducting a successful therapeutic relationship, Dr. Greene models for Victoria another failure of boundaries. He served as a healthy adult role model in her life during a period when her parents and other adults were failing her. Victoria already has endured the failure of parental boundaries and probably remains vulnerable in other significant relationships. Will the knowledge of his personal life and prior relationship with her as her treating psychologist affect Victoria's developmental tasks? Dr. Greene also will not be able to provide treatment for Victoria in the future. In both instances, Dr. Greene risks harming Victoria. In addition, a further risk of harm exists because it is unpredictable how Victoria may react to Dr. Greene's presence at future family events. After such a long, successful treatment relationship, Dr. Greene is bound to hold a great deal of influence over Victoria and her family. Should Dr. Greene become involved in a family dispute by virtue of his relationship with Kim, it would be natural to expect his sympathies to lie with Kim. Taking Kim's side in any family conflict may result in undue influence and also could be viewed as possibly exploitative.

Standard 4.01: Maintaining Confidentiality

> Psychologists have a primary obligation and take reasonable precautions to protect confidential information.

The privilege to let other people know that Victoria has been in psychotherapy with Dr. Greene is Victoria's to release. She invited Dr. Greene to the graduation party without coercion from him. However, who is to say that in a romantic relationship with Kim, he will not inadvertently let slip some piece of information that was obtained in therapy with Victoria?

Legal Issues 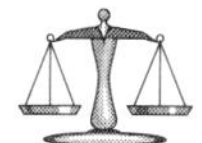

South Carolina

> *S.C. Code Ann. Regs. 100-4 (2010). Code of Ethics.*
>
> D. Impaired objectivity and dual relationships.
>
> (3) Prohibited dual relationships.
>
> (a) The psychologist, in interacting with . . . a person to whom the psychologist has at any time within the previous 24 months rendered . . . professional psychological services for the treatment or amelioration of emotional distress or behavioral inadequacy, shall not:
>
> (i) Engage in any verbal or physical behavior toward him/her which is sexually seductive, demeaning, or harassing; or
>
> (ii) Engage in sexual intercourse or other physical intimacies with him/her. . .
>
> (b) The prohibitions set out in (a) above shall not be subject to the 24-month limitation and shall extend indefinitely if the client is proven to be clearly vulnerable, by reason of emotional or cognitive disorder, to exploitative influence by the psychologist.

Texas

> *22 Tex. Admin. Code § 465.1 (2010). Definitions.*
>
> (2) "Dual Relationship" means a situation where a licensee and another individual have both a professional relationship and a non-professional relationship. Dual relationships include, but are not limited to . . . sexual relationships.
>
> *22 Tex. Admin. Code § 465.17 (2010). Therapy and Counseling.*
>
> (a) Imbalances of Power.
>
> (3) Licensees do not engage in sexual relationships with . . . any former . . . client over whom they have actual or perceived power or undue influence created through a therapeutic relationship.

Both South Carolina and Texas would consider whether Dr. Greene engaged in exploitation with Kim or whether Kim is vulnerable to being exploited. South Carolina law also calls for at least 2 years to have elapsed before the psychologist could explore a romantic relationship with a client. Based on the facts of this vignette, it is unlikely that either jurisdiction would charge Dr. Greene with violating the laws.

Cultural Considerations

Global Discussion

Code of Ethics: Netherlands

> III.1.3.8 Responsibility after termination of the professional relationship.
>
> The psychologist takes into account that after formal termination of a professional relationship there may still be a conflict of interests or an imbalance of power between himself and those involved, and that consequently his professional obligation towards those involved does not come to an end just like that.
>
> III.1.3.9 Personal relationship after termination of the professional relationship.
>
> In engaging in a personal relationship after termination of the professional relationship, the psychologist makes sure that the previous professional relationship does not have a disproportionate significance anymore. If it concerns a sexual relationship, the psychologist has the responsibility to show, if he is asked to do so, that he observed all carefulness which could be required from him, being a professional psychologist.

If Dr. Greene is practicing in the Netherlands, his responsibility to both Kim and Victoria remains even after therapy has ended, and he needs to be aware of the remaining power imbalance between them, which does not end automatically with the ending of the therapeutic relationship. Further, if he is pursuing a sexual or romantic relationship with Kim, he would need to be able to demonstrate that their therapeutic relationship does not have a "disproportionate significance" any longer, and that his therapy with Victoria does not still place him in a position of power over either one of them. What would occur, for example, if Victoria is attacked and raped at a college party, and is re-traumatized, and asks Dr. Greene for therapy again? If he should comply, what effects would that have on his relationship with both Victoria and Kim? If he refuses, and angers Kim by not helping Victoria, how would he resolve the conflict between his personal interests and professional obligations? When does a client cease being a client, especially an adolescent who may yet need therapeutic assistance? Would Dr. Greene accidentally reveal confidential information between Victoria and Kim without intending to, assuming it would be permissible, as it was "all in the family" now? Any one of these possibilities would necessitate Dr. Greene's vigilance in avoiding the previous power differential between himself and Kim and Victoria, from remaining significant, and disproportionate, long after therapy itself has ended.

American Moral Values

1. How should Dr. Greene view his professional relationships with Victoria and Kim? Are the family sessions completely over? Does he believe Victoria is phasing out of treatment, and that his dating Kim will mean the end of his work with Victoria?
2. What will it say to clients or clients of other psychologists that Dr. Greene is dating a former client? Is Dr. Greene threatening his career and reputation? Is he doing damage to the reputation of the profession?
3. Are Dr. Greene and Kim wise to date, given the therapeutic work they have done together with Victoria? How will that former relationship affect the power dynamics and communication between the two? Has Dr. Greene considered how to make the transition to personally participating in this family?
4. Is Dr. Greene open to his relationship with Kim becoming permanent? Can he become a co-guardian of Victoria (though she will be an adult) after being her therapist? How will that work?
5. Would Victoria, Kim, or Dr. Greene look back at their work in a new light now? Would Victoria eventually believe Dr. Greene had ulterior motives in the way he treated their situation and that yet again, a significant person in her life had failed her?

Ethical Course of Action

Directive per APA Code

Standard 10.08 (b) allows Dr. Greene to date Kim after 2 years have passed from the date of termination, per Standard 10.08 (a), if he can demonstrate no exploitation of Kim in the pursuit of the intimate relationship. It has been 3 years without any contact between

Dr. Greene and Kim. The primary therapeutic relationship was with Victoria, a distant cousin to Kim. The case terminated successfully and without involvement of Kim in the last year of the therapeutic relationship with Victoria. Even though there was mutual attraction between Dr. Greene and Kim, Dr. Greene did not engage in any obvious actions in regard to the attraction. And Kim is not in a vulnerable state where she could not rebuff Dr. Greene's romantic advances. It appears that Dr. Greene is able to meet the conditions outlined in Standard 10.08 (b) and thus is ethically able to pursue a sexually intimate relationship with Kim.

Dr. Greene and Kim pursuing a romantic relationship appears quite different when viewed from Victoria's perspective. The potential for harm (Principles A and B) is great because of the possibility of the romantic relationship eventually being viewed as one in which exploitation occurred, per Principle 3.05 (a).

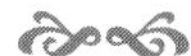

Dictates of One's Own Conscience

If you were a psychology colleague sharing office space and in a consultation group with Dr. Greene, which of these would you do?

1. Think that Dr. Greene has been alone for so many years that it is nice he has now found someone to date.
2. Think that Dr. Greene is getting desperate and will date anyone, even former clients.
3. Be alarmed about Dr. Greene's poor clinical judgment and loose professional boundaries.
4. Talk to Dr. Greene privately about the potential ethical violations.
5. Report Dr. Greene for sexual misconduct.
6. Combinations of the above-listed actions.
7. Or one that is not listed above.

If you were Dr. Greene, practicing in the Netherlands, would you:

1. Discuss the possibility of pursuing a romantic relationship with Kim with both Kim and Victoria, in order to ascertain how influential your multiple relationship from the past may be? Tell Victoria that you won't be able to treat her as her psychologist any longer if the relationship between you and Kim unfolds?
2. Tell Kim that your first allegiance is to Victoria, your client, and that you cannot risk harm to her by becoming part of her family by dating her cousin, and so you tell Kim you cannot continue to see her romantically?

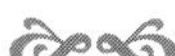

STANDARD 10.09: INTERRUPTION OF THERAPY

When entering into employment or contractual relationships, psychologists make reasonable efforts to provide for orderly and appropriate resolution of responsibility for client/patient care in the event that the employment or contractual relationship ends, with paramount consideration given to the welfare of the client/patient.

A CASE FOR STANDARD 10.09: Contractual Agreements

Dr. Chavez specialized in geriatric care when in graduate school and is happy to obtain a job with Care Ways. Care Ways contracts with nursing homes to provide allied care, which includes psychologists, physicians, social workers, nutritionists, physical therapists, and chaplains. Care Ways has assigned Dr. Chavez to four nursing homes. He makes routine rounds to these four nursing homes and has established ongoing therapeutic relationships with the residents. In one of the weekly administrative supervision sessions, Dr. Chavez is told that Care Ways has renegotiated contracts with three of his assigned nursing homes. These new contracts do not include provision of psychological services. Dr. Chavez will continue with his job at the one nursing home and may be called back if contracts are signed with other nursing homes. The new contract takes effect the first of the month, which is 1 week away.

Issues of Concern

Dr. Chavez is employed by Care Ways. Standard 10.09 requires that Dr. Chavez establish a client termination plan at the onset of his work with Care Ways. In all probability, Dr. Chavez did not negotiate a clinical exit strategy with Care Ways when he started work at each of the nursing homes. It appears that Dr. Chavez is taken by surprise at the termination of not only his work with the nursing home clients, but also of his own employment. Once having experienced the loss of a contract on such short notice, probabilities are high that he would now discuss a clinical exit strategy for the one nursing home where he will continue to work.

If, for some reason, he does not visit each of the nursing homes on a weekly basis, he might not have an opportunity to make even one last visit. What should he do now that he is given 1 week to wrap up his work with three different nursing homes?

APA Ethics Code

Companion General Principle

Principle A: Beneficence and Nonmaleficence

> When conflicts occur among psychologists' obligations or concerns, they attempt to resolve these conflicts in a responsible fashion that avoids or minimizes harm.

It is Dr. Chavez's responsibility to provide treatment, and when necessary, appropriately end the treatment relationship. It is also Dr. Chavez's obligation to comply with the terms of his employment. In this particular situation at the specific time, these two responsibilities are in conflict. Principle A tells Dr. Chavez to be guided by the value of harm reduction for patients as he negotiates a resolution.

Principle E: Respect for People's Rights and Dignity

> Psychologists are aware that special safeguards may be necessary to protect the rights and welfare of persons or communities whose vulnerabilities impair autonomous decision making.

Most nursing home patients have little or no ability to acquire mental health services independent of those provided by their nursing home facility. The status of Dr. Chavez's clients, as residents of the nursing homes, leaves them in a vulnerable position in which the decision of whether to continue or terminate treatment with Dr. Chavez is not up to them. Principle E suggests Dr. Chavez would make the effort to protect mental health services for them as he negotiates his exit strategy with Care Ways.

Companion Ethical Standard(s)

Standard 3.10: Informed Consent

> (a) When psychologists . . . provide . . . therapy[,] . . . they obtain the informed consent of the individual. . .
>
> (b) For persons who are legally incapable of giving informed consent, psychologists nevertheless . . .
>
> (1) provide an appropriate explanation . . . (2) seek the individual's assent . . . (3) consider such persons' preferences and best interests . . . and (4) obtain appropriate permission from a legally authorized person.

Regardless of whether the nursing home patients are capable of giving consent, Standards 3.10 (a) and 3.10 (b) direct Dr. Chavez to have obtained informed consent for treatment.

Standard 10.01: Informed Consent to Therapy

> (a) When obtaining informed consent to therapy as required in Standard 3.10, Informed Consent, psychologists inform clients/patients as early as is feasible in the therapeutic relationship about the nature and anticipated course of therapy.

As a part of his obtaining informed consent, Dr. Chavez was required by Standard 10.01 to have explained the nature of the therapy relationship. This means the nursing home patients should already know that he is working for Care Ways, which contracts with the nursing home for him to come to the facility.

Standard 10.10: Terminating Therapy

> . . . (c) Except where precluded by the actions of clients/patients or third-party payors, prior to termination psychologists provide pre-termination counselling and suggest alternative service providers as appropriate.

In preparation for termination of therapy, Standard 10.10 requires Dr. Chavez to hold a pre-termination session and to refer if necessary. However, in this specific situation, Dr. Chavez is excused from this requirement because of the contractual agreement between the nursing homes and his employer, Care Ways.

Standard 1.03: Conflicts Between Ethics and Organizational Demands

> If the demands of an organization for whom they are working are in conflict with this Ethics Code, psychologists clarify the nature of the conflict, make known their

commitment to the Ethics Code, and take reasonable steps to resolve the conflict consistent with the General Principles and Ethical Standards of the Ethics Code.

As discussed under Principle A, Dr. Chavez might feel a conflict between his employer's right to assign work and the need to speak up for those vulnerable nursing home patients who are unable to protect their own rights to autonomous decision making (Principle E). There may be an internal pull to call upon the directives of Standard 1.03 by voicing his objection to such an abrupt notice of termination. Are there grounds to argue that any part of the enforceable standards of the ethics code has been violated?

Legal Issues 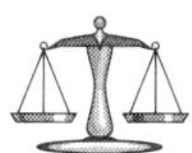

Virginia

18 Va. Admin. Code § 125-20-150 (2010). Standards of Practice.

A. The protection of the public health, safety, and welfare and the best interest of the public shall be the primary guide in determining the appropriate professional conduct of all persons whose activities are regulated by the board. Psychologists respect the rights, dignity and worth of all people, and are mindful of individual differences.

B. Persons licensed by the board shall: . . .

5. Avoid harming patients . . . for whom they provide professional services and minimize harm when it is foreseeable and unavoidable. . .

10. Make reasonable efforts to provide for continuity of care when services must be interrupted or terminated.

Washington

Wash. Admin. Code § 246-924-359 (2009). Client Welfare.

(2) Termination of services. Whenever professional services are terminated, the psychologist shall offer to help locate alternative sources of professional services or assistance if necessary.

In both jurisdictions, Dr. Chavez is directed to provide appropriate termination sessions to all of his ongoing clients. In both jurisdictions, the laws suggest that Dr. Chavez should offer assistance in finding substitute services if he cannot work out how to provide continuity of care for each of his clients at the three nursing homes where psychological services are being discontinued.

Cultural Considerations

Global Discussion

Canadian Code of Ethics for Psychologists

Principle II: Responsible caring.

II.32. Provide a client, if appropriate and if desired by the client, with reasonable assistance to find a way to receive needed services in the event that third-party payments are exhausted and the client cannot afford the fees involved.

II.33. Maintain appropriate contact, support, and responsibility for caring until a colleague or other professional begins service, if referring a client to a colleague or other professional.

II.34. Give reasonable notice and be reasonably assured that discontinuation will cause no harm to the client, before discontinuing services.

Dr. Chavez, through no fault of his own, is about to be in violation of the intent and letter of Principle II: Responsible Caring. If the renegotiated contract with the three nursing homes is considered to be an exhaustion of third-party payments, and the nursing home clients cannot afford to pay therapy fees, Dr. Chavez would then attempt to provide "reasonable assistance" to interested clients in securing needed services. This would mean that those nursing home residents who still desire psychological services would need Dr. Chavez's assistance in locating appropriate and affordable services in his absence. Further, if Dr. Chavez is making referrals to any other colleague or professional psychological service, he is obligated to maintain contact and support until the other services begin in order to ensure a smooth transition. Finally, Dr. Chavez would likely violate II.34, which demands that he give "reasonable notice" to his clients, and ensure that termination would do no harm before doing so; through no fault of his own, he has only 1 week in which to alert his clients to his pending absence, and attempt to determine any possible harm his discontinuation of therapy might cause.

American Moral Values

1. How does Dr. Chavez think of his clients at the three nursing homes now not being provided with services? What does he owe them? Does he need to explain the contract situation? Would he consider

continuing his work pro bono? Would that be allowed of a Care Ways employee? Has he signed a non-compete provision as a Care Ways employee that precludes his legally continuing to provide services to nursing homes not covered by Care Ways?

2. Does Dr. Chavez believe the new contracts are unjust? Whose decision is it? What are the considerations that factor into it? Should he protest this decision?
3. How does this form of contracting affect Dr. Chavez's work? Will he be more reluctant or careful in committing to future clients? Can he continue to do work he can accept under these conditions?
4. How does the nursing home context affect Dr. Chavez's moral view of the situation? How do the particular challenges of geriatric care shape his client–therapist relationship?

Ethical Course of Action

Directive per APA Code

If Dr. Chavez had meticulously followed the directives of Standards 3.10 (a), 3.10 (b), and 10.01 (a), his nursing home clients would not be taken by surprise if one day he did not show up for his routine visit to their facility. Dr. Chavez had negotiated a clinical exit strategy with Care Ways at the onset of employment, as directed by Standard 10.09, both Care Ways and he would know what to expect and how best to ensure appropriate termination procedures. Indeed, if Dr. Chavez had followed the directives of these standards of the ethics code, there would be no need to respond to a complaint based on Standard 1.03.

Acting with due regard for Principle E, Dr. Chavez might discuss what can be done within the next week to care for nursing home residents who do not have the ability to enact autonomous decision making regarding mental health treatment.

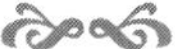

Dictates of One's Own Conscience

If you were Dr. Chavez and lacked the experience to negotiate an exit strategy, which of these would you do now?

1. Think Care Ways is callous to human suffering, and resolve to look for another job.
2. Think it is not your responsibility to ensure an appropriate termination procedure, and finish your week the best you can.
3. Offer the three nursing home residences pro bono work until appropriate termination and transition could be accomplished.
4. Negotiate with Care Ways extra time to hold appropriate pre-termination sessions with your clients in those three nursing homes.
5. Realize that hindsight is 20-20, and now negotiate a clinical exit strategy with Care Ways for the one remaining nursing home.
6. Combinations of the above-listed actions
7. Or one that is not listed above.

If you were Dr. Chavez, working for Care Ways in Canada, would you:

1. Attempt to provide each resident of the nursing homes a referral to a colleague; arrange crossover sessions for each client in order to ensure a smooth transition; and submit a bill for your hours of work to Care Ways, regardless of the contract?
2. Resolve to ensure that in the future, you will discuss termination and exit plans with all new therapy clients, apologize to your current clients, explain the situation, and offer to refer them to a colleague?

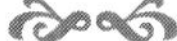

STANDARD 10.10: TERMINATING THERAPY

(a) Psychologists terminate therapy when it becomes reasonably clear that the client/patient no longer needs the service, is not likely to benefit, or is being harmed by continued service.

A CASE FOR STANDARD 10.10 (A): Strength in Numbers

Dr. Sims facilitates a 9-month-long closed women's midlife transition support group. There are eight members in this group, some of whom are divorcing, some entering their "empty nest" phase, and some who have histories of major depression. Three months into the group, it becomes clear that Sherry is seriously depressed.

Sherry's youngest child went to college the year before, and last month she and her husband separated. She has just been given notice that she will be laid off from work at the end of the year. During the session, Sherry talks about thoughts of wishing to end the pain. In the weeks that follow, Sherry has a few drinks too many one night and is killed when her car drives off an embankment. The next two sessions Dr. Sims devotes to explorations of her group's reaction to Sherry's death. The members exhibit a mixture of reactions. Regardless of the range of reactions, the group as a whole thinks Sherry committed suicide and has substantial difficulty moving beyond the guilt of being responsible for her death. It becomes clear that the group members were reinforcing each other's stuckness and guilt over Sherry's death.

Issues of Concern

Contending with an unexpected death is difficult at best. Dr. Sims is bound to suffer doubts about her own competency after Sherry's death when there is a possibility that the death was a suicide. In addition to managing her own emotions and thoughts, Dr. Sims needs to navigate and guide the inevitable difficulties in the group process and the emotional reactions of group members. Standard 10.10 (a) requires Dr. Sims to make a clinical judgment about whether the group itself could coalesce and start the healing process, or whether the continuation of the group hinders the members' ability to heal.

APA Ethics Code

Companion General Principle

Principle A: Beneficence and Nonmaleficence

> Psychologists strive to benefit those with whom they work and take care to do no harm. . . Because psychologists' . . . professional judgments and actions may affect the lives of others, they are alert to and guard against personal . . . factors that might lead to misuse of their influence. Psychologists strive to be aware of the possible effect of their own . . . mental health on their ability to help those with whom they work.

Sherry's death is bound to have an impact on Dr. Sims. Principle A suggests that Dr. Sims take care of her own psychological states so that her emotional state will not negatively impact her ability to work for the benefit of the group members.

Companion Ethical Standard(s)

Standard 2.01: Boundaries of Competence

> (a) Psychologists provide services . . . with populations . . . only within the boundaries of their competence, based on their education, training, supervised experience, consultation, study, or professional experience. . .
>
> (c) Psychologists planning to provide services . . . involving . . . areas . . . new to them undertake relevant education, training, supervised experience, consultation, or study.

Dr. Sims is no doubt retrospectively questioning her competence in providing treatment for clients who are suicidal. Of more immediate importance is her competence at conducting group therapy in which a member has met with an untimely death, one that leaves open the possibility that it might have been an accident/suicide. Upon which of the bases specified in Standard 2.01 (a) does Dr. Sims claim competency to conduct group treatment now? Should Dr. Sims find that she is working outside of her competence, per Standard 2.01 (b), how shall she best acquire the competencies needed to conduct group therapy in the current situation?

Standard 2.06: Personal Problems and Conflicts

> . . . (b) When psychologists become aware of personal problems that may interfere with their performing work-related duties adequately, they take appropriate measures, such as obtaining professional consultation or assistance, and determine whether they should limit, suspend, or terminate their work-related duties.

In compliance with the directives of Standard 2.06 (b), Dr. Sims needs to do something if her soul searching or reaction to Sherry's death interferes with her ability to provide treatment. How does Dr. Sims determine whether and when the group's conviction of Sherry's death is a suicide and whether their inability to appropriately process Sherry's death is an enactment of her own personal problems with Sherry's death?

Legal Issues 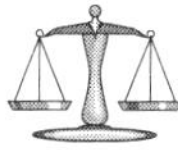

California

> *Cal. Bus. & Prof. Code § 1396 (West 2010). Competence.*
>
> A psychologist shall not function outside . . . her particular field . . . of competence as established by . . . her education, training and experience.

Cal. Bus. & Prof. Code § 1396.1. (West 2010). Interpersonal Relations.

It is recognized that a psychologist's effectiveness depends upon . . . her ability to maintain sound interpersonal relations, and that . . . problems in a psychologist's own personality may interfere with this ability and distort . . . her appraisals of others. A psychologist shall not knowingly undertake any activity in which . . . personal problems in the psychologist's personality integration may result in inferior professional services or harm to a patient or client. If a psychologist is already engaged in such activity when becoming aware of such personal problems[,] . . . she shall seek competent professional assistance to determine whether services to the patient or client should be continued or terminated.

Colorado

Colo. Rev. Stat. Ann. § 12-43-202 . (West 2010). Practice Outside of or Beyond Professional Training, Experience, or Competence.

Notwithstanding any other provision of this article, no licensee . . . psychotherapist is authorized to practice outside of or beyond . . . her area of training, experience, or competence.

Colo. Rev. Stat. Ann. § 12-43-222 .(West 2010). Prohibited Activities—Related Provisions.

(f) Has a . . . mental disability that renders such person unable to treat clients with reasonable skill and safety or that may endanger the health or safety of persons under such person's care . . .

(k) Has failed to terminate a relationship with a client when it was reasonably clear that the client was not benefiting from the relationship and is not likely to gain such benefit in the future . . .

(m) Has failed to obtain a consultation or perform a referral when the problem of the client is beyond such person's training, experience, or competence.

In both jurisdictions, as long as Dr. Sims remains competent to provide the group treatment for the impact of Sherry's suicide, Dr. Sims would comply with the laws. If for any reason Dr. Sims believed that she lacked the competence or experience sufficient to provide services to the group, she should obtain consultation, at a minimum.

Cultural Considerations

Global Discussion

Canadian Code of Ethics for Psychologists

Principle II: Responsible caring.

II.37. Terminate an activity when it is clear that the activity carries more than minimal risk of harm and is found to be more harmful than beneficial, or when the activity is no longer needed.

The first condition for termination of the group having been met, namely, that the continuation of the group carries more than minimal risk, Dr. Sims now needs to consider whether the group has become more harmful than helpful. If continuing is more harmful than helpful, she should begin to discuss ending the group in order to avoid further harm. If, however, termination of the group at this extraordinarily vulnerable time would lead to feelings of abandonment, betrayal, and loss for the members, then Dr. Sims should move to continue the group until the end of the 9 months or until the group is no longer necessary.

American Moral Values

1. How does Dr. Sims view her responsibility for the support group? To what degree can she help members mourn Sherry's death and resume full support for one another? Can the support group move on from the grieving process? Is their current discussion a kind of grieving, or is it a failure to mourn?
2. Does Dr. Sims agree with the idea that Sherry committed suicide? Does she owe it to the group to convince them it was not? Will she appear to be defending herself as the therapist by claiming it was not suicide? Will that undermine the group's trust in Dr. Sims?
3. How does the death of a group member affect the relationship between clients and therapist? Does Dr. Sims need to voice any personal grief or share her personal process of mourning? Would that build trust or erode the proper professional distance Dr. Sims needs to maintain?
4. How should Dr. Sims approach the group's "reinforcing" of one another's reactions to Sherry's death? Does this change the nature of Dr. Sims's treatment? How can she support their solidarity while pointing out a harmful group dynamic?

5. Do the group members all know the details of Sherry's death? Do Sherry's friends and family want this information shared with this group? Is there any information Dr. Sims is privy to that could be legitimately shared to help them?

Ethical Course of Action

Directive per APA Code

The question posed by Standard 10.10 (a) is whether Dr. Sims should terminate therapy with the group. Presuming Dr. Sims is not too personally impaired from Sherry's death to work (Standard 2.06), the decision for termination is to be made on the basis of Principle A: Beneficence and Nonmaleficence. Is Dr. Sims practicing within the boundaries of her competence, per Standard 2.01 (a), and thus capable of helping the group mourn and heal from the death of a group member? If Dr. Sims is not skilled enough to help the group mourn, is she capable of acquiring, as per Standard 2.01 (b), those skills quickly enough to be of benefit to the group members? Given the group's collective conviction that Sherry's death rests on their consciences, discontinuing meetings would most likely be harmful for the members.

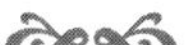

Dictates of One's Own Conscience

If you were Dr. Sims, trying to follow the directive of Standard 10.10 (a) and faced with your own doubts and seemingly intractable guilt in the group members, which of these would you do?

1. Contact Sherry's family to offer condolences and ask for more details of the car accident.
2. Contact the police department for the police report on Sherry's car accident.
3. Get supervision or therapy to process Sherry's death.
4. Get separate supervision on how best to provide group therapy in light of the development.
5. Consult a colleague on how best to proceed with the group.
6. Invite a colleague who is a skilled group therapist to cofacilitate the group.
7. Invite a colleague who specializes in suicide treatment to cofacilitate the group.
8. Discuss the pros and cons of ending the group with the group members.
9. Announce that you have decided the group is more harmful than helpful to the members now, and the group will stop meeting.
10. Combinations of the above-listed actions.
11. Or one that is not listed above.

If you were Dr. Sims running this group in Canada, you would consult with a colleague to help you determine whether continuing the group is more helpful than harmful for the group members.

STANDARD 10.10: TERMINATING THERAPY

. . . (b) Psychologists may terminate therapy when threatened or otherwise endangered by the client/patient or another person with whom the client/patient has a relationship.

A CASE FOR STANDARD 10.10 (B): Of Course I'll Keep Working With You

Through the support of Dr. Franklin, Sylvia was able to escape an abusive relationship and is now in a sequestered shelter with her two kids. She has filed for a protection order and is now beginning legal proceedings for divorce. Sylvia is worried that her soon-to-be-ex-husband, Marvin, may try to continue to harass her by intimidating Dr. Franklin since Marvin knows Sylvia is working with her. Sylvia does not want to end treatment, but tells Dr. Franklin that she would understand if she decided not to treat her. Dr. Franklin assures Sylvia that she will continue working with Sylvia through this difficult time in her life. A week after Sylvia moves into the shelter, Dr. Franklin finds a very nice card in her in-box at work. The envelope has Dr. Franklin's name with no address. Inside, the card reads,

Dear Dr. Franklin,

I really need to speak with you. I'm really concerned about where Sylvia has gone. I know you had something to do

> with this, and I know you know where she is. If you tell me where she is, get her back in your office, and fix this, then we'll be okay. By the way, I saw your son hanging out on the playground today with his friends—he looks like a nice kid.

The card is signed, "Marvin, beloved husband of Sylvia."

Issues of Concern

Standard 10.10 (b) allows Dr. Franklin to terminate therapy with Sylvia at this point, regardless of whether ending treatment with Dr. Franklin would harm Sylvia. Standard 10.10 (b) allows the psychologist to give as much weight to personal safety as she would give to clinical considerations. Dr. Franklin would be in compliance with her ethical obligation regardless of whether she decided to continue or to end treatment with Sylvia. Factors relevant to the decision for termination are whether it would be harmful to Sylvia if continuation of treatment led directly to some mishap befalling Dr. Franklin's child. Another factor is whether it would be harmful to Sylvia if Marvin were able to track her physical movements by watching Dr. Franklin's office. Would it be harmful to Sylvia if she saw that Dr. Franklin felt intimidated by Marvin? Would Sylvia give up her struggle for independence from her husband?

APA Ethics Code

Companion General Principle

Principle A: Beneficence and Nonmaleficence

> Psychologists strive to benefit those with whom they work and take care to do no harm. In their professional actions, psychologists seek to safeguard the welfare . . . of . . . other affected persons. When conflicts occur among psychologists' obligations or concerns, they attempt to resolve these conflicts in a responsible fashion that avoids or minimizes harm. . . Psychologists strive to be aware of the possible effect of their own mental health on their ability to help those with whom they work.

Principle A guides Dr. Franklin to continue working with a client for as long as the service is of benefit, or at least as long as it is not of harm. In this case, it is difficult to determine what would be harmful to Sylvia. Certainly having the safety of her child threatened is harmful to Dr. Franklin.

Principle B: Fidelity and Responsibility

> Psychologists uphold professional standards of conduct[,] . . . accept appropriate responsibility for their behavior, and seek to manage conflicts of interest that could lead to exploitation or harm.

What is the industry standard of conduct in such a situation? The conflict in this situation is between Dr. Franklin's responsibility as a mother to protect her child and her responsibility as a clinical psychologist to be of benefit to and not harm her client.

Companion Ethical Standard(s)

Standard 3.04: Avoiding Harm

> Psychologists take reasonable steps to avoid harming their clients/patients . . . and others with whom they work, and to minimize harm where it is foreseeable and unavoidable.

It may be harmful for Sylvia to witness the debilitating fear Dr. Franklin experiences if Dr. Franklin worries about the safety of her child. Depending on the age of Dr. Franklin's child and depending on the school's security, Dr. Franklin's fear for her child's safety may be sufficiently low so as not to impact treatment. Regardless of Dr. Franklin's mental status, Sylvia may come to harm by simply coming to Dr. Franklin's office for treatment, and the police not reacting swiftly to Sylvia's 9-1-1 cell phone call about Marvin violating the protective order. Marvin knows Sylvia will eventually come for an appointment with Dr. Franklin. To find Sylvia, all Marvin needs to do is to watch Dr. Franklin's office until Sylvia appears for a treatment session.

Standard 10.10: Terminating Therapy

> (a) Psychologists terminate therapy when it becomes reasonably clear that the client/patient . . . is being harmed by continued service.

Should Dr. Franklin and Sylvia decide that the risk of being found by Marvin is of more harm than the benefit Sylvia receives from treatment with Dr. Franklin, Standard 10.10 (a) directs Dr. Franklin to terminate therapy with Sylvia.

Standard 2.06: Personal Problems and Conflicts

> . . . (b) When psychologists become aware of personal problems that may interfere with their performing work-related duties adequately, they take appropriate measures, such as obtaining professional consultation or assistance, and determine whether they should limit, suspend, or terminate their work-related duties.

Having the safety of one's own child threatened by a client is certainly bound to create personal problems. Dr. Franklin may become preoccupied with the safety of her child. Such preoccupation constitutes a personal problem that interferes with her ability to focus her attention on the treatment of all of her clients. Standard 2.06 directs Dr. Franklin to decide whether to limit her work, such as communicating with Marvin that psychotherapy with Sylvia has been terminated.

Legal Issues 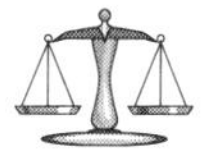

Florida

> *Florida Statute 490.009 (2010). Discipline.*
>
> (1) The following acts constitute grounds for . . . disciplinary action[:] . . .
>
> (p) Being unable to practice the profession for which he or she is licensed under this chapter with reasonable skill or competence as a result of any mental . . . condition.

Hawaii

> *Haw. Code R. § 16-98-34 (2010). Unethical Practice of Psychology.*
>
> (e) The psychologist shall respect the integrity and protect the welfare of the person . . . with whom the psychologist is working: . . .
>
> (3) The psychologist shall attempt to terminate a clinical . . . relationship when it is reasonably clear to the psychologist that the client is not benefiting from it.

In neither jurisdiction would Dr. Franklin violate the law if she withdraws from treating Sylvia, if Dr. Franklin believes that her child is at risk of harm because of Marvin's threat. Dr. Franklin would have to believe that her treatment efficacy would be impaired by her ongoing concern for her child. At that point, terminating Sylvia and finding an appropriate substitute would be viewed as reasonable conduct by both jurisdictions' licensing boards.

Cultural Considerations

Global Discussion

Canadian Code of Ethics for Psychologists

> Principle II: Responsible caring.
>
> *Values Statement*
>
> By virtue of the social contract that the discipline has with society, psychologists have a higher duty of care to members of society than the general duty of care all members of society have to each other. However, psychologists are entitled to protect their own basic well-being (e.g., physical safety, family relationships) in their work as psychologists.

The Canadian code, while clearly obligating Dr. Franklin to uphold her contract with members of society, also allows Dr. Franklin to protect herself and her child if Marvin has violated or might violate her basic well-being.

American Moral Values

1. How does Dr. Franklin weigh her respective roles as therapist and family member? When does her duty to Sylvia become too onerous for her personal safety and that of her family? Is protecting Sylvia important enough in this case to risk that safety? How important is it for Dr. Franklin to show that psychologists will not be intimidated?
2. Should Dr. Franklin contact the police about Marvin's note? Should she obtain a protective order? What will police presence mean for Sylvia's treatment? What will it mean for Dr. Franklin's family?
3. Would breaking off treatment with Sylvia be a betrayal of trust? What if the police recommended it, at least temporarily? What if the police recommend treating Sylvia in another facility? Would it send the wrong message to Marvin?
4. What kind of protection does Sylvia need now? Will Marvin be monitoring Dr. Franklin's office to see if Sylvia visits? What will this mean for other clients?
5. Does Dr. Franklin need to notify the school about possible security issues? How will that affect her son's life?
6. Would terminating treatment deter Marvin? What kind of example would it set for others (say, women in the shelter)? Does Dr. Franklin respect any aspect of Marvin's desire to reconcile with Sylvia? Does she feel any responsibility to encourage any positive emotions or impulses she sees at work in his actions?

Ethical Course of Action

Directive per APA Code

Sylvia has obviously benefited from her work with Dr. Franklin. Sylvia is now able to take steps to separate herself physically from the harm of living with someone who acts abusively. However, it is possible that continued work with Dr. Franklin may lead to harm. The harm may come from Marvin's ability to locate Sylvia through Dr. Franklin or Dr. Franklin's inability to properly attend to her client. In either case, Standards 3.04 and 10.10 (a) dictate that treatment be terminated. Standard 10.10 allows for the legitimacy of Dr. Franklin's preoccupation as sufficient reason to terminate therapy without bringing into question her competency, per Standard 2.06 (b).

Dictates of One's Own Conscience

If you were Dr. Franklin, and knowing that psychologists have a higher duty of care to society as articulated in the Canadian code, which action would you take?

1. Tell Sylvia that men like Marvin are more bluster than show, and proceed with treatment.
2. Tell Sylvia to be brave because together you will stand up to Marvin's threats, and proceed with treatment.
3. Contact the police.
4. On the weight of evidence provided by Marvin's letter, seek to obtain a restraining order that prohibits Marvin from being within 5 miles of your office or members of your family.
5. Invite Marvin in for a treatment session to explain why you are not able to comply with his requests, regardless of how much he threatens.
6. Visit your child's school with Marvin's threatening letter in hand to request a greater level of security for your child.
7. Combinations of the above-listed actions.
8. Or one that is not listed above.

If this scenario happened in Canada, the above-listed options would still apply since the directives regarding protection from personal danger are not substantially different from those listed in the APA Ethics Code.

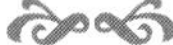

STANDARD 10.10: TERMINATING THERAPY

> . . . (c) Except where precluded by the actions of clients/patients or third-party payors, prior to termination psychologists provide pre-termination counseling and suggest alternative service providers as appropriate.

A CASE FOR STANDARD 10.10 (C): Necessary Limits

Dr. Lawson, a licensed psychologist, advertises and is clear that he is a Christian and tries to practice within the tenets of the church. Glen has requested that his minister refer him to a Christian therapist. All is well in Glen's treatment with Dr. Lawson. Then, several sessions into the therapy, Glen very hesitantly and fearfully confesses he is having an extramarital affair. His wife does not know about this long-term affair of 2 years. His mistress is pressuring him to divorce his wife and marry her. Glen is extremely ambivalent about the affair, he loves his wife, and does not want to give up his children. Dr. Lawson responds,

> As you know, when we started therapy, I am a Christian therapist. I know you are a Christian. You have just told me that you are in an extramarital affair. As a good Christian, I cannot condone or participate in this situation, so we cannot continue therapy unless you end your affair and tell your spouse. Call me when you have ended the affair and revealed your infidelity to your wife.

Issues of Concern

Dr. Lawson has introduced the idea of termination Once introduced, Standard 10.10 (c) directs Dr. Lawson to engage in two steps with his client: to provide professional advice about termination and to give a few names of other psychologists for continued treatment. The advice is of a different nature than therapy. It appears that Dr. Lawson's giving Glen the choice of continuing therapy with him or continuing his extramarital affair is a form of therapeutic intervention. Items for Dr. Lawson to consider, to act congruently with the directives of Standard 10.10 (c), include the content of a pretermination counseling session, the identities of referrals, and whether the referrals should include Glen's minister.

It is evident that Glen was fearful of Dr. Lawson's response to his extramarital affair. Was Dr. Lawson's response harmful to Glen? Was pausing treatment and demanding that Glen end the extramarital affair a failure to acknowledge Glen's struggles in an empathic manner? What is the potential harm to Glen should he not have access to treatment with Dr. Lawson?

APA Ethics Code

Companion General Principles

Principle A: Beneficence and Nonmaleficence

> Psychologists strive to benefit those with whom they work and take care to do no harm. In their professional actions, psychologists seek to safeguard the welfare and rights of those with whom they interact professionally and other affected persons.

Principle A calls for Dr. Lawson to provide therapy that is of benefit to Glen or at least does no harm to Glen. Is it more harmful to Glen, his wife, and his mistress for Dr. Lawson to continue treatment without requiring the ending of the affair? Or is it more harmful to Glen/his wife/his mistress for Dr. Lawson to end treatment in response to Glen's extramarital affair? What are the rights of Glen's wife and his mistress in terms of Principle A?

Principle D: Justice

> Psychologists exercise reasonable judgment and take precautions to ensure that their potential biases . . . do not lead to or condone unjust practices.

Dr. Lawson has a Christian perspective. Glen knew of this religious perspective. Indeed, it appears that Glen specifically chose treatment with Dr. Lawson because of his Christian approach. If Dr. Lawson's therapeutic intervention is congruent with this known approach, has Dr. Lawson violated the spirit and intent of Principle D?

Companion Ethical Standard(s)

Standard 3.04: Avoiding Harm

> Psychologists take reasonable steps to avoid harming their clients/patients . . . and to minimize harm where it is foreseeable and unavoidable.

Standard 3.04 operationalizes the Nonmaleficence part of Principle A. Standard 3.04 focuses on the avoidance of harm to Glen, not his wife or his mistress. Dr. Lawson's clinical consideration, per Standard 3.04, is to determine whether it is harmful to Glen to continue treatment without making a demand to end the affair.

Standard 10.10: Terminating Therapy

> (a) Psychologists terminate therapy when it becomes reasonably clear that the client/patient . . . is not likely to benefit, or is being harmed by continued service.

Dr. Lawson appears to equate continuing treatment of Glen with condoning extramarital affairs. If condoning extramarital affairs is determined to harm Glen, then Dr. Lawson would be obligated to end treatment.

Standard 10.01: Informed Consent to Therapy

> (a) When obtaining informed consent to therapy . . . psychologists inform clients/patients as early as is feasible in the therapeutic relationship about the nature . . . of therapy.

Standard 10.01 (a) would have had Dr. Lawson discussing the nature of therapy based on Christian values. Based on the advertisements, and the referral source, it is reasonable to expect Glen to have known about and consented to adherence to Dr. Lawson's Christian values in therapy. Indeed, it appears that Glen chose Dr. Lawson for his religion.

Standard 3.01: Unfair Discrimination

> In their work-related activities, psychologists do not engage in unfair discrimination based on . . . religion.

Standard 3.01 operationalizes Principle D: Justice, by prohibiting Dr. Lawson from discriminating against Glen on the basis of Glen's religion. It is unclear as to whether Dr. Lawson's response is based on Glen's religion or on Dr. Lawson's religious beliefs, or both.

Standard 10.10: Terminating Therapy

> . . . (b) Psychologists may terminate therapy when threatened or otherwise endangered by the client/patient or another person with whom the client/patient has a relationship.

Standard 10.10 (b) specifies that Dr. Lawson could terminate therapy with Glen without violation of the APA Ethics Code if Glen threatened Dr. Lawson. It does not appear that Glen has threatened or in any way endangered Dr. Lawson's safety. On what ethical grounds does Dr. Lawson therefore justify setting conditions for continued treatment?

Legal Issues 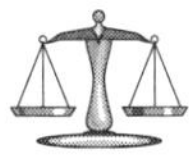

Indiana

> *868 Ind. Admin. Code 1.1-11-4.1 (2010). Relationships Within Professional Practice.*
>
> (d) The psychologist shall not undertake or continue a professional relationship with a patient or client when the objectivity or competency of the psychologist is or could be expected to be impaired because of the psychologist's: . . .
>
> (2) bias against a patient . . . because of the patient's . . . religion. . .
>
> (e) When a potentially harmful relationship becomes apparent, the psychologist shall clarify the nature of the relationship and attempt to resolve it with due regard for the best interests of the . . . client. Whenever a psychologist's objectivity . . . becomes impaired during a professional relationship with a . . . client, the psychologist shall notify the . . . client orally and in writing that the psychologist can no longer provide professional services, and the psychologist shall assist the patient or client in obtaining services from another professional.
>
> (f) If termination of the professional relationship is necessary, the psychologist shall:
>
> (1) immediately terminate the professional relationship in an appropriate manner;
>
> (2) notify the patient or client orally and in writing of this termination; and
>
> (3) assist the patient or client in obtaining services from another professional.

Kansas

> *Kan. Admin. Regs. § 102-1-10a (2010). Unprofessional Conduct.*
>
> (f) ignoring client welfare, which shall include the following acts: . . .
>
> (3) engaging in behavior that is abusive or demeaning to a client . . .
>
> (5) failing to take each of the following steps before termination for whatever reason, unless precluded by the patient's or client's relocation or noncompliance with the treatment regimen:
>
> (A) Discuss the patient's or client's views and needs;
>
> (B) provide appropriate pretermination counseling;
>
> (C) suggest alternative service providers, as appropriate; and
>
> (D) take other reasonable steps to facilitate the transfer of responsibility to another provider if the patient or client needs one immediately.

In both jurisdictions, Dr. Lawson has violated the laws related to his objectivity, competency, and the manner by which he has terminated treatment with his client. It does not appear from Dr. Lawson's abrupt ending of the session, and the directive to Glen to quit the affair before he can continue to treat, that he has been sensitive to the clinical needs of his client. He certainly has not implemented any continuity of care through an orderly termination process that is called for in both jurisdictions.

Cultural Considerations

Global Discussion

Code of Ethics for the Psychologist: Spain

> ***Article 9.*** Psychologists must respect the moral and religious beliefs of their clients, not allowing this to be a hindrance to any questioning that may be necessary in the course of his/her intervention.
>
> ***Article 10.*** In providing their services, Psychologists must never discriminate against their clients on grounds of . . . religious beliefs.

Dr. Lawson would likely be in violation of the Spanish code in this situation. First, Dr. Lawson has allowed his own religious beliefs, although he is of the same religion as Glen, to be a "hindrance" to his intervention with Glen, and has further discriminated against Glen by attempting to dictate to his client what his behavior should be on religious grounds. Further, by enforcing his own religious values on a client, attempting to coerce a specific course of action, and making continuation of Glen's therapy contingent upon his compliance, Dr. Lawson has violated the Spanish code, as well as the Principles of Autonomy: Nonmaleficence, and Beneficence.

American Moral Values

1. What does Dr. Lawson believe "Christian therapy" demands from clients? Does it mean that clients cannot disobey ethical standards thought to be Christian? To what degree does treatment of a client imply endorsement of their actions?
2. Did Dr. Lawson have an obligation to spell out from the beginning what actions would result in the ending

of treatment? Is there a moral difference between refusing treatment at the outset and stopping treatment after several sessions? Is this a betrayal of Glen or just an unforeseeable situation?

3. What is Dr. Lawson's specific objection to treating someone who is having an affair? Is he concerned about Glen's wife and children primarily? The mistress? Does ending therapy help the client to stop having an affair?

4. Is setting a condition for therapy the same thing as ending therapy? What if Glen checks back in with Dr. Lawson to report how he is doing with ending the affair? What kind of relationship will Dr. Lawson and Glen have?

5. What are the bounds that Dr. Lawson, as a Christian therapist, sets between private and public? Should Dr. Lawson tell Glen's wife about the affair, knowing what he does now?

6. How does Dr. Lawson relate the example of his practice to society's understanding of Christianity? Does his statement to Glen threaten the idea that therapy and Christian life can coexist? Could he be threatening Glen's religious life, and not just his therapy, by taking this stand?

Ethical Course of Action

Directive per APA Code

Standard 10.10 (c) requires Dr. Lawson to give Glen a pretermination counseling session and name other resources for further treatment. By giving Glen an immediate ultimatum, Dr. Lawson does not provide time for the pretermination counseling or for suggestions about alternative service providers. Dr. Lawson's response to Glen's confession of an extramarital affair is to deny treatment. It is highly probable that Glen sought out treatment to resolve the difficulties of an extramarital affair. Assuredly, termination of therapy would be harmful to Glen and is in violation of Standards 3.04 and 10.10 (a), and the value of Nonmaleficence, Principle A.

It does not appear that Glen has threatened or otherwise put Dr. Lawson in danger. Denial of treatment based on professed religion, regardless of whether Glen had knowledge of Dr. Lawson's religious values at the beginning of therapy in compliance with Standard 10.01 (a), still violates Standard 3.01 and the value of Justice, Principle D.

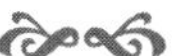

Dictates of One's Own Conscience

If you were Dr. Lawson, attempting to uphold your religious beliefs as well as maintain your professional responsibilities to Glen, which action would you take?

1. Inform Glen that this session will be his last, hoping your strong intervention will cause Glen to end his affair, return to his wife, and continue in therapy.
2. Inform Glen that this session will be his last, even if Glen decides not to return to therapy, reasoning that you cannot violate your own values and religious beliefs and maintain a congruent therapeutic alliance with Glen.
3. Inform Glen that you see his infidelity as a sign of greater psychopathology than you had at first believed, and tell him that he needs to see you more frequently.
4. Insist that Glen cannot continue in therapy with you, but if he chooses to see another therapist, you will locate an appropriate referral for him.
5. Combinations of the above-listed actions.
6. Or one that is not listed above.

If you were Dr. Lawson, practicing in Spain, would you:

1. Decide that your own religious beliefs have little bearing on therapeutic interventions, and although privately you disagree with Glen's behavior, you recognize that he will need your support more than ever before, and redouble your therapeutic efforts?
2. Inform Glen that you have strong enough negative feelings about his behavior in his marriage that continuing therapy with you may be harmful for him, or at least counterproductive.

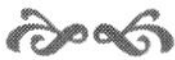

Appendices

APPENDIX A: INTERNATIONAL ETHICAL CODES OF CONDUCT

Electronic Links

British Psychological Society

http://www.scutrea.ac.uk/library/bpscode.pdf (November 2000)

http://www.bps.org.uk/the-society/code-of-conduct/code-of-conduct_home.cfm (code of conduct 2009)

Canadian Psychological Association/ Sociétié Canadienne de Psychologie

http://www.cpa.ca

Czech-Moravian Psychological Society/ Českomoravská Psychologická Společnost

http://www.cmps.ecn.cz (in Czech)
http://cmps.ecn.cz/dl/ethic-code.pdf (in English)

Association of Greek Psychologists/ Association de Psychologues Grecs

http://www.seps.gr (in Greek)

Hong Kong Psychological Society, LTD

http://www.hkps.org.hk

Psychological Society of Ireland

http://www.psihq.ie
http://www.psihq.ie/2010%20Code%20of%20Ethics.doc

Lithuanian Psychological Association

http://www.lps.vu.lt
http://www.lps.vu.lt/archyvas/index_en.php?id=code

Netherlands Institute of Psychologists (NIP)/ Nederlands Instituut van Psychologen

http://www.psynip.nl (in Dutch)

Code of Ethical Conduct Psychologists of New South Wales

http://www.psychreg.health.nsw.gov.au
http://www.stmaryspsychservices.com.au/code_of_conduct.htm
http://www.apa.org/international/directories/national-orgs.aspx#l
http://www.psychology.org.au/Assets/Files/Code_Ethics_2007.pdf

New Zealand Psychological Society

http://www.psychology.org.nz
http://www.psychologistsboard.org.nz/home

Singapore Psychological Society

http://www.singaporepsychologicalsociety.org
http://www.singaporepsychologicalsociety.org/code.cfm

Spanish Psychological Association/ Colegios Oficiales de Psicologos (COP)

http://www.cop.es (in Spanish)
http://www.cop.es/english/English.htm (English)
http://www.cop.es/English/docs/code.htm

Psychological Society of South Africa/PSYSSA

http://www.psyssa.com
http://www.psyssa.com/documents/HPCSA%20Ethical%20Code%20of%20Professional%20Conduct.pdf

APPENDIX B: UNITED STATES LAW

Legal Codes

Association of State and Provincial Psychology Boards (ASPPB): Member boards contact information for state, provincial, and territorial agencies responsible for the licensure and certification of psychologists throughout the United States and Canada

http://www.asppb.net/i4a/pages/index.cfm?pageid=3395

APPENDIX C: CREDITS

American Psychological Association Ethical Principles of Psychologists and Code of Conduct: Standards 1–10 © American Psychological Association (2010).

Association of Greek Psychologists: Ethical Codes & Guidelines © Hellenic Psychological Society.

British Psychological Society Code of Conduct, Ethical Principles & Guidelines © 2010–2011 The British Psychological Society.

California Ethical Standards © State of California Board of Psychology.

Canadian Code of Ethics © 2000 Canadian Psychological Association. Permission granted for use of material.

Code of Ethics for the Psychologist: Spain © 2010 Spanish Psychological Association.

Code of Ethics: Netherlands © 2010 Nederlands Instituut van Psychologen.

Code of Ethics New Zealand: Psychological Society © New Zealand Psychological Society Copyright Act 1994.

Code of Ethics New Zealand: Psychological Society © 1994 New Zealand Psychological Society Copyright Act.

Czech-Moravian Psychological Society Code of Ethics © © ČMPS 2009 Czech-Moravian Psychological Society Kladenská 48, 160 00 Praha 6.

Delaware Ethical Standards © State of Delaware.

District of Columbia Ethical Standards © District of Columbia Department of Health.

Florida Ethical Standards © State Department of Florida.

Georgia Ethical Standards © State of Georgia/Georgia Secretary of State.

Hong Kong Psychological Society: Professional Code of Practice © 1998 by The Hong Kong Psychological Society Ltd.

Idaho Ethical Standards © State of Idaho/Idaho Legislature.

Lithuanian Psychological Association: Ethical Codes & Guidelines © Copyright Lithuanian Psychological Association 2011.

Louisiana Ethical Standards © State of Louisiana.

Maine Ethical Standards © State of Maine.

Massachusetts Ethical Standards © Commonwealth of Massachusetts.

Michigan Ethical Standards © State of Michigan.

Minnesota Ethical Standards © State of Minnesota.

Missouri Ethical Standards © State of Missouri.

New Hampshire Ethical Standards © State of New Hampshire.

New Jersey Ethical Standards © New Jersey State Board of Psychological Examiners, The State of New Jersey, Department of Law and Public Safety.

New South Wales Code of Ethical Conduct © 2010 Australian Health Practitioner Regulation Agency.

New York Ethical Standards © State of New York.

Oklahoma Ethical Standards © State of Oklahoma.

Oregon Ethical Standards © State of Oregon.

Pennsylvania Ethical Standards © State of Pennsylvania.

Rhode Island Ethical Standards © State of Rhode Island.

South Dakota Ethical Standards © State of South Dakota.

Texas Ethical Standards © Texas State Board of Examiners of Psychologists.

Vermont Ethical Standards © State of Vermont.

Virginia Ethical Standards © Virginia Board of Psychology/ Commonwealth of Virginia.

Washington Ethical Standards © State of Washington.

West Virginia Ethical Standards © State of West Virginia.

References

American Psychiatric Association. (2000). *Diagnostic and statistical manual of mental disorders* (4th ed., text rev.). Washington, DC: Author.

American Psychological Association. (1990, August). *Guidelines for providers of psychological services to ethnic, linguistic, and culturally diverse populations.* Washington, DC: Author. Available at http://www.apa.org/pi/oema/resources/policy/provider-guidelines.aspx

American Psychological Association. (2002). *Guidelines on multicultural education, training, research, practice, and organizational change for psychologists.* Available at http://www.apa.org

American Psychological Association. (2003, May). Guidelines on multicultural education, training, research, practice, and organizational change for psychologists. *American Psychologist, 58*(5), 377–402.

American Psychological Association. (2010). *Ethical principles of psychologists and code of conduct* (2002, amended June 1, 2010). Available at http://www.apa.org/ethics/code/index.aspx

APA Task Force on Appropriate Therapeutic Responses to Sexual Orientation. (2009). *Report of the Task Force on Appropriate Therapeutic Responses to Sexual Orientation.* Available at http://www.apa.org/pi/lgbt/resources/sexual-orientation.aspx

Benjamin, G. A. H., Kent, L., & Sirikantraporn, S. (2009). Duty to protect statutes. In J. L. Werth, E. R. Welfel, & G. A. H. Benjamin (Eds.), *The duty to protect: Ethical, legal, and professional responsibilities of mental health professionals* (pp. 9–28). Washington, DC: American Psychological Association. (doi:10.1037/11866-002)

Bernard, J., & Jara, C. (1986). The failure of clinical psychology graduate students to apply understood ethical principles. *Professional Psychology: Research and Practice, 17,* 313–315.

Boysen, G. A., & Vogel, D. L. (2008). The relationship between level of training, implicit bias, and multicultural competency among counselor trainees. *Training and Education in Professional Psychology, 2*(2), 103–110.

Brabeck, M. M. (2000). *Practicing feminist ethics in psychology.* Washington DC: American Psychological Association.

D'Augelli, A. R., Grossman, A. H., Salter, N. P., Vasey, J. J., Starks, M. T., & Sinclair, K. O. (2005). Predicting the suicide attempts of lesbian, gay, and bisexual youth. *Suicide & Life-Threatening Behavior, 35*(6), 646–660.

Davidson, J. R. T., & Foa, E. B. (1993). *Posttraumatic stress disorder: DSM-IV and beyond.* Washington, DC: American Psychiatric Press.

Dell, P. F. (2001). Why the diagnostic criteria for dissociative identity disorder should be changed. *Journal of Trauma and Dissociation, 2*(1), 7–37.

Devilly, G. J. (2005). Power therapies and possible threats to the science of psychology and psychiatry. *Australian and New Zealand Journal of Psychiatry, 39*(6), 37–445.

Diaz-Lazaro, C. M., & Cohen, C. B. (2001). Cross-cultural contact in counseling training. *Journal of Multicultural Counseling and Development, 29*(1), 41–56.

Doctor, R. M., & Shiromoto, F. N. (2010). The encyclopedia of trauma and traumatic stress disorders. New York: Facts on File, Imprint of Infobase Publishing.

Ewing v. Goldstein, 120 Cal. App. 4th 807 (2004).

Fisher, C. (2009). *Decoding the ethics code: A practical guide for psychologists* (2nd ed.). Thousand Oaks, CA: Sage.

Ghaemi, S. N., & Martin, A. (2007). Defining the boundaries of childhood bipolar disorder. *American Journal of Psychiatry, 164*(2), 185–188.

Heppner, P. P., Wampold, B. E., & Kivlighan, D. M. (2008). Research design in counseling (3rd ed). Belmont, CA: Thomson Brooks/Cole.

Huang, M.-H. (2004). *Race of the interviewer and the black–white test score gap.* Institute of European and American Studies, Academia Sinica Taiwan. Available at http://tsa.sinica.edu.tw/Imform/file1/2004meeting/paper/C5-1.pdf

International Society for the Study of Dissociation. (2005). Guidelines for treating dissociative identity disorder in adults. (2005). *Journal of Trauma & Dissociation, 6*(4), 69–149.

Kitts, R. L. (2005). Gay adolescents and suicide: Understanding the association. *Adolescence, 40*(159), 621–628.

Kluft, R. P. (1999). An overview of the psychotherapy of dissociative identity disorder. *American Journal of Psychotherapy, 53*(3), 289–319.

Knapp, S. J., & VandeCreek, L. D. (2006). *Practical ethics for psychologists: A positive approach.* Washington, DC: American Psychological Association.

Koocher, G. P., & Keith-Spiegal, P. (2008). *Ethics in psychology and the mental health professions: Standards and cases* (3rd ed). New York: Oxford University.

Kulkin, H. S., Chauvin, E. A., & Percle, G. A. (2000). Suicide among gay and lesbian adolescents and young adults: A review of the literature. *Journal of Homosexuality, 40*(1), 1–13.

Lee, R. (2000). Health care problems of lesbian, gay, bisexual, and transgender patients. *Western Journal of Medicine,* 172, (6), 404–408.

Lilienfield, S. O., Lynn, S. J., & Lohr, J. M. (2003). *Science and pseudoscience in clinical psychology.* New York: Guilford Press

Neuner, F., Schauer, M., Karunakara, U., Klaschik, C., & Elbert, T. (2004). A comparison of narrative exposure therapy, supportive counseling and psychoeducation for treating posttraumatic stress disorder in an African refugee settlement. *Journal of Consulting and Clinical Psychology, 72*(4), 579–587.

Olfman, S. (2007). *Bipolar children: Cutting-edge controversy, insights, and research (childhood in America).* Westport, CT: Praeger.

Pabian, Y., Welfel, E. R., & Beebe, R. S. (2009). Psychologists' knowledge of their state laws pertaining to Tarasoff-type situations. *Professional Psychology: Research and Practice, 40,* 8–14.

Phelps, A. J., Forbes, D., & Creamer, M. (2008). Understanding posttraumatic nightmares: An empirical and conceptual review. *Clinical Psychology Review, 28*(2), 338–355.

Piper, A., & Merskey, H. (2004). The persistence of folly: A critical examination of dissociative identity disorder, Part I: The excesses of an improbable concept. *Canadian Journal of Psychiatry, 49,* 592–600.

Rubin, A. (2003). Unanswered questions about the empirical support for EMDR in the treatment of PTSD: A review of research. *Traumatology, 9*(1), 4–30.

Schubert, S., & Lee, C. W. (2009). Adult PTSD and its treatment with EMDR: A review of controversies, evidence, and theoretical knowledge. *Journal of EMDR Practice and Research, 3*(3), 117.

Singh, S., & Ernst, E. (2008). *Trick or treatment: The undeniable facts about alternative medicine.* New York: Norton.

Spiegel, D. (2001). Deconstructing the dissociative disorders: For whom the Dell tolls. *Journal of Trauma & Dissociation, 2,* 51–57.

Steele, M. C. (1997). A threat in the air: How stereotypes shape intellectual identity and performance. *American Psychologist, 52*(6), 613–629

Stringaris, A., Baroni, A., Haimm, C., Brotman, M., Lowe, C. H., Myers, F., et al. (2010). Pediatric bipolar disorder vs. severe mood dysregulation: Risk for manic episodes on follow-up. *Journal of the American Academy of Child and Adolescent Psychiatry, 49*(4), 397–405.

Sue, D. W., & Sue, D. (2007). *Counseling the culturally diverse: Theory and practice* (5th ed.). New York: Wiley.

U.S. Census Bureau. (2000). *American factfinder.* Available at http://factfinder.census.gov/home/saff/main.html?_lang=en

Walton, G. M., & Spencer, S. J. (2009). Latent ability: Grades and test scores systematically underestimate the intellectual ability of negatively stereotyped students. *Psychological Science, 20*(9), 1132–1139.

Werth, J. L.,Welfel, E. R., & Benjamin G. A. H. (2009). The duty to protect: Ethical, legal, and professional considerations in risk assessment and intervention. Washington, DC: American Psychological Association.

Index